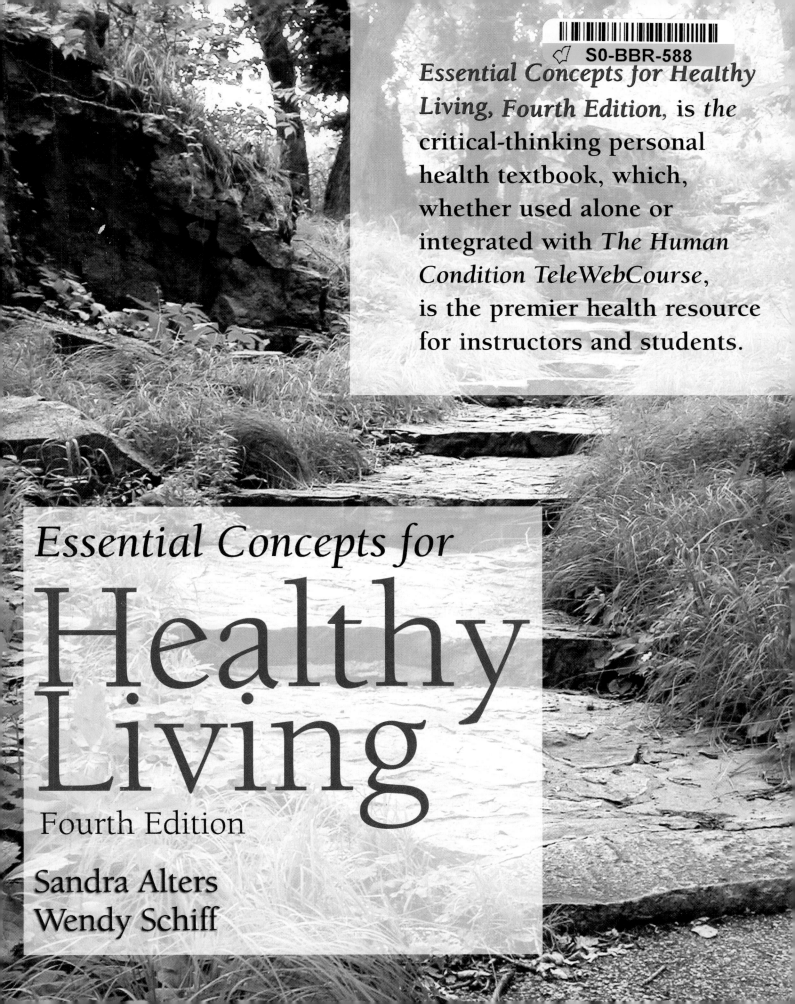

Essential Concepts for Healthy Living, Fourth Edition, is *the* critical-thinking personal health textbook, which, whether used alone or integrated with *The Human Condition TeleWebCourse,* is the premier health resource for instructors and students.

Essential Concepts for

Healthy Living

Fourth Edition

Sandra Alters
Wendy Schiff

Essential Concepts for Healthy Living, Fourth Edition, challenges students to think seriously about health-related information. The text concentrates on five key goals to help students learn and practice critical-thinking strategies. Throughout the textbook, a critical-thinking icon identifies features that focus specifically on critical-thinking skills.

What is critical thinking? What does a critical-thinking textbook do? Critical thinking encompasses a variety of cognitive skills such as:

• synthesizing

• analyzing

• applying

• evaluating information

In the health sciences, critical-thinking skills are necessary to understand and evaluate health information and then apply it to daily life. This book *teaches* critical-thinking skills that help students develop expertise in important cognitive functions:

• differentiating between verifiable facts and value statements,

• distinguishing relevant information from irrelevant information,

• determining the factual accuracy of health claims, and

• making responsible health-related decisions.

Essential Concepts for Healthy Living, Fourth Edition, and the accompanying workbook are structured to meet the critical-thinking mission. The five goals that help students learn and practice critical-thinking strategies are described on the following five pages and include the textbook features that promote each goal.

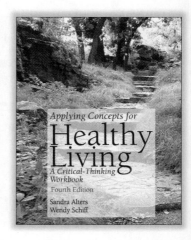

Key Goal 1: Students will understand the most recent scientifically based personal health information.

To think critically, students need a solid foundation of personal health information. *Essential Concepts for Healthy Living* has been developed from the latest scientific and medical research, relying heavily on primary sources, which are cited in the text. Because understanding health involves understanding science, this text includes basic scientific information that relates to health and presents it in an easy-to-understand manner. Additionally, Chapter 1 briefly discusses how health-related research is conducted, helping students become more critical consumers of health information.

Healthy People 2010 Updates

Students and instructors will be able to access Healthy People 2010 Updates that are pertinent to *Essential Concepts for Healthy Living, Fourth Edition,* at **http://healthyliving.jbpub.com**

CD-ROM ISBN 0-7637-1701-0
To order call 800-832-0034

key goal 1

Key Goal 2: Students will master textual material through the use of effective pedagogy.

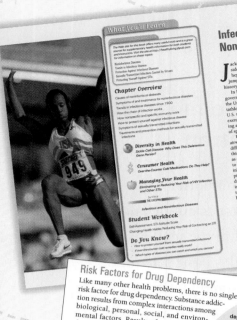

What You'll Learn

The Web site for this book offers many useful tools and is a great source for supplementary health information for both students and instructors. Visit the site at http://healthyliving.jbpub.com and explore on these topics.

Noninfectious Diseases
Trends in Infectious Diseases
Progress Against Infectious Diseases
Sexually Transmitted Infections (posed by Viruses)
Protecting Yourself Against STIs

Chapter Overview

Causes of noninfectious diseases
Symptoms of and treatments for noninfectious diseases
Trends in infectious diseases since 1900
How the chain of infection works
How nonspecific and specific immunity work
How to protect yourself against infectious disease
Symptoms of sexually transmitted infections
Treatments and prevention methods for sexually transmitted infections

Diversity in Health
Sickle Cell Disease: Why Does This Deleterious Gene Persist?

Consumer Health
Over-the-Counter Cold Medications: Do They Help?

Managing Your Health
Eliminating or Reducing Your Risk of HIV Infection and Other STIs

Student Workbook
Self-Assessment: STI Attitude Scale
Changing Health Habits: Reducing Your Risk of Contracting an STI

Do You Know?

• How to protect yourself from sexually transmitted infections?
• If over-the-counter cold remedies really work?
• Which types of infectious diseases you can catch and which you cannot?

Infection, Immunity, and Noninfectious Disease

chapter 14

Jackie Joyner-Kersee: Olympian gold, silver, and bronze medalist. Some consider Joyner-Kersee the greatest woman athlete ever. At this writing, she is the heptathlon world record holder and the American record holder in the long jump. She has won six Olympic medals, more than any woman in track and field history. Joyner-Kersee officially retired from track and field in 2001.

In late 2004, Joyner-Kersee was honored by USA Track & Field, the national governing body for track and field, citing Joyner-Kersee's breaking of her own women's heptathlon world record at the 1988 Olympic Games as the track and field history in the last 25 years. Clearly, exercise-induced asthma has not deterred this outstanding athlete from making her indelible mark in the world of sports, nor has it deterred other athletes.

Exercise-induced asthma is a condition in which the airways narrow after sustained exertion, making it more difficult than usual for a person to breathe. What triggers this problem is the cooling and reheating of the airways as a person exercises. As exercise begins, a person begins to breathe deeply and rapidly. During this deep and rapid inhalation, more air is moistened and warmed in the respiratory passageways than before exercise began, which draws moisture and heat from the airways. After a person is warmed up, the breathing rate falls, and the airways return to their normal temperature. Health scientists do not know how airway cooling and reheating triggers asthma attacks.

Asthma is one of a variety of noninfectious diseases. **Diseases** are processes that affect the proper functioning of the body and are usually accompanied by characteristic signs and symptoms. **Infectious diseases**, such as colds or the flu, are caused by **pathogens**, which are agents of infection. (Infectious diseases are discussed later in this chapter.) **Noninfectious diseases** are caused by abnormalities in the hereditary material (genetic diseases), interactions between heredity and environmental

> *Exercise-induced asthma has not deterred this outstanding athlete from making her indelible mark in the world of sports . . .*

379

Chapter-opening Pedagogy

The organization of ideas is an integral part of reading comprehension. Each chapter-opening spread shows students the organization of the chapter by means of a chapter overview and a list of the special boxed features. It also lists activities in the companion workbook and topics explored on **http://healthyliving.jbpub.com**.

Key Terms with Pronunciation Guides

Throughout each chapter, new key terms are bold-faced. In addition to the definitions and explanations in the text, these terms are defined in the margin of each two-page spread, with pronunciation guides for words that might be difficult—reinforcing students' confidence and familiarity with health-related terminology.

Risk Factors for Drug Dependency

Like many other health problems, there is no single risk factor for drug dependency. Substance addiction results from complex interactions among biological, personal, social, and environmental factors. Results of research conducted by the National Institute on Drug Abuse (NIDA) (2003) suggest that certain conditions in the home are probably the most crucial risk factors for children becoming drug abusers. Such factors include home environments in which parents abuse drugs or suffer from mental illness; ineffective parenting, particularly with children who have difficult temperaments or conduct disorders; and a lack of mutual child–parent attachments and parental nurturing. Risk factors for drug abuse that relate to a child's behavior outside of the home include inappropriately shy or aggressive behavior in the classroom; poor school performance; poor social skills; friendships with peers who use drugs; and a belief that parents, the school, peers, and the community approve of drug use. Conversely, *protective factors*, those associated with reduced potential for drug abuse, include strong family and school ties; parental monitoring of behavior with clear rules of conduct; involvement of parents

drug dependence or addiction a state in which one develops a habitual pattern of taking drugs that usually produces a compulsive need to use these substances, tolerance, and withdrawal.

tolerance an adaptation to drugs in which the usual dose no longer produces the anticipated degree of physical or psychological effects.

withdrawal a temporary physical and psychological state that occurs when certain drugs are discontinued.

Diversity in Health Essays

This feature cultivates an interest in and an appreciation for the health status and practices of various ethnic, cultural, and racial groups in the United States, as well as people in other countries. Although the diversity essays focus specifically on multiculturalism, additional multicultural information is woven throughout the book.

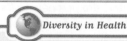
Diversity in Health

Native Americans: Culture and Psychological Health

In the United States, conventional mental health practitioners have been taught to identify normal and abnormal behaviors and diagnose mental illness by using an established set of standards. Often these health care providers do not consider the importance of culture when treating patients who are members of minority groups, particularly Native Americans.

The traditional Native American concept of health involves the *medicine wheel*, a circle divided into four equal parts representing the major aspects of health: context (natural environment and social setting), mind, body, and spirit. When the four components of the medicine wheel are balanced with each other, people enjoy wellness, or "harmony." When people are not in harmony with nature, their community, or themselves, they suffer from physical and psychological illnesses. According to some traditional Native

Figure 2-A For many Native Americans, stor[y...] spiritual and psychological health.

storytelling, and making drums and ba[...]

gives unclear responses to your questions, ask for additional information.

Across THE LIFESPAN

Sexuality

Most preschoolers masturbate. Parents who think masturbation is a healthy and normal aspect of sexuality usually let their children know that the behavior is

vey of almost 1,000 urban students in grades 6 to 8. After analyzing the results of their survey, Benson and Torpy (1995) concluded that, among other things, gender, age of puberty, and ethnic group are associated with virginity loss. Sex education, religious affiliation, grade average, and self-esteem were among the variables that were not associated, either positively or negatively, with virginity.

Results of a 2003 study conducted by the Centers for Disease Control and Prevention (CDC) across genders and races revealed that by approximately age 13, more boys reported sexual activity than girls. About 32% of male black students indicated that they were sexu-

152 **CHAPTER 6** Relationships and Sexuality

Across the Lifespan

This unique section relates the main topics of the chapter to the various stages of life, including infancy, childhood, adolescence, adulthood, and the elderly years.

Chapter Summaries

Research tells us that students learn how to identify the key ideas of stories in elementary school, but that they often have difficulty identifying key ideas in textbooks in their later schooling. Therefore, we provide chapter summaries to help students with this task. The chapter summaries follow the organization of the chapter.

CHAPTER REVIEW

Summary

Cancer is a variety of diseases that have common characteristics: Their cells exhibit abnormal growth, division, and differentiation and have the potential to spread from where they develop. These cells form masses called malignant tumors that interfere with normal body processes.

Cancer develops in cells that have damaged or mutated genes. Mutations can be inherited or can occur from exposure to low-dose radiation, drugs, toxic chemicals, or certain viruses

reduces the risk. For early cancer detection, women aged 20 to 39 years should have a breast clinical examination every 3 years, and every year at age 40 and after. Women aged 40 and older should have a mammography every year. For early detection of endometrial cancer, women at menopause should report any unexpected bleeding or spotting to their physician.

Certain viruses are implicated in the development of a variety of

Key Goal 3: Students will think critically about health information published and distributed by various sources.

The focus of education today is not just to give students information, but to teach them how to acquire and evaluate information. Unlike other personal health textbooks, the critical-thinking features discussed below teach students higher-order thinking skills and give them ways to practice these skills in every chapter.

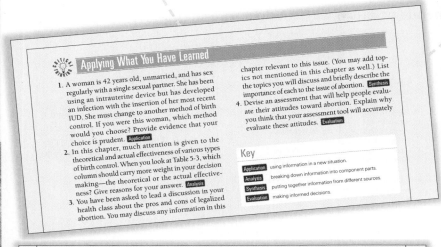

Applying What You Have Learned

This unique end-of-chapter feature is a series of questions and activities that require critical-thinking—application, analysis, synthesis, and evaluation. Each question is labeled as to what type of critical-thinking is required, and a key provides a brief explanation of the process students need to follow to answer the question or conduct the activity.

Reflecting on Your Health

This end-of-chapter journal-writing activity stimulates students to consider what they have learned and understand how their thoughts and feelings about health might have changed as a result of their new knowledge. Compiling these activities and reviewing them from time to time, especially at the end of the semester, will offer tangible evidence of changes and psychological and intellectual growth.

Analyzing Health-Related Information

This innovative feature teaches students the critical-thinking skill of analysis. Students use this skill and the model provided to determine the reliability of health-related information in articles, advertisements, Web sites, and other sources. Learning such a skill and practicing it helps students become knowledgeable consumers of health-related information and products.

Explain why you think this Web site about folic acid is a reliable or an unreliable source of information. Use the model for analyzing health-related information to guide your thinking; the main points of the model are noted below. The model is fully explained on pages 13–15. If you wish to visit this site, the Web address is http://www.cdc.gov/node.do/id/0900f3ec80010af9.

1. Which statements are verifiable facts, and which are unverified statements or value claims?
2. What are the credentials of the agency that created the Web site? If this information is available, is the agency qualified as an expert in the topic area?
3. What might be the motives and biases of the agency that created the Web site? State reasons for your answer.

key goal 3

Key Goal 4: Students will apply personal health information to their lives.

Essential Concepts for Healthy Living, Fourth Edition, encourages students to adopt healthier lifestyles and recommends practical ways to do so.

Healthy Living Practices

- If dwelling on negative self-thoughts creates stress for you, think about your strengths and develop a list of affirmative self-statements to repeat regularly.
- Consider setting aside some time to relax every day, perhaps by using the techniques discussed in this chapter.
- Try breathing slowly and deeply before or during a stressful situation as a simple but effective way to relax.
- Engaging in tai chi, yoga, and moderate exercise and physical activity on a regular basis can reduce your stress.

Healthy Living Practices

Unique to this text, these short lists of bulleted statements throughout the chapter summarize key points and concisely state concrete yet simple actions students can take to improve their health.

Managing Your Health

These features contain lists of tips or short essays that focus on ways to live a healthier life.

Managing Your Health

General Features of Reliable Weight Reduction Plans

Use the following features to judge the quality of weight loss programs.

The diet plan is medically sound if it

- provides recommendations that are safe and supported by scientific evidence.
- suggests receiving a physician's approval prior to initi-

The diet plan considers physical fitness needs if it

- recommends an exercise plan that is tailored to the individual's needs, time constraints, interests, and capabilities.
- includes practical suggestions for altering sedentary behaviors.
- encourages daily aerobic activities that last at least half an hour.
- avoids promoting costly exercise equipment, joining exercise clubs, or buying special gadgets to shed pounds.
- recommends physical activities that are safe and enjoyable.

Consumer Health

These commentaries and tips provide practical information and suggestions to help students become more careful consumers of health-related goods and services. In addition to being highlighted in this feature, consumer topics are woven throughout the book and are the subject of scrutiny in the "Analyzing Health-Related Information" activities.

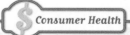

Consumer Health

Choosing a Fitness Center

Every year millions of Americans join health clubs, gyms, and exercise and fitness centers. Thousands of these people complain about their membership to states' attorneys general, Better Business Bureaus, and other consumer protection groups. The following tips can help you avoid becoming another dissatisfied health and fitness center consumer:

- Determine if you can afford to join the center.
- Inspect the center for cleanliness, type and quality of equipment, and especially staff qualifications. Ask if staff are certified as aerobics instructors, weight trainers, or athletic trainers. Are they trained in cardiopulmonary

- Ask your local Better Business Bureau about the number and nature of complaints against the organization.
- Ask for a trial period to use the facilities before joining.
- Never sign a contract under pressure at the center. Many centers use confusing and misleading advertising, including prizes or special short-term offers to spark your interest. Once you are in the facility, aggressive sales staff engage in high-pressure sales tactics to convince you to sign a contract.
- Before signing, take a few days to read the contract carefully. Make certain that you understand the details concerning payment options, membership restrictions,

Key Goal 5: Students will analyze their own health-related behavior and attitudes and change them to improve health and maintain well-being.

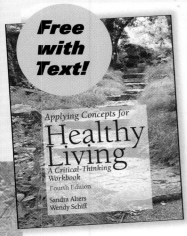

Applying Concepts for Healthy Living: A Critical-Thinking Workbook contains two types of activities that address self-assessment and changing health habits. Together, these two features help students assess their behaviors and attitudes, and provide a mechanism that will help students change health-related behaviors if they choose. We do not tell students which decisions are most valuable; instead we provide background information and guidance through the use of thought-provoking techniques to make responsible decisions.

Self-Assessments

These evaluation tools help students assess their health status, attitudes, and beliefs. Most assessments are research-based rather than derived from the popular press. Each chapter contains one or more assessments, and all relate directly to chapter topics.

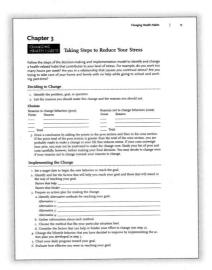

Changing Health Habits

These activities have two parts. The first helps students determine if they desire change or are ready for change; the second guides students to facilitate change if they choose. The student workbook contains one activity per chapter. This allows students to practice decision-making and the implementation model, making the transfer of these skills to their daily lives more likely.

key goal 5

Utilizing new and customary classroom resources, Jones and Bartlett Publishers and INTELECOM Intelligent Telecommunications continue to deliver a valuable health package for educators. *Essential Concepts for Healthy Living, Fourth Edition,* will serve as the basis of a college credit course when combined with *The Human Condition TeleWebCourse.*

The Human Condition

The Human Condition, produced by INTELECOM Intelligent Telecommunications, takes a visionary look at the state of health and health care today. In 26 television episodes this compelling new TeleWebCourse offers teachers and learners an up-to-the-minute look at health and health care issues–from MyPyramid guidelines to cardiovascular disease, and from the latest in HIV/AIDS treatment to changes in health-care delivery systems. *The Human Condition* combines interviews with leading health professionals, dynamic location footage, and illustrative case studies, to bring each lesson to life.

The Human Condition **takes a comprehensive view of health care, focusing on ten areas:**

- What Is Health?
- Who Is at Risk?
- The Life Cycle
- Emotional and Mental Health
- Sexual Health
- Health and Chemical Substances

- Promoting Well-Being through Fitness and Nutrition
- Health Risks: The Role of Heredity and Lifestyle
- Infectious and Non-Infectious Diseases
- The Individual in the Medical Marketplace

Contact INTELECOM at 150 East Colorado Boulevard, Suite 300 Pasadena, CA 91105-1937. (800) 576-2988. www.intelecom.org

Supplements for the Instructor and Student

The Human Condition Faculty Guide, available in electronic or print form to instructors who license the course, provides additional learning objectives linked to each lesson as well as an examination bank and answer key.

The Human Condition Study Guide combines information from both the *Essential Concepts for Healthy Living, Fourth Edition* textbook and *The Human Condition TeleWebCourse.* For each episode, the *TeleWebCourse* study guide provides learning objectives, an overview of the lesson, assignments, key terms, video viewing questions, self-test, expanded analysis questions, and the answer key for the self-test.

The Human Condition Study Guide with Essential Concepts for Healthy Living, Fourth Edition, and the critical-thinking workbook.
Order with ISBN 0-7637-4007-1.

INTELECOM Learning Resources Network–Allows instructors using *The Human Condition* to prepare integrated online components and make changes quickly and easily.

Course content from the Learning Resources Network may be downloaded and imported into course management systems such as WebCT, Blackboard, and Prometheus. This provides instructors with a framework for building online components tied to *The Human Condition*, while allowing flexibility to incorporate other information. The Learning Resources Network materials include: Learning Modules for each *Human Condition* course lesson; HTML files to copy and paste or import into a course management system; a Web-ready Faculty Guide; Instructional Activities; and Expanded Analysis Questions.

Jones and Bartlett continues to stay on the cutting edge of textbook development and the associated Internet technology that is so important in today's classrooms. In addition to *The Human Condition TeleWebCourse,* we also provide online resources and technology tools that are available for you and your students!

Applying Concepts for Healthy Living: A Critical-Thinking Workbook includes Self-Assessments and Changing Health Habits activities. (Package ISBN 0-7637-3802-6)

Transparency Set to accompany Essential Concepts for Healthy Living, Fourth Edition (ISBN 0-7637-3727-5): To enhance the classroom experience, a complete transparency set is available that contains many of the images from the text. Contact your sales representative for more information.

Healthy Living Online

Relevant and reliable health-related information can be accessed through content links on http://healthyliving.jbpub.com.

This interactive and informative web site offers students and educators an unprecedented degree of integration of their text and the online world through the following features:

eLearning for students

· Content Links
· Web Exercises
· Additional Resources
· Animated Flashcards
· Practice Quizzes
· Healthy People 2010
· Interactive Glossary
· Crossword Puzzles

Tools for instructors

· Brownstone Diploma Computerized TestBank
· PowerPoint Lecture Outline Slides
· Annotated Lecture Outlines
· Warm-up Exercises
· Transparency Masters

Instructor's ToolKit
(ISBN 0-7637-3723-2)

The Instructor's ToolKit CD-ROM contains a variety of programs and files to help you teach your course. All of the materials are cross-platform for Windows and Macintosh systems. The ToolKit CD-ROM includes:

The Kaleidoscope Media Viewer program offers full-color art files of more than 100 of the text's illustrations in formats appropriate for computer projection and for printing overhead transparencies.

The Brownstone Diploma Computerized TestBank helps you choose an appropriate variety of questions organized by chapter, create multiple versions of a test, and even administer and grade tests online.

PowerPoint Lecture Outline Slides provide a template for each chapter that includes the chapter outline for building your lecture presentation.

Annotated Lecture Outlines are complete, ready-to-use lesson plans that outline all of the topics covered in the text. They are provided in an electronic format that can be easily modified.

Warm-up Exercises are designed to promote creative classroom discussions among students and instructors.

Transparency Masters contain tables and bulleted lists that can be used as handouts or overhead transparencies.

healthy living online

Brief Contents

brief contents

Essential Concepts for
Healthy Living
Fourth Edition

Sandra Alters
Wendy Schiff

JONES AND BARTLETT PUBLISHERS

Sudbury, Massachusetts

BOSTON   TORONTO   LONDON   SINGAPORE

World Headquarters
Jones and Bartlett Publishers
40 Tall Pine Drive
Sudbury, MA 01776
978-443-5000
info@jbpub.com
www.jbpub.com

Jones and Bartlett Publishers
Canada
6339 Ormindale Way
Mississauga, Ontario L5V 1J2
CANADA

Jones and Bartlett Publishers
International
Barb House, Barb Mews
London W6 7PA
UK

Jones and Bartlett's books and products are available through most bookstores and online booksellers. To contact Jones and Bartlett Publishers directly, call 800-832-0034, fax 978-443-8000, or visit our website, www.jbpub.com.

Substantial discounts on bulk quantities of Jones and Bartlett's publications are available to corporations, professional associations, and other qualified organizations. For details and specific discount information, contact the special sales department at Jones and Bartlett via the above contact information or send an email to specialsales@jbpub.com.

Production Credits

Chief Executive Officer: Clayton Jones
Chief Operating Officer: Don W. Jones, Jr.
President, Higher Education and Professional Publishing: Robert W. Holland, Jr.
V.P., Sales and Marketing: William J. Kane
V.P., Design and Production: Anne Spencer
V.P., Manufacturing and Inventory Control: Therese Connell
Acquisitions Editor: Jacqueline Ann Mark-Geraci
Senior Production Editor: Julie Champagne Bolduc
Associate Editor: Nicole L. Quinn
Editorial Assistant: Amy L. Flagg
Associate Marketing Manager: Wendy Thayer
Interactive Technology Manager: Dawn Mahon Priest
Composition: Graphic World
Text and Cover Design: Anne Spencer
Senior Photo Researcher: Kimberly Potvin
Cover Image: © Judy Drietz/Shutterstock
Printing and Binding: Courier Kendallville
Cover Printing: John Pow Company

Library of Congress Cataloging-in-Publication Data
Alters, Sandra.
  Essential concepts for healthy living / Sandra Alters, Wendy Schiff.
 -- 4th ed.
    p. ; cm.
  Includes index.
  ISBN 0-7637-2952-3
  1. Health.   I. Schiff, Wendy. II. Title.
  [DNLM: 1. Health--Popular Works.   QT 255 A4664e 2006]
  RA776.5.A596 2006
  613--dc22   2005021644

Printed in the United States of America
09 08 07 06 05   10 9 8 7 6 5 4 3 2 1

CONTENTS

FEATURES

Diversity in Health

Consumer Health

Managing Your Health

Across
THE LIFESPAN

ACKNOWLEDGMENTS

The authors' writing is only one small portion of the work that goes into the development and production of a textbook. Many people work long hours with a shared goal: to produce a visually appealing, error-free, up-to-date, high-quality textbook for students. We would like to acknowledge the dedication and hard work of these individuals, for without them this project never would have been realized.

Our thanks to Jacqueline Mark-Geraci, acquisitions editor, and Nicole Quinn, associate editor, for their contributions to the project. Julie Bolduc, senior production editor, along with John May and Trudi Elliott of Graphic World, managed the production of *Essential Concepts for Healthy Living,* doing an amazing job to keep an incredibly complex process running smoothly. Anne Spencer is responsible for the outstanding cover and interior design. Anne is a true professional who created a dynamic and fresh look for the fourth edition. A heartfelt thanks to you all.

Jones and Bartlett is a company on the cutting edge of integrating technology with print materials for learning. The superb web-based materials that are a part of the *Essential Concepts for Healthy Living* program could not have been developed without Wayne Hoang.

Other key members of the Jones and Bartlett team are Wendy Thayer and Amy Flagg. These members of the Marketing and Editorial group have helped all involved in the book's development to remain focused on the needs of our audience.

Two of our opening narratives introduced individuals who allowed us to explore their healthy lifestyles. Our thanks to Justin Godin, the formerly obese college student, who discussed his experiences in achieving a healthy body weight, and to Mary Blum, a centenarian who embodies healthy living.

And finally a special acknowledgment to Sally Beatty and Judy Sullivan of INTELECOM. We are thrilled that *Essential Concepts for Healthy Living* is an integral part of the telewebcourse *The Human Condition.*

REVIEWERS

Many health teachers and researchers have made significant contributions to the development of this book. Our gratitude goes to the following reviewers whose expertise gave invaluable direction to the development of *Essential Concepts for Healthy Living:*

Martin Ayim, *Grambling University*
Charles Baffi, *Virginia Technical Institute*
M. Patsy Bergen, *Kansas State University*
Roberta Donahue, *University of Alabama*
Lea Fields, *Cerritos College*
Cathy Kennedy, *Colorado State University*
Karen King, *University of North Carolina, Greensborough*
Jennifer McLean, *Corning Community College*
Kadee Murray, *Cerritos College*
Mark Oliver, *University of Central Arkansas*
Roseanne Poole, *Tallahassee Community College*
Jeff Schulz, *Mississippi State University*
Andrew Shim, *Southwestern College*
Carol Weideman, *Grand Valley State University*
Terry Wessell, *James Madison University*

We would also like to acknowledge the reviewers of the first edition of *Essential Concepts for Healthy Living,* whose advice helped us move on to the next editions:

Donna Jean Allis, *Seattle Pacific University*
Judy B. Baker, *East Carolina University*
Deborah Banebini, *Grand Valley State University*
Gene Barnes, *University of South Alabama*
Rick Barnes, *East Carolina University*
Lois Beach, *SUNY–Plattsburgh*
Luana J. Beeson, *Oregon State University*
Robert J. Bensley, *Western Michigan University*
David R. Black, *Purdue University*
Jill M. Black, *Cleveland State University*
David L. Blievernicht, *Wayne State University*
Mary Ann Borysowicz, *Purdue University*
Bob Bowers, *Tallahassee Community College*
Ruth C. Bragg, *University of Tampa*
James Brik, *Willamette University*
Gary W. Brinkman, *Oxnard College*
Susan Burge, *Cuyahoga Community College*
Lorraine D. Campbell, *California State University, Bakersfield*
Marion T. Carr, *University of South Carolina*

James Lester Carter, *Montana State University*
John S. Carter, *Health and Physical Education*
Dan Connaughton, *University of Florida*
Lori L. Dewald, *Shippensburg University*
Lawrence G. Doty, *Linfield College*
Marvin Druger, *Syracuse University*
Jack Ellison, *University of Tennessee*
Jule Gast, *Utah State University*
Stephen C. Goodwin, *University of Delaware*
John Gratton, *Bee County College*
Jack E. Hansma, *Baylor University*
Joanna Hayden, *William Paterson College of New Jersey*
David Hines, *Ball State University*
Stephanie Hupp, *Southern Illinois University-Carbondale*
Chester Jones, *University of Arkansas*
Arnold W. Joyce, *Virginia Military Institute*
Walt Justice, *El Camino College*
Greg Kandt, *Fort Hays State University*
Catherine A. Kennedy, *Colorado State University*
Jean Levitan, *William Paterson College of New Jersey*
Loretta M. Liptak, *Youngstown State University*
J. Lisk, *University of South Carolina–Aiken*
Beverly Saxton Mahoney, *Pennsylvania State University*
Terry M. Manning, *University of North Carolina–Charlotte*
Larry K. Olsen, *Pennsylvania State University*
Christopher S. Ousley, *North Carolina State University*
John Paxman, *Portland Community College*
Sally A. Radmacher, *Missouri Western State College*
Linda L. Rankin, *Idaho State University*
Richard S. Riggs, *University of Kentucky*
Jim Sartoris, *Glendale Community College*
Mary Schutten, *Calvin College*
John Sciacca, *Northern Arizona University*
Melinda J. Seid, *California State University, Sacramento*
John C. Smith, *Springfield College*
Harry Specht, *Pennsylvania College of Technology*
Sue Viscomi, *SUNY–Oswego*
J. Dale Wagoner, *Chabot College*
David M. White, *East Carolina University*
Susan Yeager, *Mesa State College*

Sandra Alters
Wendy Schiff

ABOUT THE AUTHORS

Essential Concepts for Healthy Living, Fourth Edition, was written by an author team with extensive credentials and backgrounds in biology, health, and education. Sandra Alters holds a Ph.D. degree in Science Education and a Master's degree in biology. Formerly of the University of Missouri–St. Louis and Salem State College (Massachusetts), Dr. Alters has authored several textbooks in addition to *Essential Concepts for Healthy Living,* a laboratory manual, a children's science book, many articles in professional literature, and over sixty chapters and features in books. Additionally, she has written the instructional design for a variety of science-related software products for students. With twenty-five years of teaching experience, Dr. Alters brings her educational expertise, background in biology and human biology, and extensive writing experience to the author team.

Wendy Schiff holds a Master's degree in Human Nutrition. She is an Adjunct Instructor in the Department of Physical Education at the St. Louis Community College-Meramec Campus. Ms. Schiff has authored a college health textbook, two health education manuals, a low-calorie cookbook, and published articles in professional journals. She has served as a consulting nutritionist, reviewer of health education and nutrition materials, and a freelance health essayist. With her educational background in health and her experience teaching college health, nutrition, stress management, and sexuality classes, Ms. Schiff complements Dr. Alters' expertise in biological sciences and science education.

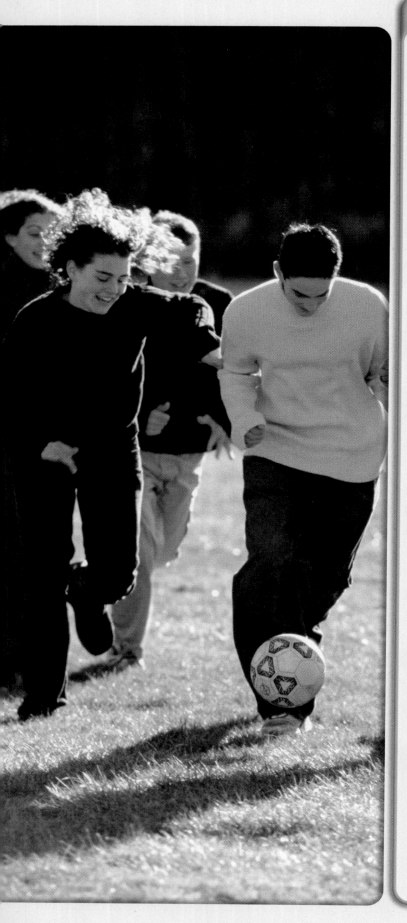

What You'll Learn

http://healthyliving.jbpub.com

The Web site for this book offers many useful tools and is a great source for supplementary health information for both students and instructors. Visit the site at http://healthyliving.jbpub.com for information on these topics:

The Nation's Health
Analyzing Health Information
Conventional versus Complementary and Alternative Medicine
Consumer Health: Consumer Protection

Chapter Overview

How the dimensions of health influence your well-being

The major health concerns of our nation

How your decisions affect your health

How to analyze health-related information

The differences between conventional and alternative treatment methods

Diversity in Health
Minority Health Status in the United States

Consumer Health
Consumer Protection

Managing Your Health
Routine Health Care for Disease Prevention

Across
THE LIFESPAN

Health

Student Workbook

Self-Assessment: Healthstyle

Changing Health Habits: Altering Your Behavior for Better Health

Do You Know?

· *How your lifestyle affects your health?*

· *How to make responsible health-related decisions?*

· *How to analyze health-related information?*

Health: The Foundation for Life

What is the status of health in the United States? *Healthy People 2000: Final Review,* a report issued by the Centers for Disease Control and Prevention (CDC) in Atlanta, indicates that since 1985 many Americans have altered their lives to improve their health (U.S. Department of Health and Human Services [USDHHS], 2001). Between 1985 and 2000 more adults exercised regularly and ate the recommended amounts of fruits and vegetables. During this period, fewer adults smoked cigarettes and drank alcohol, and fewer people died as a result of alcohol-related motor vehicle accidents than before 1985. The number of deaths from AIDS, heart disease, cancer, and homicides dropped dramatically.

Recent findings about certain aspects of Americans' current health status, however, are less encouraging. In 2000, about one in ten adults reported never being physically active (Barnes & Schoenborn, 2003). Moreover, approximately 40% of adults did not engage in physical activity during their leisure time. Physically inactive people are more likely to be overweight than active people. In the period from 1999 to 2002, 65% of American adults and 16% of children and adolescents were too fat (Hedley et al., 2004). Excess body fat is associated with many serious diseases, including type 2 diabetes, high blood pressure, heart disease, and certain cancers.

> **Between 1985 and 2000, more adults exercised regularly . . .**

Among young Americans, cigarette smoking and alcohol abuse are widespread practices that have negative effects on health. At the present time, cigarette smoking is the most preventable cause of disease and death in the United States. About 22% of Americans who are 18 years of age and older smoke cigarettes (National Center for Health Statistics [NCHS], 2004). Young adults between 18 and 24 years of age are more likely to be current smokers than are members of other age groups (Woollery et al., 2003). Binge drinking, that is, consuming five or more alcoholic drinks in a row, is common among high school and college students. Nearly three in ten high school students binge drink (Centers for Disease Control and Prevention [CDC], 2004). Approximately 44% of college students engaged in this risky behavior on at least one occasion during the 2 weeks that preceded a national survey that was conducted in 2001 (Wechsler et al., 2002). About one in four college students indicated that their drinking behaviors contributed to serious academic problems, including missing classes, performing poorly on exams, and lowering their grade point averages (National Institutes of Health [NIH], 2002). Clearly, people living in the United States have more lifestyle changes to make if they are to live longer and healthier lives.

Lifestyle is a way of living. As a college student, your lifestyle includes a variety of behaviors that promote or impair good health and longevity. Although you may be unable to prevent severe birth defects or inherited disorders from affecting your health, you can modify many health risk factors, reducing the likelihood that you will develop serious medical problems. A **risk factor** is a characteristic that increases an individual's chances of developing a health problem. For example, physical inactivity, tobacco use, emotional stress, and a high-fat diet are risk factors for heart disease, hypertension, and certain types of cancers. You can dramatically lower your chances of developing these conditions by incorporating exercise into your daily schedule, choosing not to use tobacco products, practicing relaxation techniques, and eating a low-fat diet. Of course, the decision to adopt a healthier lifestyle is up to you.

To evaluate the impact of your lifestyle on your health, answer the questions in the "Healthstyle" assessment in the student workbook that accompanies this textbook.

Are you concerned about your health? What are you doing to protect it? What steps can you take to enhance your state of health so you can enjoy life more fully? Where can you find reliable information concerning health? The information and recommendations in this textbook can help you make choices that will improve your health.

lifestyle
a way of living, including behaviors that promote or impair good health and longevity.

risk factor a characteristic that increases an individual's chances of developing a health problem.

health good health is the ability to function adequately and independently in a constantly changing environment.

■ The Dimensions of Health

What Is Health?

Most people can describe how it feels to be healthy or ill, but trying to define *health* is not an easy task. In 1948 the World Health Organization (WHO) constitution defined health as "a state of complete physical, mental, and social well-being and not merely the absence of disease or infirmity" (p. 2). This definition, however, is too limited. Consider the person in Figure 1-1. Although he is in a wheelchair, he is able to compete as an athlete. If you judged his state of health using WHO's 1948 definition, you might conclude that he is unhealthy. Many physically disabled people are able to function adequately in society and do not consider themselves ill or infirm.

The Ottawa Charter for Health Promotion (WHO, 1986) defined *health* as "a resource for everyday life . . . a positive concept emphasizing social and personal resources, as well as physical capabilities." According to this charter, health requires "peace, shelter, education, food, income, a stable ecosystem, sustainable resources, social justice and equity." In addition to these conditions, most healthy adults want to function independently; enjoy eating, sexual, and physical activities; feel good about themselves; and be with family and friends.

Behavioral scientist Godfrey Hochbaum (1979) proposed a simple definition for *health*: "Health is what helps me be what I want to be . . . do what I want to do . . . [and] live the way I would like to live." Using Hochbaum's definition, you might conclude that the wheelchair-bound athlete in Figure 1-1 is as healthy as a person who is capable of running.

Health and Wellness

Health and wellness are related concepts. Good **health** enables one to function adequately and independently in a constantly changing environment; **wellness** is a sense that one is functioning at his or her best level. Figure 1-2 illustrates the concept of health as a continuum; there are degrees of health. The absence of

Figure 1-1 **Wheelchair Athletes.** Many physically disabled people do not consider themselves ill or infirm because they can function well in society. According to Hochbaum's definition of *health*, individuals with physical disabilities can be healthy and enjoy life.

Figure 1-2 **A Health Continuum.** Some people view health as a continuum; that is, there are degrees of health. Premature death is at one end of this continuum, and optimal well-being is at the other end. Source: Adapted from Ebersole, P., & Hess, P. (1994). *Toward healthy aging.* St. Louis: Mosby-Year Book, Inc.

functioning (premature death) is at one end of this continuum, and the highest level of functioning (optimal well-being) is at the other end. Many people accept responsibility for the quality of their health and well-being. These people are willing to take various steps to improve their health, achieving a higher degree of wellness in the process.

Most health educators agree that health and wellness are **holistic**, that is, they involve all aspects of the individual. Thus, the holistic concept of health encompasses not only the physical, psychological, and social aspects, but also the intellectual, spiritual, and environmental dimensions of a person. Each dimension is an integral part of a person's health, and any change in the quality of one component of health affects the others. For example, individuals who exercise with others to increase their level of physical health often report a sense of improved psychological and social health.

The Components of Health

Physical Health Physical health refers to the overall condition of the organ systems, such as the cardiovascular system (heart and blood vessels), respiratory system (lungs), reproductive system, and nervous system. When certain organs do not function adequately, a person has various signs and symptoms of illness. **Signs** are the observable and measurable features of an illness such as fever, rash, and abnormal behavior. **Symptoms** are the subjective complaints of an illness, such as reports of fatigue, headaches, and numbness. A healthy person's systems function properly; the individual feels well and is free of disease.

Psychological Health Psychological (mental) health involves the ability to deal effectively with the psychological challenges of life. Psychologically healthy people accept responsibility for their behavior, feel good about themselves and others, are comfortable with their emotions (feelings), and have positive, realistic outlooks on life. Although experiences such as losing a job or a family member cause stress or grief, psychologically healthy people are able to limit the extent to which crises affect their lives.

Social Health Social health is the sense of well-being that one achieves by forming emotionally supportive and intellectually stimulating relationships with family members, friends, and associates. Living in communities rather than in isolation, identifying with social groups, and belonging to organizations strengthen the social dimension of health. When social networks break down, health declines.

Intellectual Health Intellectual health is the ability to use problem-solving and other higher-order thinking skills to deal effectively with life's challenges. Healthy people analyze situations, determine alternative courses of action, and make decisions. After making decisions, intellectually healthy individuals are able to judge the effectiveness of their choices and learn from their experiences. Effective intellectual skills enable people to feel in control of their lives.

Spiritual Health Spiritual health is the belief that one is a part of a larger scheme of life and that one's life has purpose. Identifying with a religion and having religious beliefs influence the spiritual health of many people. However, spirituality is not confined to those who belong to organized religious groups or have religious beliefs. People can develop spirituality without practicing a particular religion or believing in the power of a supreme being. Whatever the nature of their spirituality, many individuals achieve a sense of inner peace and harmony as well as emotional fulfillment by believing that their lives have a purpose. As in the other wellness dimensions, a breakdown in spiritual health can have a negative impact on one's well-being.

Environmental Health Nothing affects the quality of wellness components as much as the state of the environment—the conditions where people live, work, and play. Environmental concerns that influence wellness include the provision of clean water and air, the management of wastes, and the control of distressing social problems such as crime and family violence. Humans cannot achieve a high degree of wellness if their environment is polluted or unsafe (Figure 1-3). Chapter 16 discusses environmental health concerns.

wellness a sense that one is functioning at his or her best level.

holistic (hole-IS-tic) a characteristic involving all aspects of the person.

signs observable and measurable features of an illness.

symptoms subjective complaints of illness.

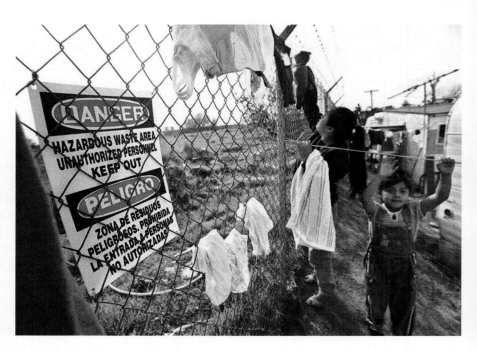

Figure 1-3 **Environmental Health.** The state of the environment in which people live, work, and play affects the quality of their health. People cannot achieve a high degree of wellness if their environment is polluted or unsafe.

Figure 1-4 is a model that illustrates how these six components of wellness are related and integrated into a holistic approach to understanding health. This model has the physical and psychological health components at the core of the larger environmental component. The social, intellectual, and spiritual components involve thought processes; therefore, they are found in the psychological health dimension. When the components of health integrate and function well, the individual has a sense of well-being.

■ The Nation's Health

Many people fail to recognize that health involves more than just personal health—health is a national concern, too. Many of the crucial social, political, and economic issues facing this country are health-related, such as domestic violence, health care reform, terrorism, and care of the aged.

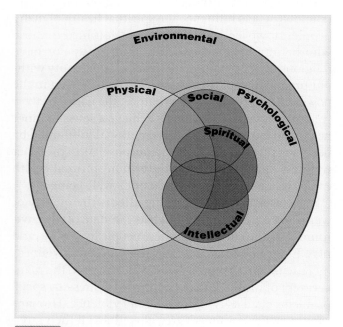

Figure 1-4 **The Components of Health.** The components of health are interrelated. According to this model, the social, intellectual, and spiritual components of health are in the larger spheres of physical and psychological health, which are in the largest sphere of environmental health.

Tracking the Nation's Health

The U.S. government, particularly the Public Health Service of the Department of Health and Human Services, monitors the nation's health in a variety of ways. One way is by recording cases of certain diseases and causes of death. Table 1-1 shows the ten leading causes of death for all Americans in 2002. In the United States, heart disease is the leading cause of death, followed by cancer and strokes.

Table 1-1	The Ten Major Causes of Death in the United States	
Rank	Cause	Percentage of Deaths
1	Heart disease	28.4
2	Cancer	22.8
3	Stroke	6.7
4	Chronic lung diseases	5.1
5	Accidents/unintentional injuries	4.2
6	Diabetes mellitus	3.0
7	Pneumonia/influenza	2.7
8	Alzheimer's disease	2.4
9	Kidney disease	1.7
10	Septicemia (blood infection)	1.4
—	Other causes	21.6

Kochanek, K. D., & Smith, B. L. (2004). Deaths: Preliminary data for 2002. *National Vital Statistics Reports, 52*(13):1–48.

Table 1-2	Causes of Death: All Races, Selected Age Groups of Americans

Ages 15–24

Rank	Cause
1	Unintentional injuries
2	Homicide
3	Suicide
4	Cancer
5	Heart disease

Ages 25–44

Rank	Cause
1	Unintentional injuries
2	Cancer
3	Heart disease
4	Suicide
5	AIDS/HIV

Kochanek, K. D., & Smith, B. L. (2004). Deaths: Preliminary data for 2002. *National Vital Statistics Reports, 52*(13):1–48.

The major causes of death differ for members of various age groups. Table 1-2 shows the leading causes of death in two age categories: 15 to 24 years and 25 to 44 years. Unintentional injuries (accidents), homicide, and suicide are the leading causes of death of people between 15 and 24 years of age. Note that unintentional injuries, cancer, and heart disease are the leading causes of death of people between 25 and 44 years of age.

Over the past 100 years, Americans made great progress toward improving their health, well-being, and longevity. In 1900 the life expectancy of a newborn baby was less than 50 years. **Life expectancy** is the average number of years that an individual of a particular age can look forward to living. Compared to people who lived in the first half of the twentieth century, many Americans can now expect to live longer and healthier lives. In 2002 the average life expectancy of a newborn American was 77.4 years (Kochanek & Smith, 2004). This progress occurred largely because various government agencies provided greater access to health care, conducted health education and research programs, and regulated the safety of the environment. For example, childhood vaccination programs have removed the threat of polio and controlled other infectious diseases such as measles, diphtheria, rubella, and tetanus. Food fortification programs have nearly eliminated nutritional defi-

ciency diseases such as goiter, rickets, and pellagra. Efforts to educate the public concerning the hazards of tobacco use and drinking and driving have reduced the prevalence of smoking among adults and made motor vehicle travel safer.

Although the life expectancy of Americans has increased, many people die prematurely, that is, before they reach 75 years of age. According to health experts at the Centers for Disease Control and Prevention in Atlanta, *actual causes* of death are the underlying reasons that are not reported on death certificates. In 2000, for example, about 18% of all deaths were the result of tobacco use, including secondhand exposure to tobacco smoke; poor diet and lack of physical activity accounted for over 16% of deaths (Mokdad et al., 2004). Leading-causes-of-death tables such as Table 1-1, however, integrate those deaths within the number of deaths resulting primarily from heart disease, cancer, and stroke. Health experts predict that the combination of poor diet and physical inactivity will soon replace tobacco use as the leading actual cause of death in the United States. In many instances, actual causes of death are associated with lifestyle choices, such as tobacco use or physical inactivity. By changing these and other health-related behaviors, people may be able to avoid dying prematurely.

Federal, state, and local governments can help individuals develop healthy lifestyles by providing educational and professional services. How does the federal government monitor the health of its citizens? What is being done to improve the nation's health?

Health Promotion: *Healthy People 2000* and *Healthy People 2010*

Health promotion is the practice of helping people become healthier by encouraging them to change their lifestyles. In the late 1980s, a team of concerned health experts, health educators, and U.S. government officials analyzed the results of recent studies, reports, and recommendations that summarized the health status of Americans. In 1991 these experts published their findings in a report called *Healthy People 2000* (USDHHS, 1991).

Healthy People 2000 had three general goals: increase the healthy life span of Americans, improve the health status of American minorities, and extend the accessibility of preventive health services to all Americans. The overall goal was for Americans to achieve the health objectives by the year 2000; as more *Healthy People 2000* objectives were met, the overall health status of Americans would improve.

life expectancy the average number of years that an individual can expect to live.

Staff of various federal, state, and local agencies developed and implemented health educational efforts that supported *Healthy People 2000* goals. Additionally, they monitored Americans' progress in meeting these health objectives. The U.S. Public Health Service published progress reports to show national trends in achieving the goals. The information concerning the state of Americans' health that was given in the beginning of this chapter is from the final *Healthy People 2000* progress report. Several chapters of this textbook also highlight findings from this report.

By 1997 members of the original *Healthy People 2000* team focused their attention on preparing a national health promotion and disease prevention plan that would be relevant for the year 2010. Today, differences in death and illness rates between the nation's rich and poor, men and women, as well as among its diverse ethnic and racial groups are major public health concerns. For example, American men generally do not live as long as American women, and they are more likely to die from each of the ten leading causes of death. Additionally, more African Americans die of cancers and diseases of the heart and blood vessels than members of other ethnic and racial groups. The reasons for these differences are unclear, but lifestyle choices, environmental conditions, and socioeconomic situations are major contributing factors. The Surgeon General of the United States' *Healthy People 2010* strategy is to increase the years and quality of healthy life by eliminating the differences in health among population groups.

To monitor the population's progress in meeting the targeted goals of the 467 objectives of *Healthy People 2010,* health experts condensed the objectives into a smaller group of health concerns, the ten *Leading Health Indicators*, and identified 21 key objectives for the indicators (see Appendix A). The Leading Health Indicators, which include physical activity and substance abuse, were selected because of their importance to personal and community health as well as their relevance to individual health-related behaviors, environmental health problems, and health system issues. Developing health promotion strategies that focus on the indicators, such as programs to encourage seat belt use, childhood immunizations, and smoking cessation, can increase the quality and years of life as well as eliminate health disparities among Americans.

Minority Health Status

For hundreds of years, immigrants from around the world have been changing the face of the United States as they settle in this country. Each new group of immi-

Figure 1-5 **An American Family.** Culture consists of the unique social characteristics of a population, such as its customs, rituals, and health practices. Immigrants who settle in the United States from regions such as Southeast Asia contribute much to the racial, ethnic, and cultural diversity of the population.

grants brings different cultural traditions and various ethnic identities with them (**Figure 1-5**). Culture consists of the unique social characteristics of a population, such as its customs, rituals, and health beliefs and practices, which are passed down from generation to generation. An ethnic group is one that shares a common national, religious, racial, or ancestral identity. According to the U.S. Department of Health and Human Services, the major American racial/ethnic subpopulations are Caucasians (whites), African Americans (blacks), Latinos (Hispanics), Native Americans (American Indians), and Asian and Pacific Islanders. The same terms, however, are not used by all agencies. Throughout this textbook, terms such as *Caucasian* may be used in one context and *whites* in another; we reflect the language of the agency or researcher when reporting statistics or results of research studies.

Today in the United States, the majority of Americans have European ancestry, particularly Northern European. The National Center for Health Statistics refers to this population as "white, non-Hispanic." About 30% of the U.S. population identifies itself as a member of an ethnic or racial minority, such as African American, Hispanic, or Asian American.

Throughout this textbook, the Diversity in Health essays feature topics that concern a variety of populations in the United States as well as around the world. The Diversity in Health essay in this chapter, "Minority Health Status in the United States," discusses differences in the overall health of certain minority groups in the United States.

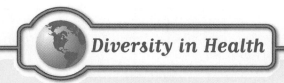

Minority Health Status in the United States

Did you know that African Americans are more likely to die of cancer than whites? Were you aware that Native American males are more likely to be murdered than American males with Asian/Pacific Islander ancestry? Did you know that Hispanics are more likely to die in accidents than as the result of strokes? The differences in death and illness rates for various population subgroups reflect numerous factors, such as socioeconomic status and access to health insurance and medical care. By investigating reasons for these differences, health scientists have learned a great deal about the health of American minorities. A major goal of the U.S. Department of Health and Human Services is improving the health of *all* Americans through research, education, and better access to health care.

Hispanic or Latino People

Hispanic, or Latino, people have immigrated to the United States or have ancestors from Spanish-speaking countries, especially Mexico, Puerto Rico, Central and South America, and Cuba. Currently, Hispanics make up the largest minority group in the United States (NCHS, 2003).

In 2001, the leading causes of death for Hispanics were heart disease, cancer, and accidental injuries. Compared to white non-Hispanics, Hispanics were more likely to die from accidents, diabetes, and chronic liver disease (NCHS, 2003). Although Latinos are less likely to commit suicide or die from kidney and Alzheimer's disease than non-Hispanic whites, their homicide rate is considerably higher than that of non-Hispanic whites.

Poverty, lack of health insurance, and poor education are barriers to good health for many Hispanics. One of four members of this minority lives in poverty (NCHS, 2003). Health disorders associated with poverty, such as tuberculosis and malnutrition, are more common in certain Spanish-speaking subgroups. In 2001, about 16% of all Americans younger than 65 years did not have health insurance. Hispanic persons, especially those of Mexican ancestry, are more likely to be uninsured than non-Hispanic whites. Regardless of one's ethnic/racial background, not having health insurance is a major obstacle to obtaining good health care in the United States.

African Americans

In the United States, African Americans are the second largest minority group. Despite recent improvements, the health status of black Americans is generally poorer than that of other minorities. The life expectancies of whites and blacks reflect their health status. In 2002, the life expectancy of African American females was 75.7 years; the life expectancy of white American females was 80.3 years (Kochanek & Smith, 2004). At the same time, the life expectancy for African American males was 68.9 years, and that of white males was 75.3 years.

The major causes of death of black Americans are similar to those of non-Hispanic whites. Although black Americans are less likely to die from chronic lung diseases, Alzheimer's disease, and suicide, death rates for 9 of the 11 leading causes of death are higher than for whites. Black women are more likely to die of breast and cervical cancer than white women (Office of Minority Health, 2004). Black men are more than twice as likely as white men to die of prostate cancer (Gargiullo et al., 2002). HIV/AIDS is the leading cause of death for black Americans who are 34 to 44 years of age (Office of Minority Health, 2004). The homicide rate for African Americans is very high: Blacks are six times more likely to be murdered than whites.

Childbearing is riskier for an African American woman; in 2001, she was over three times more likely to die during pregnancy or childbirth than a white woman (Arias et al., 2003). Additionally, black infants are more likely to die during the first month of life than other babies. The infant death rate among black infants is more than twice that of white babies.

Hypertension (chronic high blood pressure) is twice as common in blacks compared with whites. The reason for this high prevalence is unclear, but scientists think diet, genetics, stress, and smoking play roles. Overweight increases the risk of hypertension. Black women are more likely to have excess body fat than other Americans. In the period from 1999 to 2000, more than 80% of black women who were 40 years of age and older were too fat (Flegal et al., 2002).

Asian and Pacific Islanders

As one of the fastest-growing minority groups, Asian Americans and Pacific Islanders (APIs) are a diverse group of people who immigrated to the United States from China, Japan, Vietnam, Korea, India, the Philippines, and other Pacific Islands. In general, Americans with Chinese and Japanese ancestry are healthier than other Americans (Office of Minority Health, 2004). Vietnamese American women, however, are five times more likely to develop cervical cancer than white women. Additionally, people who immigrated recently from Asia and the Pacific Islands are more likely to suffer from hepatitis, a serious liver disease, and tuberculosis than people who have lived in the United States for longer periods of time.

Continued

■ Understanding Health-Related Behavior

Regardless of their cultural and ethnic background, not all Americans share the same level of concern for their health. How many times have you heard a smoker say, "I can stop smoking whenever I want to; now is just not a good time" or "You've got to die of something; it might as well be lung cancer." You may know people who eat too many fatty foods, do not exercise regularly, and smoke cigarettes. You may know other people who follow a low-fat diet, walk at a brisk pace for 45 minutes nearly every day, and avoid drugs such as alcohol and tobacco. Why do some people adopt more positive health-related behaviors than others?

Changing Health-Related Behavior

"I wish I had the willpower to stop smoking." "I just can't seem to find the motivation to exercise more often." Do these statements sound familiar? Is having a lot of willpower the key to becoming healthier?

Health educators often refer to willpower as **motivation**, the force or drive that leads people to take action. Past experiences, perceived needs, and personal values influence one's motivation. For example, a person who has tried unsuccessfully to stop smoking several times and claims to enjoy smoking may have little motivation to make another attempt to quit.

Efficacy enhances motivation. **Efficacy** is the belief that one is capable of changing behavior. Various barriers such as poor education or lack of support from family members can interfere with someone's motivation to change behaviors.

Having knowledge about risky behaviors and the seriousness of a health-related condition does not necessarily motivate individuals to take appropriate actions. For example, most people know that seat belts reduce the possibility of a serious injury in an automobile accident and that most states require them to wear seat belts in a car. Nevertheless, individuals often make a variety of excuses to explain why they fail to buckle up. Additionally, many students enrolled in personal health classes can correctly identify behaviors that promote optimal health, yet they do not practice what they know. Acquiring knowledge about health is important, but becoming motivated to adopt a healthier lifestyle is essential if individuals are to make long-term changes that can benefit their health.

Taking an active role in achieving and maintaining good health depends on certain personal factors: degree of vulnerability, level of motivation (*willpower*), sense of control, and perceived value of the behavior. People are motivated to take action if they feel that a sufficient threat to their health exists and that the consequences of changing the behavior are worthwhile.

Assume, for example, that diabetes affects several members of your family. You have heard that diabetes may be inherited; therefore, you are aware that you have a good chance of developing this condition (*vulnerability*). You know that family members who have diabetes suffer from kidney damage, blindness, and premature heart disease. Since you want to avoid these consequences, you are motivated to change certain behaviors (*motivation*). Additionally, you believe that

motivation
the force or drive that leads people to take action.

efficacy (EF-fih-ka-see) regarding health education, the belief that one is capable of changing his or her behavior.

your actions influence the quality of your health (*sense of control*). Concerned, you decide to learn more about diabetes and determine what actions can reduce your risk of developing the disease. You now have a reason to take action because you believe it is important (*value*) to prevent this disease, even if it means making lifestyle changes now while you are still healthy.

Making Positive Health-Related Decisions

How I Quit Smoking

About a month ago I was a smoker—about 10 cigarettes a day during the week and up to a pack a day on weekends. After thinking about quitting for about a year, it happened. Without even giving it any consideration, I was able to not buy a pack for 2 days. On day 3, I realized my success and told myself I would never buy a pack again. I miss it, especially after a drink or a meal, but I'm glad I've gone this far. There have been times when I've really wanted one, but that's when you realize how powerful of a drug it is. At least that's how I talk myself out of having one. Before, I never thought of myself as being addicted—too harsh of a word—but I was just like all of the other smokers out there. It's a filthy habit—I'm glad I stopped.

Although this college student smoked less than a pack of cigarettes a day, he took about a year to quit smoking. He made the final decision to stop smoking while listening to other students' habit-breaking experiences in his health class. Some people take less time to make health-related decisions than others, and some people have less difficulty making lifestyle changes than others. Figure 1-6 illustrates the complex process of decision making.

Stages of Behavioral Change According to many health education experts, the process of changing behaviors involves the five stages shown in Figure 1-7 (Norcross & Prochaska, 2002). We will use the example of smoking to illustrate this process. The first stage is *precontemplation*. In this stage, smokers show no interest in quitting tobacco use, do not see a need to quit, and may avoid discussing their smoking behavior with others. Smokers move into the *contemplation* stage when they realize or admit tobacco use is unhealthy, and they intend to quit smoking in the next 6 months. In the *preparation* stage of change, smokers may have made unsuccessful attempts to quit smoking, yet they express the desire to stop within the next month. Smokers in the *action* stage of change take steps to quit smoking, such as "going cold turkey" or using a nicotine patch. They succeed in quitting for up to 6 months. Finally, smokers in the *maintenance* stage develop practices to avoid relapsing into using tobacco. Former smokers, for example, might socialize with nonsmokers or use exercise as a substitute for smoking. According to

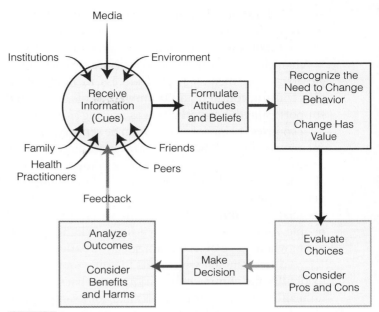

Figure 1-6 **Decision-Making Model.** Decision making can be a complex process. Information, personal attitudes, and personal experiences influence your decision-making process. To change health-related behaviors, you must recognize the need to change, that the change has personal value, and that it is consistent with your beliefs.

health education researchers, 40% of people who engage in risky behaviors such as smoking, being physically inactive, and eating high-fat diets are in the precontemplation stage, 40% are in the contemplation stage, and the remaining 20% are preparing to change the unhealthy behaviors (Prochaska & Velicer, 1997).

When people relapse, they return to the precontemplation stage of change and usually feel like failures as a result of their inability to maintain the new behaviors. In the case of smokers, they may even return to the precontemplation stage in which they stop thinking about quitting. However, the majority of people who relapse eventually decide to stop smoking again, and they tend to try a different method of quitting.

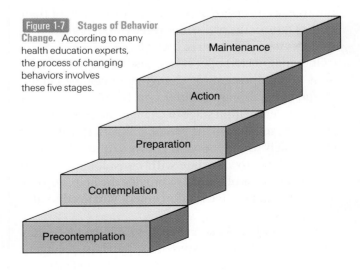

Figure 1-7 **Stages of Behavior Change.** According to many health education experts, the process of changing behaviors involves these five stages.

People who seriously want to quit smoking, for example, typically make three to four efforts to stop before they actually succeed (Norcross & Prochaska, 2002).

When changing a behavior, people use various strategies to increase their chances of success, including stimulus control, counterconditioning, rewards, and social support. *Stimulus control* involves altering *cues* to modify responses (behaviors). Cues can be sensory triggers, such as seeing a billboard advertisement for cigarettes or smelling someone else's cigarette smoke. Cues can also be emotional states or thoughts. For example, a person may smoke to relieve stress or because he or she associates smoking with celebrities or sophisticated people. As a result, this person is likely to light up a cigarette when tense or in certain social situations.

If you are a smoker who wants to quit, you may need to identify and eliminate the various cues that signal this unhealthy behavior. You may realize, for example, that seeing ashtrays and lighters are your smoking cues. Throwing out or giving away your ashtrays and lighters are ways of avoiding these cues. If feeling tense triggers your desire to smoke, then learning and practicing relaxation techniques whenever you feel stressed out may help you resist the urge to buy a pack of cigarettes.

Counterconditioning involves replacing unhealthy behaviors with less destructive or healthier ones. When you desire a cigarette, you may be able to eliminate the craving by walking, taking a warm bath, or calling someone who supports your efforts to quit. Chewing sugarless gum, eating raw vegetables or fruit, or drinking a glass of water whenever you feel the urge to smoke may also reduce the craving.

Rewards are incentives for positive behaviors. Some former smokers keep a jar in which they save the money that would have been used to buy cigarettes. At the end of a week or two, they spend that money on something fun such as a movie, DVD, or another type of reward to help maintain the new behavior. Other former tobacco users are rewarded by the return of their sense of taste or the praise they receive from nonsmokers for adopting a smoke-free lifestyle.

Obtaining social support by enlisting the help of others is very important for changing a negative behavior and maintaining a positive one. If you are a smoker in the contemplation stage of change and most of your friends are smokers in the precontemplation stage, they are not likely to support your efforts to quit. Therefore, you may have to associate with nonsmokers or people in later stages of change to provide the help, encouragement, and positive reinforcement you need to quit tobacco use.

A Decision-Making Model In *Applying Concepts for Healthy Living: A Workbook*, the student activities' supplement that accompanies this textbook, you will find a Changing Health Habits feature for each chapter. This feature uses a systematic model for the decision-making process that can help you improve your health and well-being. The first part of the process involves identifying a problem behavior that you want to change, a goal that you'd like to reach, or a question that you'd like to answer. For example, you might want to quit smoking, lose 20 pounds, or determine whether you are ready to end an abusive relationship. Because the process of altering a behavior can have its unpleasant aspects, particularly if you have to overcome side effects or cravings, it is important to determine your level of commitment. To determine if you are ready to change a behavior or situation, it is helpful to make a list of the benefits, or pros, as well as the harms, or cons, of changing. After you make the list, think about each pro and con's value or importance to you. Assign a point value from 1 to 5 to each pro and con; a rating of 5 points would be the highest value. Then find the sums of each list. If the sum of the cons list is greater than that of the pros list, you are probably in the precontemplation stage and not ready to make the change. On the other hand, if the sum of your pros is higher, you are likely in the contemplation stage and ready to make the change.

The second part of the process used in the decision-making model describes steps you can take to implement the change and evaluate your progress. After you decide to make a change, set a target date to begin the new behavior, reach the goal, or modify the situation. Mark that date on a calendar that is in an obvious place for you to notice, such as by your computer monitor or on your refrigerator or mirror. Then make a list of factors that will increase the chances that you will be successful in making the change, such as enlisting the help of friends or obtaining advice from a medical expert. Because there are often barriers to making changes, make another list of factors that will hinder your chances for success, such as having little time to practice new behaviors or friends who won't support your decision to change.

The third major step in the process involves preparing an action plan that provides specific steps you will take to change your behavior or situation. You should be able to identify more than one way to reach your goal. To quit smoking, for example, you might quit "cold turkey," gradually reduce the number of cigarettes smoked over a 4-week period, or use a medically approved nicotine-containing product. At this point, you need to learn about the pros and cons of each method and consider the factors that can help or hinder your effort to change. How are you going to handle cravings or social situations that promote the behavior you're trying to change? Now you are ready to make the change by implementing your action plan. Keep a daily record of your progress, including strategies that are helpful and your feelings about the process. When you reach the goal date, analyze your success in attaining the goal. How well did your plan work? What can you learn from the experience?

To enjoy a long, healthy, and productive life, it is important for you to make numerous health-related decisions every day. If you act impulsively and base these decisions simply on cues, attitudes, and emotions, you may make poor choices. However, you are likely to make responsible choices if you follow a systematic method of decision making such as the one we have described. Changing habits often requires learning new information and practicing new skills. To prac-

tice making responsible health-related choices, complete the decision-making activities in *Applying Concepts for Healthy Living: A Workbook.*

The Goal of Prevention A primary component of health promotion is preventing diseases, infections, injuries, birth defects, and other health problems. Preventing a health problem is a far better and less costly option than trying to treat it. In addition to adopting healthy lifestyle practices, you can take responsibility for preventing serious health problems by having routine physical examinations. The Managing Your Health box below provides recommendations for the frequency of routine screening procedures such as blood pressure, cholesterol, and

Managing Your Health

Routine Health Care for Disease Prevention

The following recommendations concerning routine screening and immunizations apply to adults who have low risks of disease. People who have higher risks may need more frequent testing and to begin testing at an earlier age. Consult your personal physician for advice about routine health care.

Medical Test/ Preventive Measure	Recommended Frequency*
Blood pressure	At least every 2 years.
Height/weight	Periodic.
Cholesterol	At least every 5 years for men aged 35 and older; regularly for women aged 45 and older; younger people who smoke, have diabetes, or have a family history of heart disease should be screened beginning at age 20.
Glucose (diabetes screening)	Routine for people with high blood pressure or cholesterol.
Prostate (PSA) and digital rectal exam	Annually after 50 years of age (men); at-risk men should be tested earlier.
Testicular examination (cancer)	Men with average risk can perform monthly self-exam.
Skin examination (cancer)	Every 3 years for people between 20 and 39 years of age; annual screening after age 40.
Breast examination (cancer)	American Cancer Society recommends annual screening mammography and clinical breast exams for healthy women aged 40 years and older; women between 20 and 39 years of age should undergo clinical breast exam every 3 years. Breast self-exam is an option for women.

Medical Test/ Preventive Measure	Recommended Frequency*
Pap test (cervical cancer)	Begin screening within 3 years of first sexual intercourse or by 21st birthday; yearly Pap test, or every 2 years if liquid form of the test is used.
Colon/rectal examination (cancer)	Have test at age 50; physician can decide which test is appropriate.
Sexually transmitted infections	Sexually active people who are 25 years of age or younger should be screened for chlamydial infection; physician and patient can decide which other tests are appropriate such as for HIV.
Depression screening	Patients who have felt sad, hopeless, or no interest in usual activities for at least 2 weeks should be screened.
Immunizations	
Rubella	All women of childbearing age should be screened for rubella susceptibility at their first health care checkup; nonpregnant women who have not been exposed to rubella should be offered rubella vaccination.
Influenza (flu)	Annually for those who wish to be vaccinated.
Tetanus-diphtheria	Every 10 years.
Hepatitis B and other infectious diseases	Consult personal physician.

*Recommendations vary somewhat among medical organizations. Sources: U.S. Preventive Services Task Force, Department of Health and Human Services, http://www.ahcpr.gov; U.S. Department of Health and Human Services, Centers for Disease Control and Prevention, http://www.cdc.gov/nchstp/dstd/personal_Health_Questions.htm; American College of Preventive Medicine, http://www.acpm.org; American Cancer Society, http://www.cancer.org. Accessed June 14, 2004.

body weight and height measurements; mammograms; pelvic, skin, and prostate exams; and Pap smears. Note that some examinations, such as testicular and breast self-exams, are easy enough to be done in the privacy of your home. Many college students think they are healthy and do not see the need for routine physical evaluations. Having regular medical checkups, however, enables you and your physician to monitor your physical and psychological health status. Furthermore, your physician may be able to identify a problem before it results in serious damage to your health and well-being.

Can Good Health Be Prescribed?

No one has a crystal ball that predicts future health, nor can anyone guarantee good health. Numerous factors contribute to one's chances of enjoying a long and productive lifetime of good health. Several of these factors are the result of lifestyle choices that people can make, while they are still young, to prevent or delay disease. You may know someone or have heard about individuals who avoided exercise, smoked a pack of cigarettes, and consumed a six-pack of beer each day, yet lived to a ripe old age. Such behavior defies nearly every reasonable prescription for good health. Perhaps these people inherited the hardiness to withstand the effects of their risky lifestyles. You might wonder if these people enjoyed good health throughout their lives, or if they spent their last years in poor health. Would their lives have been even longer if they had followed more health-conscious behaviors?

Health experts generally base their recommendations for healthier lifestyles on scientific information collected from numerous studies that involved large numbers of people and not on reports of individual cases. This textbook presents findings from current research for you to use in your own health decision-making process.

Healthy Living Practices

- To change your health-related behaviors, you must determine that you need to change and that you value the change.
- Use a decision-making plan as a tool to help you make responsible decisions.

■ Analyzing Health Information

"Take natural antioxidants to live longer." "Drink red wine to prevent heart attacks." "Improve your memory with ginkgo biloba." Every day Americans are barraged with a confusing array of health-related information in newspapers; magazines; and television and radio talk shows, commercials, and infomercials. In addition to the media, family members, friends, teachers, health care professionals, and the Internet supply information about health and health-related products. Are these sources reliable? Not necessarily. There are no laws that prevent anyone from making statements or writing books about health, even if their information is false. The First Amendment to the U.S. Constitution protects freedom of speech and freedom of the press. This protection extends to talk-show guests, authors, and salespeople in health food stores who might provide health misinformation.

Companies and individuals make considerable amounts of money by selling untested remedies, worthless cures, toxic herbal preparations, unnecessary nutrient supplements, and books filled with misinformation. Health frauds include the promotion or sale of substances or devices that are touted as being effective to diagnose, prevent, cure, or treat diseases or other conditions but that lack scientific evidence of their safety and effectiveness. Despite the regulatory activities of the Food and Drug Administration (FDA) and the Federal Trade Commission (FTC), the sale of fraudulent products and services and the circulation of misleading or false health information continue to be concerns of medical experts and public health officials.

Keep in mind that if the claim sounds too good to be true, it probably is not true. Some other telltale signs that information about a health-related product or service is questionable include

- Claims that a secret formula or ingredient gives the product its beneficial effects on health
- Promotional techniques that rely heavily on Internet or mail-order outlets, radio ads, televised home shopping channels, or infomercials
- Claims that the product or service is the result of a miraculous scientific discovery
- Claims that the product or service provides "quick," "painless," "effortless," or "guaranteed" cure or other desirable result
- Details of the product's or service's benefits are given, but no mention of its risks
- Testimonials and personal experiences are cited as supporting evidence
- Few scientific references to indicate that the product has been tested for safety and effectiveness
- Discrediting of scientific studies or conventional medical practices

Assessing Information on the Internet

The Internet can be a valuable source of health-related information. Many Web sites, however, are sources of inaccurate and potentially harmful information, because anyone with a computer and the appropriate software can produce and post a Web page. Moreover, there is no organization that regulates the quality or edits the content of health information on the Internet. Therefore, you need to analyze the reliability of health information from Web sites as critically and carefully as you analyze health information from other sources. One way is to use the model for analyzing health-related information that is discussed on page 16. Additionally, determine answers to the following questions.

What is the source of the information? The Web site should identify its sponsors. Is the site sponsored by an individual or newsgroups? Does the site have a chat room or message board? Individuals who sponsor sites, visit chat rooms, or post messages often give advice that is based on personal experiences, biases, or opinions instead of medical expertise and scientific evidence. Furthermore, some message boards and newsgroups do not have moderators who act as "gatekeepers" by checking messages and eliminating questionable postings. Is it a commercial site (".com")? Commercial sites may or may not contain misinformation and are likely to be biased toward their product, treatment, or service. Is the site sponsored by a nationally known health/medical organization such as the American Heart Association or the American Medical Association? Such organizations use health experts to write and review their Web site content, which is usually reliable. Is the site staffed by medical experts who are affiliated with major research institutions or universities? These sites usually provide accurate and timely health information. Does the site include up-to-date references for articles from journals with scientific-sounding titles? It may be difficult to determine if these journals are reliable. Finally, is the information at the Web site current? Health information is constantly changing; the site should indicate when the information was posted and updated.

At healthyliving.jbpub.com, we provide Web sites that are pertinent to the content of each chapter. The U.S. government maintains Web sites for health-related information, including the sites of the Centers for Disease Control and Prevention (www.cdc.gov), Food and Drug Administration (www.fda.gov), and National Institutes of Health (www.nih.gov). Additionally, the Department of Health and Human Services maintains www.healthfinder.gov, a general health information Web site that provides links to reliable sources such as government agencies (Web sites denoted by ".gov"), information clearinghouses, nonprofit organizations (".org"), and universities (".edu").

Reliable health Web sites generally follow standards and codes established by nonprofit organizations such as the Health on the Net Foundation and TRUSTe. Eventually, the Internet industry may adopt standards for publishing health information on Web sites. Until then, consumers should be careful when choosing Internet sources for health information. When researching a health topic, seek information from more than one Internet source, and consult a medical professional before following advice from the Web.

Healthy Living Practices

- Use the model for analyzing health-related information to evaluate information from the media and other sources.
- To obtain reliable answers for your health-related questions, consult experts at clinics or hospitals, state and local health departments, universities and colleges, federal health agencies, and nationally recognized health associations and foundations.

Becoming a Wary Consumer of Health Information

Maybe you've read an article or ad about the health benefits of an herbal supplement that you might buy. How do you know if the information in the article or advertisement is true? Will the supplement do what the author or manufacturer claims? Or will you merely be wasting your money?

As shown in Figure 1-6, information is a crucial element of decision making. Although health information from some sources is based on scientific evidence and can be extremely useful, that from other sources may be unreliable. Relying on flawed information can waste time and money and can even be dangerous. To be a wary consumer of health information, you need to learn how to analyze it.

Analysis Model Analyzing something simply means breaking it down into its component parts for study. Analyzing information is easier to do if you follow a particular model of analysis. A model is a plan or pattern that can be used as a guide. The following model is a series of questions that will help you evaluate health information and determine if it is reliable, regardless of its source.

1. **Which statements are verifiable facts, and which are unverified statements or value claims?** In the context of this model, *verifiable facts* are conclusions drawn from scientific research or statements supported with other types of credible evidence. *Unverified statements* are conclusions that have no such support. *Value claims* are statements suggesting that something is useful, or effective, or has other worthwhile characteristics. Unverified statements and value claims may or may not be true.

   Look for *disclaimers* in advertisements, such as "This statement has not been evaluated by the FDA," "This product is not intended to diagnose, treat, cure, or prevent disease," or "Results are not typical." In written ads, disclaimers usually appear in small print near the end of the ad. Disclaimers generally indicate that the value claims in the ad are not based on well-designed scientific studies.

2. **What are the credentials of the person who wrote the article or advertisement? Does the author have appropriate background and education in the topic area? If it is difficult to tell if the author has specific health expertise, what can you do to check his or her credentials?** Although advertisements usually do not indicate who wrote the ad, people with appropriate credentials may have supplied the information. Articles usually state the name and credentials of the author. In some cases, however, the author's credentials may be fraudulent. Anyone can call himself or herself a "nutritionist," "doctor," or "health expert." Therefore, a Ph.D. or the title "Certified . . ." after someone's name is no guarantee that this person has had extensive training in a health or science field from an accredited educational institution. Individuals can buy certain doctorate degrees through the mail from unaccredited colleges called "diploma mills." If the information is extremely important to your health, you can check the author's credentials by contacting the institution to which he or she claims to be affiliated. To determine if a college or university is accredited, contact the U.S. Department of Education (http://www.ed.gov).

3. **What might be the motives and biases of the author?** *Motive* is the incentive, purpose, or reason why someone writes an article or advertisement. Ads are always written to motivate the consumer to buy the product. Even if a person with bona fide health credentials supplies information for an advertisement, that person may have also developed the product and may profit from its sale. Therefore, this researcher may be biased.

A *bias* is the tendency to have a particular point of view. A researcher may be biased toward a particular outcome of his or her work. In analyzing health-related information, it is important to try to determine the biases of the people writing the information so that you can take their inclinations into account as you draw conclusions from the information.

4. **What is the main point of the ad or article? Which information is relevant to the issue, main point, or product? Which information is irrelevant?** The main point may be to provide practical information, but in many instances, it may be to encourage you to buy a product or service. Look for *red-flag* terms, expressions that indicate the possibility of misinformation, such as "patented formula," "all-natural," "chemical-free," "scientifically proven," "guaranteed to work," or "everyone is using." Look for anecdotes and testimonials. *Anecdotes* are personal reports. A young woman, for example, may state that she feels more "vitalized" after drinking a certain brand of herbal tea. *Testimonials* are claims individuals make concerning the value of a product. Advertisers often rely on celebrities such as sports figures to provide testimonials. The celebrities usually receive money or other types of compensation from promoters of the products; therefore, they are not likely to provide negative feedback. Anecdotes may be interesting and testimonials may be persuasive, but these sources of information are not scientific. Ignore terms and information that are not pertinent to the point; they will only confuse your analysis.

5. **Is the source reliable? Does it have a reputation for publishing misinformation? Does the article or ad present the pros and cons of the topic discussed or the benefits and risks of the advertised product?** Professional organizations or educational institutions generally publish scientific or medical journals that have articles written and reviewed by health care professionals. Articles that appear in scientific journals have been *peer reviewed,* meaning their content was critiqued by experts in that field before it was accepted for publication. If peer reviewers think a study was poorly designed or provides questionable conclusions, the article describing the study is likely to be rejected by the journal's editor. Although peer-reviewed scientific journals are usually credible sources of information, their articles often include jargon, graphs, charts, and statistical information that can be challenging for lay people to understand.

Some health magazines and journals look like bona fide sources of health information, but they are actually designed to sell products or services. Be wary of publications that have articles about the benefits of health care products and include advertisements for these products. Furthermore, be skeptical of articles or ads that do not present the risks along with the benefits of using a health product or service. For example, a reliable article about taking bee pollen supplements should present scientific evidence from peer-reviewed journals to support as well as refute health claims. Moreover, reliable sources of information often caution people about the hazards of using treatments, and they may include recommendations to seek the advice of medical experts.

6. **Does the ad or article attack the credibility of conventional scientists or medical authorities?** In some instances, writers of advertisements or articles try to confuse readers by implying that the Western scientific establishment is unreliable. For example, the ad may state, "unknown to Western medicine" or "used for centuries in China" to suggest that U.S. scientists lag behind others in finding cures or treatments. Statements that attack the reliability of conventional medical practitioners are usually indications that the information in the ad or article is unreliable.

Finding reliable sources of health-related information can be challenging. Be wary of references to magazines or journals to which your local medical school library does not subscribe. Reference librarians at medical school libraries can help you determine whether such journals are credible sources of health information. If you need additional help to determine the validity of information that concerns health, pose your questions to people trained in specific health-related fields. If you have a question about a psychological condition, for example, contact a mental health professional at a local hospital. You can usually obtain reliable answers to your health-related questions from experts at state and local health departments, universities and colleges, local hospitals, and federal health agencies.

The Analyzing Health-Related Information features in this textbook provide examples of ads, articles, and Web sites to help you determine the value of health-related information. To sharpen your critical thinking skills, analyze the information in these features using the six points of the analysis model. Additionally, the Consumer Health features in this and other chapters provide tips to help you become a better consumer of health information.

Consumer Protection

The U.S. government has some laws and agencies to protect consumers against health fraud. As a result of the Federal Food, Drug, and Cosmetics Act passed in 1938, manufacturers may not place false or misleading claims on the labels of food, medicinal, or cosmetic products. Later legislation protects consumers by requiring that manufacturers of medications and medical devices prove the safety and effectiveness of their products before they can be marketed.

The federal agencies that enforce consumer protection laws include the Food and Drug Administration (FDA) and the Federal Trade Commission (FTC). The FDA protects consumers by regulating the information that manufacturers can place on food or drug product labels. In addition, FDA personnel alert consumers about fraudulent health practices and can seize untested or unsafe medical devices and drugs. The manufacturers of such products can be punished (usually fined) for their illegal practices. The FTC reg-

ulates claims made in advertisements for products and services. Both agencies only regulate products and services involved in interstate commerce.

Besides government agencies, various voluntary organizations such as the American Council on Science and Health and the American Association for Retired Persons (AARP) provide consumers with reliable health information. The National Council Against Health Fraud investigates and evaluates health claims, supports laws that protect consumers against quackery, and provides educational materials to help people combat deceptive health practices.

To avoid being victims of health frauds, people must take the initiative and be very critical when judging the reliability of health-related information. If you suspect fraudulent activity, you can file a complaint with the local office of the FDA or your state's attorney general. You can also file a lawsuit if you have been injured as a result of following the advice or using the services or products of unscrupulous practitioners and manufacturers.

Analyzing
Health-Related Information

Sample Analysis of Health-Related Information

This statement has value claims that are supported with evidence.

No treatment contains everything each person needs to improve his or her health.

"Clinical proof" is a red flag. The medical experts, the medical schools, or journals where their research has been published are not identified. Objective testing could show the product is neither safe nor effective. The ad should cite the specific effects of the product, including negative ones.

"Chemical-free" is a red flag; all matter, including herbs and other plants, is chemical. Furthermore, scientific studies should be cited to provide evidence for these value claims. These statements are not verifiable facts.

A testimonial from an individual is not scientific evidence. This student's G.P.A. my have risen for a variety of reasons. Studies conducted to show that a treatment is useful in particular ways should contain at least 30 subjects.

"Potency" is a vague and undefined red-flag term. Again, this testimonial is a value claim that is unsupported by scientific evidence.

This is irrelevant information. Where the product is sold has nothing to do with its quality or characteristics. The authors of the ad are simply trying to make their product look superior to other similar products.

This statement gives people the impression that there is no time to investigate the product thoroughly. It is intended to make consumers think that the product will sell out if they wait, and they will miss out on a good thing. Again, this information is irrelevant.

For centuries, doctors in the Orient have known about the wonders of herbal medicines—nature's botanical cures for human ailments.

PANACEA

All Natural

Finally, American scientists are recognizing the healthful benefits of these herbs.

A PANACEA PILL A DAY KEEPS THE EXPENSIVE DOCTORS AWAY!

* These statements have not been evaluated by the FDA.

SwayCon Pharmaceuticals has developed a capsule that contains everything you need to reduce suffering, enhance health, and regain youthful vigor.

A team of medical experts from three major medical schools in the United States have clinical proof that the ingredients of Panacea are effective! Panacea contains a chemical-free mixture of natural enzymes and exotic herbs that
* relieve up to 80% more arthritis pain than aspirin;
* lower blood pressure by up to 20%;
* lower cholesterol by up to 45%;
* reduce lung cancer risk by as much as 50%, even in smokers;
* and reduce the risk of heart attack by 75%.*

Other remarkable findings

Taking Panacea for a few months can improve intelligence. R.P., a college student at a large East Coast university reports, "At the beginning of the fall semester, I started taking three capsules of Panacea a day. My G.P.A. went from a 1.8 to a 3.4! Panacea has helped me get all A's!"

Reports are coming into our offices that Panacea acts as a sexual stimulant, increasing potency. S.D., a computer programmer in St. Louis, writes, "Thanks for saving my marriage. Before taking Panacea, my husband complained about my lack of interest in sex. One of my friends told me that Panacea can help. Just a few days after taking the capsules, our marriage turned into a perpetual honeymoon."

Panacea is only available in fine health food stores. Order a three-month supply now, while supplies last

---

This suggests that American scientists do not understand that medicines can be derived from plant sources, when, in fact, American researchers often rely on plants as sources of chemicals that have medicinal uses. No scientific evidence is cited to show that the herbs in Panacea have the touted properties. These two sentences, then, contain only value claims; thus, the information may be unreliable.

No scientific evidence is cited that a daily Panacea pill prevents serious illness. Additionally, this statement attacks conventional medical practitioners by implying that they are interested only in making money, which suggests that physicians can't be trusted.

Disclaimer

Conclusion: This ad is merely a collection of value claims that are not supported by scientific research. The ad further attempts to encourage the reader to purchase the product by suggesting that it is better (and less expensive) than conventional therapies. It claims to relieve a wide range of health conditions. The red-flag phrases and testimonials rather than scientific evidence, the lack of details concerning the medical experts' credentials, and the lack of caution about the hazards of using the product all suggest the ad is an unreliable source of health-related information.

Conventional versus Complementary and Alternative Medicine

Conventional medicine (scientific medicine) relies on modern scientific principles, modern technologies, and scientifically proved methods to prevent, diagnose, and treat health conditions. The notion that certain agents of infection such as bacteria and viruses cause many health disorders is accepted by conventional medical practitioners. To practice in their professions, *conventional health care practitioners*, such as physicians, nurses, and dentists, must meet established national and/or state standards concerning their education and pass licensing examinations. To maintain their professional certification or licensing, certain types of conventional health care practitioners must update their medical backgrounds regularly by participating in continuing education programs. Most Americans use the services of conventional medical practitioners.

Before adopting a method of treatment, conventional medical practitioners want to know if it is safe and effective. To determine the safety and effectiveness of a treatment, medical researchers usually conduct studies on animals before testing humans in *clinical studies*. A clinical study should contain at least 30 subjects, preferably hundreds or thousands, if possible. The greater the number of participants in the study, the more likely the findings did not occur by chance and are the result of the treatment.

In designing clinical studies, researchers take a group of volunteers with similar characteristics and randomly divide them into two groups: a treatment group and a control group. Subjects in the treatment group receive the experimental treatment; members of the control group are given a placebo. A **placebo**, often referred to as a "sugar pill," is a sham treatment that has no known physical effects. Since a person's positive expectations can result in positive findings, placebos help rule out the effects of such wishful thinking.

Researchers give subjects placebos to compare their responses to responses of subjects who receive the actual treatment. In double-blind studies, subjects and researchers are unaware of the identity of those taking placebos. Placebos can temporarily relieve subjective complaints, such as pain, lack of energy, and poor mood. Thus, subjects who are given placebos often report feeling better even though the placebo has no known physical effects. Scientists refer to these reports as the *placebo effect*. The placebo effect may be responsible for many claims of beneficial results from using complementary and alternative medical therapies.

Complementary and alternative medicine (CAM) is an unconventional and diverse system of preventing, diagnosing, and treating diseases that emphasizes spirituality, self-healing, and harmonious interaction with the environment (Eskinazi, 1998). A treatment is complementary when it is used along with conventional medical care. A young man with liver cancer, for example, may use yoga and meditation to accompany the conventional medical treatments prescribed by his physician. An alternative therapy replaces conventional medical therapy (Vickers, 2004). If the patient with liver cancer stops his prescribed treatments and substitutes fasting and coffee enemas in hopes of a cure, he is relying on alternative forms of medical care.

Certain CAM therapies have positive effects on the body and mind. For example, acupuncture (Figure 1-8) can relieve nausea and vomiting associated with early pregnancy and certain cancer treatments (Kaptchuk, 2002). Although difficult to test scientifically, aromatherapy and therapeutic massage can be soothing and relaxing. Table 1-3 provides information about popular CAM practices, including homeopathy and reflexology.

Promoters of certain CAM practices claim diseases can be prevented or cured by "cleansing" tissues, "eliminating toxins" from the body, and "balancing chi." To support claims of their method's effectiveness, promoters often use anecdotal reports and testimonials. Nevertheless, well-designed clinical studies to determine the effectiveness of most CAM therapies have not been conducted.

placebo
a sham treatment that has no known physical effects; an inactive substance.

Figure 1-8 **Acupuncture.** Some physicians combine acupuncture with conventional forms of medical care.

Table 1-3　Common Alternative Medical Practices

Type	Claims and Principles of Practice	Results of Scientific Research
Acupuncture	Used to treat a variety of common ailments. Based on an ancient Chinese medical practice in which thin needles are inserted into the skin or underlying muscles at specific places and stimulated to regulate the flow of "chi," the life force.	Although testing acupuncture is difficult, most studies fail to support its usefulness when not combined with conventional therapies. It may relieve nausea and vomiting associated with "morning sickness" and cancer chemotherapy. Acupuncture may stimulate the body to release natural pain-relieving compounds.
Ayurvedic medicine	According to ancient Hindu religious beliefs, one achieves good health by meditating; eating grains, *ghee* (a form of butter), milk, fruits, and vegetables; and using herbs. Lack of balance between "energies" causes health problems. Fasting and enemas are used to treat severe ailments.	Meditation relieves stress; fruits, vegetables, and dairy products are nutritious foods; and some herbs have medicinal value. Ghee, however, can be fattening, and fasting is not a healthy practice. Enemas are unnecessary for good health and should be used only under a physician's instructions.
Chiropractic medicine	According to some chiropractors, misaligned spinal bones cause disease. Spinal manipulation prevents or cures disease by correcting the spine. Other practitioners use spinal manipulation, but accept the germ theory of disease.	Can be effective in treating certain types of back pain, but some spinal conditions require medications and surgery that only a physician can provide. There is no scientific evidence that all diseases can be treated by spinal adjustment.
Homeopathy	Use of extremely dilute solutions of natural substances to treat specific illness symptoms.	Studies do not indicate that homeopathy is effective.
Naturopathy or natural medicine	Practice based on natural healing. Practitioners believe diseases occur as the body rids itself of wastes and toxins. Treatments include fasting, enemas, acupuncture, and "natural" drugs.	No standardized training for practitioners called "naturopaths." They may recommend patients ignore conventional medical advice and practices, which can be harmful.
Reflexology or zone therapy	Specific areas of the hands and feet correspond to certain organs. To alleviate pain or treat certain diseases, practitioners press on the area that is related to the affected tissues.	Scientific evidence does not indicate that pressing on body parts is an effective method of diagnosing or treating ailments.

Herbs as Medicines

An increasing number of Americans ingest pills or teas made from herbs and other plants because they think these products are natural and harmless ways to cure various disorders or achieve optimal health and well-being. The U.S. government classifies herbal products as *dietary supplements*, which are not regulated like medications by the U.S. Food and Drug Administration (FDA). As a result, the FDA does not require dietary supplement manufacturers to register their products and submit clinical evidence indicating that the products have been tested for safety and effectiveness prior to being marketed. Manufacturers are responsible for ensuring that their products are safe and properly labeled, but at present, the FDA does not require dietary supplements' manufacturers to control the purity, quality, potency, and composition of ingredients in their products. Additionally, the FDA does not regulate the composition of dietary supplements; therefore, consumers cannot be certain that these products are identified properly and have the ingredients listed on the label. For example, pills taken from ten different samples of a company's herbal product labeled "kava" may contain different amounts of the herb or none at all.

When the FDA determines that an ingredient contained in dietary supplements is dangerous, the agency can ban its use. Furthermore, the FDA can remove a dietary supplement from the market if its label states claims about the product's health benefits that are not supported by scientific evidence. The FDA permits herbal supplement manufacturers to include certain structure/function claims on the product's label. For example, the claims "maintains a healthy circulatory system" and "improves urine flow" describe how supplements can affect body functions. Unless given prior approval by the FDA, herbal supplement manufacturers cannot indicate on the label that a supplement can prevent, diagnose, treat, improve, or cure diseases.

Results of clinical studies indicate that specific herbs can provide measurable physical benefits such as reducing inflammation, improving urine flow, and increasing alertness. Other herbs can improve psychological health. St. John's wort, for example, can relieve symptoms of mild to moderate depression and appears to be relatively safe when not combined with prescription medications (Ernst, 2002).

Not every herbal product has measurable beneficial effects on health. Ginseng is one of the leading-selling dietary supplements in the United States; people use the herb for a variety of purposes, including as a sedative, antidepressant, and aphrodisiac. The results of well-designed clinical studies, however, do not indicate that ginseng has any beneficial uses (Ernst, 2002). Furthermore, a "natural" therapy is not necessarily a safe one. Many plants, including comfrey, chaparral, pennyroyal, kava, and germander, contain chemicals that can be harmful and even deadly when consumed. Aristolochic acid, a naturally occurring chemical in Chinese herbs such as birthwort and snakeroot, is known to cause cancer and kidney failure ("Dangerous Supplements," 2004). Ingesting kava, an herb that is promoted for relieving anxiety, can result in serious liver damage (FDA, 2002). In 2004, the FDA banned the sale of dietary supplements that contained *ephedra*, a naturally occurring stimulant drug that is often called ma huang. Early in 2005, a court ruled that the FDA could not enforce the ban against certain ephedra-containing products. Consuming ephedra can result in stroke, heart attack, and death (Rados, 2004). In 2003, a weight loss supplement that contained the toxic herb contributed to the sudden death of Steve Bechler, a 23-year-old professional pitcher for the Baltimore Orioles baseball team.

Consumers need to be aware that medicinal herbs may interact with prescription medications or other herbs, producing serious side effects. Additionally, these products may be contaminated with pesticides or highly toxic metals. Many dietary supplements are expensive and useless in promoting good health. Table 1-4 includes information about the safety and effectiveness of some popular herbal supplements. Chapters 9 and 11 also

Table 1-4 Popular Herbal Supplements

Supplement	Common Claims	Research Findings	
		Uses	Risks
St. John's wort	Relieves depression	Can reduce mild to moderate depression symptoms; no value for major depression	Can interfere with birth control pills and other prescribed medicines, increase sensitivity to sunlight, and cause stomach upset
Saw palmetto	Improves urine flow	May reduce symptoms of prostate enlargement that are not caused by cancer	May interfere with PSA test to detect prostate cancer
Feverfew	Relieves headaches, fever, arthritis pain	Contains a chemical that may prevent migraines or reduce their severity	May cause dangerous interactions with aspirin or Coumadin (a prescribed drug)
Echinacea	Prevents colds and influenza	Does not prevent colds or reduce their severity	May cause allergic response and be a liver toxin
Ginkgo biloba	Enhances memory and sense of well-being; prevents dementia	May mildly improve mental performance but is ineffective as a treatment for Alzheimer's disease	May interfere with normal blood clotting, cause intestinal upset, and increase blood pressure
Ginseng	Enhances sexual, mental, and exercise performance; increases energy; relieves stress and depression	Has no mood-enhancing effects. Asian ginsengs may improve immune system functioning and reduce fatigue. Lack of scientific findings to support benefits in humans.	Can cause "jitters," insomnia, hypertension, and diarrhea and can be addictive; can be contaminated with pesticides and the toxic mineral lead
Yohimbe	Enhances muscle development and sexual performance	Dilates blood vessels but has no beneficial effects on muscle growth or sex drive of humans	Can produce abnormal behavior, high blood pressure, and heart attacks
Ma huang (ephedra)	Enhances weight loss and muscle growth	Increases heart rate and blood pressure; contains stimulant ephedrine	Has been linked to headaches, heart attacks, strokes, and deaths.
Guarana	Boosts energy and enhances weight loss	Acts as a stimulant drug	May cause nausea, anxiety, and irregular heartbeat
Kava	Relieves anxiety and induces sleep	Acts as a depressant drug	May cause serious liver damage; do not use when driving

provide information about dietary supplements. For reliable information about herbs and other dietary supplements, check the following FDA Web sites:

www.cfsan.fda.gov/~dms/ds-savvy.html

www.cfsan.fda.gov/~dms/hclaims.html

Herbal supplements are not *standardized*, which means the amount of active ingredients in each dose may vary considerably. An herbal tea, for example, may contain too much or too little of the chemicals that have medicinal effects. The active ingredients in pharmaceutical products that have *USP* (United States Pharmacopeia) on the label, however, are standardized for strength, identity, and purity. When you buy a bottle of aspirin, you can feel assured that each pill contains about the same amount of salicylic acid, the active ingredient.

Some herbal supplement manufacturers claim their products have been clinically tested and shown to provide health benefits. The reliability of these claims may be questionable, however, since they are often based on results obtained from animal research or few, poorly controlled human studies. Given the lack of standardization and scientific evidence that most medicinal herbs are safe and effective, the amount of money consumers pay for these products is astonishing. In 1998, for example, Americans spent over $150 million just on products that contain ginkgo biloba and almost $100 million on products containing ginseng (Ernst, 2002).

CAM Therapies in Perspective

A recent national survey provided estimates of the extent to which Americans use unconventional medical therapies. According to this survey, 62% of adults used forms of CAM that included prayer in 2002 (Barnes et al., 2004). Other commonly used CAM treatments were natural products, deep breathing exercises, meditation, and chiropractic care. In most cases, CAM was used to treat back, neck, and joint problems; colds; anxiety; and depression.

The natural or exotic nature of many alternative therapies such as herbal pills and teas, coffee enemas, shark cartilage, and reflexology may appeal to people who distrust modern technology or have lost faith in conventional medical care. Others use alternative therapies to prevent or treat ailments because they want to take more control over their health. Conventional medical practitioners are concerned when persons with serious conditions forgo or delay conventional treatments and rely instead on questionable alternative therapies. These could be life-threatening decisions. Many forms of cancer, for example, respond well to conventional treatments, particularly if the disease is in an early stage.

The majority of people who use alternative medical therapies choose them to complement rather than replace conventional treatments (Barnes et al., 2004).

Regardless of treatment, people suffering from acute conditions such as low back pain, common colds, and gastrointestinal disturbances generally recover with time. Individuals with chronic health problems such as osteoarthritis and multiple sclerosis often report remissions, times when their conditions improve. If people use alternative therapies when they are recovering or their illnesses are in remission, they are likely to think the nonconventional treatment cured or helped them. Additionally, people who combine alternative therapies with conventional medical care may attribute any improvement in their health only to the alternative treatments.

Conventional medical practitioners are likely to be skeptical of CAM techniques if they have not been shown scientifically in large-scale clinical studies to be safe or more helpful than placebos. The National Center for Complementary and Alternative Medicine within the National Institutes of Health funds research to determine the safety and effectiveness of alternative medical practices. Until supportive data are available from these and other controlled studies, consumers should be wary of CAM practices.

Before using alternative therapies, discuss your options with your physician and consider taking the following steps to protect yourself:

- Contact a variety of reliable sources of information to determine the risks and benefits of the treatment. For example, ask persons who have used the treatment to describe its effectiveness and side effects. Conduct a review of medical literature, and recognize that popular sources of information such as health magazines and the Internet are often unreliable. Be suspicious of sources that promote miracle cures or provide information about the benefits of alternative treatments without describing their harmful aspects. Instead, look for articles in medical journals or news magazines that have information concerning the usefulness of conventional as well as alternative medical approaches to care.

- Ask persons who are administering the treatment to provide proof of their medical training. Investigate the validity of their educational credentials. People who promote certain alternative medical practices often have little or no medical and scientific training.

- Determine the cost of treatment and whether your health insurance covers the particular alternative therapy. If it does not, find out why. You may find that your health insurer considers the treatment risky or ineffective.

- Ask your primary care physician for his or her opinion of the treatment.
- If you decide to use an alternative therapy, do not use it along with conventional therapy or abandon conventional treatment for any medical problem without consulting your physician.
- Investigate the possibility that the alternative medicine or herbal supplement can interact with conventional medications that you take and produce serious side effects. Additionally, investigate the possibility that taking combinations of herbal supplements can be harmful.
- If you are pregnant or breast feeding, do not use herbal supplements or alternative therapies without consulting your physician.
- Do not give herbal supplements or alternative therapies to children.

The Health Care Practitioner–Patient Relationship

Scientific research, technological advancements, and a systematic approach to medical education make the health care system in the United States among the best in the world. Conventional medicine, however, has its limitations; not every condition can be prevented, managed, or cured. To help ensure high-quality health care, consumers should choose knowledgeable health care practitioners who have appropriate training and credentials. Ideally, people should be able to form a trusting relationship with their practitioners, including physicians. To develop these relationships, patients need to acknowledge that they are largely responsible for their health status. For example, patients should adopt healthy lifestyles, obtain regular checkups, and seek medical attention for ailments that do not improve within a reasonable time or have serious signs or symptoms. Moreover, patients should follow their health care practitioners' advice and communicate with their practitioners should concerns about their medical care arise.

Health care practitioners can foster positive relationships with patients by spending adequate time with them, listening to their concerns carefully, and showing an interest in knowing more about them, not just their physical signs and symptoms. Additionally, it is important for practitioners to be caring, sensitive, and understanding; to modify treatment to meet the patient's concerns and values; and to enlist the patient's active participation in health-related decisions.

Across THE LIFESPAN

Health

Although the focus of this text is adult health, the Across the Lifespan feature in each chapter briefly describes health concerns that are specific to other stages of life, such as infancy, childhood, adolescence, and the elderly years. Table 1-5 indicates the approximate age groupings for these life stages. Why should college students learn about health conditions that can affect very young or very old members of the population? This information is relevant because many college students have younger siblings, some students have children, and those who are not parents may have children in the future. Additionally, many college students are middle-aged or have elderly parents and grandparents. The following information highlights some major life-cycle health concerns of Americans.

In the United States in 2002, about 7 babies in 1,000 died during the first year after birth. Most of these deaths were due to birth defects, low birth weights, and breathing difficulties that arose from prematurity, being born too early (Figure 1-9). Public health efforts aimed at educating and providing medical care for pregnant women can reduce the number of infant deaths.

Unintentional injuries (accidents) are the major health threat to children between 1 and 14 years of age.

Table 1-5	Life Stages
Stage	**Approximate Age**
Prenatal period	Conception to birth
Infancy	Birth to 1 year
Childhood	1 to 12 years
Adolescence	13 to 20 years
Adulthood	21 to 65 years
Older adult	Older than 65 years

Source: Based on Smith, R. E. (1993). *Psychology.* Minneapolis/St. Paul: West Publishing Company, p. 120.

Premature Newborns. Infants born prematurely have a greater risk of serious health problems than healthy full-term infants.

Most deaths from unintentional injuries are preventable, such as deaths due to motor-vehicle crashes, drownings, and house fires. Today, children are less likely to die as a result of these causes than in 1990 (USDHHS, 2001). Appendix B, "Injury Prevention and Emergency Care," provides information concerning safety.

Adolescence is a time when youngsters establish behaviors that may last a lifetime and when experimentation with risky behaviors usually begins. In 2003, nearly one-third of high school students had ridden in a car with a driver who had consumed alcohol shortly before taking the wheel; one-third had been in a physical fight; and over one-fifth smoked cigarettes during the 30 days preceding the survey (Grunbaum et al., 2004). Over 13% of these students reported being too fat. Unintentional injuries, homicide, and suicide are major causes of death for people aged 15 to 24. Three-fourths of the preventable deaths in this age group involve motor-vehicle crashes (NCHS, 2003).

Although teenage birth rates have been declining since 1991, unplanned pregnancies and sexually transmitted infections (STIs) continue to be major health problems for adolescents. About one million teenage girls become pregnant each year. In 2000, people between 15 and 24 years of age contracted about 50% of all new cases of sexually transmitted infections in the United States (Weinstock et al., 2004). AIDS is primarily a sexually transmitted infection; sexually active adolescents are at risk of becoming infected with HIV, the virus that causes AIDS. In 2002, HIV infection was the seventh leading cause of death for people between 15 and 24 years of age (Kochanek & Smith, 2004).

In 2000, people 65 years of age and older made up 12.4% of the U.S. population; this percentage is expected to increase rapidly (NCHS, 2003). Americans are living longer, but a growing number of people over 70 years of age report difficulty performing daily activities such as bathing and dressing. Furthermore, the number of deaths attributed to falls and motor vehicle crashes is increasing among members of this age group. Chapter 15 discusses the health-related concerns of elderly Americans.

CHAPTER REVIEW

Summary

Lifestyle includes behaviors that promote or deter good health and longevity. Wellness is an optimal degree of health. The holistic approach to health integrates physical, psychological, social, intellectual, spiritual, and environmental dimensions. Contemporary definitions of *health* reflect not only how one functions, but also what one can achieve, given his or her circumstances.

Heart disease and cancer are the major killers of Americans. Lifestyle choices contribute to the development of these and many other life-threatening diseases. *Healthy People 2000* established key objectives for improving the overall health of Americans by the year 2000. *Healthy People 2010* sets additional goals for the future. The distribution of health problems differs among the various ethnic and racial groups in the United States.

Experiences, knowledge, needs, and values affect one's motivation to change health-related behaviors. People are motivated to take action if they feel that a sufficient threat to their health exists and that the results of changing their behavior will be worthwhile.

Although no one can guarantee good health, many factors contribute to one's chances of enjoying a long and productive lifetime of good health. Several of these factors are the result of lifestyle choices that people can make, while they are still young, to prevent or delay disease. Responsible health-related lifestyle choices involve a systematic approach to decision making.

People can become more careful consumers of health-related information, products, and services by learning to recognize misinformation. To obtain reliable health-related information, check with experts in federal, state, and local agencies and organizations.

Conventional medicine relies on modern scientific principles, modern technologies, and scientifically proved methods to prevent, diagnose, and treat health conditions. Complementary and alternative medicine (CAM) is an unconventional and diverse system of preventing, diagnosing, and treating diseases that emphasizes spirituality, self-healing, and harmonious interaction with the environment. Conventional medical practitioners are likely to be skeptical of CAM techniques that have not been shown scientifically to be safe and effective. Until supportive data are available, consumers should be wary of CAM practices.

Throughout the life span, health concerns vary. The most common causes of infant deaths are birth defects, low birth weights, and prematurity. Preventable injuries are the major causes of death for children and youth. Additional serious public health concerns for adolescents are suicide, homicide, drug abuse, obesity, pregnancy, and sexually transmitted infections (including HIV). Americans are living longer, but a growing number of persons over 70 years of age report having difficulty performing daily activities such as bathing and dressing.

 ## Applying What You Have Learned

1. Develop a plan to improve your health. **Application**
2. Analyze a health-related advertisement or article to determine the validity of its information. **Analysis**
3. Identify sources of health information that you have used in the past year. Explain why you think each source is reliable or unreliable. **Synthesis**
4. Think of a health-related decision that you made recently. For example, did you decide to turn down an offer to use a mind-altering drug, wear a helmet while riding a motorcycle, lose a few pounds, or use an herbal product to treat a condition? When you made this decision, did you use the decision-making process described in this chapter or did you act impulsively? Explain why you would or would not make the same decision today. **Evaluation**

Key

Application   using information in a new situation.

Analysis   breaking down information into component parts.

Synthesis   putting together information from different sources.

Evaluation   making informed decisions.

Reflecting on Your Health

A reflective journal is a personal record of your thoughts and expressions of your feelings. The purposes of keeping this journal are to stimulate your thinking about what you have learned about health and to help you understand how your thoughts and feelings about your health might have changed over the semester. Thinking about new information can help you determine its usefulness, which can influence your attitudes and behaviors.

The Reflecting on Your Health questions at the end of each chapter are designed to guide your thinking. If you want to write about something else that is related to the contents of the chapter, feel free to do so, but make sure to identify the topic in your opening sentence. Write your journal entries in the first person, using "I" statements to express your thoughts, as though you were talking to a close friend. Don't worry about your spelling, punctuation, or grammar—just let your thoughts flow.

Some instructors make journal writing an optional activity; others require that you respond to all of the questions, and they grade journals. Still other instructors simply check to see if students are doing the assignment. Refer to the course syllabus or ask your instructor about his or her grading practices and other instructions concerning the journal.

Journal Questions

1. What does the term *health* mean to you?
2. What do you think of the idea that people should strive to achieve optimal health?
3. What impact does spiritual health have on your sense of well-being? If spiritual health is important to you, describe the role it plays in your life.
4. Do you agree with the idea presented in the chapter that social health influences your physical health? Why or why not?
5. Under what circumstances would you consider using alternative therapies?

References

Arias, E., Anderson, R. N., Kung, H. C., Murphy, S. L., & Kochanek, K. D. (2003). Deaths: Final data for 2001. *National Vital Statistics Reports, 52*(3):1–115.

Barnes, P. M., Powell-Griner, E., McFann, K., & Nahin, R. L. (2004). *Complementary and alternative medicine use among adults: United States, 2002* (CDC Advance Data Reports No. 343). Hyattsville, MD: National Center for Health Statistics.

Barnes, P. M., & Schoenborn, C. A. (2003). *Physical activity among adults: United States, 2000* (PHS Publication No. 2003-1250). Washington, DC: U.S. Department of Health and Human Services, Centers for Disease Control and Prevention, National Center for Health Statistics.

Centers for Disease Control and Prevention. (2004). Surveillance summaries. *Morbidity and Mortality Weekly Report, 53*(SS-2):1–95.

Dangerous supplements still at large. (2004). *Consumer Reports, 69*(5):12–17.

Ernst, E. (2002). The risk-benefit profile of commonly used herbal therapies: Ginko, St. John's wort, ginseng, echinacea, saw palmetto, and kava. *Annals of Internal Medicine, 136*:42–53.

Eskinazi, D. P. (1998). Factors that shape alternative medicine. *Journal of the American Medical Association, 280*(18):1621–1623.

Flegal, K. M., Carroll, M. D., Ogden, C. L., & Johnson, C .L. (2002). Prevalence and trends in obesity among US adults, 1999–2000. *Journal of the American Medical Association, 288*:1723–1727.

Food and Drug Administration, Center for Food Safety and Applied Nutrition. (2002). *Kava-containing dietary supplements may be associated with severe liver injury* [Consumer advisory]. Washington, DC: U.S. Food and Drug Administration. Retrieved from http://www.cfsan.fda.gov/~dms/addskava.html.

Gargiullo, P., Wingo, P. A., Gates, R. J., & Thompson, T. D. (2002). Recent trends in mortality rates for four major cancers, by sex and race/ethnicity—United States, 1990–1998. *Morbidity and Mortality Weekly Report, 51*(3):49–53.

Grunbaum, J. A., Kann, L., Kinchen, S., Ross, J., et al. (2004). Youth risk behavior surveillance—United States, 2003. *Morbidity Mortality Weekly Reports Surveillance Summaries, 53*(2):1–96.

Hedley, A. A., Ogden, C. L., Johnson, C. L., Carroll, M. D., Curtin, L. R., & Flegal, K. M. (2004). Prevalence of overweight and obesity among US children, adolescents, and adults, 1999–2002. *Journal of the American Medical Association, 291*(23):2847–2850.

Hochbaum, G. M. (1979). An alternative approach to health education. *Health Values, 3*:197–201.

Kaptchuk, T. J. (2002). Acupuncture: Theory, efficacy, and practice. *Annals of Internal Medicine, 136*(5):374–383.

Kochanek, K. D., & Smith, B. L. (2004). Deaths: Preliminary data for 2002. *National Vital Statistics Reports, 52*(13):1–48.

Mokdad, A. H., Marks, J. S., Stroup, D. F., & Gerberding, J. L. (2004). Actual causes of death in the United States, 2000. *Journal of the American Medical Association, 291*(10):1238–1245.

National Center for Health Statistics. (2003). *Health, United States, 2003.* Retrieved June 11, 2004, from http://www.cdc.gov/nchs/hus.htm.

National Center for Health Statistics. (2004). Early release of selected estimates based on data from the National Health Interview Survey. Retrieved June 10, 2004, from http://www.cdc.gov/nchs/about/major/nhis/released200403.htm.

National Institutes of Health, Task Force of the National Advisory Council on Alcohol Abuse and Alcoholism. (2002). A call to action: Changing the culture of drinking at U.S. colleges. Retrieved June 8, 2004, from http://www.collegedrinkingprevention.gov.

Norcross, J. C., & Prochaska, J. O. (2002). Using the stages of change. *Harvard Mental Health Letter, 18*(11):5–7.

Office of Minority Health. (2004). Disease burden and risk factors. Retrieved February 1, 2005, from http://www.cdc.gov/omh/AMH/dbrf.htm.

Prochaska, J. O., & Velicer, W. F. (1997). The transtheoretical model of health behavior change. *American Journal of Health Promotion, 12*(1):38–48.

Rados, C. (2004). Ephedra ban: No shortage of reasons. *FDA Consumer, 38*(2):6–7.

U.S. Department of Health and Human Services, Public Health Service. (1991). *Healthy people 2000: National health promotion and disease prevention objectives.* Washington, DC: Government Printing Office.

U.S. Department of Health and Human Services, National Center for Health Statistics, Public Health Service. (2001). *Healthy people 2000: Final review.* Washington, DC: Government Printing Office.

Vickers, A. (2004). Alternative cancer cures: "Unproven" or "disproven"? *CA: Cancer Journal for Clinicians, 54*(2):110–118.

Wechsler, H., Lee, J. E., Kuo, M., Seibring, M., Nelson, T. F., & Lee, H. (2002). Trends in college binge drinking during a period of increased prevention efforts. *Journal of American College Health, 50*(5):203–217.

Weinstock, H., Berman, S., & Cates, W. Jr. (2004). Sexually transmitted diseases among American youth: Incidence and prevalence estimates, 2000. *Perspectives on Sexual and Reproductive Health, 36*(1):6–10.

Woollery, T., Trosclair, M. S., Husten, C., Caraballo, R. C., & Kahende, J. (2003). Cigarette smoking among adults—United States, 2001. *Morbidity and Mortality Weekly Report, 52*(40):953–956.

World Health Organization. (1948). *Official records of the World Health Organization, no. 2. Proceedings and final acts of the international health conference held in New York from 19 June to 22 July 1946.* New York: United Nations WHO Interim Commission.

World Health Organization. (1986). *Ottawa Charter for Health Promotion.* Copenhagen, Denmark: World Health Organization.

http://healthyliving.jbpub.com

The Web site for this book offers many useful tools and is a great source for supplementary health information for both students and instructors. Visit the site at http://healthyliving.jbpub.com for information on these topics:

Adjustment and Growth
Understanding Mental Illness
Common Psychological Disorders
Suicide

Chapter Overview

How your nervous system affects your psychological health

How biological, social, and cultural forces interact to mold your personality

How psychological adjustment leads to psychological growth

How to identify common psychological disorders

How to recognize suicidal behavior and prevent suicide

Diversity in Health
Native Americans: Culture and Psychological Health

Consumer Health
Locating and Selecting Mental Health Therapists

Managing Your Health
Resolving Interpersonal Conflicts Constructively

Across
THE LIFESPAN

Psychological Health

Student Workbook

Self-Assessment: The Self-Esteem Inventory

Changing Health-Related Behaviors: Are You Ready to Improve Your Psychological Health?

Do You Know?

· *If you are psychologically healthy?*

· *Why emotions are useful?*

· *How to resolve conflicts in a healthy manner?*

Psychological Health

Observing newborn infants in a hospital nursery is a fascinating experience. While some of the babies sleep peacefully, others are awake, calmly gazing around at their surroundings while gently sucking their pacifiers. A few of the newborns are restless. Although tightly wrapped in swaddling, one infant tries to stretch her hand into the air as though she were reaching for something hanging above the bassinet. Another fussy baby frowns and closes his eyes tightly, before spitting out his pacifier, kicking his feet, and howling in pain. Moments later, several other babies begin to grow fussy. Soon a chorus of crying babies shatters the calmness of the nursery. The infants' caretakers scurry to each bassinet, trying to determine which babies are truly in need of their attention and the reasons why. Why do some newborns respond differently when all of them are in the same situation?

Each newborn is a unique person. All infants, however, have basic physical needs that must be met if they are to survive. These needs include nutritious food and a safe environment. Additionally, children have psychological needs for belonging, love, social acceptance, and respect that must be met if they are to mature into healthy adults. What if there were a crystal ball in the nursery that would enable you to predict each baby's future? Which of these infants will be psychologically healthy, achieving personal fulfillment and being satisfied with themselves and their lives? Which ones will be emotionally distressed and lead troubled lives?

> **Why do some newborns respond differently . . .?**

Psychological (mental) health is dynamic, becoming more positive or negative as one responds to a constantly changing environment. Many individuals, however, manage to maintain high degrees of positive psychological functioning throughout their lives. People with positive mental health are able to deal effectively with the psychological challenges of life. Such people accept themselves, have realistic and optimistic outlooks on life, function independently, form satisfying interpersonal relationships, and cope effectively with change (Table 2-1). In addition to these traits, psychologically healthy individuals resolve their problems without resorting to substance abuse or violence, and they assert themselves in social situations.

The quality of one's psychological health often affects the other components of health, such as social, spiritual, and physical health. This chapter discusses factors that influence positive psychological health as well as those that contribute to the development of psychological disorders. Chapter 3 examines the impact of psychological stress on health; Chapter 4 focuses on the effects of violence on health.

The Basics of Psychological Health

Understanding psychological health involves learning about **physiology**, the study of body functions, and **psychology**, the study of the mental (cognitive) processes that influence human behavior. Cognitive processes such as thinking, decision making, and remembering rely on the functioning of the nervous system. The nervous system is an elaborate biological communications network that contains billions of nerve cells, or neurons, which are designed to receive, send, and interpret messages in your body by means of electrical and chemical signals. As you can see in Figure 2-1, this network consists of two interrelated parts: the **central nervous system (CNS)**, the brain and spinal cord; and the **peripheral nervous system (PNS)**, nerves that relay information to and from the CNS.

Most nerves produce and release **neurotransmitters**, chemicals such as acetylcholine, dopamine, and serotonin that convey information between nerve cells. By altering the levels of various neurotransmitters, the nervous system transmits information and produces physical responses, thoughts, and emotions.

Emotions are a way of communicating our moods to others. Emotions are associated with typical behavioral and physical responses, including changes in speech patterns as well as facial expressions and other forms of body language. Happiness, sadness, anger, and fear are among the basic emotions that we often call *feelings*. A psychologically healthy person is able to express his or her emotions appropriately. Much of the disability that is associated with psychological illness results from abnormal or extreme emotional responses to situations.

Parts of the brain, collectively referred to as *the mind*, process various types of information received from the rest of the body and the environment. As a result, the mind thinks about what takes place, finds meaning in events, considers actions, makes decisions, directs responses, evaluates and remembers consequences, and plans for the future. These activities involve neurotransmitters in the brain. Certain conditions can negatively affect the mind by altering neurotransmitter levels and disrupting normal brain chemistry. As a result, inappropriate moods, unrealistic thoughts, and *maladaptive* behaviors occur. Maladaptive behaviors interfere with one's ability to be productive, interact socially, and adjust to the demands of everyday living. In many instances, treating these conditions involves taking medication that corrects abnormal neurotransmitter levels as well as learning how to change distorted ways of thinking.

physiology the study of bodily functions.

psychology the study of the mental processes that influence human behavior.

central nervous system (CNS) of the two primary divisions of the nervous system, the one that consists of brain and spinal cord.

peripheral nervous system (PNS) of the two primary divisions of the nervous system, the one that consists of nerves, which relay information to and from the CNS.

neurotransmitters chemicals produced and released by nerves that convey information between most nerve cells.

Personality Development

Personality is a set of distinct thoughts and behaviors, including emotional responses, that characterizes the way a person responds to situations. Many factors, including biological, cultural, social, and psychological forces, interact to mold personality.

Biological Influences **Heredity** is the transmission of biological information, coded within genes, from parents to offspring. This information determines, in part, an individual's physical, emotional, and intellectual characteristics. Much of a person's **temperament**, the predictable way an individual responds to the environment, is inherited. Soon after birth, parents can usually describe their chil-

Figure 2-1 **The Nervous System.** The nervous system consists of the brain, the spinal cord, and peripheral nerves.

Labels: Brain, Spinal cord, Nerves

dren's temperamental styles, such as irritable, fearful, or pleasant. As children mature, social and cultural influences modify their temperaments.

Social and Cultural Influences From the moment of birth, the social environment, such as interactions with parents and other family members, influences the psychological development of an individual. Most people learn how to respond to situations in socially and culturally acceptable ways when they are children. The circumstances surrounding a situation influence the kind and extent of an emotional display. Consider, for example, emotions that are appropriate to express while attending the funeral of a child.

A person's cultural and ethnic background can influence his or her responses to situations and perceptions of mental health disturbances. Although psychological problems affect people from every culture, symptoms of these problems may differ among cultures. The Diversity in Health essay "Native Americans: Culture and Psychological Health" discusses a traditional Native American concept of health, the *medicine wheel*, and healing methods.

personality a set of distinct thoughts and behaviors that characterizes a person's response to situations.

heredity the transmission of biological information, coded within genes, from parents to offspring.

temperament the predictable way an individual responds to situations and others, such as being pleasant, outgoing, or shy.

Diversity in Health

Native Americans: Culture and Psychological Health

In the United States, conventional mental health practitioners have been taught to identify normal and abnormal behaviors and diagnose mental illness by using an established set of standards. Often these health care providers do not consider the importance of culture when treating patients who are members of minority groups, particularly Native Americans.

The traditional Native American concept of health involves the *medicine wheel*, a circle divided into four equal parts representing the major aspects of health: context (natural environment and social setting), mind, body, and spirit. When the four components of the medicine wheel are balanced with each other, people enjoy wellness, or "harmony." When people are not in harmony with nature, their community, or themselves, they suffer from physical and psychological illnesses. According to some traditional Native American beliefs, an emotionally disturbed individual is in a state of disharmony with the rest of nature or in a hopeless state of health. In other Native American traditions, the symptoms of mental illnesses result from supernatural forces exerting control over the person.

The Diversity in Health essay in Chapter 1 discussed major health concerns affecting Native Americans, including problems associated with poor mental health, such as alcoholism, suicide, and accidents. Traditionally, Native Americans view alcohol abuse and other mental health problems as imbalances in the spiritual component of the medicine wheel. Because spiritual health is linked closely with psychological health, treatments are spiritual in nature and may include prayer, sweat lodges, or purification ceremonies led by natural healers. Efforts to restore spiritual balance may also include participation in activities that increase cultural identity and self-esteem, such as crafts,

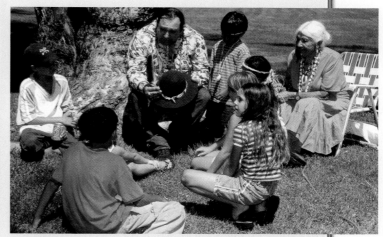

Figure 2-A For many Native Americans, storytelling is a way to restore spiritual and psychological health.

storytelling, and making drums and baskets. In addition to relying on traditional healing methods, many Native Americans will accept conventional forms of treatment for serious mental health problems.

Medical practitioners need to recognize the importance of cultural traditions when treating a Native American or any individual. Furthermore, mental health care providers can often gain the trust and respect of clients from various cultural backgrounds by learning about traditional healing methods. As a result, patients are more likely to accept the health care provider's advice and suggestions for conventional treatment.

Source: Cross, T., Earle, K., Echo-Hawk Solie, H., & Manness, K. (2000). Cultural strengths and challenges in implementing a system care model in American Indian communities. *Systems of care: Promising practices in children's mental health* (2000 series, Vol. 1). Washington, DC: Center for Effective Collaboration and Practice, American Institutes for Research.

Table 2-2   Common Defense Mechanisms

Defense Mechanism	Behavior	Example
Repression	Blocking unpleasant thoughts or feelings	A woman suppresses the memory of being sexually abused as a child.
Rationalization	Making up false or self-serving excuses for unpleasant behavior or situations	A man makes excuses for not being hired for a job.
Denial	Refusing to acknowledge unpleasant situations or feelings	A young man does not accept the fact he has been diagnosed with a terminal illness.
Projection	Attributing unacceptable thoughts, feelings, or urges to someone else	A woman accuses her boyfriend of being unfaithful while repressing her desire to have an affair.
Displacement	Redirecting a feeling or response toward a target that usually is less of a threat	An abused wife does not fight back but mistreats her child instead.
Avoidance	Taking action to prevent situations that produce powerful feelings	A woman will not date because she is afraid of falling in love.
Regression	Reducing anxiety by acting immature to feel more secure	A 6-year-old child begins to suck his thumb after the birth of his baby brother.

Theories of Personality Development

Freud's Framework of Personality More than one hundred years ago, physician Sigmund Freud pioneered modern approaches to the diagnosis and treatment of psychological disturbances. Freud observed that people have an element of the mind that lacks awareness of certain thoughts, feelings, and impulses. He proposed that this "unconscious" component of the mind influences much of one's behavior. The unconscious mind, for example, engages various defense mechanisms such as repression and avoidance to cope with anxiety and guilt.

defense mechanisms
ways of thinking and behaving that reduce or eliminate anxious and guilty feelings.

Defense mechanisms are ways of thinking and behaving that reduce or eliminate anxiety and guilty feelings by altering the individual's perception of reality. Nearly everyone uses defense mechanisms to protect their minds against psychological conflicts and threats. A basic defense mechanism is *repression,* the unconscious forgetting of anxiety-producing feelings, thoughts, or impulses. For example, adults who were sexually or physically abused as children may repress the memories of the abuse. Students who blame teachers for their lack of academic success, instead of themselves for skipping classes or not studying, may be using *rationalization* as a defense mechanism. Table 2-2 lists repression, projection, and some other common defense mechanisms and describes instances in which the unconscious mind employs them. Although these strategies may protect the mind and reduce anxiety in the short run, defense mechanisms usually do not provide long-term solutions to problems.

Freud believed that unconscious desires or drives, particularly the *libido,* or sex drive, control human behavior by creating psychological tension. Relieving this tension produces pleasurable sensations. However, members of society establish *moral values,* rules for good and bad behavior, that often prevent individuals from satisfying all of their desires. If a person who accepts the moral values of society acts or thinks in ways that conflict with these rules, he or she usually feels anxious and guilty. Many people use moral values as guidelines to judge their behavior, themselves, and others.

Erikson's Psychosocial Stages of Development Erik Erikson (1982) modified Freud's ideas by proposing that social influences play a greater role in shaping personalities than do sexual drives. According to Erikson, individuals progress through eight psychosocial stages during their lifetimes (Table 2-3). Each stage has major social crises or conflicts that people must manage or resolve to achieve a sense of emotional well-being.

Infants require a considerable amount of care and nurturing from adults to survive and to develop normally. Erikson thought that babies learn to *trust* other individuals if their parents or other caretakers meet their basic physical and emotional needs. Establishing trusting relationships with caring and loving adults enables infants to begin the process of developing high degrees of psychological well-being later in life.

Erikson viewed adolescence as a critical period in which youth develop a sense of *identity*. During this stage, adolescents become increasingly responsible for making their own decisions. They begin to function separately from their families and define who they are as well as what their future roles will be. According to Erikson, the three major areas of concern that adolescents must clarify relate to their sexuality, future occupation, and social conduct. Adolescents begin to establish their identities when they begin to clarify their feelings and positions about their roles in life. Identity confusion results when they are unable to develop sound self-concepts and function independently of their families.

As adolescents mature into young adulthood, they face the challenge of *intimacy*, forming close and loving relationships with others. Adults who did not develop a sense of trust earlier in their lives or have not clarified their identities may be unable to establish intimate relationships and thus feel isolated. During middle age, individuals who have mastered previous developmental tasks focus on meeting the needs of others through activities such as raising families and performing community service. Erikson coined the term *generativity* to refer to these psychosocial tasks. In the final stage of life, people seek *integrity*, a feeling that their lives have been fulfilling and complete.

Maslow's Hierarchy of Human Needs According to Abraham Maslow (1968), individuals behave in response to their values rather than to their unconscious drives. Maslow thought that healthy people value the freedom to achieve personal fulfillment by developing their talents and competencies. This freedom becomes a psychological need that drives personality development. Maslow created a hierarchy of five human needs, from the most basic biological requirements that contribute to human survival to the one that is most essential for psychological fulfillment, *self-actualization* (Figure 2-2). To achieve self-actualization, each level of needs from the base to the top of the hierarchy must be met, in order. Self-actualized persons are psychologically healthy and mature. They feel free to pursue their creative and intellectual capabilities. The possibility of self-actualization exists in all people, but unless the prerequisite needs are met, individuals can never fully realize their potentials. According to Maslow and others, only about one person in a hundred will reach the top of the human needs hierarchy. Nevertheless, Maslow admitted that many people are satisfied with their lives even if they have not achieved self-actualization.

Figure 2-2 **Maslow's Hierarchy of Human Needs.** Maslow created a hierarchy of five human needs, from the basic biological survival requirements to psychological fulfillment (self-actualization). Before achieving self-actualization, a person must satisfy all of the preceding needs.

Self-Actualization
A need for achievement and mastery

Esteem Needs
A need to have a high self-image

Love Needs
A need to give love and receive love

Safety Needs
The need for a secure environment in which one can live, work, and play

Physiological Needs
The most basic human needs for air, water, food, housing, sleep, and sexual activity

Table 2-3	Erikson's Psychosocial Stages of Personality Development

Conflicts	Approximate Age Ranges
Trust vs. mistrust	Birth to 1 year
Autonomy vs. doubt and shame	1 to 3 years
Initiative vs. guilt	3 to 6 years
Industry vs. inferiority	6 to 12 years
Identity vs. identity confusion	12 to 18 years
Intimacy vs. isolation	Young adulthood
Generativity vs. stagnation	Middle age
Integrity vs. despair	Old age

Healthy Living Practices

- Seek practical solutions to your problems rather than avoid them by using defense mechanisms.

■ Adjustment and Growth

Each day, individuals respond to the demands of other people, their physical environment, and themselves. Throughout life, these demands are changing constantly. Being in college is especially demanding, but consider how your life will change after you graduate. What do you think your life will be like 10, 20, or 30 years after graduation? What kinds of adaptations do you expect to make over your lifetime?

Adapting to change, which is called *adjustment*, involves the responses people make to cope with the demands of life. **Psychological adjustment** occurs when an individual learns that certain responses meet these demands more effectively than others. For example, one way a new student might psychologically adjust to college life is by scheduling time each week for various tasks, such as studying, attending classes, and going to work. Maintaining the new schedule may be challenging, particularly if the student followed a less structured lifestyle in the past.

Psychological growth occurs when a person discovers that certain adjustment strategies, such as studying more or planning for the future, enhance one's sense of freedom and control over oneself and the environment. To adjust in beneficial ways and to experience psychological growth, an individual needs to obtain reliable information, set realistic goals, plan effective ways to achieve those goals, take actions that are based on reasonable judgments and decisions, and evaluate the consequences of his or her choices.

If not managed effectively, interpersonal conflicts can hinder psychological adjustment and growth. Such conflicts often arise when people do not share opinions, values, needs, or beliefs. In these situations, many individuals respond by expressing anger or aggression. *Aggressive* reactions often injure other people physically or psychologically; therefore, these responses do not facilitate social interactions.

Assertiveness is a way of reacting to social situations by maintaining one's rights without interfering with the rights of other people and without harming them. Consider how students respond to an instructor who failed to consider certain possible answers to an essay question. An aggressive student might take class time to argue a point, verbally lashing out at the teacher. An assertive student might arrange to meet with the instructor after class, using the time to discuss his or her case in a more thoughtful and rational manner.

Another way healthy people constructively resolve interpersonal conflicts is by using compromise. An individual who disagrees with a friend over an issue, for example, may decide that preserving the friendship is more valuable in the long run than "winning" the argument. This person is willing to compromise by modifying his or her attitudes. The Managing Your Health feature in this chapter provides additional suggestions for resolving conflicts constructively.

Psychological growth fosters the development of **autonomy**, or self-control. People with a high degree of autonomy function independently. Autonomy is associated with **self-esteem**, the extent to which a person feels worthy and useful.

psychological adjustment changing one's thoughts, attitudes, and behaviors to cope effectively with the demands of the environment.

psychological growth the process of learning from one's experiences.

autonomy sense of independence and self-control.

self-esteem the extent to which a person feels worthy and useful.

Managing Your Health

Resolving Interpersonal Conflicts Constructively

In addition to compromise, consider using the following tips to resolve conflicts constructively:

1. Focus on one issue; state your perception of the problem as clearly as possible.
2. Consider the feelings of others; avoid criticizing, name-calling, threats, or sarcasm.
3. Use "I feel" statements. "You" statements make others defensive. For example, say "I feel angry when you . . ." instead of "You make me angry."
4. Do not assume how other people feel, what they believe, or how they will react.
5. Discuss the current concern; avoid dredging up past arguments.
6. Think before you speak; choose your words carefully to avoid confusion.
7. Listen carefully to others; avoid interrupting them while they talk.
8. Offer reasonable solutions.
9. Give others time to consider, accept, or reject your ideas.
10. Be patient; keep the door open for future communication.

Self-Esteem

Self-esteem is a key component of personality that influences one's thoughts, actions, and feelings. Positive self-esteem is a characteristic of psychologically healthy people. Individuals who have positive or high self-esteem have a high degree of autonomy, are self-confident, have self-respect, and are satisfied with themselves. These people work well with others, accept challenging tasks and responsibilities, seek supportive and loving relationships, and adjust easily to change. When they make mistakes, they accept responsibility for their actions without blaming others or making excuses. People with low self-esteem have difficulty making decisions, resist changing their behavior, and resent any form of criticism, even if it is constructive. These individuals tend to put down others to make themselves look or feel better. The "Self-Esteem Inventory" in the workbook that accompanies this textbook can help you assess your self-esteem.

People begin developing self-esteem early in childhood. Parents play a crucial role in determining their children's level of self-esteem. By interacting with parents and other family members, for example, young children learn that certain behaviors are good or bad. Children use this information to begin forming their *self-image*, the way they view themselves. Positive relationships between children and their caretakers are essential for the youngsters to become psychologically well-adjusted adults. Children with positive self-images have high self-esteem because they see themselves as being good, lovable, and possessing many worthwhile and valuable characteristics such as honesty and sensitivity.

When children enter school, their social environment enlarges to include more children, teachers, and other members of the community. These individuals provide new learning experiences that can have positive or negative impacts on the personality, self-image, and self-esteem of children. If a child who has a negative self-image enters school and has experiences that reinforce this perception, emotional disturbances can develop that persist into adulthood. With the help of others, children can develop positive self-concepts that establish the foundation for a lifetime of wellness. Parents and other adults help children feel good about themselves by spending time with them, listening to their concerns, and treating them with respect.

During adulthood, experiences at school, work, and home and a variety of social factors, including relationships, influence self-esteem. Relationships and experiences that are rewarding, enriching, and satisfying support positive self-esteem. In addition to having self-respect, people with a high degree of self-esteem gain the respect and approval of colleagues and others.

Self-esteem is a deep-rooted aspect of an individual. Although self-esteem may rise or fall over the course of a day, its basic nature remains fairly stable over longer periods. Individuals with persistent low self-esteem can improve their negative thoughts and feelings about themselves. By analyzing their situations, these people can determine factors that contribute to their poor self-concepts. For example, working in a dull job or remaining in an abusive relationship can affect self-esteem negatively. In these instances, people may improve their situations and feelings of self-worth by finding new jobs or ending the self-destructive relationships.

To feel better about themselves, persons with low self-esteem can learn to identify and appreciate their positive traits and abilities, instead of focusing on their negative characteristics and shortcomings. It can also help if the individual recognizes that not all criticism is destructive and insensitive. Accepting constructive criticism can support personal growth. Making a few lifestyle changes, such as developing new interests, changing some bad habits, or taking an assertiveness training class, can improve one's psychological outlook. To overcome low self-esteem, psychological counseling may be necessary to help individuals develop the ability to evaluate themselves realistically and form accurate self-perceptions.

Improving Your Psychological Health

What can you do to improve your psychological health? You can enhance the quality of your mental health primarily by improving the other dimensions of your health. Exercising regularly can boost your mood (Dunn et al., 2001; Kritz-Silverstein et al., 2001). Getting enough sleep, eating a nutritious diet, and maintaining a healthy weight for your height also enhance psychological health by improving physical health. In addition to taking good care of your physical needs, fostering positive social contacts, whether with family, friends, or colleagues, is very important. Everyone needs to communicate with other people on a regular basis. For example, one goal to improve your psychological health could be to make and maintain at least one new social contact each year. You can improve your intellectual health by reading challenging books, playing stimulating games such as crossword puzzles or chess, or serving as a tutor. Some people find that keeping a journal or diary in which they record their most private feelings helps them cope with daily life. Attending to your spiritual needs can provide personal fulfillment also. For example, you can volunteer to serve as a mentor for troubled children or become involved in your religious organization. Finally, taking an active role in ensuring and protecting the quality of your environment will support all dimensions of your health.

■ Understanding Psychological (Mental) Illness

Having "the blues," feeling "scared to death," or being "worried sick"—perhaps you can recall situations in which you experienced these strong emotions or uncomfortable sensations. Occasionally, healthy people have disturbing thoughts, experience unpleasant feelings, or display inappropriate behaviors. In most instances, these are normal responses and adaptive reactions to unpleasant or threatening situations. For example, it is normal to be sad after learning about the death of a friend or to be afraid when a snake crosses your path. Given a reasonable amount of time, however, the strong emotional responses or unpleasant thoughts and feelings resolved, and you regained your sense of well-being.

The observable physical and behavioral changes that signal an emotional state are referred to as **affect**, or mood. Expressing emotions appropriately is a characteristic of a psychologically healthy individual; extreme or improper emotional responses can indicate a serious psychological disturbance. The key features that distinguish a normal emotional response from an abnormal one are the *intensity* and *duration* of the feelings. Mentally ill individuals experience abnormal feelings, thoughts, and behaviors that persist, interfere with daily life, and hinder psychological adjustment and growth.

A *psychosis* is a severe type of mental illness characterized by disorganized thoughts and unreal perceptions that result in strange behavior, isolation, delusions, and hallucinations. **Delusions** are inaccurate and unreasonable beliefs that often result in decision-making errors. For example, a person suffering from a delusion might think that he or she can fly, so this individual jumps off a tall building. **Hallucinations** are false sensory perceptions that have no apparent external cause, but they are real to the psychotic individual. Examples of hallucinations include hearing instructions from pictures, seeing ghostly images, or feeling insects crawling underneath skin. Psychotic conditions (psychoses) can be acute or chronic, and they can result from brain damage, chemical imbalances in the brain, or substance abuse.

Situations and cultures provide the context in which behaviors are judged as normal or abnormal. If a person who is living in a country torn apart by civil war bombs a crowded marketplace, people may view this individual as a terrorist or a hero, but not necessarily mentally ill. However, if this bombing occurs in an American shopping mall, and the bomber says that a dog gave the order to perform the deed, you might suspect that this person is psychotic. Only a small percentage of psychotic people become violent, and they are most likely to attack family members or other individuals who set limits on their behavior (Binder, 1999).

The Impact of Psychological Illness

Why is it important to learn about psychological illness? Most Americans have one or more family members who suffer from a psychological illness. About one in five Americans experience some form of mental illness annually (U.S. Department of Health and Human Services [USDHHS], 1999). According to data from the National Comorbidity Survey (Kessler et al., 1994), depression and alcohol dependence are the most common psychological disturbances that affect Americans (Table 2-4). Throughout the world, mental illnesses are prevalent and often not treated adequately (Demyttenaere et al., 2004).

The emotional and economic costs of mental illness are high not only for affected individuals and their families but also for society. People may drop out of

affect observable expressions of mood.

delusions inaccurate and unreasonable beliefs that often result in decision-making errors.

hallucinations false sensory perceptions that have no apparent external cause.

Table 2-4 Lifetime Prevalence of Mental Health Disorders

Disorder	Percentage of Americans Affected*
Any mood disorder	19.3
Major depressive episode	16.2†
Any anxiety disorder	24.9
Panic disorder	3.5
Simple phobia	11.3
Social phobia	13.3
Generalized anxiety disorder	5.1
Any substance abuse/dependence	26.6
Alcohol dependence	14.1
Drug dependence other than alcohol	7.5
Any mental health disorder	48.0

*Many individuals reported suffering from more than one disorder.
Source: Based on Kessler, R. C., et al. (1994). Lifetime and 12-month prevalence of DSM-III-R psychiatric disorders in the United States: Results from the National Comorbidity Survey. Archives of General Psychiatry, 51:8–19.
†Source: Kessler, R. C., et al. (2003). The epidemiology of major depressive disorder. Results from the National Comorbidity Survey Replication (NC5-R). Journal of the American Medical Association, 289(23):3095–3105.

college or abuse alcohol and other drugs because of unresolved emotional problems or underlying psychological disorders. Mental illness frequently has a negative impact on the quality of life and the productivity of workers.

In the past, psychologically disturbed individuals were often misunderstood and mistreated. Having a mental illness was considered disgraceful by people who associated the condition with bizarre behaviors, violent acts, and long stays in mental health care facilities. Today, being diagnosed with a psychological disorder is no longer a hopeless situation, because scientists are understanding more about the various biological, environmental, and social factors that influence behaviors. Nevertheless, these disorders do not receive the kind of interest and concern from public health officials that conditions such as heart disease, cancer, and stroke generate. Why? Richard Neugebauer (1999) thinks mental illnesses do not get much attention because of the stigma associated with them and the lack of major risk factors that can be modified to prevent them.

Although mental health disorders are common and can be quite disabling, many of these conditions can be managed effectively with medications and other forms of therapy. According to the *Healthy People 2000* final review (USDHHS, 2001), in 1993 about 14% of Americans 18 years of age and older sought help for their emotional problems; in 1998, that number increased to over 22%. The target for the year 2000 was to increase to at least 20% the proportion of American adults who seek such help. Because negative attitudes toward mental illness persist, many psychologically disturbed people are reluctant to seek beneficial therapy; they live in misery, hiding their illness from others. Seeking professional help for psychological problems is a sign of personal strength, not weakness.

What Causes Psychological Disorders?

There are numerous psychological disorders, and in each case, it may be impossible to determine a single cause. Alterations in the normal chemical and physical environment of the brain often produce mental illness. In many instances, these alterations are the result of genetic defects that adversely affect neurotransmitter levels. Additionally, people whose brains have been physically damaged by injuries, tumors, or infections often display abnormal behavior. When introduced into the body, drugs such as cocaine can interfere with the brain's ability to produce, use, or eliminate neurotransmitters. Furthermore, pollutants such as pesticides and toxic minerals, including lead, mercury, and arsenic, can damage the brain.

Scientists note that certain mental illnesses such as schizophrenia and most major mood disorders tend to occur within the same family. These observations support the role of inheritance in their development. Genetic factors alone, however, do not explain the development of every psychological disorder. Several members of a family could develop similar forms of mental illness because they are more likely to experience the same physical, economic, and social environments than unrelated individuals.

Environmental conditions influence the expression of many inborn traits, including psychological responses. Children, for example, often learn ways of reacting to situations by observing their parents. Think about how you respond when angered or frustrated. Are your responses like those of your mother or father?

Personal experiences can trigger the onset and influence the severity of some psychological disturbances. Some experts think that a child's brain can be altered by exposure to extremely stressful situations, increasing the youngster's risk of developing depression later in life. Even psychologically healthy individuals can develop *post-traumatic stress disorder,* a severe anxiety disorder, after surviving life-threatening experiences (Figure 2-3). Researchers have yet to understand completely the extent to which biological, social, and environmental factors interact to influence psychological health.

Figure 2-3 **Surviving a Disaster.** After surviving life-threatening situations, such as the September 11 terrorist attack on the Pentagon, individuals can develop post-traumatic stress disorder.

Table 2-5 lists the major types of mental health therapists and some information concerning their qualifications.

Many people learn to cope with various psychological problems, such as drug addictions or the loss of loved ones, by joining *support groups*. The support group is an informal approach to treatment. Support group participants have regular meetings in which they can discuss personal adjustment problems. Group members usually conduct these meetings rather than mental health therapists. In addition to attending regular meetings, some group members may need to obtain professional counseling.

Mental health therapists can offer a variety of effective psychotherapies (treatments) that enable many individuals with psychological disorders to lead normal, productive lives. Psychotherapy often includes counseling, including *cognitive behavioral therapy*; group therapy; and medications. Cognitive behavioral therapy can help anxious, angry, or depressed people identify and change negative or inaccurate ways in which they think about themselves and their situations. As mentioned earlier, medication can correct neurotransmitter imbalances in the brain. Table 2-6 lists some medications that are commonly prescribed to treat various psychological disorders.

More than one form of treatment may be necessary to alleviate or control the disorder. In severe cases, psychologically disturbed people may require hospital-

Treating Psychological Disorders

Many people with psychological disorders respond well to treatment. Treating these conditions involves the cooperation of the affected individuals and their families and, in many instances, the assistance of mental health therapists who have specialized training.

Table 2-5 Major Types of Mental Health Therapists

Therapist	Training and Degrees
Counseling and clinical psychologists	M.A., Ph.D., or Psy.D. in psychology; 5 or more years in psychotherapy methods, research, and assessment
Psychiatrists	Medical (M.D. or O.D.) degree and at least 3 years of specialized training in psychiatry
Psychoanalysts	Have undergone personal psychoanalysis and completed 7 to 10 years of part-time psychoanalytic training (most are psychiatrists)
Psychiatric social workers	MSW; most states require certification by the Academy of Certified Social Workers
Clinical mental health counselors	Master's degree (or equivalent) and 2 years of counseling experience; certified by National Academy of Certified Clinical Mental Health Counselors
Psychiatric nurse practitioners	Registered nurses with additional education and experience working in psychiatric settings
Marital and family therapists	Master's degree. Licensed or certified in about one-half of the states; member of the American Association for Marriage and Family Therapy
Sexual therapists	Minimum of a master's degree, a license in related field, specialized sex education and sex-therapist training, extensive supervised individual and group therapy experience; the American Association of Sex Educators, Counselors and Therapists provides certification
Abuse counselors	Substance abuse training; often counselors are recovering substance abusers
Clergy	Religious training; may have spiritual and family counseling training

Source: Cornacchia, H. J., & Barrett, S. (1993). *Consumer health.* St. Louis: Mosby.

Consumer Health

Locating and Selecting Mental Health Therapists

The following tips can help you find and select qualified mental health specialists:

- Discuss psychological health concerns with your general medical practitioner or with medical staff at your student health center. These individuals can assess your health and refer you to qualified mental health specialists if necessary.
- Contact local mental health associations or agencies for information about psychological health. Members of these associations can give you information about local support groups and mental health services.
- Contact your state's social welfare department or the social services department of a local hospital to identify qualified therapists.
- Interview therapists before making any agreements for services.
- Ask therapists about treatment philosophies, methods, insurance coverage, and payment expectations before agreeing to use their services.

Table 2-6 Medications Frequently Prescribed for Psychological Disorders

Type of Medication	Medications (brand names)	Disorders
Antianxiety	Xanax, Librium, Paxil, Buspar, Ativan, Serax, Valium	Anxiety, obsessive-compulsive, psychosomatic disorder
Antidepressants	Elavil, Prozac, Zoloft, Luvox, Wellbutrin, Effexor, Celexa, Lexapro	Depression, eating disorders, obsessive-compulsive disorder
Mood stabilizers	Eskalith, Lithane, Trileptal	Certain types of depression, especially bipolar disorder
Antipsychotics	Thorazine, Haldol, Prolixin, Zyprexa, Seroquel	Schizophrenia
Nonamphetamine stimulants	Ritalin, Adderal, Concerta	Attention deficit disorders

ization for treatment and to prevent self-injury or harm to others. If you or someone you know needs mental health care, the Consumer Health box titled "Locating and Selecting Mental Health Therapists" provides some suggestions for finding and choosing qualified help.

Healthy Living Practices

- Many psychological problems respond well to treatment. If you think you may have a mental health disorder, ask your personal health care practitioner or the medical staff at your campus health center for help.

■ Common Psychological Disorders

Anxiety Disorders

Do you feel uneasy when you ride in an elevator, enter a classroom to take a test, or give a speech? Nearly everyone experiences anxiety, the uncomfortable feeling of apprehension or uneasiness that results while expecting a vague threat. The physical changes associated with anxiety states include increased heart rate, rapid breathing, and elevated blood pressure. Anxious people may report feeling tense, distressed, or worried; and they may be emotionally upset, sweating, and trembling. Anxiety disorders are common; according to the results of the National Comorbidity Survey, nearly one in four Americans suffers from these conditions at some time in their lives (Kessler et al., 1994).

Generalized Anxiety Disorder When you perceive a threat, it is normal to feel mildly anxious as your body physically prepares to deal with the danger. However, if the anxiety interferes with your ability to perform daily activities, the condition is abnormal. During their lifetimes, as much as 5% of the population suffers from **generalized anxiety disorder**, a condition characterized by uncontrollable chronic worrying, anxiousness, and nervousness. People with this disorder have unrealistic and excessive concerns about their jobs, children, health, or minor situations such as making home repairs. They are tense, irritable, and restless, and they often experience sleeping problems. Treatment usually includes antianxiety and antidepressant medications as well as cognitive behavioral therapy.

generalized anxiety disorder a condition characterized by uncontrollable chronic worrying and nervousness.

phobia an intense and irrational fear of an object or a situation.

panic disorder psychological condition that features panic attacks, unpredictable episodes of extreme anxiety, and loss of emotional control.

Phobias A **phobia** is an intense and irrational fear of a situation or object. *Agoraphobia* is the fear of open places or public areas. *Social phobias* are fears of performing in situations that involve people, such as giving speeches or taking tests. *Specific phobias* (formerly called simple phobias) are fears of certain objects or situations, such as snakes or flying. According to the results of the National Comorbidity Survey, phobias are among the most common psychological disturbances in the United States (Kessler et al., 1994). About 13% of Americans report having social phobias, and about 11% of Americans report experiencing specific phobias. It is not uncommon for a person to be affected by more than one phobia. Although people who suffer from phobias know that their behavior is irrational, they still become anxious in the situations that arouse their fears (Figure 2-4).

Most cases of phobia are mild; affected individuals often learn to live with this condition by avoiding situations that arouse the anxiety. Severe phobias can interfere with normal social functioning. For example, people with agoraphobia may refuse to leave their homes. Individuals who are severely affected by phobias can seek professional treatment that includes behavioral therapy and medications to control irrational feelings and reduce anxiety.

Panic Disorder An estimated 3 million Americans suffer from **panic disorders** that feature *panic attacks,* unpredictable episodes of extreme anxiety and loss of emotional control. During a panic attack, people usually experience shortness of breath, shakiness, faintness, nausea, and a rapid, pounding heartbeat. Affected individuals often feel terrified because they think they are becoming insane or having a heart attack. Severe

Figure 2-4 | **Phobias.** Phobias are intense and irrational fears of certain situations or objects that can interfere with everyday functioning. This woman has a fear of heights.

phobias, certain drugs, or frightening experiences may trigger panic attacks, but they can occur spontaneously.

Therapists often combine cognitive behavioral therapy and medications to treat panic disorders. People who have frequent panic attacks should seek medical help because studies indicate that they are at risk of committing suicide.

Post-traumatic Stress Disorder Individuals who survive extraordinary life events such as a sexual assault, natural disaster, or combat may develop *post-traumatic stress disorder (PTSD)*. Nevertheless, some people suffer from PTSD even after being in an auto accident or abusive relationship. Nearly 1 in 10 Americans experiences PTSD during their lifetime (Lamberg, 2001).

Symptoms of PTSD may take months to develop fully and include having disturbing recollections or nightmares of the event as well as being emotionally "numb." Affected people often avoid thinking about or discussing the traumatic experiences, and they may smoke heavily, overeat, or abuse drugs as a way of coping. Treatment of PTSD includes antianxiety medication and counseling that encourages survivors to talk about the traumatic events with others (Davidson, 2001).

Obsessive-Compulsive Disorder Although the experts disagree, *obsessive-compulsive disorder (OCD)* is generally classified as an anxiety disorder. An **obsession** is a persistent, inappropriate, and repetitive thought or impulse that produces anxious feelings. Obsessions are often related to self-doubt or fears. A **compulsion** is the behavior that usually follows the obsessive thoughts or impulses. Compulsive behaviors reduce the obsessed individual's anxiety. A young person, for example, might have recurring thoughts of injuring a family member. This individual may wash his or her hands hundreds of times a day and take numerous long showers to reduce anxious feelings. Other typical compulsive behaviors include hoarding cats and dogs or useless items like plastic containers or making repetitive actions such as checking the oven frequently to see if it is turned off. Affected individuals often think that their obsessions and compulsions are repulsive or troublesome, but efforts to stop create more anxiety. Treatment includes medication and psychological counseling. In most cases, the longer the obsessive-compulsive behavior pattern has been in place, the more difficult the disorder is to treat.

Unclassified Impulse Control Disorders

Some psychologists consider frequent gambling, promiscuous sexual activity, and certain eating disorders to be subtypes of obsessive-compulsive disorder. These activities, however, are distinguished from true compulsions because the affected person enjoys the activity, at least until the persistent behavior interferes with his or her well-being, relationships, or job (Hollander et al., 1999).

Problem Gambling Nearly every state permits some form of gambling, such as lotteries, track racing, or casinos. For most people who place bets, the activity is entertaining, occasional, and controllable. However, an estimated 1% to 4% of adult Americans are problem gamblers who gamble compulsively, excessively, and at the expense of their families, jobs, and relationships ("Problem Gambling," 2004). Men are more likely to be compulsive gamblers than women. Psychological disorders, including depression, anxiety disorders, and alcohol and other drug abuse, often accompany problem gambling behavior, but it is not known if gambling losses caused the disorders or the disorders led to the compulsive gambling. Table 2-7 lists typical features of problem gamblers.

In college students, problem gambling often accompanies other risky behaviors, such as binge drinking and illegal drug use. At one time, the rate of problem gambling among college students was thought to be increasing, but results of a more recent survey indicate that the percentage of college students who gamble compulsively is about the same as the rest of the adult population (LaBrie et al., 2003).

Gamblers Anonymous is a self-help group that can enable problem gamblers to control their troublesome behavior, but many participants in the program do not remain in treatment. Some counselors have certification to treat compulsive gambling, but health insurance providers may not cover their services. More research is needed to determine effective ways to prevent as well as treat this condition.

Table 2-7	Typical Features of Problem Gambling

The problem gambler

- Seems to think only about gambling or how to get money to gamble
- Loses friends, family members, and jobs because of his or her behavior
- Gambles more often over time
- Has no control over the impulse to gamble
- Becomes restless, angry, or agitated when he or she tries to gamble less often (withdrawal)
- Gambles to escape problems or cope with depression, guilt, or anxiety
- Gambles again, trying to recover losses
- Lies to cover up the behavior
- Has others financially bail him or her out
- Resorts to illegal acts, such as forging checks and stealing money, to obtain money for gambling
- Abuses mind-altering drugs

Mood Disorders

Until a few years ago, the two words that best described my life were fear *and* loneliness. *As a child, I experienced physical, emotional, and verbal abuse from my parents. There were some instances when the beatings were so severe, I just forgot about them. I married a man who also physically abused me. Having no savings or college degree, I lacked the self-confidence to walk out of the marriage. I felt trapped. Deep depression set in; I cried a lot of the time and felt guilty because I was unable to carry out the normal daily responsibilities of cooking and cleaning the house. I began to think suicidal thoughts.*

Finally, I entered a hospital that had a stress unit. Between the group sessions and private therapy, I learned a lot about those who abuse others and how to handle stress. However, spending three weeks in the hospital did not cure my depression. I realized that the only thing that would do that would be to remove myself from its cause. I separated from my husband and started college.

It has been a struggle financially, but I am determined to make it. I am preparing to graduate this semester with a Bachelor of Arts degree, and I plan to continue on to get a Master of Arts degree. The best change is my new self-confidence gained from overcoming the obstacles and becoming independent.

This middle-aged college student's case not only illustrates the harsh origins of her depression, but also how an emotionally resilient person can recover from depression, resolve problems, and regain self-esteem. How can you distinguish a normal period of sadness from one that signals a major depressive disorder?

obsession a repetitive thought that produces anxious feelings.

compulsion the behavior that follows obsessive thoughts and reduces anxiety.

It is normal for people to feel "down" after a loss or disappointment. After a significant loss, such as the death of a close friend or relative, one normally feels *grief,* an intense sadness that may persist up to a year after the loss. Most grieving individuals soon recover their emotional balance and resume their usual activities. Grieving people are probably severely depressed if they become so profoundly sad that they withdraw and isolate themselves for several months and harbor feelings of guilt, low self-worth, and suicide. Enduring other stressful experiences can trigger the first episode of depression in susceptible persons.

major depressive disorder a mood disorder characterized by persistent and profound sadness, hopelessness, helplessness, and feelings of worthlessness; lack of energy; loss of interest in usual activities; loss of the ability to concentrate; suicidal thoughts; and appetite and sleep disturbances.

Major depressive disorder is a mood disorder characterized by persistent and profound sadness, hopelessness, helplessness, and feelings of worthlessness. Depressed people often report a lack of energy, loss of interest in usual activities, inability to concentrate on tasks, and appetite disturbances. These symptoms last for 2 weeks or more and interfere with relationships and responsibilities related to school, work, and home. Insomnia is a common complaint of depressed individuals; the most reliable sign of early depression is waking up too early in the morning (Rakel, 1999). Depressed people may be anxious and irritable, and they often use alcohol or illegal drugs to alter their emotional state. An estimated 2% to 9% of people diagnosed with depression commit suicide (Bostwick & Pankratz, 2000).

According to a recent survey, about 16% of U.S. adults reported experiencing major depression during their lifetimes (Kessler et al., 2003). Physicians, however, often fail to diagnose the condition in their patients. As a result, about half of the individuals who suffer from depression do not obtain treatment (Gelenberg, 1999). Although a small percentage of these untreated persons recover spontaneously and never experience another bout with the disorder, the remaining untreated individuals suffer from chronic depression or recurrent episodes of depression (Glass, 1999).

Researchers have detected abnormal blood flow and chemical responses in the emotional centers of depressed people's brains (Vastag, 2002). Moreover, the parts of a person's brain that manage emotions shrink considerably during depressive episodes, which may explain why the individual has difficulty "snapping out of it." These changes often persist, and as a result, a person who recovers from one episode of depression has a high risk of experiencing future bouts of the condition.

Like diabetes and high blood pressure, depression is a chronic but treatable disease. Many severely and chronically depressed people can obtain dramatic relief from their disabling symptoms by receiving therapies that include prescribed antidepressant medications (Gelenberg, 1999). Compared to the late 1980s, significantly more depressed Americans are receiving conventional treatments, particularly antidepressant medications (Olfson et al., 2002). To treat chronic severe depression, however, physicians usually combine cognitive behavioral therapy with antidepressant medication.

Alternative remedies for depression are becoming popular in the United States. The herb St. John's wort may be helpful as a treatment for mild to moderate depression (Ernst, 2002). SAMe, a compound that is made in the body and sold as a dietary supplement, has antidepressant properties also (Fugh-Berman & Cott, 1999). St. John's wort and SAMe have been reported to interact with certain prescription drugs and cause side effects, so one should not take these substances without consulting a physician.

Some affected individuals feel better by engaging in regular physical activity. According to the Surgeon General's Report on Physical Activity and Health (Centers for Disease Control and Prevention, 1996), a moderate amount of physical activity each day may reduce symptoms of anxiety and depression and improve mood and a sense of well-being.

Bipolar depression, formerly called manic depression, is characterized by periods of depression followed by episodes of extremely elevated mood called *mania.* Individuals with mania typically brag about themselves and their accomplishments, engage in excessive physical activity and rapid talking, and sleep very little. Another characteristic of mania is excessive participation in pleasurable and risky activities that can lead to unwelcome consequences, such as careless sexual encounters or costly shopping sprees. During each phase of the bipolar illness, the mood of the affected person gradually reaches an extreme level, which is maintained sometimes for weeks before it swings gradually to the opposite mood. These cyclic mood shifts may recur several times during one's life. Medications, such as lithium carbonate, and hospitalization are often used to treat persons with mania.

Besides bipolar depression, other mood disorders occur in cycles. People with *seasonal affective disorder (SAD)* become depressed around mid- to late fall, and their depression ends in late winter or early spring. Besides feeling depressed and tired, people with SAD also report craving sweets and gaining weight. Since these symptoms resolve when the daylight period lengthens or when people with the condition spend time in sunnier climates, medical experts think SAD may be related to a lack of exposure to bright light. Light therapy is an effective form of treatment for this disorder (Terman et al., 2001).

Disordered Eating and Eating Disorders

A female college athlete habitually skips breakfast. For lunch, she typically drinks an 8-ounce canned milkshake that is marketed as a weight loss supplement. By the time dinner is served in her dormitory, she describes herself as "starving." A male college student whose height is 5′9″ and weight only 125 pounds also skips breakfast. Nearly every day, he eats cheeseburgers and french fries from a fast-food restaurant that's within walking distance of his campus. He rarely eats fruits or green vegetables. A young man who describes himself as a vegetarian eats only brown rice, fruit, and tea. Are these behaviors examples of disordered eating or signs of eating disorders?

Occasionally, most people engage in unusual eating practices, such as skipping meals, fasting, or avoiding sweets in an effort to lose a few pounds. *Disordered eating* practices are mild and often temporary changes in one's otherwise normal food-related behaviors. In many instances, a person uses these behaviors to improve health or appearance. Disordered eating practices, however, can become eating disorders. *Eating disorders* are persistent, abnormal eating patterns that can threaten a person's health and well-being. The three major eating disorders—bulimia nervosa, anorexia nervosa, and binge eating disorder—affect an estimated 5 million Americans each year (Becker et al., 1999). These conditions often develop in adolescence or young adulthood, and they are more likely to affect females than males. An estimated 85% to 95% of the people with anorexia nervosa and 65% of those suffering from bulimia nervosa are female.

Hormonal, genetic, psychological, and sociocultural factors influence the development of eating disorders. Risk factors include family history, childhood abuse, depression and anxiety, low self-esteem, and family conflict (American Psychiatric Association, 2000; Lamberg, 2003). Additionally, homosexual males have a higher risk of eating disorders than heterosexual males (Russell & Keel, 2002).

Although it is true that excess body fat is not healthy, a society that emphasizes thinness as a sign of physical attractiveness makes many young people overly concerned about and dissatisfied with their body size, even when it is normal. As a result of societal influences, many American females admire the bodies of fashion models, actresses, and ballet dancers who look as though they are starving (Figure 2-5). Young males, on the other hand, may equate optimal health and

Figure 2-5 In 2004, actress Mary-Kate Olsen entered a treatment center to obtain help for an undisclosed health condition that was later reported to be anorexia nervosa.

attractiveness with the massive, well-defined muscles of action heroes that are typically portrayed in comic books and movies. Such efforts to achieve an ideal body shape can evolve into a disastrous and obsessive preoccupation with body weight and composition, food intake, and physical activity level. It is interesting to note that eating disorders are uncommon in regions of the world where the food supply is limited and starvation is an everyday occurrence.

Although usually considered nutritional problems, eating disorders are often associated with psychological disturbances, including obsessive-compulsive and mood disorders as well as substance abuse. Goals of counseling include encouraging patients to cooperate in their recovery and change their unhealthy attitudes toward food and their bodies. Treating underlying psychological and family-related problems may help resolve the eating disorder or reduce the frequency of the abnormal eating behavior, but many people with severe eating disorders do not respond to treatment.

Anorexia Nervosa Occasionally nearly everyone has *anorexia*, appetite loss that can occur under various circumstances, such as excitement or fever. **Anorexia nervosa**, however, is a severe psychological disturbance in which an individual refuses to eat enough food to maintain a healthy body weight. People with anorexia nervosa (*anorexics*) have an irrational fear of becoming fat, usually maintain strict control over their food intake, and are preoccupied with calorie counting and food preparation. As mentioned earlier, females are more likely to suffer from anorexia nervosa than males. During their lifetime, an estimated 0.5% to 3.7% of American females suffer from anorexia nervosa (National Institute of Mental Health [NIMH], 2001).

People with anorexia nervosa have a distorted image of their bodies. They deny that they are severely underweight even though they weigh 15% or more below normal for their height. Typically, females with this condition do not have normal menstrual cycles and feminine body contours. Without an adequate supply of fat to insulate their bodies against heat loss, anorexics feel cold easily and often wear layers of clothing to provide extra warmth.

Some people suffering from anorexia nervosa occasionally lose control over their food intake and eat excessive amounts of food (*bingeing*). To avoid gaining weight, these individuals induce vomiting, give themselves frequent enemas, or abuse laxatives (*purging*). Additionally, anorexics often exercise excessively to "burn up" calories. Table 2-8 lists these and other typical signs of anorexia nervosa.

Table 2-8   Typical Signs of Anorexia Nervosa

In addition to refusing to gain weight despite weighing 15% or more below that which is healthy, a person who has anorexia nervosa typically

- Has an intense drive to achieve a thin body
- Seems unaware that body size has changed
- Denies malnourished appearance
- Derives little satisfaction from his or her body shape
- Fears losing control over appetite
- Becomes full after eating small amounts of food
- Is a "picky" eater; avoids foods that contain fat, starch, or sugar
- Exercises excessively
- Lacks menstrual periods (females)
- Is depressed
- Has low self-esteem
- Has perfectionist tendencies

Source: Based on Garfinkel, P. (1992). Classification and diagnosis. In K. A. Halmi (Ed.), *Psychobiology and treatment of anorexia nervosa and bulimia nervosa.* Washington, DC: American Psychiatric Press.

Treatment for anorexia nervosa includes individual and family counseling; patients must reach about 85% of their normal body weight before antidepressant therapy is useful. In severe cases, people with anorexia nervosa can die unless they are given special feedings and monitored closely in hospitals. Earlier estimates of the percentage of deaths that resulted from anorexia nervosa may have been too high. According to a review of studies in which the long-term outcomes of nearly 5,600 anorexics were analyzed, about 5% of people suffering from the condition died, in most instances from suicide, and less than 50% recovered (Steinhausen, 2002). The remaining individuals with anorexia nervosa were improved or remained chronically ill with the disorder.

Bulimia Nervosa While people with anorexia nervosa are so thin they are easy to identify, those with bulimia nervosa may be more difficult to recognize because their weights are often normal. **Bulimia** is a craving for food that is difficult to satisfy; bulimic people typically eat excessive amounts of food at one time because they are depressed or anxious rather than hungry. Some bulimic persons are able to maintain normal body weights because after bingeing, they purge by fasting, practicing self-induced vomiting, taking laxatives and diuretics, or exercising. Vomiting prevents the body from absorbing and using the nutrients in food and beverages. Laxatives speed up the movement of the intestinal tract and can lead to watery diarrhea; diuretics increase urine production and elimination. Vomiting and abusing laxatives and diuretics can seriously disrupt the body's normal fluid and chemical balance, which can be life-threatening.

Occasional episodes of bulimic behavior are common among young women who are trying to control their weight. It is estimated that about 1% to 4% of females suffer from bulimia nervosa during their lifetimes (NIMH, 2001).

Many young women, especially on college campuses, accept and openly practice bingeing and purging. Other bulimic individuals are disgusted with their disordered eating behavior, hiding it from roommates, friends, and family members. Some people practice bingeing and purging twice a week; in severe cases, affected individuals engage in these behaviors several times a day. Severely bulimic people can become so preoccupied with eating that they shoplift food to supply their binges and experience legal problems as a consequence. College students with bulimia frequently encounter academic problems after they neglect to attend their classes.

An estimated 40% of binge eaters are boys or men (Becker et al., 1999). Men, for example, may be affected by bulimia nervosa if they regularly consume too much food or excessive amounts of alcohol and then vomit afterwards. Furthermore, some young men who participate in sports that require maintaining low weight, such as wrestling and gymnastics, practice the behaviors associated with bulimia nervosa to remain competitive.

Typically, bulimic individuals are more socially outgoing than people with anorexia nervosa, yet they experience low self-esteem, anxiety, and depression. Eating temporarily relieves the bulimic person's anxiety. Although antidepressant medications and psychotherapy are useful treatments, people with bulimia nervosa often do not seek help for their behavior. Affected women tend to improve over time, but 10 years following diagnosis, about 30% still suffer from the condition (Keel et al., 1999).

Binge Eating Disorder About one-third of overweight people engage in regular episodes of binge eating that are rarely followed up with purging or heavy exercise (deZwaan, 2001). This behavior is called **binge eating disorder**. Some binge eaters report *blackouts*, periods of time that they cannot recall when they had overeating episodes, but empty food containers provide them with evidence of the incidents. Like persons with bulimia nervosa, binge eaters have poor self-esteem, and they often feel disgusted, depressed, and guilty about their eating behavior and physical appearance. These feelings may trigger additional episodes of overeating. *Night eating syndrome*, which is more common among obese than normal-weight persons, may be a variation of binge eating disorder. People with night eating syndrome are not hungry during the day, but have difficulty staying asleep at night; they awake often and frequently get out of bed to eat large amounts of food.

If you or someone you know suffers from an eating disorder such as bulimia nervosa or binge eating, ask the staff at your campus health center or your personal physician to recommend mental health practitioners who specialize in treating these conditions. Additionally, check hospitals in your area, because many have self-help groups for people with eating disorders.

Other Disordered Eating Conditions Athletes involved in sports that often emphasize leanness and low body weight, such as gymnastics, wrestling, light-weight rowing, horse racing, figure skating, body building, and distance running, have an increased risk of developing eating disorders. An estimated 15% to 62% of female college athletes suffer from the *female athlete triad*, a condition characterized by disordered eating, absence of menstruation, and premature osteoporosis (Kazis & Iglesias, 2003). Osteoporosis weakens bones and may result in serious spinal and hip fractures. Osteoporosis is generally associated with post-menopausal women, not young women.

Although most females with the female athlete triad do not show every sign of illness associated with anorexia nervosa or bulimia nervosa, their food-related practices, such as bingeing and self-induced vomiting, are similar. To prevent this condition, it is important to teach young athletes about healthy eating practices and body weights. Furthermore, parents need to be aware of factors that contribute to the triad, such as having low self-esteem and few friends, identifying thin physiques with ideal body shapes, being preoccupied with weigh-ins, and having overly demanding coaches who criticize the young athlete for being "fat" and insist on weight loss.

In the United States, many men experience social pressure to attain larger, more muscular body builds. *Muscle dysmorphia* is a newly recognized condition that affects weightlifters, including female bodybuilders (Choi et al., 2002). Despite their very muscular body builds, people suffering from this condition are not satisfied with the size of their bodies, and as a result, they spend hours working out each day, particularly lifting weights. Moreover, they are ashamed of their bodies and reluctant to expose themselves in public places such as beaches. Individuals with muscle dysmorphia are obsessed with the need to gain muscle without adding body fat; they have a high risk of eating disorders and abuse of *anabolic steroids*, drugs that can increase muscle size. At this point, little is known about the prevalence of muscle dysmorphia or effective ways to treat the condition.

binge eating disorder a pattern of eating excessive amounts of food in response to distress such as anxiety or depression.

dementia impaired cognitive functioning, particularly memory loss, confusion, disorientation, and delusions.

schizophrenia a form of psychosis.

Dementia

People who suffer from **dementia** experience impaired cognitive functioning, particularly memory loss, confusion, and disorientation. Dementia can be a temporary or progressive condition, and it occurs in young as well as aged persons. Brain injuries or tumors, Parkinson's disease, exposure to certain drugs, and infection with human immunodeficiency virus (HIV) can produce dementia. Insufficient blood flow to the brain and *strokes*, bleeding within the brain that results in tissue destruction, frequently produce senile dementia in the elderly. However, about 50% of senile dementia cases involve Alzheimer's disease (see Chapter 15).

Schizophrenia

An estimated 2 million Americans suffer from **schizophrenia**, a type of psychosis. Lay people often believe schizophrenia means split or multiple personalities, but actually, people with schizophrenia experience extremely disorganized thought processes, including hallucinations and delusions. These individuals often display strange behavior and inappropriate emotions. Communicating with some affected individuals is difficult because their speech often consists of words strung together into meaningless sentences. The causes of schizophrenia are unknown, but the brains of people with the disorder tend to have biochemical or structural defects that many medical experts think are inherited.

Schizophrenia usually develops during adolescence and young adulthood; the disorder affects about 1% of the population (Sawa & Snyder, 2002). Some affected persons have one schizophrenic episode and recover, but others experience recurrent episodes and require long-term treatment. By taking special medications, many people with this form of dementia experience relief from their symptoms and live as productive members of society. Some people with severe forms of schizophrenia must live in mental health care facilities because their behavior is unmanageable or dangerous to themselves or others.

Healthy Living Practices

- If you or someone you know has an eating or other psychological disorder, seek help from the medical staff at the campus health center or from your personal health care provider.

■ Suicide

Suicide, the deliberate ending of one's own life, is not a mental illness. However, such extreme violence against oneself is often the behavioral consequence of a severe psychological disorder. Most people who choose to end their lives feel overwhelmed by the demands of life; they are unable to solve their problems or adapt to their situations.

Overall, suicide accounts for only a small percentage of deaths in the United States. In 2001 about 1% of deaths were attributed to suicide; males were over four times more likely to kill themselves than females (Arias et al., 2003). Suicide was the second leading cause of death for whites and Native Americans between 20 and 24 years of age and the third leading cause of death for their black or Hispanic counterparts (Anderson & Smith, 2003).

A goal of *Healthy People 2000* was to reduce the overall suicide rate to 10.5 per 100,000 Americans by the year 2000. According to the *Healthy People 2000* final review (USDHHS, 2001), the suicide rate is down slightly from the 1987 rate.

Alcohol consumption is associated with suicide. An estimated one-third to two-thirds of teenagers consumed alcohol prior to taking their lives. According to Birckmayer and Hemenway (1999), efforts to lower the minimum legal drinking age to 18 in the United States could increase the number of suicides in the 18-to-20-year-old population by nearly 10%.

In spite of what many people believe, the Christmas holiday season is not the time that suicide rates peak; intentional deaths are generally low in winter, and high in late spring (Lambert et al., 2003). Although women are more likely to attempt suicide, men are more likely to complete the act of killing themselves. Most people use a firearm to end their lives; however, taking drug overdoses and crashing motor vehicles are also frequent suicide methods. Thus, it is difficult to determine the actual number of suicides that occur each year. Taking one's own life places a social stigma on surviving family members, and some medical practitioners may want to protect them by ruling that the death was unintentional rather than a suicide.

Preventing Suicide

Most suicide victims suffered from a psychological disturbance, particularly a major depressive condition that included alcohol abuse (Cheng et al., 2000). Other characteristics associated with a high risk of committing suicide are previous suicide attempts; a family history of suicide; excessive grieving over the death of a loved one; marital or financial problems; and schizophrenia, an eating disorder, or a terminal illness. Some persons with severe or terminal health problems seek the help of others, particularly family members or physicians, to commit suicide. (Chapter 15 discusses the "right to die" and physician-assisted suicide.) People who know or treat individuals with these characteristics or conditions should be aware of their suicide risk and initiate intervention methods to prevent them from ending their lives.

Suicidal persons usually feel intense emotional strain, are preoccupied with thoughts of death, and often communicate their intentions to others. These individuals might say "everyone would be better off if I were dead" or "I am going to kill myself," discuss the pros and cons of various suicide methods, and make unsuccessful suicide attempts. After deciding to kill themselves, suicidal individuals often seem cheerful and relaxed. When survivors recall the positive emotional state of the victims, they may report that these persons showed no

Analyzing
Health-Related Information

The following ad promotes a series of compact discs designed to improve the functioning of the mind. Read the advertisement and evaluate it using the model for analyzing health-related information. The main points of the model are noted below; the model is fully explained on pages 13–15.

1. Which statements are verifiable facts, and which are unverified statements or value claims?
2. What are the credentials of the person who wrote the ad? Does the author appear to have appropriate background and education in the topic area? If it is difficult to tell if the author has specific health expertise, what can you do to check his or her credentials?
3. What might be the motives and biases of the author?
4. What is the main point of the ad? Which information in the ad is relevant to the product? Which information is irrelevant?
5. Is the source reliable? Does it have a reputation for publishing misinformation? Does the ad present both the pros and cons of this product?
6. Does the ad attack the credibility of conventional scientists or medical authorities?

Based on your analysis, do you think that this ad is a reliable source of health-related information? Explain why you would or would not buy the CDs. Summarize your reasons for coming to this conclusion.

ADVERTISEMENT ADVERTISEMENT ADVERTISEMENT ADVERTISEMENT ADVERTISEMENT

Can't seem to learn new tricks? Getting forgetful? Having memory lapses?

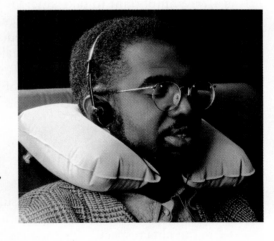

As you age, mental functioning declines. Before you know it, you can't seem to follow even the simplest instructions, you can't remember your children's names, and you can't keep your mind from wandering when you should be paying attention.

"How can I ever thank you? I've tried three other neurotechnology products, but BRAINFIT was the only one that worked."
B. J., London, England

"Please send another copy of the miraculous BRAINFIT CD—my sister took mine and won't return it!"
S. A., New Delhi, India

Fortunately, you can learn how to prevent your mind from slipping away from you. Now you can benefit from the latest discovery in subliminal microtechnology that produces phenomenal advances in brain functioning. Scientists from around the world are predicting that this incredible breakthrough will be the greatest medical discovery of the 21st century!

Our amazing new **BRAINFIT CD** can increase your mental capacity without the need for potentially harmful drugs. Listening to the CD has been scientifically proven to improve learning by up to 35%, enhance memory by up to 28%, and boost awareness by up to 55%. Millions of people in 60 countries report that **BRAINFIT** really works!

For the first time, BRAINFIT is available in the United States. Order your copy now. We guarantee that BRAINFIT will improve your mental functioning. BRAINFIT is easy to use at home, work, or even as you drive your car!

FOR YOUR PERSONALIZED COPY OF BRAINFIT, SEND A MONEY ORDER FOR $39.95 TO: BRAINFIT

Table 2-9	Behavioral Warning Signs of Suicide

Behavior and examples

- Discussing, joking, or writing about suicide or death
- Giving away prized possessions
- Making final arrangements: planning a will or making funeral plans
- Displaying severe depressive symptoms
- Reporting feelings of hopelessness and helplessness
- Performing risky behaviors: playing with guns, driving while drunk, or performing daredevil stunts
- Injuring oneself by cutting, burning, or hitting
- Behaving in a manner that is different from usual: showing no interest in usual activities or becoming socially withdrawn
- Planning the suicide: buying a gun or hoarding a supply of barbiturates
- Expressing anxiety over an impending action: worrying about a divorce, dropping out of school, or losing a job
- Showing physical signs of a previous suicide attempt: cut or scarred wrists, neck bruises

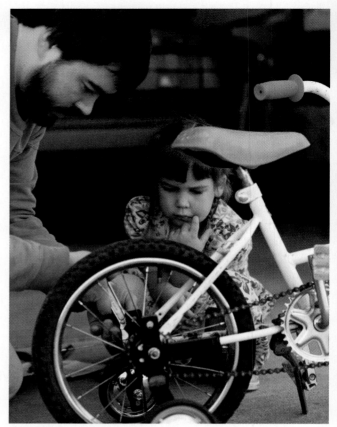

Figure 2-6   **Establishing Good Mental Health.** Parents can help their children feel good about themselves by spending time with them.

signs of distress prior to dying. Table 2-9 lists these and other behavioral warning signs of suicidal persons.

It is always important to take suicidal conversations or gestures seriously and obtain suicide prevention counseling for these individuals immediately. Most major metropolitan areas have mental health centers with trained counselors who provide 24-hour crisis intervention services. The Yellow Pages of local telephone books usually list these facilities under "suicide prevention centers."

Healthy Living Practices

- If you are or someone you know is suicidal, immediately contact a suicide prevention center to obtain specific instructions concerning ways to prevent yourself or another from committing this act.

Across
THE LIFESPAN

Psychological Health

Children and adolescents establish the foundation for a lifetime of good mental health by developing positive self-concepts. Parents can help their children feel good about themselves by spending time with them, listening to their concerns, and helping them learn to adjust to a changing world (Figure 2-6).

School-age children who live in dysfunctional families are vulnerable to developing emotional disorders such as depression and school anxiety. However, childhood depression can occur in any child who experiences a traumatic event, such as the loss of a parent through death or divorce. Children who are anxious about going to school often complain of morning headaches and stomach upsets before leaving for school, and they return home in a distressed state. Parents and teachers need to recognize the symptoms of childhood depression and anxiety. By receiving individual and family counseling, many distressed children and their families can learn positive ways of handling crisis situations.

Attention-deficit hyperactivity disorder (ADHD) is the most common childhood behavioral disorder; about 8% of American school-age children, mostly boys, meet strict criteria for ADHD (Barbaresi et al., 2002). This condition is characterized by an inability to focus and maintain attention on tasks, such as doing homework or following simple instructions. Children with ADHD also display excessive levels of physical activity and restlessness. They cannot sit still; they rush through meals, dash away from their caretakers, and resist efforts to relax or fall asleep. Their attention spans are so short, they are often unable to follow instructions or complete tasks. Additionally, children with this condition demonstrate impulsive behaviors such as interrupting conversations, talking when inappropriate, and acting before thinking. Some children with ADHD are aggressive, argumentative, and defiant. These behaviors often persist through adolescence and adulthood. Not surprisingly, children with ADHD frequently have low self-esteem and conflicts with their family members, peers, and teachers.

In addition to prescribing stimulants and other medications, many physicians recommend behavioral and family counseling to treat the disorder. Recently, some mental health practitioners expressed concerns that ADHD is overdiagnosed and that too many children are being treated with stimulants in the United States. Additionally, questions were raised about the negative effects of stimulants on children's growth and the potential for substance abuse among children treated with these medications. Although some studies indicate stimulants can mildly suppress the growth rates of children with ADHD, more long-term research is needed. On the other hand, children with ADHD who are treated with stimulants have a lower risk of smoking cigarettes and substance abuse than those who did not receive medication for the disorder (Daley, 2004).

During the maturation process, an adolescent undergoes numerous hormonal, physical, social, and other changes necessary to become an independent adult. Many youth make this transition smoothly with a minimum of problems, but for some, the teenage years are filled with emotional turmoil and family conflict. Certain forms of mental illness, including major depression and eating disorders, are likely to develop during this period. As mentioned earlier, suicide is a major cause of death for adolescents.

By the time people reach late adulthood, they may have raised a family, retired from working outside of the home, and maintained a network of friends and family. Elderly people who approach the end of their lives with a sense of satisfaction with their accomplishments are more likely to feel emotionally fulfilled. Many elderly people, however, suffer from sleep disturbances and depression after the death of a spouse and friends, family separation or disintegration, financial instability, or a disabling physical illness. Americans over 75 years of age are more likely to commit suicide than younger persons (Arias et al., 2003). It is important for elderly persons and their families to recognize the symptoms of depression and obtain professional help. Chapter 15 discusses the health concerns of elderly individuals in detail.

CHAPTER REVIEW

Summary

A person's psychological health affects and is affected by other wellness components such as one's physical and social health. Psychological health is dynamic, becoming healthier or unhealthier as one responds to a constantly changing environment. Psychologically healthy people accept themselves, are assertive, have realistic and optimistic outlooks on life, function independently, form satisfying interpersonal relationships, cope with change, and find effective solutions to their problems.

Understanding mental health involves the study of physiology and psychology. Biochemical changes in the brain elicit myriad human responses, including thoughts, emotions, and behaviors. Conditions that alter normal brain chemistry can disrupt the mind, producing negative moods or abnormal behaviors.

Personality is a set of distinct thoughts and behaviors, including emotional responses that characterize the way one responds to situations. Biological, cultural, social, and psychological forces interact to mold one's personality.

Over the past 100 years, numerous psychologists, including Freud, Erikson, and Maslow, provided valuable insights into human behavior, laying the foundation for our present understanding of personality development. Freud thought unconscious drives control human behavior. Erikson identified eight stages of the life span in which different social forces influence personality. Maslow believed that the freedom to achieve personal fulfillment is a psychological need that motivates human behavior.

Psychological adjustment and growth occur when one adapts effectively to the demands of life by altering one's thoughts, attitudes, and responses. Self-esteem, a feeling of self-worth, is a key component of personality. Positive self-esteem is a characteristic of psychologically healthy people.

Intensity and duration are the key features that distinguish a normal emotional response from an abnormal one. Mentally ill individuals experience abnormal feelings, thoughts, and behaviors that persist, interfere with daily life, and hinder psychological adjustment and growth.

There are numerous psychological disorders; each may have multiple causes. Alterations in the normal chemical and physical environment of the brain often produce mental illness. These alterations may be the result of genetic defects, injuries, tumors, infections, or exposure to certain drugs or pollutants. Additionally, social interactions, including those with one's family, contribute to the quality of an individual's psychological health.

In many cases, medications and/or behavioral therapies are effective treatments for mental health problems. People can learn to cope with various problems by seeking the help of mental health therapists or by joining self-help groups.

It is common for individuals to experience phobias, anxiety, panic attacks, or mood disorders at some time in their lives. In many cases, these disorders are mild and do not interfere with the affected person's ability to function in society. In other instances, psychological illnesses such as schizophrenia, generalized anxiety, or major depression impair functioning to the extent that affected individuals require professional treatment.

Eating disorders are often symptoms of underlying mental illnesses, particularly depression and obsessive-compulsive disorders. Self-imposed starvation and denial of thinness characterize anorexia nervosa. Bulimic individuals and some people with anorexia nervosa engage in food bingeing and purging practices. Binge eaters overeat but rarely follow up with purging.

When it is progressive, dementia is a devastating mental illness. Impaired thought processes, particularly memory loss, disorientation, and confusion, characterize dementia. Schizophrenia is a serious form of mental illness that usually begins during adolescence or young adulthood.

Suicide is not a mental illness, but in many instances, suicide is the behavioral consequence of a major depressive illness that included substance abuse. Individuals who are contemplating suicide often discuss their feelings and intentions with others. Thus, people should take someone's suicidal conversations or gestures seriously and assist the individual by obtaining immediate intervention.

Parents can help their children feel good about themselves by spending time with them, listening to their concerns, and helping them learn to adjust to a changing world. Some children develop psychological disturbances, particularly anxiety and depression. Attention-deficit hyperactivity disorder is the most common childhood behavioral disorder. Most adolescents experience relatively few emotional problems as they mature into adults, but for some, the teenage years are filled with turmoil. Certain forms of mental illness, including major depression and eating disorders, are likely to develop during this period of life. Elderly persons who approach the end of their lives with a sense of satisfaction with their accomplishments are likely to feel emotionally fulfilled.

Applying What You Have Learned

1. Develop at least three recommendations for parents to follow that would build their children's self-esteem. Application

2. Analyze your present situation to determine your position on Maslow's human needs hierarchy. Explain how you determined your position. Analysis

3. Many persons have negative feelings about people with mental illness. Explain how the media contribute to these feelings. Synthesis

4. Consider your current state of psychological health. Rate your psychological health as excellent, good, fair, or poor. Explain how you determined this rating. Evaluation

Key

Application	using information in a new situation.
Analysis	breaking down information into component parts.
Synthesis	putting together information from different sources.
Evaluation	making informed decisions.

Reflecting on Your Health

1. As described in this chapter, self-esteem develops during childhood. When you were a child, how did your interaction with family members influence the development of your self-esteem?

2. Using Table 2-1, "The Characteristics of Psychologically Healthy People," identify the characteristics that describe you best. Why did you choose those traits?

3. What have you done to improve your psychological health by improving your physical, social, intellectual, spiritual, and environmental health? How did your actions help?

4. As mentioned in this chapter, people often have negative feelings toward psychologically disturbed persons. How would you feel if you, a close friend, or a family member were diagnosed with a psychological disorder? If you, a close friend, or a family member has a serious psychological disorder, how does it affect you?

5. People over 65 years of age have a high risk of depression. What could you do or have you done to enhance the psychological health of an elderly person whom you know, such as a grandparent?

References

American Psychiatric Association Work Group on Eating Disorders. (2000). Practice guideline for the treatment of patients with eating disorders (revision). *American Journal of Psychiatry, 157*(1 Suppl):1–39.

Anderson, R. N., & Smith, B. L. (2003). Deaths: Leading causes for 2001. *National Vital Statistics Reports, 52*(9):1–85.

Arias, E., Anderson, R. N., Kung, H. C., Murphy, S. L., & Kochanek, K. D. (2003). Deaths: Final data for 2001. *National Vital Statistics Reports, 52*(3):1–115.

Barbaresi, W. J., Katusic, S. K., Colligan, R. C., Pankratz, V. S., et al. (2002). How common is attention-deficit/hyperactivity disorder? *Archives of Pediatric and Adolescent Medicine, 156*(3):217–224.

Becker, A. E., Grinspoon, S. K., Klibanski, A., & Herzog, D. B. (1999). Eating disorders. *New England Journal of Medicine, 340*(14):1092–1098.

Binder, R. L. (1999). Are the mentally ill dangerous? *Journal of the American Academy of Psychiatric Law, 27*(3):189–201.

Birckmayer, J., & Hemenway, D. (1999). Minimum-age drinking laws and youth suicide, 1970–1990. *American Journal of Public Health, 89*(9):1365–1368.

Bostwick, J. M., & Pankratz, V. S. (2000). Affective disorders and suicide risk: A reexamination. *American Journal of Psychiatry, 157*(12): 1925–1935.

Centers for Disease Control and Prevention. (1996). *Physical activity and health: A report of the Surgeon General.* Atlanta, GA: Author.

Cheng, A. T. A., Chen, T. H. H., Chen, C. C., & Jenkins, R. (2000). Psychosocial and psychiatric risk factors for suicide. *British Journal of Psychiatry, 177*:360–365.

Choi, P. Y. L., Pope, H. G. Jr., & Olivardia, R. (2002). Muscle dysmorphia: A new syndrome in weightlifters. *British Journal of Sports Medicine, 36*(5):375–377.

Daley, K. C. (2004). Update on attention-deficit/hyperactivity disorder. *Current Opinion in Pediatrics, 16*(2):217–226.

Davidson, J. R. T. (2001). Recognition and treatment of posttraumatic stress disorder. *Journal of the American Medical Association, 286*(5):584–587.

Demyttenaere, K., Bruffaerts, R., Posada-Villa, J., Gasquet, I., et al. (2004). Prevalence, severity, and unmet need for treatment of mental disorders in the World Health Organization world mental health surveys. *Journal of the American Medical Association, 291*(21):2581–2590.

de Zwaan, M. (2001). Binge eating disorder and obesity. *International Journal of Obesity and Related Metabolic Disorders, 25*(Suppl 1):S51–S55.

Dunn, A. L., Trivedi, M. H., & O'Neal, H. A. (2001). Physical activity dose-response effects on outcomes of depression and anxiety. *Medicine & Science in Sports & Exercise, 33*(6 Suppl):S587–S597.

Erikson, E. H. (1982). *The life cycle completed.* New York: Morton. (Original work published 1964)

Ernst, E. (2002). The risk-benefit profile of commonly used herbal therapies: ginko, St. John's wort, ginseng, echinacea, saw palmetto, and kava. *Annals of Internal Medicine, 136*:42–53.

Fugh-Berman, A., & Cott, J. M. (1999). Dietary supplements and natural products as psychotherapeutic agents. *Psychosomatic Medicine, 61*:712–728.

Gelenberg, A. (1999). Depression is still underrecognized and untreated. *Archives of Internal Medicine, 159*:1657.

Glass, R. M. (1999). Treating depression as a recurrent or chronic disease. *Journal of the American Medical Association, 281*(1):83–84.

Hollander, E., Simeon, D., & Gorman, J. M. (1999). Anxiety disorders. In R. E. Hales, S. C. Yudofsky, & J. A. Talbott (Eds.), *Textbook of psychiatry* (3rd ed., pp. 567–633). Washington, DC: American Psychiatric Press.

Kazis, K., & Iglesias, E. (2003). The female athlete triad. *Adolescent Medicine, 14*(1):87–95.

Keel, P. K., Mitchell, J. E., Miller, K. B., Davis, T. L., & Crow, S. J. (1999). Long-term outcome of bulimia nervosa. *Archives of General Psychiatry, 56*:63–69.

Kessler, R. C., Berglund, P., Demler, O., Jin, R., et al. (2003). The epidemiology of major depressive disorder: Results from the National Comorbidity Survey Replication (NCS-R). *Journal of the American Medical Association, 289*(23):3095–3105.

Kessler, R. C., McGonagle, K. A., Zhao, S., Nelson, C. B., Hughes, M., Eshleman, S., Wittchen, H. U., & Kendler, K. S. (1994). Lifetime and 12-month prevalence of *DSM-III-R* psychiatric disorders in the United States: Results from the National Comorbidity Survey. *Archives of General Psychiatry, 51*:8–19.

Kritz-Silverstein, D., Barrett-Connor, E., & Corbeau, C. (2001). Cross-sectional and prospective study of exercise and depressed mood in the elderly: The Rancho Bernardo study. *American Journal of Epidemiology, 153*(6):596–603.

LaBrie, R. A., Shaffer, H. J., LaPlante, D. A., & Wechsler, H. (2003). Correlates of college student gambling in the United States. *Journal of American College Health, 52*(2):53–62.

Lamberg, L. (2001). Psychiatrists explore legacy of traumatic stress early in life. *Journal of the American Medical Association, 286*(5):523–526.

Lamberg, L. (2003). Advances in eating disorders offer food for thought. *Journal of the American Medical Association, 290*(11):1437–1442.

Maslow, A. H. (1968). *Toward a psychology of being* (2nd ed.). New York: Van Nostrand Reinhold.

National Institute of Mental Health. (2001). Eating disorders: Facts about eating disorders and the search for solutions. Retrieved June 20, 2004, from http://www.ni,h.nih.gov/publicat/eatingdisorders.cfm

Neugebauer, R. (1999). Mind matters: The importance of mental disorders in public health's 21st century mission. *American Journal of Public Health, 89*(9):1309–1311.

Olfson, M., Marcus, S. C., Druss, B., Elinson, L., Tanielian, T., & Pincus, H. A. (2002). National trends in the outpatient treatment of depression. *Journal of the American Medical Association, 287*(2):203–209.

Problem gambling. (2004). *Harvard Mental Health Letter, 20*(9):1–4.

Rakel, E. (1999). Depression. *Primary Care, 26*(2):211–224.

Russell, C. J., & Keel, P. K. (2002). Homosexuality as a specific risk factor for eating disorders in men. *International Journal of Eating Disorders, 31*:300–306.

Sawa, A., & Snyder, S. H. (2002). Schizophrenia: Diverse approaches to a complex disease. *Science, 296*(5568):692–695.

Steinhausen, H. C. (2002). The outcome of anorexia nervosa in the 20th century. *American Journal of Psychiatry, 159*(8):1284–1293.

Terman, J. S., Terman, M., Lo, E. S., & Cooper, T. B. (2001). Circadian time of morning light administration and therapeutic response in winter depression. *Archives of General Psychiatry, 58*(1):69–75.

U.S. Department of Health and Human Services. (1999). *Mental health: A report of the surgeon general*. Retrieved May 14, 2002, from http://www.surgeongeneral.gov/library/mentalhealth/chapter1/sec4.html#.

U.S. Department of Health and Human Services, National Center for Health Statistics, Public Health Service. (2001). *Healthy people 2000: Final review*. Washington, DC: Government Printing Office.

Vastag, B. (2002). Decade of work shows depression is physical. *Journal of the American Medical Association, 287*(14):1787–1788.

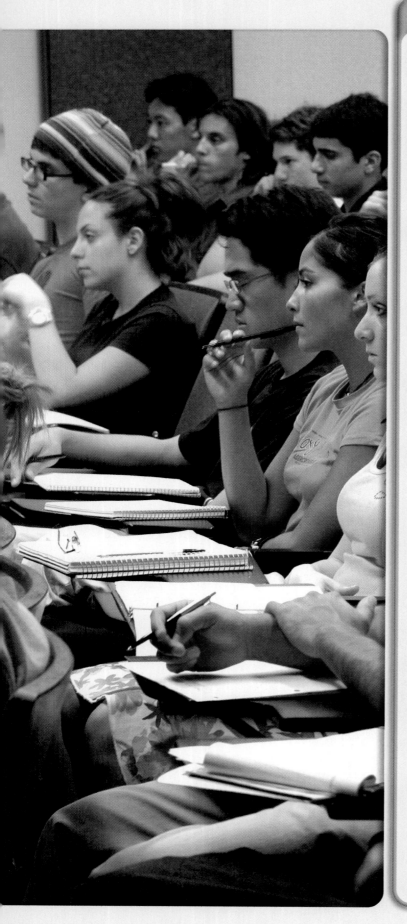

What You'll Learn

http://healthyliving.jbpub.com

The Web site for this book offers many useful tools and is a great source for supplementary health information for both students and instructors. Visit the site at http://healthyliving.jbpub.com for information on these topics:

What Is Stress?
The Impact of Stress on Health
Stress Management Skills

Chapter Overview

The different meanings of *stress*
The ways your body responds to stress
How stressful life events can affect your health
Strategies for coping with stress
Skills that can help you manage stress

Diversity in Health
Stress and Asian Americans

Consumer Health
Herbal Remedies for Stress Symptoms

Managing Your Health
A Technique for Progressive Muscular Relaxation

Across
THE LIFESPAN

Stress

Student Workbook

Self-Assessment: How Much Stress Have You Had Lately?
Changing Health Habits: Taking Steps to Reduce Your Stress

Do You Know?

· *An easy way to manage your time more effectively?*
· *If having a pet can reduce stress?*
· *How to relax within just a few minutes?*

Stress and Its Management

*I*f you ask students to identify what makes college life stressful, you will receive a long list of situations, including taking exams, preparing term papers and lab reports, applying for loans, and juggling hours to fit part-time jobs into their class schedules. College students probably cannot imagine any other period in their lives that will place as many demands on their emotional well-being as well as their time, energy, and finances.

How would you respond to the question, "What was the most stressful situation that you've experienced in the past year?" Three college students enrolled in a health course wrote the following answers to this question.

The most stressful situation I've encountered in the past twelve months must be the discovery that my wife was pregnant and our financial security was at risk because the only source of income for us is her wages. I'm wondering if I will be able to continue pursuing my degree after the baby is born—this adds to my stress day by day.

I went away to a university last year and was the victim of a rape. The whole ordeal of talking to the police, confronting the man who did it, and telling my boyfriend was horrible, but the most stressful part was having to tell my parents.

The most stressful situation was the death of both of my grandparents within six months of each other. I watched them suffer as they passed away. It was very difficult. Also, my choice of a major was a mistake; I've had to change it.

Each of these students had to cope with a different stressful situation. You may have had to cope with similar distressing events. Although going to college places considerable demands on your time and mind, you can expect stressful situations to arise during every phase of your life.

What is stress? What effects can it have on your health and well-being? Can stress be good for you? What factors make a situation stressful? Is it possible to reduce the negative effects that stress can have on your health? This chapter examines the nature of stress, how it can affect you, and how you can manage your stress.

> "*Going to college places considerable demands on your time and mind...*"

What Is Stress?

Stress can have different meanings. *Stress* can refer to the situations that threaten or place demands on your mind and body. Stressful situations can be real, such as being confronted by an angry dog, or imaginary, such as worrying over your future employment possibilities. *Stress* can also describe your responses to a threatening situation; you feel stress. Imagine that a vicious dog attacks you. How would you feel?

Many experts define **stress** as a complex series of psychological and physical reactions that occur as a person responds to a demanding or threatening situation. Each person views and appraises the situation to determine whether it will have positive, negative, or neutral consequences. Additionally, an individual determines his or her ability to manage the situation according to his or her previous experiences and personality characteristics. Thus, it is possible that several individuals form different appraisals of the same event and that each person can, as a result, have a different response.

Stressors

Stressors are situations that create stress by placing physical or psychological demands on an individual. *Physiological* (physical) *stressors* include engaging in exercise; experiencing illness, pain, or injury; and being exposed to dangerous pollutants or extreme temperature changes. *Psychological stressors* include managing extreme emotions, handling difficult social situations, and dealing with troublesome thoughts and relationships. Psychologically demanding situations can add just enough stress to make life more challenging and interesting, but enduring too much stress, physical or psychological, can make life miserable. This chapter focuses on the effects that psychological stressors can have on health and well-being.

The nature of a stressor has a major role in determining its impact on health. When people think of stress, they usually think of **distress**, that is, events that are difficult to control and that have unwanted or negative outcomes. Distressing experiences include having problems with one's education, job, family, and relationships. Other situations create *positive* stress, or **eustress**. Becoming a new parent, competing in an athletic event, and accepting a desired job are examples of events that can have positive outcomes by making

stress
a complex series of psychological and physical reactions that occur as one responds to a situation.

stressors events that produce physical or psychological demands on an individual.

distress events or conditions that produce unwanted or negative outcomes.

eustress (YOU-stress) events or conditions that create positive effects, such as making one feel happy, challenged, or successful.

people feel happy, challenged, or successful. Experiencing stressors with positive physical or psychological consequences may reduce the unhealthy effects of negative stressors.

Some stress experts point out that eustress still has negative effects on the body and mind, because any event that creates stress requires specific physical and psychological adjustments. These changes can damage the body and disturb the mind. Burnout is a common result of too much stress. In this chapter, the terms *stress* and *distress* are used interchangeably when referring to negative psychological stressors.

Stress Responses

Physical Responses

The environment constantly exposes organisms to stressful situations; to survive, they must deal physically with these stressors. In emergencies a person's nervous system instantly activates the adrenal glands to release certain hormones: cortisol, epinephrine (adrenaline), and norepinephrine (noradrenaline). **Hormones** are chemical messengers that convey information from a gland to other cells in the body. The glands of the **endocrine system** produce several different hormones and secrete them directly into the bloodstream (Figure 3-1). Some endocrine hormones regulate

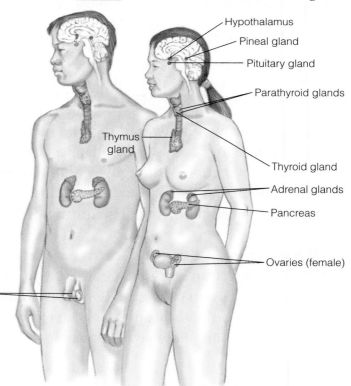

Hypothalamus
Pineal gland
Pituitary gland
Parathyroid glands
Thyroid gland
Adrenal glands
Pancreas
Ovaries (female)
Thymus gland
Testes (male)

Figure 3-1 **The Endocrine System.** The glands of the endocrine system produce chemical messengers called hormones, which enter the bloodstream via small ducts.

Table 3-1 Physical Adaptations to Stress

Physical Change	Effect
Pupils enlarge	Improves vision
Energy nutrients released from storage	Supplies fuels for muscular activity
Heart rate increases	Pumps more blood and faster
Blood pressure increases	Provides more pressure to circulate blood
Blood clots more easily	Prevents bleeding
Skeletal muscles become tense and can work longer	Allows for fighting or escaping threats
Sweating increases	Removes extra heat created by muscular activity
Saliva flow decreases	Avoids wasting valuable body fluids
Respiratory tract (the smaller airways) dilates	Allows more air to move into and out of lungs, supplying more oxygen for energy and removing more carbon dioxide waste
Gastrointestinal tract movements decrease	Shifts blood to skeletal muscles for their more critical needs
Endorphin levels increase	Reduces sensations of pain

body processes, growth, and development. Cortisol, epinephrine, and norepinephrine are often called the "stress hormones" because they prepare the body to respond when danger threatens.

The stress hormones increase heart rate, central nervous system activity, and blood flow to the heart and skeletal muscles, the muscles that move the body. At the same time, the blood flow to the skin, kidneys, and intestinal organs decreases. Under the influence of stress hormones, certain cells release a supply of fuels (fats and blood sugar) into the bloodstream, which transports these fuels to the active muscle or nerve cells. The nervous system produces and releases chemical messengers called

endorphins. Endorphins interfere with the brain's ability to sense pain. Being less able to feel pain may be a valuable adaptation, especially if an injured person has to react quickly in a dangerous situation. These and other adaptations enable the person's body to confront or leave a dangerous situation (the *fight-or-flight* response). Table 3-1 lists the major physical adaptations to stress and their possible survival value.

Selye's General Adaptation Syndrome

The classic research of Hans Selye (1976) paved the way for our understanding of the relationship between the mind and body. Selye first used the term *stress* to describe the responses that allow a person to adapt physically or psychologically to any demand. As a result of his classic observations, Selye developed a three-stage description of the physical responses to stressors, the **general adaptation syndrome (GAS)**. Selye identified the three GAS stages as alarm, resistance, and exhaustion and described the physical status of the body in each stage (Figure 3-2).

hormones chemical messengers that convey information from a gland to other cells in the body.

endocrine system a group of glands that produce hormones.

general adaptation syndrome (GAS) the three-stage manner in which the human body responds to stress: alarm, resistance, and exhaustion.

(a)

Figure 3-2 **The Three Stages of General Adaptation Syndrome.** (a) In the alarm stage, the adrenal glands release stress hormones, preparing the body to deal physically with the stressful event. (b) In the resistance/recovery stage, the body maintains its protective reactions to the stressor, and as the threatening situation eases, the body recovers its normal physical state. (c) The exhaustion stage occurs if the level of stress persists and the body's defense mechanisms weaken.

(b)

(c)

When you think of or see a stressor, your brain sends an alarm through your nerves to your adrenal glands. Almost immediately, the adrenal glands release their stress hormones, preparing your body to deal with the stressful event. This activity is called the *alarm* stage. In the alarm stage, your entire body undergoes the dramatic physical changes listed in Table 3-1. Consider, for example, how quickly you respond to an unexpected loud noise.

If you manage to survive the initial encounter but the stressor persists, your body enters the *resistance phase* of the response. During this stage, your body maintains its protective physical reactions to the stressor. As the threatening situation eases, recovery of your body's normal physical state occurs. Generally, by resting and avoiding additional exposure to stressors, your body can repair any damage that has occurred. However, if the stressful situation persists, your body will not be able to maintain its resistance, and it will enter the *exhaustion* stage. In this stage, your physical stress

defenses are weakened, and you become more susceptible to infections. Prolonged exposure to stress can even lead to death if the body depletes its response mechanisms. The Diversity in Health essay "Stress and Asian Americans" discusses the effects of severe stress on the physical and psychological health of Asian immigrants in the United States.

The stress response evolved to enable humans to react immediately to physical threats to their well-being. Indeed, when people are in life-threatening situations, these dramatic physical changes may be essential for their survival. The same dramatic adaptations, however, take place when people deal with everyday hassles and worries. Although these situations usually do not represent direct or serious threats to people's physical well-being, they elicit the release of stress hormones into the bloodstream. People with higher than normal levels of the stress hormones and energy-supplying compounds in their blood are likely to develop high blood pressure and other diseases of the heart and blood

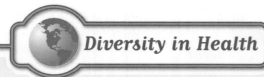

Diversity in Health

Stress and Asian Americans

Before leaving their homelands, many immigrants experience the extreme stresses of civil war, religious persecution, political uncertainty, starvation, and poverty. As immigrants adjust to life in a foreign country, they must cope with the loss of friends and family support, learning an unfamiliar language, and being exposed to a very different culture. Life in the United States is especially challenging for new Asian immigrants because they often experience discrimination, unemployment, racial stereotyping, language barriers, and social isolation.

Asian Americans are a diverse minority group that includes people from Japan, China, Korea, and Vietnam. About 4% of the U.S. population has Asian ancestry; the number of Asian Americans is expected to nearly double by 2020. More than half of the Asian American population are not naturalized citizens (U.S. Census Bureau, 2001). The majority of recent Asian American immigrants are from China, the Philippines, India, Korea, and Vietnam.

Asian Americans who espouse traditional beliefs think that fate determines much of what occurs in their lives, and they typically deny or hide feelings of sadness, disappointment, and anxiety. As a result, they avoid expressing negative feelings. Moreover, recent Asian immigrants tend to follow traditional gender-specific roles; men are accustomed to having a dominant role over women, especially in making decisions, and they expect their wives to main-

tain households and take care of children. Although wives may work outside the home, their incomes often are not crucial for supporting their families. In the United States, most people accept more equitable roles at work and home for men and women. Therefore, many Asian American women perceive their status in society as very low, and they experience much psychological stress as a result (Ibrahim & Ohnishi, 2001). Instead of seeking treatment for anxiety or depression, distressed Asian American women often visit conventional medical practitioners for treatment of various physical symptoms such as appetite loss, headaches, and fatigue (Ro, 2002). The effects of unrecognized and untreated stress can be devastating. Compared to women of other ethnic/racial minorities, Asian American women between 20 and 24 years of age have a higher risk of suicide (Anderson, 2001).

After leaving their homelands, people usually face a variety of unfamiliar situations and new demands. The cultural "shock" that occurs may create numerous psychological conflicts for the immigrants. Regardless of one's ethnic/racial background, the unwillingness to reveal conflicting feelings can produce stress. The serious effects of stress on the health and well-being of Asian American immigrants underscore the need for conventional medical practitioners to be culturally sensitive and recognize symptoms of emotional distress in members of this minority group.

$\mathcal{A}$nalyzing
Health-Related Information

The following article appeared in *FDA Consumer.* Read the article and explain why you think it is a reliable or an unreliable source of information. Use the model for analyzing health information to guide your thinking; the main points of the model are noted below. A full explanation of the model can be found on pages 13–15.

1. Which statements are verifiable facts, and which are unverified statements or value claims?
2. What are the credentials of the person writing the article? If this information is available, does the author's background and education qualify him or her as an expert in the topic area?
3. What might be the motives and biases of the person writing the article? State reasons for your answer.
4. Which information is relevant to the issue or main point of the article; which information is irrelevant?
5. Is the source reliable? Does it have a reputation for publishing misinformation?
6. Does the article attack the credibility of conventional scientists or medical authorities?

Based on your analysis, do you think that this article is a reliable source of health-related information? Summarize your reasons for coming to this conclusion.

Sleepless Society

Tamar Nordenberg, staff writer for FDA Consumer

Millions of Americans undersleep by choice, burning the candle at both ends because of hectic work and family schedules. Recent surveys show that Americans sleep 7 hours each night on average, down from 9 hours in 1910 when, without electricity, people generally went to sleep as darkness fell.

"People don't respect sleep enough," says Daniel O'Hearn, a sleep disorders specialist at Johns Hopkins University. "They feel they can do more—have more time for work and family—by allowing themselves less time for sleep. But they do sleep; they sleep at work, or driving to work."

Nodding off at work isn't just unproductive; in the worst cases, it causes serious industrial accidents. The 1989 Exxon Valdez Alaskan oil spill, for example, was reportedly due at least in part to the severe fatigue of the tanker's sleep-deprived third mate.

Also, like drunk driving, drowsy driving can kill. The National Highway Traffic Safety Administration estimates that more than 200,000 crashes each year involve drivers falling asleep at the wheel, and that thousands of Americans die in such accidents annually.

"Besides being an unpleasant sensation, when we're tired, we're less alert and less able to respond," says FDA drug reviewer Bob Rappaport, M.D.

Lack of sleep can cause memory and mood problems, too, Rappaport says, and may affect immune function, which could lead to an increased incidence of infection and other illnesses. In studies performed on rats, prolonged sleep deprivation resulted in death.

Beyond the observable consequences of sleep deprivation, why humans—or any animal, for that matter—need sleep remains largely a mystery. "What happens in the brain while we're sleeping is what we're trying to untangle," says James Kiley, director of the National Center for Sleep Disorders Research of the National Institutes of Health. "We're just beginning to understand why a third of our life is spent sleeping. What we do know is that sleep is an important biological need, like food and drink, and that the brain is very active while we're sleeping."

The leading sleep theories focus on "rest and resuscitation for the body and psyche," says Rappaport. During sleep, the brain may recharge its energy stores and shift the day's information that has been stored in temporary memory to regions of the brain associated with long-term memory.

So just how much nightly R and R does a person need? That can change throughout one's life based on age and other factors. For most people, though, 7.5 to 8.5 hours of sleep each night fulfills the basic physical need, Rappaport says, adding that this is "very individual" and can range from as few as 4 or 5 hours to as many as 9 or 10.

The Mayo Clinic of Rochester, Minnesota, defines an adequate amount of sleep as whatever produces daytime alertness and a feeling of well-being. People should not need an alarm clock to wake them if they are getting enough sleep.

Source: Nordenberg, T. (1998). Sleepless society. *FDA Consumer*, 32(4):11.

vessels. Genetic and lifestyle factors, however, can benefit health by modifying the way people respond to stress. For example, a group of men with heart disease who participated in a stress management program experienced fewer complications during a 5-year study than men who did not receive stress reduction training (Blumenthal et al., 2002).

Psychological Responses Stressful situations affect the mind as well as the body, but the psychological impacts are not easy to test, observe, or measure. Chapter 2 describes several mental health conditions, including depression and anxiety disorders, that have direct links to stressful life events. Distressed individuals are more likely to report psychological symptoms such as frustration, anxiety, and anger. They may be irritable most of the time, eat too much food, or abuse drugs. "Stressed-out" people often have difficulty focusing their attention, making decisions, and sleeping.

Stress can have positive effects on the mind. Low levels of psychological stress can enhance performance by increasing one's effort and attention to the task. As the degree of stress increases, however, the individual may respond by worrying too much about performance, which creates even more psychological stress. This response can reduce the ability of actors, athletes, and college students to concentrate on and perform tasks. Stage fright affects the best veteran actors, and many superb athletes "choke" under competitive pressure.

Taking tests is stressful for many college students, but students with test anxiety overreact emotionally to the testing situation and have difficulty recalling information and concentrating on test questions. To avoid becoming overwhelmed by task-related anxiety, students can learn to use the stress management skills presented later in this chapter.

■ The Impact of Stress on Health

The Mind–Body Relationship

Certain health problems are associated with psychological stress (Table 3-2). For example, people with chronic conditions such as asthma, rheumatoid arthritis, migraines, and genital herpes report that the signs and symptoms of their illness tend to worsen or recur during stressful periods (Levenson, 2003). Stress slows wound healing, increases susceptibility to infection, and may stimulate the body's immune response when it's not necessary, resulting in inflammation that is associated with heart disease, Alzheimer's disease, and arthritis (Kiecolt-Glaser et al., 2002).

Table 3-2	Common Disorders Linked to Psychological State
Eating disorders	Itchy skin
Tension headaches	Rapid or irregular heart rate
Migraines	Intestinal ulcers
Muscle spasms	Nausea and vomiting
Chest pains	Frequent urination
Excessive menstrual cramps	Irritable bowel syndrome
Acne	Rheumatoid arthritis flare-ups
Recurring herpes simplex	Asthma attacks
PMS	Chronic fatigue syndrome
	Fibromyalgia syndrome

Anxiety and stress also worsen the signs and symptoms of *irritable bowel syndrome (IBS)*. People with IBS have recurrent bouts of intestinal cramps, constipation, diarrhea, and mucus in bowel movements. Medical testing and physical examination, however, fail to find a physical cause for the condition. IBS is a common health problem in the United States; 10% to 17% of adults report suffering from the disorder (Heitkemper et al., 2004).

Irritable bowel syndrome often occurs with *fibromyalgia syndrome (FMS)*, a condition characterized by extreme fatigue, muscle and joint pain, headaches, and sleep disturbances for which no physical cause can be found. In many instances, stress triggers FMS (Shaver, 2004). People suffering from FMS tend to be depressed and anxious; however, these negative psychological states may be the result of the symptoms of the disorder, rather than the cause.

Psychoneuroimmunology, the study of the relationships between the nervous and immune systems, is a new and exciting field of medical research that explores the connection between mind and body. Scientists have discovered links between the nervous and immune systems that explain how some emotional responses affect physical health.

The **immune system**, which includes the red bone marrow, spleen, lymph nodes, white blood cells, and thymus gland, defends the body against disease-causing agents (Figure 3-3). The white blood cells are the key soldiers of the immune system, serving as the body's internal scouts and commandos. These special cells find, identify, and destroy many agents that can endanger one's health.

Recently, scientists discovered that the immune system does not function independently of the other body systems. Using nerves and neurotransmitters, the brain

Thymus

Lymph node

Spleen

minutes to 2 hours after eating, or they feel bloated and nauseated after meals.

In some persons, the protective lining of the stomach may be chronically infected with the bacterium *Helicobacter pylori* (*H. pylori*). This organism is thought to weaken the stomach lining and make the person more susceptible to ulcers. However, not all infected individuals have ulcers. Cigarette smoking, alcohol, and certain medications may also make the stomach lining susceptible to developing an ulcer (Levenstein, 2000).

The avoidable risk factors associated with ulcers are cigarette smoking, chronic alcohol use, and chronic use of anti-inflammatory drugs such as aspirin and ibuprofen. These drugs may damage the stomach lining. Unavoidable risk factors are age and family history. As you age, your risk for ulcers increases; most ulcers are diagnosed in persons over 40 years of age. Infection with *H. pylori* is an additional risk factor, although most people do not know if they are infected.

relays information about the person's emotional state to the places where white blood cells are made and located in the body. These specialized cells produce their own chemical messengers that enable them to communicate information about the state of the body back to the brain and the endocrine system.

Stress alters the normal balance and functioning of the immune system, leading to changes that can increase susceptibility to infections and damage other systems in the body. Immune cells produce *cytokines*, a group of compounds that regulate the immune response and communicate with the nervous system. Medical researchers are particularly interested in studying the cytokines that stimulate inflammation, because stress increases the production of these compounds in the body. Proinflammatory cytokines may be associated with serious health problems, including rheumatoid arthritis, inflammatory bowel disorders, type 2 diabetes, heart and other blood vessel diseases, certain cancers, and osteoporosis (Kiecolt-Glaser et al., 2003; Wong, 2002).

Ulcers You probably know someone who has a stomach or intestinal ulcer—about 10% of the population will have an ulcer at some time in their lives. An **ulcer** is a sore in the lining of the esophagus (the food tube), stomach, or duodenum, which is the first part of the small intestine that leads from the stomach (see Figure 9-1). Ulcers may form in the stomach when its protective lining and overlying mucous layers do not resist the normal amount of certain chemicals, including hydrochloric acid, secreted by the stomach. Ulcers can develop in the esophagus when the acidic contents of the stomach chronically splash back into the food tube. This "splash-back" (*acid reflux*) is often due to a relaxed muscle that serves as the "doorway" to the stomach from the esophagus. Cigarette smoking, alcohol, chocolate, fats, and peppermints relax this muscle. In addition, lying down immediately after eating or overeating promotes acid reflux. People with ulcers experience burning or aching sensations in the middle of their abdomens from 30

psychoneuro-immunology (SIGH-ko-NEW-ro-im-mu-NOL-lo-gee) the study of the relationships between the nervous and immune systems.

immune system the specific defenses of the body that include combatting infectious agents.

ulcer a sore in the lining of the esophagus, stomach, or duodenum.

Many people think that the "typical" individual who develops an ulcer has a hard-driving personality and endures a great deal of stress. Although stress contributes to the occurrence of ulcers, an ulcer-prone personality may not exist. A distressed person, however, may smoke, drink too much alcohol, and not get enough rest; such behaviors can negatively affect the immune system, making ulcers more likely (Levenstein, 2000).

Ulcers can be serious, especially if they bleed. Signs and symptoms of a bleeding ulcer include dark, tarry stools; a bloating sensation; and weakness. If you think you have a bleeding ulcer, seek medical attention immediately.

Headaches Nearly everyone has had a headache at one time or another. People who drink caffeinated beverages regularly may get headaches when they do not consume them, and physical ailments such as sinus infections often cause headaches. The most common type of headache is the *tension-type* headache. People suffering from tension-type headaches report that the pain feels like a tight band has been placed around their forehead. The mechanisms that result in tension-type headaches are unknown, but in many instances, stress triggers tension-type headaches. Additionally, smoking cigarettes and abnormal tension in the muscles of the head, face, and neck are thought to contribute to their development (Millea & Brodie, 2002). The typical tension-type headache is not accompanied by visual problems, stiff neck, nausea, vomiting, or fever.

Migraines are another type of recurring headache. Nearly 30 million Americans suffer from migraines; about 18% of women and 6% of men reported having a migraine during the previous year (Silberstein, 2004). Migraine headaches are thought to result from inflammation of the nerves in the *meninges*, the layers of tissues that surround and protect the brain. Migraine attacks are often preceded or accompanied by *aura*, a nerve-related symptom that usually lasts for less than an hour. In most cases, the aura includes visual disturbances such as flashing lights or zigzag lines, but "pins and needles" sensations, numbness, and speech problems may occur as well. The pain of a migraine is moderate to severe in intensity, usually throbbing, and felt on one side of the head. In addition to being disabled by the headache, migraine sufferers often experience nausea and vomiting. Because their headaches are aggravated by light, sound, and routine physical activity, people with a migraine usually retreat to a darkened, quiet room to rest and recover. The headaches usually persist for 4 to 72 hours.

The first line of defense against migraines is identifying and avoiding their triggers. Some people develop migraines, for example, from insufficient sleep or disrupted sleep patterns. In these cases, maintaining a regular, sufficient sleep schedule is crucial to avoiding attacks. Others have migraines triggered by certain foods. Keeping a food diary to determine which foods bring on headaches and then avoiding those foods are important. In addition to avoiding their triggers, people who suffer from migraine headaches can take various over-the-counter and prescription medications. Certain headache medications can be taken before migraines begin to lessen the chances that they will develop. The Consumer Health feature in this chapter discusses the usefulness of feverfew as a natural means to prevent migraines.

Over-the-counter painkillers are usually effective for relieving tension-type headaches. For some people, simply applying hot packs to the head or neck and relaxing by having a massage are helpful. It is important to note that "rebound headaches" can occur when remedies that contain caffeine are used regularly to

| Table 3-3 | Serious Headache Symptoms |

Consult a physician if a headache

- Is accompanied by confusion, unconsciousness, or convulsions
- Involves pain in the eye or ear
- Is accompanied by fever
- Is accompanied by nausea
- Occurs after a blow to the head
- Is persistent in someone previously free of headaches
- Is recurrent, especially in children
- Interferes with normal life

Source: Farley, D. (1992, September). Headache misery may yield to proper treatment. *FDA Consumer*, p. 31.

treat headaches. Headaches rarely signal life-threatening conditions. Table 3-3 describes circumstances under which you should seek immediate medical attention for a headache. If you suffer from frequent headaches, seek help from your physician.

Healthy Living Practices

- To reduce the risk of ulcers, avoid cigarette smoking, chronic alcohol use, lying down after eating, overeating, and chronic use of anti-inflammatory drugs.
- If you experience a burning or aching sensation in the middle of your abdomen after eating, or feel bloated and nauseated after meals, you may have an ulcer. See your health care provider for diagnosis and treatment.
- To reduce the risk of tension-type headaches, learn to relax. Consult a physician if you have a severe headache.

Stressful Life Events

In 1967 Thomas Holmes and Richard Rahe introduced the Social Readjustment Rating Scale (SRRS), maintaining that people who experience numerous major life events within a short time span are likely to develop illnesses (Holmes & Rahe, 1967). Holmes and Rahe developed this scale by asking nearly 400 people to rate life events according to the average amount of social change the individuals thought would be needed to deal with the situation. Death of a spouse, for example, received the maximum score of 100 points (see Table 3-4). In studies using the SRRS, Rahe found that

Herbal Remedies for Stress Symptoms

Since ancient times, people have treated their stress symptoms with herbs and other plants. Many plants contain chemicals that have medicinal properties. Recently, many Americans have tried kava, valerian, and feverfew to relax or treat their stress-related symptoms. Does kava induce relaxation? Is valerian effective for treating insomnia? Can feverfew prevent migraines? Are these alternative therapies safe?

For hundreds of years, a ceremonial beverage made from the roots of the kava plant has been used by South Pacific Islanders to reduce anxiety, relax muscles, and induce sleep. Conventional medical experts, however, are concerned about the herb's growing popularity among Americans because the long-term safety of kava, including its potential for addiction, is unclear. It is known that kava produces serious, potentially life-threatening side effects when consumed in very large doses (FDA, 2002). Furthermore, the herb can intensify the effects of depressant drugs, including alcohol. Therefore, check with

your physician before consuming products made from this herb.

Ancient Romans were aware of the medicinal value of the heliotrope plant, commonly known as valerian. Roots of the plant are dried, then brewed into a tea that is used to induce sleep. Valerian is available in pills or mixed with alcohol to make a tincture. Valerian may have usefulness as a mild tranquilizer (Fugh-Berman & Cott, 1999). In a few studies, however, the herb had toxic side effects (Wong et al., 1998). You should consult your physician before taking valerian.

Feverfew has been used for centuries to treat headaches, menstrual problems, and fever. Before supplements were available, people would chew the leaves of the plant, but this practice caused sores in the mouth. Feverfew may reduce the risk of migraines. The herb does not seem to be toxic when consumed in recommended amounts, but it may cause allergic responses and even headaches in some people ("Herbal Rx," 1999). As in the case of all herbal treatments, check with your physician before trying feverfew. Be aware that feverfew can upset the stomach, and stop taking it (or any herbal product) if you have adverse reactions.

Table 3-4 Social Readjustment Rating Scale

Rank	Life Event	Value	Rank	Life Event	Value
1	Death of spouse	100	23	Son or daughter leaving home	29
2	Divorce	73	24	Trouble with in-laws	29
3	Marital separation	65	25	Outstanding personal achievement	28
4	Jail term	63	26	Wife begins or stops work	26
5	Death of close family member	63	27	Begin or end school	26
6	Personal injury or illness	53	28	Change in living conditions	25
7	Marriage	50	29	Revision of personal habits	24
8	Fired at work	47	30	Trouble with boss	23
9	Marital reconciliation	45	31	Change in work hours or conditions	20
10	Retirement	45	32	Change in residence	20
11	Change in health of family member	44	33	Change in schools	20
12	Pregnancy	40	34	Change in recreation	19
13	Sexual difficulties	39	35	Change in religious activities	19
14	Gain a new family member	39	36	Change in social activities	18
15	Business readjustment	39	37	Mortgage or loan less than $10,000	17
16	Change in financial state	38	38	Change in sleeping habits	16
17	Death of close friend	37	39	Change in number of family get-togethers	15
18	Change to different line of work	36	40	Change in eating habits	15
19	Change in the number of arguments with spouse	35	41	Vacation	13
20	Mortgage over $10,000	31	42	Christmas	12
21	Foreclosure of mortgage or loan	30	43	Minor violations of the law	11
22	Change in responsibilities at work	29			

Source: Holmes, T. H., & Rahe, R. H. (1967). The social readjustment rating scale. *Journal of Psychosomatic Research, 11*:213–218. Reprinted with permission from Elsevier Science.

subjects who accumulated higher scores, because they had experienced more major life events in a year, were more likely to become ill at some time in the following year.

Although a few items on the original SRRS are outdated, such as "mortgage over $10,000," this scale has been a popular measurement of stress levels. Many stress experts, however, question the scale's ability to predict the onset of illness. Using the SRRS as a model, Marx and his colleagues (1975) developed the College Schedule of Recent Experience to assess the level of stress experienced by college freshmen (see the assessment activity "How Much Stress Have You Had Lately?" in the workbook). First-year college students often have difficulty coping with the unfamiliarity and demands of college life. Not surprisingly, these individuals have a high dropout rate. Concerned with the negative impact of change on first-year students, college administrators often establish academic, social, and counseling programs to ease the stress that new students feel during their first year in school.

Medical experts generally agree with the idea that stressful life events are related to illness. However, observing an association between stressful events and the onset of illnesses does not mean that stress *causes* poor health. Distressed people may follow unhealthy lifestyles. They may not exercise, eat nutritious foods, or get enough sleep. Such behaviors are likely to result in poor health. Psychological, environmental, and biological forces can influence health in complex ways. Scientists need to collect more information before they can understand fully how psychological stress affects the body.

Personality, Disease, and Stress

Although exposure to any stress can increase one's susceptibility to illnesses, the same stressful situation can have a different impact on different individuals. Why do people often respond differently to a stressor? Each person's unique combination of personality traits and background experiences contributes to his or her stress response.

People who see only the negative aspects of a stressor may view a difficult situation as impossible to overcome and be more vulnerable to stress than those who make positive appraisals of the situation. As a result, vulnerable people are more likely to become anxious, angry, and depressed and to make poor decisions. By making poor decisions, people often create more stress for themselves. Additionally, distressed individuals may adopt lifestyles that undermine their health, such as obtaining insufficient sleep, smoking cigarettes, or abusing drugs.

People who are less vulnerable to the negative effects of stress may have personalities that act as buffers. These individuals generally have more positive outlooks on life, and they are more likely to appraise stressors as having positive outcomes (Brissette et al., 2002). Stress-resistant people view the need to change as a challenge, but they recognize that it is a part of life. Although some aspects of the stress-resistant personality may be inherited, children learn various ways of handling stressful situations by observing and copying the behaviors of relatives in challenging situations. These youngsters often continue to employ the same positive behaviors to deal with stressors as they mature.

Are there specific personality types that increase one's risk of heart disease? For years, it has been popularly believed that people who have a type A personality (ambitious, restless, competitive, impatient, and hostile) are more likely to develop heart disease than people who do not have these characteristics. During the 1980s, medical researchers recognized that many people with type A personalities did not develop heart disease. More recently, scientists have associated certain personality traits with the development of heart and blood vessel diseases (cardiovascular disease). People who harbor negative feelings, such as anger, hostility, resentment, suspicion, and mistrust are more likely to develop cardiovascular disease than people who do not (Williams et al., 2000; Williams et al., 2001; Williams et al., 2003).

Chronic stress increases the risk of cardiovascular disease, particularly stroke (Ohlin et al., 2004; Iso et al., 2002). The minds of some people overreact to stressors, and their bodies respond by releasing excessive amounts of stress hormones into the bloodstream. This response may lead to high blood pressure and other physical changes that damage the inside walls of certain blood vessels. Additionally, scientists have found that *platelets,* cell fragments that participate in the blood-clotting process, become stickier when a person is distressed (Camachoe & Dimsdale, 2000). When a blood vessel is damaged and bleeding occurs, platelets clump together and form a plug that may stop blood loss. If a person is injured during a fight for survival, the ease with which the platelets form blood clots can be lifesaving. Many stressful encounters, however, do not include the risk of bleeding, yet the enhanced ability for blood clotting still occurs. In these instances, blood clots can be life-threatening, particularly when a clot forms and blocks the blood flow to the heart muscle or the brain.

The stress response can reduce the effectiveness of the immune system, possibly interfering with its ability to detect and destroy cells that become cancerous. Most scientific studies, however, do not show an association between personality and cancer onset ("Cancer and the Mind," 1998). *After* being diagnosed with cancer, people who have optimistic outlooks and fighting spirits survive longer than those who do not have these characteristics (Faller et al., 1999; Lillberg et al., 2002). Chapter 12 presents more information concerning the development of cardiovascular disease; Chapter 13 discusses the development of cancer.

■ Coping with Stress

Stress is a consequence of living. In today's world, many people cannot fight or escape some of their stressors because the sources of this stress are difficult to pinpoint and control. In other instances, distressed individuals can identify their stressors, but they lack the resources to improve their situations. By learning ways to lessen the overall impact of everyday stressors on their health, many persons can live with their stress. To become more stress-resistant, for example, one can adopt a lifestyle that may reduce the negative effects of stress on the immune system, such as getting enough rest, exercising regularly, or becoming involved with spiritually uplifting activities.

Coping strategies are behavioral responses and thought processes that individuals use to deal actively with sources of stress. Coping strategies can be problem-focused, emotion-focused, or social-support methods of managing stressful situations. Although many coping strategies are useful, some can be harmful to health.

Problem-Focused Strategies

Problem-focused strategies, such as planning, confronting, and problem-solving activities, are behaviors that can directly reduce or eliminate the negative effects of stressors. For example, setting priorities, managing money and time, planning for retirement, or retraining for a career change are strategies that can make people feel more in control of stressful situations. When individuals identify the sources of their stress and think that they have some control over their stressors, they feel less distress and experience fewer health problems. The Changing Health Habits activity in the workbook can help you identify and change a distressing health-related habit.

Managing Your Time One of the most useful stress-reduction skills that you can learn is effective time management. Begin by making a list of all work, school, family, and leisure activities that you perform in a day. Then analyze the list so you can rank the activi-

ties according to level of priority. High-priority activities are those that must be accomplished if you are to meet your goals. Are some activities, such as watching television, chatting online, or talking on the phone, relatively unimportant or "time wasters"? These activities have low priority. In order to allocate and use time well, you may decide to eliminate some activities from your daily schedule.

After analyzing and ranking the activities, determine the amount of time that is needed to carry them out. Allow more time to complete the high-priority tasks than for those of lesser importance. Perform the high-priority tasks first. Putting off an important task (*procrastination*) often results from fear—fear of failure or doing a less-than-perfect job. If the task appears overwhelming, break it into smaller jobs that can be checked off as they are completed. Additionally, consider when is your "best time" of the day; plan to do the most challenging tasks during that period. To be successful in college, for example, you should allow time to attend all classes and prepare for each class, which includes setting some time aside for studying daily.

coping strategies behavioral responses and thought processes that people use to deal with stressors.

To manage time, using a calendar or handheld computer to record appointments or when papers are due or exams are given can be helpful. Many people also make daily lists of "things to do," especially on very busy days. Allow some time for unexpected situations; it is not necessary to lock yourself into a rigid work schedule. Of course, you also need time to relax, eat, exercise, socialize, and sleep. Allow 7 to 8 hours for rest each night. Many college students are sleep deprived, and to stay alert, they often drink caffeinated beverages. Since excess caffeine can interfere with relaxation, you may need to reduce your consumption of these drinks.

If you work or have family responsibilities while you are in school, planning your time carefully is even more crucial. Individuals who balance the time that they spend performing task-centered responsibilities with that spent engaging in pleasurable activities are able to improve their performance and feel a sense of accomplishment.

Journal Writing

In the past, I have seen a psychiatrist. There were times when I didn't want to go, either because I didn't have anything to say or I was in a good mood. But, I learned that no matter how I felt, it made me feel better just to talk about my life. Journaling acts somewhat like a psychiatrist or even a friend. It allows you to "get it off your chest" . . . by writing down your feelings, you receive feedback from yourself.

Coping with daily stressors may be easier if you keep a written record of personal events, thoughts, and feelings. Entering your thoughts in a journal regularly can help you focus on your emotional responses to situations. There are no rules to writing effective therapeutic journals. You do not have to write the passages in prose; some people express their feelings in poetry or as letters that are not to be mailed. Identify distressing problems or situations and then write your thoughts concerning them, including ways to resolve these problems or manage the troublesome situations (see the Reflecting on Your Health activity in this chapter).

Emotion-Focused Strategies

Instead of directly dealing with stressors, many individuals use *emotion-focused* strategies to alter their appraisal of stressful situations. Such alterations can make the events less threatening. Chapter 2 describes various defense mechanisms, such as denial and projection, that serve as coping strategies to defend one's mind against threats. In addition to using defense mechanisms, some distressed individuals overeat or make poor food choices (Oliver et al., 2000). Others abuse alcohol. These unhealthy lifestyles often create even more stress. Emotion-focused strategies can have harmful consequences for individuals and those who must live or work with them. People need to recognize that stress is a part of life; trying to avoid stressors and denying the need to manage stress usually do not reduce its long-term impact on health.

Not all emotion-focused strategies are counterproductive; some are helpful, especially if the strategy aids in mental relaxation or encourages more positive thinking. Humor can serve as a "stress buffer," lessening the impact of both daily hassles and major life events (Kelly, 2002). For example, the homeowners who post a "For Sale" sign in front of their hurricane-damaged house are using humor to relieve some of their distress. Additionally, forming constructive rather than destructive appraisals of stressful situations is a useful emotion-focused strategy. Many successful athletes cope with the stress of competition by appraising each competitive event as an opportunity to challenge themselves and achieve excellence in their sport. By viewing the competition as a challenge rather than a threat, athletes are less likely to experience the emotionally and physically destructive effects of stress on their performance.

Social-Support Strategies

Besides these strategies, many individuals use *social-support strategies* to cope with stressful situations. Social-support strategies include seeking the advice, assistance, or consolation of close friends and relatives; partici-

Figure 3-4 **Pets as Friends.** People who love animals often find comfort in the companionship of their pets.

pating in support groups; and obtaining spiritual help from members of the clergy or religious congregations.

When a major disaster occurs in a community, relief organizations like the Red Cross provide valuable social and financial support services that reduce the impact of the catastrophe on peoples' lives. The knowledge that other people, even strangers, are willing to provide assistance is comforting and reassuring for many distressed individuals. Humans are not the sole providers of social support; lonely people who love animals often find comfort in the companionship of their pets (**Figure 3-4**).

People can use rest and relaxation to redirect their attention away from stressors. By learning how to relax, most people can manage the stress in their lives more effectively. The following section examines ways to cope with stress through relaxation and other activities.

Healthy Living Practices

- Accepting stress as a part of life and finding some positive aspects of stressful situations can reduce the negative or harmful impact of stress on your health.
- Planning for the future, setting priorities, and managing time can help you feel more in control of your life.
- Recording your thoughts and feelings in a journal can help you manage stress.
- Viewing challenging situations as opportunities to experience psychological growth can help you manage your stress.
- Seeking the companionship and social support of others can reduce your stress.

■ Stress Management Skills

Although no one can eliminate stress, you can use a variety of relaxation techniques to reduce its impact on your health. As you relax, your intestinal functioning becomes normal, your breathing and heart rate slow, and your blood pressure declines. Practicing relaxation techniques can restore many body processes to normal, and reverse the potentially damaging responses to stress that may have occurred in your body. The major objective of many relaxation activities is learning how to relax your skeletal muscles while remaining mentally alert.

Deep Breathing

While having panic attacks, people often *hyperventilate* (pant for air) and feel as though they are suffocating. Hyperventilation alters the chemistry of the blood, which increases the heart rate and causes dizziness. By deliberately breathing more slowly and deeply, distressed people can feel more relaxed as their blood chemistry values return to normal. Concentrating on breathing more deeply allows people to shift their attention away from stressors and toward the breathing activity.

Under normal conditions, you breathe an average of 12 to 18 times per minute, but to relax, you need to breathe only 8 to 10 times per minute. The key is to take several deep breaths, using your abdominal muscles, and recognize how deep breathing feels different from your usual breathing pattern. Results from studies show that deep breathing is a quick and simple method to reduce the impact of stress on your health. You can use this breathing technique whenever you begin to feel excited or stressed; so before your next exam, speech, or job interview, relax by simply breathing deeply.

Of all the relaxation techniques we learned this semester, the deep breathing method was the most helpful. I can remember many situations when I've had to use it. While driving home from school, somebody pulled out in front of me and I had to make a ridiculous move to avoid hitting him head on. I didn't turn my car around and try to find him, which I would have done six months ago; I simply took some deep breaths and was thankful that no one, including myself, was injured.

 Managing Your Health

A Technique for Progressive Muscular Relaxation

1. Choose a quiet location and sit in a comfortable position, hands down at your sides, and both feet flat on the floor.
2. Close your eyes and take a few deep breaths; concentrate on becoming as relaxed as possible.
3. With your arms at your sides, make a fist with one of your hands. Hold your clenched fist for about 5 seconds, release your hand from this position, and concentrate on the feeling as the muscular tension "drains" out of your hand.

This basic exercise is repeated as you tense muscles, hold the tensed position for 5 seconds, and then relax the major muscle groups in your body. It is important to focus on recognizing the difference between muscular tension and relaxation sensations. Continue breathing normally as the activity progresses. Begin with your head.

4. Tense your forehead and scalp muscles; feel the tight muscular sensations as you hold this position for 5 seconds; relax these muscles.
5. Tense your facial muscles; hold this position for 5 seconds; relax.
6. Tense the muscles of your neck and jaw; hold this position; relax.
7. Tense your back muscles—but not too tight; hold this position; relax.
8. Tense your right arm; hold; relax.
9. Tense your left arm; hold; relax.
10. Tense your chest muscles; hold; then relax.
11. Tense your stomach muscles; hold; relax.
12. Tense your buttocks; hold; relax.
13. Tense your right leg—but not too tight; hold; relax.
14. Tense your left leg—but not too tight; hold; relax.

Now, imagine traveling back through your body searching for muscles that are not relaxed. As you find tense muscles, relax them. Maintain this position for several minutes, concentrating on your breathing. In this relaxed state, you may practice tranquil imagery and positive self-talk. To regain your normal physical activity, open your eyes, stand, and stretch your muscles.

Progressive Muscular Relaxation

Although some degree of skeletal muscular tension is necessary to maintain a comfortable body posture, excess tension in forehead, scalp, jaw, and neck muscles may contribute to the development of tension-type headaches. Distressed individuals often look tense because of their tightened facial muscles or clenched fists. Even when they are resting, stressed people still report feeling excess muscle tension. Teeth grinding is a common sign of stress that often occurs during sleep and may lead to headaches and pain in the **temporomandibular joint**, the joint where the lower jaw attaches to the skull in front of the ear (Figure 3-5).

The *progressive muscular relaxation* technique teaches people how to recognize the differences between a tensed muscle and a relaxed one. Individuals learn how to voluntarily release muscle tension, becoming aware of the relaxed sensations. When a person's skeletal muscles are completely relaxed, the individual is limp and feels calm. People often use the technique to fall asleep. The Managing Your Health tip entitled "A Technique for Progressive Muscular Relaxation" highlights the steps of this particular relaxation method.

temporo-mandibular joint (TEM-pe-row-man-DIB-you-ler) the place where the lower jaw bone (mandible) attaches to the temporal bone of the skull.

meditation an activity in which one relaxes by mentally focusing on a single word, object, or thought.

Temporomandibular joint

Figure 3-5 **The Temporomandibular Joint.** The temporomandibular joint is the point at which the lower jaw attaches to the skull in front of the ear. Pain in the temporomandibular joint may result from grinding teeth during sleep, a common sign of stress.

Meditation and the Relaxation Response

For some people, praying or meditating reduces stress. **Meditation** is an activity in which one relaxes by mentally focusing on a single word, object, or thought. *Mindfulness meditation* involves a variety of relaxation methods that focus your attention completely and in a nonjudgmental way on what you are doing or experiencing at the moment (Proulx, 2003). Instead of repeating one word or thinking about a single thing or object, you allow your thoughts to flow and experience as much as you can about what you are sensing and thinking. Some people include deep breathing and yoga postures as part of their mindfulness meditation practice. You can engage in mindfulness-based stress reduction while performing ordinary activities such as eating or walking, or by studying an interesting photograph, painting, or object such as a seashell. By practicing this relaxation technique regularly, you can learn to regulate your attention and reduce your negative reactions to stress.

Current medical interest in the value of meditation as a stress management technique began with the transcendental meditation (TM) movement of the 1960s. Herbert Benson (1975) incorporated features of TM into his *relaxation response*, claiming that this method is effective for reducing blood pressure and drug abuse. To practice Benson's method, find a quiet place where you can sit comfortably for 10 to 20 minutes. Close your eyes, breathe normally, and concentrate on repeating a simple word or maintaining a pleasant thought. Progressively relax groups of muscles, starting at your feet and moving up your body to your face. After relaxing your muscles, maintain this pose for at least 10 minutes. When you are ready to regain your usual degree of alertness, open your eyes, stand up, and stretch.

Imagery

Imagery is a mental activity that is often combined with progressive muscular relaxation exercises to enhance physical relaxation. The technique is simple. After relaxing their muscles, individuals think of peaceful, pleasurable scenes, using their imaginations or past experiences to guide them. As these persons "see" the scenes in their minds, they imagine other sensations as well. For example, a person who enjoys outdoor activities might recall floating down a small stream in a canoe. This individual would imagine the peaceful feeling of floating gently on the water as well as the sound of birds singing and water flowing. Imagery, or visualization, can be a creative and enjoyable way to relax as it disengages the mind from thinking about problems. Relaxation tapes or CDs often incorporate nature sounds with slow-tempo music to facilitate imagery.

Athletes, actors, and other performers often use imagery to reduce their stress and enhance their performance. Before an event, for example, a pole vaulter often visualizes the entire sequence of events that takes place when approaching and vaulting over the pole. Although imagery is not a substitute for actually practicing the required skills, the technique is a useful training activity for many competitive athletes.

You do not have to be an athlete or an actor to use imagery to reduce your stress levels. Before facing a stressful situation, like giving a speech or interviewing for a job, imagine the setting. Then imagine the other people's responses and your own behavior. Mentally rehearsing the situation can reduce your anxiety by making you feel better prepared.

Self-Talk

At times, people may have irrational or negative thoughts concerning their abilities to deal effectively with their stressors. Individuals can reduce their stress levels by identifying these self-defeating thoughts and replacing them with positive self-talk statements. Positive self-talk reflects a person's attributes and boosts self-confidence. However, thinking about oneself in a positive manner may be difficult for individuals who have low self-esteem. People with poor self-esteem often have self-degrading or self-critical thoughts, and they are unaccustomed to acknowledging their positive characteristics.

To practice positive self-talk, think of at least three affirmative statements to say about yourself, including your feelings, accomplishments, skills, and characteristics. Self-talk can be personal compliments ("I look great today"), statements of encouragement ("I can handle this problem"), or statements that reflect personal strengths ("I know I can ace that test"). Write these positive statements on a small card and place the card where you will see it daily. Repeat these statements to yourself every day and when you are feeling "stressed out." You can begin your daily relaxation sessions with progressive muscular relaxation followed by imagery, and then complete the stress management activity by repeating your positive self-statements.

Most relaxation methods are relatively easy to learn, but to be effective, the individual needs a high degree of motivation, self-control, and willingness to practice the skills. You can learn each technique and determine which one is the most effective. Regardless of the relaxation technique chosen, you will need to reserve about 10 to 20 minutes each day to practice the activity. At first, learning to relax may be difficult, but by practicing at least one of these techniques every day, you should be able to master the activity within a couple of weeks.

Physical Exercise

Whether it is ballroom dancing or gardening, physical activity can reduce stress by shifting one's attention away from stressors and toward the enjoyable aspects of the activity. Besides this psychological benefit, physical activity can metabolize the extra energy released during the stress response, lessening the impact of stress on the body. Additionally, engaging in physical activity with others can enhance social and spiritual well-being. Nearly everyone can think of at least one physical activity that they can enjoy on a regular basis.

According to a position statement issued by the International Society of Sport Psychology (1992), regular exercise improves mood and self-image, while reducing anxiety and stress. Scientists have found that moderate physical activity or exercise enhances the functioning of the immune system, and this degree of activity can often reduce symptoms of depression and anxiety. Too much physical activity, however, can cause muscle exhaustion or damage, creating emotional stress. Thus, athletes who engage in endurance activities and extensive physical training may have less effective immune systems. During strenuous physical activity, like running, the nervous system releases *endorphins* that may be responsible for creating the "runner's high," the heightened sense of well-being that long-distance runners often experience. As mentioned earlier in this chapter, endorphins can reduce the activity of certain components of the immune system. Chapter 11 describes how most people can gain far more health benefits than harmful effects from regular, moderate exercise.

Tai Chi and Yoga Tai chi, a form of martial art that originated in China, emphasizes relaxation of the mind while the body is in motion. As people perform the gentle, gliding movements of tai chi, they focus their attention on this physical activity and disregard all other thoughts. In addition to tai chi, the other martial arts can be effective in reducing stress, increasing the body's flexibility, and boosting self-confidence. Tai chi, however, may be preferred by less physically active older adults because the exercises are less strenuous.

Figure 3-6 **Managing Stress with Yoga.** Yoga includes specific physical exercises, breathing techniques, meditation activities, and dietary restrictions to promote a healthier body. After practicing yoga, trained individuals usually report feeling relaxed and refreshed.

Yoga, a philosophy of living that originated in India thousands of years ago, includes specific physical exercises, breathing techniques, meditation activities, and dietary restrictions to promote a healthier body and manage stress (Figure 3-6). As individuals practice the yoga exercises, they slowly move their bodies into positions that stretch their skeletal muscles. After maintaining these positions, trained individuals usually report feeling relaxed and refreshed. Although some of yoga's teachings concerning nutrition and the health benefits of stretching organs are not based on modern medical concepts, these exercises can enhance the body's muscular flexibility and reduce stress.

Interest in tai chi and yoga is increasing in the United States; if you would like to learn the exercises, check with the physical education department on your campus or the local YMCA/YWCA to determine if they offer classes in these activities. Before beginning any new physical activity program, especially the martial arts and yoga, it is advisable to receive approval from a qualified health care practitioner.

Across
THE LIFESPAN

Stress

Distressed adults may recall images of a carefree childhood, but children also experience stress. Common stressors for children include separation from a parent through divorce or death, moving to a new neighborhood and changing schools, and illness of a close family member.

When children are distressed, they often exhibit regressive behaviors, like clinging to and acting more dependent on their parents. In addition to acting immature, distressed youngsters may become depressed and withdrawn; suffer sleep disturbances, headaches, and stomachaches; or experience problems at school. Parents can help their children learn healthy ways to cope with stressful situations by teaching them problem-solving skills and relaxation exercises.

As mentioned in Chapter 2, the adolescent years are stressful because individuals undergo numerous physical and social changes during this time. Distressed youth who do not have effective and healthy coping mechanisms are likely to suffer from depression, abuse drugs, have serious traffic accidents, and experience problems with parents and school authorities. If an adolescent's stress response persists or is severe, professional counseling is necessary.

For many people, the elderly years can be very stressful. Aging individuals often feel bored or useless, especially if they have retired from the responsibilities of a job or raising a family. On the other hand, many older adults are distressed because they must work to supply an income, or they must raise their grandchildren because their own children are unable, unwilling, or unavailable to do so. Older adults frequently experience distress when they must care for spouses with debilitating mental or physical illnesses.

Coping with loneliness and the deaths of friends or close family members is especially difficult for aging individuals as they face the reality of their own mortality. Suffering from disabling illnesses creates additional distress for many elderly people. The inability to cope with stress can have serious results; rates of depression and suicide are high among the isolated elderly. To enhance the well-being of elderly people, communities often have programs that encourage social interaction among aged members of the population. Additionally, elderly residents of most nursing homes can participate in social and physical activities that combat the stress of isolation (Figure 3-7).

Figure 3-7　Social Interaction among the Elderly.　To enhance the well-being of elderly people and combat the stress of isolation, communities often offer programs that encourage social interaction among aged members of the population.

CHAPTER REVIEW

Summary

Stress can refer to a threatening or demanding situation, a person's responses to a situation, or the interactions that take place between a person and a situation. Various situations or conditions, referred to as stressors, create stress. Individuals, however, can appraise the same situation differently. Situations with unwanted or negative outcomes produce distress, those with positive outcomes produce eustress. Stress can make life more challenging and interesting, but too much can make life miserable.

In a combined response, the nervous and endocrine systems prepare the body to confront or leave dangerous situations. Hans Selye proposed the general adaptation syndrome to describe the three stages of the body's adaptive physical responses to stressors. The stress response produces physical changes that include altering the activity and effectiveness of the immune system. As a result, enduring too many stressful life events can increase one's susceptibility to disease.

People often use either problem-focused, emotion-focused, or social-support coping strategies to deal actively with stressful situations. Although these strategies can be effective methods of helping people take control over their stressors, some coping methods can be harmful to health. For example, avoiding and denying stressors are coping mechanisms that usually do not eliminate the sources of stress. Adopting healthy lifestyles can help one manage stress effectively.

Many stress management activities involve learning skills that enable one to relax. Relaxation can reverse many of the normal but damaging physical responses to stress. Relaxation techniques include deep breathing exercises, progressive muscular relaxation, meditation, and mental imagery. Journal writing, effective time management, positive self-talk, and moderate physical activity can also reduce stress.

Common childhood stressors include separation from a parent through divorce or death, moving to a new neighborhood and changing schools, and the illness of a close family member. Older distressed youths are often depressed, abuse drugs, and experience problems with parents and school authorities. Aging people often find that coping with loneliness, disability, and the deaths of friends or close family members is especially stressful.

Applying What You Have Learned

1. Using the techniques described in this chapter, develop a personal stress-reduction program that you can incorporate into your daily schedule. `Application`

2. You have two final exams scheduled for the same day. Describe how you could use a negative coping strategy to reduce your stress. Describe how you could use a positive coping method to deal with the same situation. `Application`

3. Plan a program that uses social support as a coping strategy to help distressed elderly people who live in your community. `Synthesis`

4. Evaluate your present situation. Identify and list the sources of distress in your life. `Evaluation`

Key

`Application` using information in a new situation.

`Synthesis` putting together information from different sources.

`Evaluation` making informed decisions.

Reflecting on Your Health

1. Review the physical adaptations to stress that are listed in Table 3-1. The last time you were faced with a stressful situation, did you experience these changes? How did you feel?

2. Recall that stress can have positive outcomes. Reflect on a stressful experience that made you feel happy, challenged, or successful. Why did the experience make you feel this way?

3. Each person can appraise a situation differently; what is distressing to one can be thrilling to another. Choose a situation that distresses you. Why do you think it affects you in this manner? Do you think other people would find this situation distressing? Why or why not?

4. Chronic stress can have negative effects on health. What was the most stressful situation that you had to endure in the past year? How did this experience affect your health and well-being?

5. How do you usually react when faced with stressful situations? Are your responses positive or negative? How do you think you could reduce the impact of stress on your health?

References

Anderson, R. N. (2001). Deaths: Leading causes for 1999. *National Vital Statistics Report, 49*(11):1–88.

Benson, H. (1975). *The relaxation response*. New York: William Morrow & Company.

Blumenthal, J. A., Babyak, M., Wei, J., O'Connor, C., et al. (2002). Usefulness of psychosocial treatment of mental stress-induced myocardial ischemia in men. *American Journal of Cardiology, 89*(2):164–168.

Brissette, I., Scheier, M. F., & Carver, C. S. (2002). The role of optimism in social network development, coping, and psychological adjustment during a life transition. *Journal of Personality and Social Psychology, 82*(1):102–111.

Cancer and the mind. (1998). *The Harvard Mental Health Letter, 14*(9):1–5.

Camacho, A., & Dimsdale, J. E. (2000). Platelets and psychiatry: Lessons learned from old and new studies. *Psychosomatic Medicine, 62*(3):326–336.

Food and Drug Administration, Center for Food Safety and Applied Nutrition. (2002). Kava-containing dietary supplements may be associated with severe liver injury [Consumer advisory]. Washington, DC: U.S. Food and Drug Administration. http://www.cfsan.fda.gov/~dms/addskava.html.

Faller, H., Bülzebruck, H., Drings, P., & Lang, H. (1999). Coping, distress, and survival among patients with lung cancer. *Archives of General Psychiatry, 56*:756–762.

Fugh-Berman, A., & Cott, J. M. (1999). Dietary supplements and natural products as psychotherapeutic agents. *Psychosomatic Medicine, 61*:712–728.

Heitkemper, M., Jarrett, M., & Bond, E. F. (2004). Irritable bowel syndrome in women: A common health problem. *Nursing Clinics of North America, 39*(1):69–81.

Herbal Rx: The promise and pitfalls. (1999). *Consumer Reports, 64*(4): 44–49.

Holmes, T. H., & Rahe, R. H. (1967). The Social readjustment rating scale. *Journal of Psychosomatic Research, 11*:213–218.

Ibrahim, F. A., & Ohnishi, H. (2001). Posttraumatic stress disorder and the minority experience. In Pope-Davis, D. B., & Coleman, H. L. K. (Eds.), *The intersection of race, class, and gender in multicultural counseling* (pp. 89–126). Thousand Oaks, CA: Sage Publications.

International Society of Sport Psychology. (1992). Physical activity and psychological benefits: A position statement. *The Sport Psychologist, 6*:199–203.

Iso, H., Date, C., Yamamoto, A., & Toylshima, H., et al. (2002). Perceived mental stress and mortality from cardiovascular disease among Japanese men and women. *Circulation, 106*(10):1229–1236.

Kelly, W. E. (2002). An investigation of worry and sense of humor. *The Journal of Psychology, 136*(6):657–666.

Kiecolt-Glaser, J. K., McGuire, L., Robles, T. F., & Glaser, R. (2002). Psychoneuroimmunology and psychosomatic medicine: Back to the future. *Psychosomatic Medicine, 64*(1):15–28.

Kiecolt-Glaser, J. K., Preacher, K. J., MacCallum, R. C., & Atkinson, C., et al. (2003). Chronic stress and age-related increases in the proinflammatory cytokine IL-6. *Proceedings of the National Academy of Sciences, 100*(15):9090–9095.

Levenson, J. L. (2003). Psychological factors affecting medical conditions. In R. E. Hales, S. C. Yudofsky, & J. A. Talbott (Eds.), *Textbook of psychiatry* (3rd ed., pp. 635–661). Washington, DC: American Psychiatric Press.

Levenstein, S. (2000). The very model of a modern etiology: A biopsychosocial view of peptic ulcer. *Psychosomatic Medicine, 62*(2):176–185.

Lillberg, K., Verkasalo, P. K., Kaprio, J., Helenius, H., & Koskenvuo, M. (2002). Personality characteristics and the risk of breast cancer: A prospective cohort study. *International Journal of Cancer, 100*(2):361–366.

Marx, M. B., Garrity, T. F., & Bowers, F. R. (1975). The influence of recent life experiences on the health of college students. *Journal of Psychosomatic Research, 19*:87–98.

Millea, P. J., & Brodie, J. J. (2002). Tension-type headache. *American Family Physician, 66*(5):797–804, 805.

Ohlin, B., Nilsson, P. M., Nilsson, J. A., & Berglund, G. (2004). Chronic psychosocial stress predicts long-term cardiovascular mortality in middle-aged men. *European Heart Journal, 25*(10):867–873.

Oliver, G., Wardle, J., & Gibson, E. L. (2000). Stress and food choice: A laboratory study. *Psychosomatic Medicine, 62*(6):853–865.

Proulx, K. (2003). Integrating mindfulness-based stress reduction. *Holistic Nursing Practice, 17*(4):201–208.

Ro, M. (2002). Moving forward: Addressing the health of Asian American and Pacific Islander women. *American Journal of Public Health, 92*:516–519.

Selye, H. (1976). *The stress of life* (2nd ed.). New York: McGraw-Hill.

Shaver, J. L. (2004). Fibromyalgia syndrome in women. *Nursing Clinics of North America, 39*(1):195–204.

Silberstein, S. D. (2004). Migraine. *Lancet, 363*(9406):381–391.

U.S. Census Bureau. (2001). Table 8. Foreign-born population by sex, citizenship status, year of entry, and race and Hispanic origin: March 2000. Retrieved May 17, 2002, from http://www.census.gov/population/socdemo/race/api/ppl-146/tab08.txt.

Williams, J. E., Nieto, F. J., Sanford, C. P., & Tyroler, H. A. (2001). Effects of temperament on coronary heart disease risk: The atherosclerosis risk in communities study. *American Journal of Epidemiology, 154*(3):230–235.

Williams, J. E., Paton, C. C., Siegler, I. C., Eigenbrodt, M. L., et al. (2000). Anger proneness predicts coronary heart disease risk. *Circulation, 101*(17):2034–2039.

Williams, R. B., Barefoot, J. C., & Schneiderman, N. (2003). Psychosocial risk factors for cardiovascular disease: More than one culprit at work. *Journal of the American Medical Association, 290*(16): 2190–2192.

Wong, A. H. C., Smith, M., & Boon, H. S. (1998). Herbal remedies in psychiatric practice. *Archives of General Psychiatry, 55*:1033–1044.

Wong, C. M. (2002). Post-traumatic stress disorder: Advances in psychoneuroimmunology. *Psychiatric Clinics of North America, 25*(2):369–383.

Violence and Abuse

"**M**ost of the campus security notices seemed to be for women, and I had a high school letter in wrestling, so I wasn't worried. Late one night, I was walking across campus, hardly watching where I was going, when a guy with a gun jumped out of some bushes and demanded my money. I gave him my watch and wallet, but he still hit me in the face with the gun barrel. I needed several stitches to close the wound."

According to the Federal Bureau of Investigation (FBI), one violent crime happened every 22 seconds and one aggravated assault occurred nearly every 35 seconds in the United States during 2002. One forcible rape took place almost every 5.5 minutes. One murder happened nearly every 32 minutes (U.S. Dept. of Justice, 2003).

In 2002 an estimated 896,000 children were abused or neglected in the United States, and an estimated 1,400 children died as a result (U.S. Dept. of Health and Human Services [USDHHS], 2004). Partner-against-partner violence is common in the United States. During their lifetimes, 1 in every 4 American women and 1 in every 14 American men suffer sexual and/or physical abuse at the hands of their intimate partners (Tjaden & Thoennes, 2000). For many Americans, violence is a way of life.

Every society tolerates certain controlled uses of force, for example, spanking a misbehaving child or playing contact sports. In this chapter, **violence** refers to interpersonal uses of force that are not socially sanctioned. Such violence occurs when at least one person intentionally applies or threatens physical force against one or more people. These incidents are usually one-sided—for example, a perpetrator attacking a victim—but they are sometimes mutual, such as in a barroom brawl, a schoolyard scuffle, or a fight between a husband and wife.

No one is exempt from violence; it may be directed against infants, children, adolescents, and the elderly. Certain groups of people, such as African Americans, homosexuals, and Jews, are often targets of violence (*hate crimes*). Recently, Americans became victims of violence as foreign terrorists waged deadly attacks in the United States.

> **. . . one aggravated assault occurred nearly every 35 seconds in the United States during 2002.**

Most physical violence in America could be regarded as nonsexual crimes against persons, primarily assault, robbery, and homicide. **Assault** is the intentional use of force to injure someone physically. **Abuse** occurs when one takes advantage of a relationship to mistreat a person, often by using frequent threats of force. Examples of abuse include spouse abuse, child abuse, elder abuse, and sexual harassment.

At some time in your life, you may have been a victim of violence or have been indirectly involved in violent incidents. As a child, you may have been punched or kicked by a playground bully. As a teenager, you may have been slapped, shoved, or forced to have sex by someone you dated. As an adult, you may have been threatened or assaulted by a person with a weapon, as was the male college student in the chapter opener. Moreover, you are likely to become a victim of violence or abuse in the days to come.

Many Americans feel that their lives are more dangerous than in the past, but rates of violent crimes have declined dramatically since 1994, reaching the lowest level ever in 2002 (U.S. Dept. of Justice, 2004). Nevertheless, males, blacks, and young people experienced higher rates of violent crime than others in 2002 (Rennison & Rand, 2003). This chapter explores the causes of violence and describes its effects on health. Additionally, this chapter provides practical steps you can take to reduce your risk of being a victim.

violence interpersonal uses of force that are not socially sanctioned.

assault the intentional use of force to injure another person physically.

abuse taking advantage of a relationship to mistreat a person.

How Violence Affects Health

Many patients who seek treatment in hospital emergency rooms are victims of violence. Although some victims just need medical attention for minor cuts or bruises, others have more serious injuries such as lost teeth, broken bones, and firearm or knife wounds that may require hospitalization (Figure 4-1). Additionally, victims of rape or attempted rape may need immediate treatment to reduce the risk of sexually transmitted infections (STIs) and unintentional pregnancies.

In some cases, victims of violence suffer serious permanent physical disabilities such as blindness, brain damage, and loss of body movement (*paralysis*). Additionally, the stress of fighting or living in an abusive situation alters the functioning of the immune system, which can lower one's resistance against infectious illnesses. Death is, of course, the most serious consequence of violence. Homicide is the leading cause of death for black American males who are 15 to 34 years

Figure 4-1 **The Aftermath of Violence.** Injuries resulting from violence often require medical treatment.

of age, and the second leading cause of death for Hispanic males in that age group (Anderson & Smith, 2003).

Even if they do not have physical injuries, victims of violence or abuse usually experience some degree of psychological damage that often includes anxiety and depression. Anxious or depressed people have a high risk of abusing drugs, developing eating disorders, and having suicidal thoughts. When people encounter violence outside their homes, it can create serious problems for the victims' family life. Family relationships may become strained, suspended, or even ended as a consequence. Violence that occurs within a family setting is very harmful. Cases of marital separation or divorce often involve violence against a spouse or child. Another possible social effect is the *intergenerational* transmission of violence, in which abused children mature and become abusive parents, perpetuating family violence (Pears & Capaldi, 2001). This particular effect, however, occurs with only some abused children; others have personality factors that buffer them from the long-term effects of child abuse. Overall, the financial costs of violence on physical, psychological, and social health are staggering; the cost in human misery is immeasurable.

What Causes Violent Behavior?

Violence is complex; there is no single cause of violence, nor is violent behavior limited to a particular group of people. Nevertheless, several factors contribute to violence, including poverty, substance abuse, availability of guns, psychological problems, and poor self-esteem. In many instances, however, violence is learned behavior. Each year, more than 3 million American children witness acts of abuse or violence between their parents (Eisenstat & Bancroft, 1999).

As mentioned earlier, children who are exposed to violence in their homes are more likely to be abusive or violent as adults than children who do not witness violence.

Does exposure to violent media, particularly television programs, contribute to violent behavior? The average American child watches 23 to 27 hours of television per week (Willis & Strasburger, 1998). According to a landmark long-term study, 14-year-old boys who viewed at least 3 hours of television daily had twice the risk of getting into a serious fight by the time they reached young adulthood than boys who watched less television (Johnson et al., 2002). The link between television viewing and violence was observed in girls also, but not as much as in boys. Furthermore, the results of this and other studies show that the association between viewing televised violence and behaving aggressively continues into adulthood. How do television shows and other media contribute to violence in America?

The visual media, including violent computer games and movies, offer opportunities for young people to learn violent behavior. Watching violent movies, for example, provides indirect ways to participate in the violence, experience emotional states associated with being violent, and observe the outcomes of violence. Television programs and movies often glamorize violent and abusive people, and the perpetrators may avoid punishment. If violence is portrayed as an effective way of getting what one wants, an impressionable young observer may resort to violence when he or she is in similar situations.

New televisions are equipped with "V-chips" that enable adults to block certain programs from being viewed by children (Muscari, 2002). The television industry provides a rating system to help parents select nonviolent programs for their children. Some children, however, misuse the ratings to find violent programs to watch. Thus, parents should exercise good judgment concerning which programs are appropriate for their children as well as monitor their offspring's viewing habits.

■ Major Types of Violence and Abuse

Sexual Violence

My first sexual experience was very unpleasant. It happened on San Padre Island over Spring Break when I was a freshman. I was 18, and he was 25 years old. He took me to an area where no one could see him or hear me. I was naive and thought I could stop him, but I couldn't. I had wanted to wait until I was married, or at least in love with the person.

Sexual violence involves some type of sexual activity gained through force, threat of force, or coercion. **Rape** is sexual intercourse by force or with a person who is not able to give legal consent, such as a 12-year-old child. Both men and women can be the perpetrators or targets of rape and sexual assault. Nevertheless, females are the targets of most attempted or completed rapes. One of 6 American women and 1 of 33 American men have been victims of an attempted or completed rape at some time in their lives (Tjaden & Thoennes, 1998).

College campuses are not safe havens for women. Results of a recent survey indicate that nearly 3% of female college students reported being the victim of a completed and/or attempted rape during the past academic year (Fisher et al., 2000). Most of the completed rapes occurred in campus residential housing; the remainder of these assaults took place in fraternity houses.

sexual violence gaining sexual activity through force or threat of force.

rape sexual intercourse by force or with a person who is incapable of legal consent.

In most cases, a woman is raped by someone she knows, particularly a current or former husband, current or ex-boyfriend, a date, classmate, or live-in (*cohabiting*) partner. Although men are not as likely to be raped as women, they are usually raped by male strangers and acquaintances (Tjaden & Thoennes, 1998). *Marital rape* generally refers to the use or threat of violence against one's spouse to force sexual activity. *Acquaintance rape* is forced sexual activity that occurs between unmarried adults who know each other. If the couple is involved in a dating relationship, it is called *date rape*. In acquaintance rape, the rapist has a need to demonstrate his dominance over women, but he is sexually motivated as well. He intends to have sex with a woman he has met, not sexually assault her. When she declines his sexual advances, however, he rapes her. In other instances, a man may expect sex as repayment for money spent for dinner or entertainment. He may think it is acceptable to insist on having sex, even if his date says "no" and physically resists. Survey data suggest that many men who rape do not think of themselves as rapists, especially if the victim is someone they know.

The use of alcohol or other drugs may weaken a person's inhibitions and alter his or her usual behavior. While intoxicated, a man may act more sexually aggressive toward his partner, and an intoxicated woman may be less able to prevent forced sex. The deliberate use of *Rohypnol* and other so-called date-rape drugs to sexually assault unsuspecting women is a growing problem in the United States. Rohypnol causes not only loss of consciousness but also loss of memory concerning events that occurred when the drug was taken.

Chapter 7 includes information concerning date-rape drugs.

Reporting Sexual Assault Data from crime surveys suggest that sexual crimes occur more often than previously suspected. Rape victims frequently feel ashamed and embarrassed, and are often reluctant to report their experiences to the authorities. Moreover, they may fear further victimization by the assailant or negative reactions from family, friends, and coworkers. Some victims, however, fail to report the assault because they simply do not want to become involved in the criminal justice system. Many victims of acquaintance rape are often unwilling to report the incidents because they feel partially to blame. For example, a female college student may feel that if she had consumed less alcohol at a party, she would have been able to resist the sexual advances of others.

Sexual assault victims should obtain immediate medical attention for their injuries. Hospital emergency rooms often have staff who are trained to manage rape cases. In addition to receiving treatment for physical injuries, many rape victims need testing for sexually transmitted infections, medication to prevent pregnancy, and counseling to cope with the situation.

If the victim chooses to prosecute the rapist, she should preserve all physical evidence because it might assist the police. For example, she should not wash any part of her body or change clothes. Semen and pubic hair from the attacker can be used to identify this individual. Victims who are unsure if they want to take legal action against their assailant can contact a rape crisis center for free advice from trained counselors. Most major metropolitan areas have rape crisis centers; their phone numbers may be listed under "Rape Hotline" or "Women Self-Help" in phone books. The Managing Your Health feature on page 79 provides some suggestions to lower your risk of becoming a sexual assault victim.

Family Violence

Family (domestic) violence is a pattern of behavior characterized by physical assaults, psychological abuse, or threats that occur between family members, couples in intimate relationships, or unrelated individuals who live together. Such violence includes spouse, child, and elder abuse. Nearly 30% of all violence occurs in family settings, and in most instances, females are the victims of such offenses (U.S. Dept. of Justice, 1998). Child abuse and elder abuse are often classified as forms of family abuse; the Across the Lifespan section of

family violence violence or abuse between family members, people who are involved in intimate relationships, or unrelated individuals who live together.

this chapter provides information concerning these forms of family violence.

Intimate Partner Violence *Intimate partner violence* involves actual or threatened physical or sexual violence, as well as emotional abuse, by a spouse, ex-spouse, lover, former lover, or date. According to a recent survey, nearly 1 in 5 intimate couples experienced at least one episode of partner-against-partner violence during the previous year (Schafer et al., 1998). Results of a survey of men who have sex with men indicated 22% had experienced physical battering from their partners at some time during the previous 5 years (Greenwood et al., 2002). Domestic violence between lesbian couples is quite high; according to various surveys, 17% to 52% of lesbians reported they had been physically abused by their partners (Ristock, 2003).

Violent acts may range from slapping, shoving, and punching to beating and murder. Typically, verbal and emotional abuse accompany the physical violence. *Dating violence,* the threat or use of force against one's partner during courtship, is quite common. About 1 in 5 high school students and 1 in 3 college students have experienced some form of nonsexual violence in a dating relationship (Centers for Disease Control, 2000).

Compared to women, men are far more likely to injure seriously or murder their intimate partners (Figure 4-2). In 2002 nearly a third of female murder

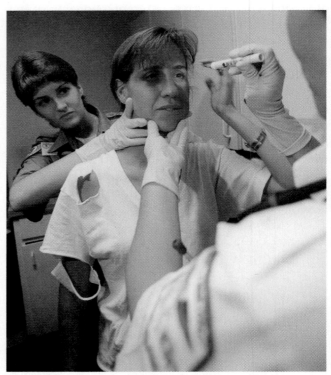

Figure 4-2 **A Case of Domestic Violence.** A woman is far more likely than a man to be seriously injured as the result of domestic violence.

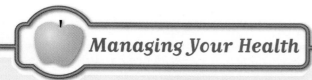

Sexual Assault: How to Prevent Becoming a Victim

To avoid stranger rape:

- Avoid high-risk situations such as being alone in isolated areas or using drugs that affect your physical responses to a threat or your decision-making abilities.
- Walk with your head up, looking alert and confident.
- Consider carrying pepper spray. (See the Consumer Health box on page 86.)
- Have your keys or remote carlock device in your hand as you approach your parked vehicle so you do not have to stand outside your car looking for them. Check the area around your parked car and in the back seat before you enter it.
- If your car becomes disabled, do not accept a stranger's help. Place a "Help, call police" sign in the window. Stay inside of the car until police arrive. Do not hitchhike. Carry a cell phone and keep it on for quick use in an emergency.
- Keep the doors and windows of your car and home locked. Install deadbolt locks and peepholes on all outside doors of your home.
- Be wary of strangers who want you to open your door to them; they may intend to harm you. If they ask to use your phone, tell them you will make the call for them. Even if they appear to be from a business, do not open the door.

If you are attacked:

- Yell or scream "Fire" instead of "Help" to get people's attention. Do not stop screaming; making a loud commotion may scare your attacker away.

- Do not allow yourself to be moved to another location. Resist being forced into a car. If you leave the original scene of the assault, it becomes more likely that you will be seriously injured or murdered.
- Avoid kicking a man's groin area; men are wary of this maneuver and guard their genitals. Instead, making a swift, hard kick across the attacker's kneecap can disable the person, allowing you to escape.
- If your attacker has a weapon, he may intend to kill you regardless of whether you comply with his demands. In this instance, rape prevention experts often recommend that you use extreme actions to confuse or intimidate the criminal such as throwing up, acting psychotic, or pretending to have a heart attack or other life-threatening condition. In other instances, you may pretend to cooperate with your attacker, waiting until his guard is down to make a surprise move in your defense.

To avoid date rape:

- Agree to meet a "blind date" at a crowded location, or agree only to a group dating situation until you feel comfortable going out with the individual.
- Be wary of dates who show unreasonable or inappropriate behaviors in public, such as aggressiveness, rudeness, dominance, or hostility in social situations that do not involve sex. These individuals may display the same behaviors when alone with you.
- Do not send mixed sexual messages that confuse your date. Clearly say "no" to unwanted sexual advances.

victims were killed by their intimate partners; only about 3% of male murder victims were killed by their intimate partners (U.S. Dept. of Justice, 2003). Although both sexes commit violent acts against their dates or partners, women usually engage in violence against their male partners as acts of self-defense.

What factors contribute to violence between intimate partners? Such violence exists within every racial, ethnic, socioeconomic, and religious group. The rates of intimate partner violence, however, are higher among the poor, the unemployed, and those with low-status occupations. Additionally, children who are exposed to violence between their parents have a greater risk of abusing their lovers later in life. Moreover, girls who witness their fathers' abusive treatment of their

mothers have a high risk of becoming the victim of partner abuse themselves when they mature (Coker et al., 2000). As a result of their childhood experiences, these women may think such abuse is a "normal" aspect of intimate relationships.

Another major factor that contributes to intimate partner violence is drug use. Often, one or both partners have consumed alcohol or used other mind-altering drugs when the violence between them erupts. Both perpetrators and victims tend to have low self-esteem and be highly dependent on their partners. Some men and women have difficulty asserting themselves without becoming angry and resort to aggressive behavior to control and intimidate their partners. The student workbook activity "Am I in an Abusive

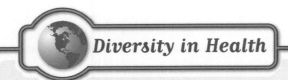

Diversity in Health

Spouse Abuse: An International Problem

Throughout the world, women of all cultural, religious, ethnic, and socioeconomic groups are abused by their intimate partners. According to a report of the World Health Organization, 20% to 50% of women in 24 countries on four continents were physically abused by their husbands at one time in their relationships (Afkhami, 1999). Severe psychological and verbal abuse usually accompanies the physical violence, and the victim is often blamed for her mistreatment.

Why does spouse abuse persist? Certain non-Western cultures ascribe low status to women. Men living in these societies do not consider wife battering and other forms of mistreatment of their spouses as violence or abuse.

Additionally, certain practices in such cultures increase the financial dependence of women on their spouses, which makes it difficult for them to leave their abusive husbands. For example, women living in some countries lose their inheritance or the opportunity to earn an income outside of the home when they marry. The economic power in these countries is unequally distributed in favor of men, and as a result, husbands feel entitled to control their wives and families. Male domination continues at community and state levels as women are often denied access to education and government positions. Thus, they lack the knowledge and political power necessary to change public policy. To eliminate violence against women, people from around the world must work to change the attitudes, behaviors, and laws that negatively affect the status of women (Afkhami, 1999).

Relationship?" can help you determine if your partner is abusive. Furthermore, Table 4-1 lists certain behaviors and attitudes that often characterize physically abusive individuals. Since dating violence is often a precursor of marital violence, you should leave a relationship if your partner displays any of these characteristics.

Why do men and women stay in abusive relationships, sometimes for decades? Women often remain in these situations because of their emotional attachment to and economic dependency on the abuser. They feel trapped and isolated (Frank & Rodowski, 1999). Furthermore, an abusive partner may be apologetic and loving after episodes of violence, raising the victim's hopes that the violence has ended. Spouse abuse is not just an American phenomenon; the Diversity in Health feature "Spouse Abuse: An International Problem" discusses the nature of this behavior in non-Western societies.

sexual harassment
intentional use of annoying sexually related comments or behaviors to intimidate or coerce people into unwanted sexual activity.

Sexual Harassment

Sexual harassment is the intentional use of annoying and offensive sexually related comments or behaviors to intimidate people or coerce them into unwanted sexual activity. Such abusive behavior can include unwelcome requests for dates, sexually offensive jokes, lewd comments, or touching and fondling. It is difficult to determine the scope of the problem because

Table 4-1	Signs of Danger in a Relationship

A partner who is likely to become physically abusive:

- Insists that you do things that you do not want to do and prevents you from doing things that you would like to do
- Argues with you over any issue
- Does not accept responsibility for his or her mistakes and blames you or other persons for his or her problems
- Prevents you from associating with your family and friends and threatens to end the relationship if you do not stop interacting with others
- Displays excessive jealousy or is too possessive
- Attempts to control your behavior, for example, tells you how to dress or wear your hair
- Is verbally abusive, for example, criticizes you or says degrading things to you either in private or in public
- Expects you to do everything perfectly and according to his or her wishes, and expects you to know what they are even without being told
- Reacts violently when things go wrong, he or she loses control, or he or she is embarrassed
- Exhibits cruelty to other persons or animals, usually without remorse

Source: Mariani, C. (1996). *Domestic violence survival guide.* Flushing, NY: Looseleaf Law Publications.

surveys often use different definitions of *sexual harassment.* Furthermore, sexual harassment is not always easy to recognize. For example, if someone tells a sexually offensive joke, under what circumstances would you consider this sexual harassment?

Sexual harassment can happen anywhere. College instructors, for example, engage in sexual harassment if they provide special treatment, such as awarding a passing grade, to students who submit to their sexual advances. In addition to schools, sexual harassment frequently occurs in the workplace, where it creates stress and reduces employees' job satisfaction, performance, and loyalty. It is especially devastating for individuals who feel that their grade, job, or career depends on enduring the harassment or submitting to the intimidating person.

How can one handle a person who engages in sexual harassment? Some people simply avoid or ignore harassing persons; others choose to confront their tormentors by telling them, verbally or in writing, to stop the annoying and unprofessional comments or behaviors. If the harassment persists, victims can pursue more aggressive steps, including reporting the behavior to management or taking legal action. Many educational institutions and businesses have policies concerning sexual harassment that follow guidelines established by the federal government's Equal Employment Opportunity Commission (EEOC). These policies usually identify steps that people can take to file harassment-related complaints. Before initiating such action, a person should document episodes of sexual intimidation, recording the date and nature of the unwanted comments or behaviors. In many instances, the abusive person has harassed other workers or students; therefore, a victim may be able to strengthen his or her case against this person by asking other victims to serve as witnesses.

Stalking

Sensational stories about celebrities who are pursued relentlessly by overly aggressive, obsessive fans have led to interest and research into stalking behavior. Anyone, however, can be the victim of a stalker. A stalker willfully and repeatedly follows and harasses another individual. Examples of harassment include making unwanted phone calls, sending unwanted gifts, and making unwelcome visits to the targeted person's home or workplace. In a national survey, 8% of American women and 2% of American men reported that they had been stalked at some point in their lives (Tjaden & Thoennes, 1998).

Most stalkers are males; the largest group of stalkers is comprised of lonely, emotionally disturbed men who have been rejected by their partners (Lamberg, 2001). Despite his ex-partner's efforts to avoid him, the stalker often hopes to convince her to rekindle the relationship. In many instances, however, he is angry with her and wants to harm her emotionally or physically. Stalkers physically attack one-third of their victims (Lamberg, 2001). Even if she is not physically threatened or harmed, the victim usually experiences extreme emotional distress and often seeks legal means to make the stalker stop harassing her. Victims often continue to suffer severe emotional effects long after the stalking ends, and they may need treatment for depression and post-traumatic stress disorder.

If you are being stalked, what can you do to discourage the stalker and end his or her terrifying behavior? If the stalker is a former intimate partner, experts advise confronting the stalker, telling him or her that the relationship is over and you have no interest in renewing it. After that, avoid all communication with the person but keep records of his or her harassing behavior. If the stalker persistently telephones you, have an answering machine record calls on that line and get a separate, unlisted phone number for other callers. If the stalker uses emails or instant messages to annoy you (*cyberstalking*), contact your Internet service provider (ISP) for help. Additionally, seek support and help from family, friends, neighbors, and coworkers by telling them about the stalking incidents. Finally, make sure your home is secure, and if you feel threatened by this person, notify the police.

Community Violence

Community violence refers to violence that happens in public settings such as street corners, bars, and public places. Among youths, community violence often occurs as gang violence. Although many people think gangs are a recent development, gangs have been a feature of urban life in American cities for more than a century. In the late 1800s, cities such as St. Louis had groups of adolescents who wore differently colored clothing to identify their particular gang membership (Decker, 1997). Today, typical members of a gang are males between 8 and 24 years of age who share similar racial or ethnic backgrounds. Such gangs are prevalent in certain neighborhoods of American cities and are becoming more common in many suburbs.

community violence violence between strangers or acquaintances that occurs in public settings.

Violence is a characteristic of gang activities—gang members often resort to violence to defend their territory. The most common kinds of gang violence include homicides, attempted homicides, assaults, shootings, and robberies. Violent gang activities are more likely to occur on city streets during weekend evenings. The late-night drive-by shooting, for example, has come to be associated with gang violence.

Why are some youths attracted to gangs, placing themselves at high risk for serious injury and even death? Adolescents may join gangs for social reasons, especially if their communities offer few opportunities for safe social activities. Additionally, gang membership provides an opportunity for some youths to belong to a group and find self-identity, that is, to "be someone." Involvement with gangs, however, dramatically increases one's risk of being murdered. In 2001 homicide was the second leading cause of death for persons between 15 and 24 years of age and the number one cause of death for African American men and women in this age group (Anderson & Smith, 2003).

Institutional Violence

School Violence Most acts of **institutional violence** occur in schools, where students attack their peers or even their teachers and school administrators. Earlier generations of students may have shoved and punched to settle arguments; today's students may use guns and knives.

In the past few years, several incidents in which students used guns to kill their classmates and teachers made headline news (Figure 4-3). Such terrible events, however, are rare. Less than 1% of murders involving youth take place on school property. Youth are less likely to carry weapons to school and engage in fighting than in 1990 (Brener et al., 1999).

What can be done to reduce the risk of violence at school? Many urban schools now resort to using metal detectors and hiring uniformed police in an attempt to curb school violence. Other steps to manage the problem include training elementary school teachers and administrators to identify potential troublemakers in their classrooms. Children who are prone to become violent often model the aggressive behaviors of their parents. Such high-risk children have difficulty controlling their anger; tend to poke, shove, or annoy other people; act impulsively; bully other children; and defy authorities, including parents and teachers. In many communities, schools now offer conflict resolution classes for children that emphasize socially acceptable ways of settling disputes.

Violence on College Campuses According to a recent report, college students are less likely to be victims of violent crime than nonstudents of the same age (Hart, 2003). The majority of rapes, robberies, and assaults occurred to students living off campus. As in the general population, violence on American campuses is associated with the availability of guns and widespread use of drugs, especially alcohol.

The Student Right to Know and Campus Security Act requires administrators of colleges and universities that receive federal funds to report information concerning the number of murders, assaults, rapes, and other specific crimes that take place on their campuses. Additionally, the administrators must develop programs that are designed to educate students about personal safety and campus security. To reduce the violence on their campuses, many college administrators have adopted security measures such as restricting access to campus buildings, setting up emergency call boxes on campus, improving lighting near walkways and parking lots, limiting visitation hours in residence halls, and initiating escort services for

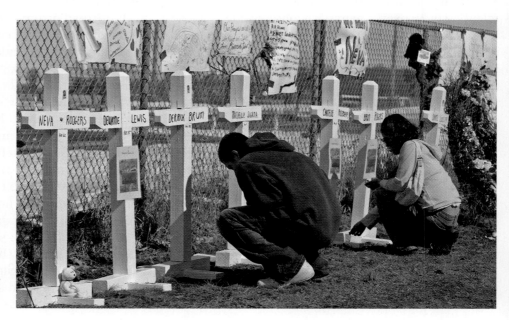

Figure 4-3 **School Violence.** Red Lake, Minnesota, high school students mourn the deaths of five classmates, a teacher, and a security guard who were shot by a 16-year-old male student. The young man later shot himself to death. Despite incidents such as this, youth are less likely to carry weapons to school today than in 1990.

female students. For information about the types and extent of violent crime at your college or university, contact staff at the campus police department.

Workplace Violence

Workplace violence is any act of violence or abuse directed toward an individual who is performing his or her job. Although most people will never experience the most dangerous types of workplaces, such as psychiatric hospitals and prisons, any workplace can be a setting for violence. In 1998, homicide was the second leading cause of death for American workers (Sygnatur and Toscano, 2000). The stereotype of workplace violence as vengeful acts committed by disgruntled former workers is misleading. Work-related homicides are most likely to occur during armed robberies of retail businesses such as grocery stores, restaurants, bars, and gas stations. Employees with the highest risk of being murdered while working are cab drivers, convenience store attendants, police, and security guards.

Certain workers have a high risk of becoming violent, particularly when they are laid off, fired, or not promoted. Persons most likely to resort to workplace violence are men between the ages of 25 and 40 who are loners, have marital and other family problems, appear angry and paranoid, abuse alcohol and/or other drugs, and blame others for their problems. Women are less likely to commit violent acts in workplaces, but they are more likely to be victims.

Terrorism

Terrorism is intentional violent acts against civilians to produce extreme fear, severe property damage, and numerous deaths. Terrorists may attack specific cultural or political symbols, such as the World Trade Center or the Pentagon, or more random targets, such as restaurants, airplanes, and places of worship (Figure 4-4). Regardless of whether terrorists are citizens of the country they attack or foreigners, a major purpose of terrorism is to frighten the general population and make them feel vulnerable and helpless.

The use of conventional bombs by terrorists is not new, but recently, terrorists adopted more sinister methods of killing civilians and destroying property. The arsenal of terrorist weapons now includes poisonous chemicals, life-threatening infectious agents such as the bacterium that causes anthrax, hijacked airplanes as guided missiles, and explosives strapped to suicidal individuals who intentionally blow themselves up in crowded places.

In addition to physical injuries, survivors of a terrorist attack often experience long-term psychologi-

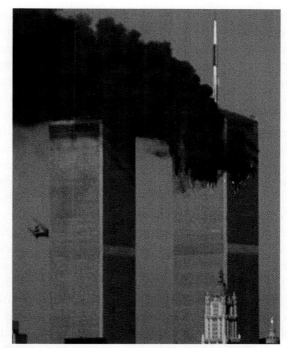

Figure 4-4 New York City, September 11, 2001. On this day foreign terrorists used commercial jets to attack the World Trade Center and the Pentagon.

cal consequences such as post-traumatic stress disorder (PTSD) and depression. Extensive media reporting of the disastrous event, however, indirectly affects the psychological health of those outside the zone of destruction. A national survey conducted a few days after September 11, 2001, indicated that 90% of adult Americans suffered from stress symptoms as a result of the attacks on the United States (Schuster et al., 2001). Personal efforts to cope with the events included talking with others, practicing religious rites, and reducing time spent watching television, especially news programs that repeatedly showed shocking scenes of the disaster. Additionally, some Americans donated blood or money for people directly affected by the attacks. After the September 11 attacks, U.S. government officials took steps to reduce the risk of terrorism by, for example, increasing airport security. Nevertheless, many Americans think additional terrorist attacks in the United States are likely (Schuster et al., 2001). Living with such fear increases the risk of stress-related health problems such as those discussed in Chapter 3.

■ Assessing Your Risk of Violence

What are the chances that you, or some of the people you care about deeply, are at risk for violence? The risk is difficult to determine because many violent incidents, especially rapes and spouse battering, are never reported to the police. Nevertheless, some people are more likely to suffer serious or fatal injury than others. The likelihood of a particular person experiencing such harm depends on specific risk factors, including his or her family situation, living conditions, personality, and activities.

Family disruption is a major risk factor for family and community violence. Parental conflict that leads to separation, divorce, or desertion contributes to family disruption, as does the presence of criminal or drug-addicted parents. Neighborhood conditions, such as high rates of unemployment, can lead to high rates of family disruption. Other risk factors for family violence are social isolation, the presence of children with special needs, and a large number of children in the family. Conditions that contribute to school violence are poor discipline in the classroom, weak administrators, poor enforcement of rules, and low levels of student and parent interest in academic achievement.

As mentioned earlier in this chapter, the availability of alcohol, other drugs, and guns dramatically escalates the likelihood of serious injury or death in violent situations. A significant percentage of people who commit serious crimes test positive for alcohol, marijuana, cocaine, or combinations of mind-altering drugs at the time of their arrest. In 2002, guns were involved in 7% of violent crimes and nearly 70% of murders (U.S. Dept. of Justice, 2004).

Certain individuals are more likely than others to find themselves in places and situations in which violence is likely to occur. Age is a major risk factor. Americans younger than 25 years old are more likely to become involved in violence than older persons. Teens experience the highest rates of violent crimes, and young adults between 18 and 24 years of age have the highest homicide rate (U.S. Dept. of Justice, 2004). Another key risk factor is gender. While in their homes, women are as likely as men to use force, but in community settings they are far less likely to do so. Men are more likely than women to be arrested for perpetrating crimes of violence, and they are more likely to be the victims of such crimes. Women, however, have a greater risk of being killed by their spouses than men.

Race and ethnicity are two other characteristics strongly associated with involvement in violent incidents. A striking feature of American violence is the volume and concentration of violence within minority populations, particularly homicides among young African American males living in urban areas. Blacks are seven times more likely to commit murder than whites (Fox & Zawitz, 2001). In most instances, murderers and their victims are members of the same racial group. An objective of *Healthy People 2000* (USDHHS, 1999) was to reduce the homicide rate from 8.5 per 100,000 (the rate in 1987) to 7.2 per 100,000 Americans. This is one national health indicator in which progress is being made; the rate declined to 5.6 murders per 100,000 Americans in 2002 (U.S. Dept. of Justice, 2003).

■ Preventing and Avoiding Violence

Although many Americans doubt that violence can be prevented, they do think it can be controlled. To reduce violent crime, communities are turning increasingly to environmental measures such as improved street lighting, neighborhood watch organizations, and surveillance by closed-circuit cameras. Many large companies have taken specific steps to reduce workplace violence, such as hiring security staff, controlling access to offices, requiring employees to wear identification badges, and offering employee assistance programs that provide referrals for counseling services.

There are numerous practical steps you can take to reduce your personal risk of victimization. Many avoidance measures are simple and inexpensive, and they work. To be effective, however, these measures must become part of your routine. The most effective action is staying away from high-risk situations and people. For example, a woman who does not attend a binge drinking party cannot be date raped by another participant; a man who stays out of a high-crime district is unlikely to be a victim of a drive-by shooting. Simply put, people should avoid high-risk places and dangerous persons.

Home security is another avoidance measure that can discourage and prevent criminals from victimizing you. In many break-ins, the intruder simply came through an unlocked door or window. The most important home or dorm safety measure is to have and always use good deadbolt locks on doors. Also, keep windows securely locked, especially when you are not home. Contact your police department or the campus security center to see if they will perform a free safety inspection of your residence.

If you live in a dangerous neighborhood, consider moving to a safer one if you can. This is the most effective measure you can take to avoid violence. If you cannot leave the neighborhood, look for a place to live that is farther away from the most dangerous streets. If the new area looks safer, ask a few residents, and even local police, if they would prefer to live elsewhere. The police may have local crime statistics so you can compare crime rates of various neighborhoods.

Daily life is filled with people and situations that cannot be avoided, but you can use certain tactics to reduce your chances of victimization. If your usual routine requires traveling through dangerous neighborhoods, remove yourself from these high-risk areas by taking safer routes, even if they are out of your way. Avoid isolated places, especially when you are alone. Deserted buildings, infrequently used sections of libraries, and nearly empty parking lots and garages are places where violent incidents are likely to occur.

A considerable percentage of violent crimes, especially sexual assaults, happen between 6 P.M. and midnight. Thus, if you must go out at night, do not go alone. If you are driving and someone in another car threatens you, do not stop, but drive to a well-lit public place; obviously, police stations or fire stations are the best choices. Additionally, stay in places where you can see other people. Being in the presence of others greatly reduces your risk of violence. If you are alone at night and on campus, use the college's escort service or use the "buddy system" when walking to and from buildings.

Regardless of the time of day, as soon as you enter your car, lock the doors. Keep your car doors locked, and take the keys with you, even when you leave the car for a minute. Do not give rides to strangers or stop to help others. If you spend a lot of time in your car, obtain a cellular phone to call for assistance in any emergency. If you are involved in a minor accident, stay in your car; keep the doors locked and the windows rolled up until the police arrive. If someone demands that you surrender your car, do not argue with or resist the person: Get out of the car, move away

from the area quickly, and contact the police. If you are driving and someone drives aggressively and irresponsibly, avoid getting angry with the person. If a driver tailgates your car, flashes high beams at you, or makes angry gestures, do not stop to discuss the matter. Avoid making eye contact with this individual, and discourage him or her from harming you by driving to a secure, well-lit area, preferably a police station. The Managing Your Health feature lists some other important personal safety tips.

Family and workplace ties are difficult to end, but you can excuse yourself from situations that have the potential to become dangerous. In the workplace, learn your company's security measures, for example, the locations of fire alarms so you can activate one in case of any trouble. Perhaps most important, strive to get along with coworkers and the public. Help create a positive working environment and relationships by displaying a friendly attitude, good manners, tact, and diplomacy. The Changing Health Habits activity for this chapter in the workbook can help you identify and change habits that may increase your risk of becoming a victim of violence.

Relying on destructive responses such as angry verbal exchanges to manage interpersonal conflicts can lead to physical violence. Arguments are the most frequently cited circumstances that result in murder. In 2002, for example, arguments were involved in almost 4 out of 10 murders in which the circumstances were known (U.S. Dept. of Justice, 2003). If you become involved in a heated dispute or threatening situation, keeping calm may prevent the situation from escalating into a violent one. For example, breathe

 Managing Your Health

Going Out: Safety Tips

To reduce your risk of being victimized, practice the following security rules:

- Before you leave, check to see if your home or dorm is secure. Make sure windows are locked. Leave some lights and a radio on to give the impression that someone is there.
- When riding in a car, keep doors locked at all times, and windows rolled down no more than one inch. If using public transportation, sit near the driver or conductor.

- If violence erupts anywhere near you, run away if you can.
- Look alert.
- Park in a well-lit area. Check inside and underneath the car before entering. If you need to use public transportation, choose well-populated stops.
- As you approach your home or dorm room, do not enter if you see signs of a break-in or suspicious persons in the area. Go instead to a neighbor or public phone and call the police. If surprised, burglars often become assailants.
- Lock the door immediately after entering your home or dorm room.

deeply, count to ten, "bite your tongue," or make some excuse and quickly leave the scene. The relaxation techniques described in Chapter 3 can help you maintain your composure in such situations. The student workbook activity "Assessing Your Anger" can help you identify situations that make you angry. If you have a "short fuse," counseling can help you learn conflict management strategies such as impulse control, anger management, and negotiation techniques.

Self-Protection

When faced with the threat of force, your actions can influence the outcome of the situation. For example, you may obtain help from others by calling the police, pressing an alarm button, blowing a whistle, or screaming to attract attention. When cornered and facing a threatening person alone, a person might try to defuse the situation verbally by reasoning with his or her assailant. If you become overwhelmed by fear or conclude that you cannot escape, your response may be to offer no resistance. However, the gut responses to danger are the flight-or-fight reactions described in Chapter 3. Sometimes flight—simply running away—is the best means of escaping threatening situations. The opposite response is to fight by making counterthreats or by physically attacking another person. Many Americans carry with them, or keep handy in their homes, a weapon for self-defense such as a gun, knife, or chemical spray (see the Consumer Health feature). When danger threatens, other people may rely on improvised weapons such as car keys, scissors, or a flashlight. Some people seek training in personal

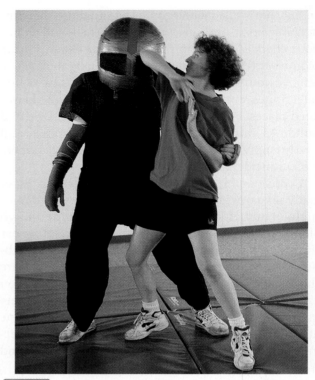

Figure 4-5 **In Self-Defense.** Fighting back is one way of responding to violent situations.

defense or in firearm use to enhance their ability to defend themselves (**Figure 4-5**).

Should victims always resist their attackers? No uniform answer can be given. Each potential victim must assess each situation to decide how to respond under the circumstances. In situations involving partner abuse

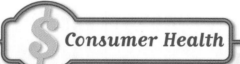

Consumer Health

Natural Defense: Pepper Spray

One way to protect yourself against an aggressor is to use pepper spray. Pepper spray contains capsaicin, a compound that is found in hot chili peppers. When sprayed in an assailant's eyes, pepper spray produces a painful burning sensation. Almost immediately, the person's eyelids swell shut and tears begin to flow. The spray also causes the attacker to experience difficulty breathing and lose control over body movements. These effects last about 20 to 30 minutes, which gives you time to escape the situation and call police. Pepper spray is an effective and safe way to subdue an attacker, but it may take a few seconds to work on enraged or drugged individuals.

Hardware or variety stores often sell pepper spray in small canisters that can be carried in a coat pocket or purse. Persons under the age of 18, however, are not permitted to possess pepper spray. Some states may impose other restrictions concerning the use of pepper spray. Therefore, before buying the product, check with local law-enforcement agencies to determine if it is legal to use pepper spray. Always follow the package directions when using it as a defense and keep the canister out of the reach of children and irresponsible persons.

Source: Buster, R. W., & van Helden, H. P. M. (1998). Toxicological evaluation of pepper spray as a possible weapon for the Dutch police force. *American Journal of Forensic Medicine and Pathology* *19*(4):309–316.

or stalking, civil protection orders that separate and prohibit contact between the abuser or stalker and the victim can be effective in preventing further abuse (Wathen & MacMillan, 2003).

■ Reporting Violence

If you are attacked, you must decide whether to report the incident. You should report any attempted or completed crime of violence by strangers or acquaintances to the police. Most large police departments include specially trained family violence and sexual assault units that provide sympathetic and appropriate responses. A 911 call usually gains access to the appropriate emergency services.

In certain instances, you may feel reluctant to inform police about what happened to you. Consider reporting the incident to an agency, such as a rape crisis center or a women's self-help service, that can assist you in dealing with legal authorities and medical establishments. Nationwide, a 24-hour, toll-free family violence hotline can be reached at 1-800-799-SAFE. Seeking help is beneficial to one's recovery from violence.

Managing the short- and long-term effects of the violent incident on the victim's family and friends also is important. Useful services include marital counseling, couple therapy, financial and legal aid, and family therapy. Access to such services and information concerning local self-help groups can usually be arranged through your campus student health center or through social service agencies in your community.

Healthy Living Practices

- To reduce your risk of violence, avoid high-risk places and dangerous people.
- If a dispute turns into a heated argument, try to keep calm to prevent the threatening situation from escalating into a violent one.
- Conflict management skills can help defuse tense, angry situations. Some college campuses offer courses in conflict management; consider taking a class to learn these techniques.
- There is no single way to react whenever someone threatens your safety; therefore, assess each situation to decide how to respond under the circumstances.
- If you are a victim of violence, report the attack to police. In addition, obtain prompt treatment of your physical injuries and emotional distress.

Violence and Abuse

Child physical abuse includes beating, squeezing, burning, cutting, suffocating, binding, and poisoning a child who is under 18 years of age. Although child physical abuse takes place in institutional settings, such as day-care centers and schools, homes are by far the most common setting. Most physical violence against children is not committed by strangers or casual acquaintances but by parents and other adults known to the victims, such as neighbors, baby-sitters, and family friends. Abused children under 2 years of age are at greatest risk of fatalities, primarily from head injuries. Many children, however, receive less severe injuries on a regular basis. Such violence is not confined to impoverished families or to any particular racial or ethnic group. In the United States, the actual prevalence of child abuse is not known; fatal cases often are not identified as child mistreatment (Herman-Giddens et al., 1999).

Why do some parents abuse their children? Parents who are physically abusive to each other have a high risk of abusing their children. Additionally, abusive parents generally lack effective parenting skills and frequently have faulty or unrealistic expectations about their children's behavior. For example, a parent may shake a 3-month-old infant to make it stop crying or kick a 2-year-old child for not using the toilet. Abusive parents tend to be under tremendous stress and often are isolated from people who could provide helpful advice and social support. Regardless of the parents' situation, suspected or observed cases of child neglect or abuse can be reported anonymously by calling the Childhelp National Child Abuse hotline (1-800-422-4453). In some states, a person must report suspected cases of child abuse or neglect to authorities.

Data from various studies indicate that many adults were victims of sexual abuse during childhood. **Child sexual abuse** refers to sexual activity with a child that takes place as a result of force or threat, or by taking advantage of an age difference or a caretaking relationship. A **pedophile** is an individual who is sexually attracted to children and fantasizes about having physical contact with them. A *child molester* acts on his or her urges by having sexual activity with vulnerable children. The abuse usually involves fondling a child's body, but it may include completed or attempted

child physical abuse physical violence against a child who is under 18 years of age.

child sexual abuse sexual activity involving a child that takes place as a result of force or threat.

pedophile (PEE-doe-file) an individual who is sexually attracted to children.

vaginal, anal, or oral sex. As many as 15% of children, primarily girls, are sexually abused (Weiss et al., 1999). Most molesters are heterosexual males who generally target girls between 8 and 10 years old.

Many people think that child molesters are strangers who are mentally ill, looking for children to kidnap, rape, and murder. In fact, most cases involve adults whom the children know and trust, such as babysitters, family friends, relatives, teachers, camp counselors, coaches, and clergy. Only 3% of murdered children under 5 years of age were killed by strangers (Fox & Zawitz, 2001). However, the increasing number of children who have access to personal computers provides a new method for sophisticated child abusers to communicate with vulnerable children through Internet chat rooms or electronic bulletin boards.

Incest, sexual experiences between family members who are not spouses, is the most serious form of sexual abuse. Victims may be boys, although girls are at much greater risk. Incest is often nonviolent, but forced, and it typically escalates over time. The risk factors for incest are similar to those of nonsexual abuse: childhood victimization of the perpetrator and high levels of stress within the family.

To prevent child sexual abuse, parents should teach their young children how to recognize and report sexual abuse. Since most cases involve people the youngsters know, simply telling children "Don't talk to strangers" is not sufficient advice. Very young children need to learn which parts of their bodies are private. Additionally, these children need to learn that if any-

incest sexual relations between family members who are not spouses.

elder abuse use of physical or sexual violence against an elderly person.

one touches them in ways that make them feel uncomfortable, they should report the incidents to parents.

Studies show that abused children behave more aggressively at every stage of the life span. As adults, they are more likely to be violent against dates, spouses, their children, and, later, their elderly parents. Furthermore, a significant percentage of women who suffer from depression were sexually abused as children (Weiss et al., 1999).

Elder abuse is the use of physical or sexual violence against an elderly person; some researchers include verbal threats and neglect in their definitions. Physical and psychological abuse of elderly individuals takes place not only in institutional settings such as hospitals and nursing homes, but especially in family settings. Such abuse occurs in all racial and ethnic groups and at all socioeconomic levels. As many as 2.5 million Americans over 65 years of age are abused annually (Kleinschmidt, 1997). As the average age of the American population increases, many experts expect that the prevalence of elder abuse will increase as well.

The causes of elder abuse are complex. Elderly persons are most likely to be victimized by their spouses or adult children who must care for them. Caring for frail, aged relatives can be frustrating and stressful. Furthermore, the caretaker may depend on the elderly person for his or her housing and income. In such situations, resentful caretakers may resort to abusive behavior. In severe cases, violence against the elderly is associated with certain mental illnesses and drug (usually alcohol) abuse. If you observe an elderly person being abused or neglected, you can report the situation to a local adult protective services agency.

CRITICAL THINKING

The following article promotes an herbal tea formulated to reduce a person's level of anger. Read the article and evaluate it using the model for analyzing health-related information. The main points of the model are noted below; the model is fully explained on pages 13–15.

Aunt Annie's Tranquillity Tea

As you know, I've been using herbs all my life to treat everything from acne to zinc deficiency. Most of my knowledge about herbs didn't come from books or the Internet, it was passed down to me in my Great Aunt Annie's diary. Annie had a fabulous herb garden in the back of her house. One afternoon in 1914 she made the most amazing discovery, which she later recorded in her diary. She had dug up some comfrey root and picked a bunch of pennyroyal and lobelia leaves from the garden. Since coltsfoot was blooming, she thought it might be a nice change to add some of its leaves to her usual tea recipe. She brewed a pot of tea from the mixture and drank about 2 cups of it. The tea was delicious. Very soothing.

Less than an hour later, Great Uncle Jeb came in from the barn, tracking dirt all over Aunt Annie's new carpet. Now I need to tell you that Annie had a terrible temper—she was only 4' 8" tall, but she used to push big old Jeb around a lot. Needless to say, Uncle Jeb was expecting the worst from his wife. But this time, instead of flying off the handle and kicking Jeb, as she was prone to do, Aunt Annie laughed and hugged him. Happy as a kitten rolling in catnip, Annie cleaned up the mess. Uncle Jeb suspected Annie had added something different to her usual tea recipe, so he had her sit down and recall the herb mixture. Using her recipe, Jeb made a pot of that tea for Annie to drink every day for the rest of her life. When Uncle Jeb began making whiskey in the barn and staying out late with his friends, Annie never raised a fuss. She just sat in the bent oak rocking chair, sipping her tea.

If you want to try Aunt Annie's Tranquillity Tea on someone you know who's got a bad temper, I'll send the recipe to you. I'm the editor of this magazine, so just send $10 for shipping and handling to my address, which is on the inside of the front cover. I'd love to hear about your experiences with the tea; be sure and let me know how it worked for you.

Your friend

Herb
Herb Z. Gardenia

1. Which statements are verifiable facts, and which are unverified statements or value claims?
2. What are the credentials of the person writing the article? Does the author appear to have appropriate background and education in the topic area?
3. What might be the motives and biases of the person writing the article? State reasons for your answer.
4. Which information is relevant to the issue or main point of the article, and which information is irrelevant?
5. Is the source reliable? Does it have a reputation for publishing misinformation?
6. Does the article attack the credibility of conventional scientists or medical authorities?

Based on your analysis, do you think that this article is a reliable source of health-related information? Summarize your reasons for coming to this conclusion.

CHAPTER REVIEW

Summary

Violence refers to interpersonal uses of force that are not socially sanctioned. A violent social incident occurs when at least one person intentionally applies or threatens physical force on others. Violence is a major public health problem because it produces staggering physical, psychological, and social consequences. For many Americans, violence is a way of life; no one is exempt from violence.

Assault is the intentional use of force to injure someone physically; abuse occurs when one takes advantage of a relationship to mistreat a person. Examples of abuse include spouse abuse, child abuse, and sexual harassment.

Regardless of whether physical harm occurs, violent victimization always damages psychological health. Psychological effects of violence include anxiety, depression, and suicidal thinking. Anxious or depressed people have a high risk of drug abuse and eating disorders. Family relationships may become strained or end as a result of violence. Furthermore, intergenerational transmission of violence occurs when abused children mature and abuse their own children. To recover from the psychological effects of violence, one should seek help from health care professionals.

Violence is complex; there is no single cause of violence, nor is violent behavior limited to a particular group of persons. Factors that contribute to violence include poverty, substance abuse, certain psychological disorders, and poor self-esteem. In many instances, violence is learned behavior. Watching violent media, for example, contributes to violent behavior.

Sexual violence involves areas of the body that are sensitive to sexual arousal. Such violence involves sexual activity gained through force, threat of force, or coercion. The majority of sexual assaults are committed not by strangers but by acquaintances, friends, family members, and spouses. Family (domestic) violence encompasses both friends and family members and usually takes place in homes. Community violence includes acts that occur between strangers or acquaintances, usually in public places. Institutional violence occurs mainly within institutional environments such as schools, workplaces, or prisons. Terrorism involves violent acts against civilians to produce extreme fear, severe property damage, and numerous deaths.

To reduce the likelihood of becoming a victim of violence, one should limit exposure to risky situations. When faced with a violent situation, obtain help from others by attracting attention, defuse the situation by reasoning with an assailant, or simply run away. In some instances, a person may need to defend himself or herself physically.

Most physical violence against children is committed by adults known to the victims, such as relatives, neighbors, or baby-sitters. Most violence against children occurs in their homes. Girls, especially those between the ages of 8 and 10, are more likely to be targets of sexual abuse than boys. Parents should teach their young children how to recognize and report sexual abuse. Children who experience violence often suffer emotional and social injuries that remain long after physical injuries have healed.

Elder abuse occurs in all racial and ethnic groups and at all socioeconomic levels. Family members are responsible for the vast majority of abuse directed toward elderly persons. As the average age of the American population increases, many experts predict that the incidence of elder abuse will also increase.

Applying What You Have Learned

1. If your friend reports being sexually harassed by a college professor, what advice could you give to him or her? **Application**
2. You have to attend classes or work at a job in the evenings. Determine at least two steps you can take to reduce your risk of violence on campus or at work. **Analysis**
3. Plan a program to increase security in your dorm or on your campus. Consider forwarding it to an official at the university who might be interested in your plan, such as the Dean of Student Affairs. **Synthesis**

4. Evaluate your present security situation. Determine situations in your life that provide some risk of violence and describe ways in which you can reduce these risks. **Evaluation**

Key

Application using information in a new situation.

Analysis breaking down information into component parts.

Synthesis putting together information from different sources.

Evaluation making informed decisions.

Reflecting on Your Health

1. As mentioned in this chapter, visual media can influence a person's attitudes toward violence. Choose a violent movie or television show that you watched recently. What impact, if any, did it have on your feelings about violence?
2. Do you like to play violent computer games? If so, how does this activity affect your attitudes toward violence?
3. What could you do to avoid getting into an abusive relationship with an intimate partner? If you are already in an abusive relationship, what are

your feelings about your partner? What would make you change your current situation?
4. How safe do you feel at home or in the dorm? What worries you most about the safety of your environment? What steps could you take to make your residence more secure?
5. If you were out walking alone at night and realized someone was following you, describe what you would do to reduce your risk of being attacked. Do you think that it is safe for you to walk alone at night? Why or why not?

References

Afkhami, M. (1999). An AMEWS/MESA special session on violence against women. *Middle East Women's Studies Review, 13*(4):5+.

Anderson, R. N., & Smith, B. L. (2003). Deaths: Leading causes for 2001. *National Vital Statistics Reports, 52*(9):1–86.

Brener, N. D., Simon, T. R., Krug, E. G., & Lowry, R. (1999). Recent trends in violence-related behaviors among high school students in the United States. *Journal of the American Medical Association, 282*(5):440–446.

Centers for Disease Control and Prevention. (2000). *Fact sheet: Dating violence.* Retrieved from http://www.cdc.gov/ncipc/factsheets/datviol.htm.

Coker, A. L., Smith, P. H., McKeown, R. E., & King, M. J. (2000). Frequency and correlates of intimate partner violence by type: Physical, sexual, and psychological battering. *American Journal of Public Health, 90*(4):553–559.

Decker, S. H. (1997, March 27). Getting a grip on gangs. *St. Louis Post-Dispatch, 119*(86):1G–2G.

Eisenstat, S. A., & Bancroft, L. (1999). Domestic violence. *New England Journal of Medicine, 341*:887–892.

Fisher, B. S., Cullen, F. T., & Turner, M. G. (2000). *The sexual victimization of college women* (NCJ 182369). Washington, DC: National Institute of Justice, Bureau of Justice Statistics, U.S. Department of Justice.

Fox, J. A., & Zawitz, M. W. (2001). *Homicide trends in the United States.* Bureau of Justice Statistics, Washington, DC: United States Department of Justice. Retrieved from http://www.ojp.usdoj.gov/bjs/homicide/homtrnd.htm.

Frank, J. B., & Rodowski, M. J. (1999). Review of psychological issues in victims of domestic violence seen in emergency settings. *Emergency Medical Clinics of North America, 17*(3):657–677.

Greenwood, G. L., Relf, M. V., Huang, B., Pollack, L. M., et al. (2002). Battering victimization among a probability-based sample of men who have sex with men. *American Journal of Public Health, 92*(12):1964–1969.

Hart, T. C. (2003). *Violent victimization of college students* (NCJ-196143). Office of Justice Programs, U.S. Department of Justice. Retrieved from http://www.ojp.usdoj.gov/bjs/abstract/vvcs00.htm.

Herman-Giddens, M. E., Brown, G., Verbiest, S., Carlson, P. J., Hooten, E. G., Howell, E., & Butts, J. D. (1999). Underascertainment of child abuse mortality in the United States. *Journal of the American Medical Association, 282*(5):463–467.

Johnson, J. G., Cohen, P., Smailes, E. M., Kasen, S., & Brook, J. S. (2002). Television viewing and aggressive behavior during adolescence and adulthood. *Science, 295*:2468–2471.

Kleinschmidt, K. C. (1997). Elder abuse: A review. *Annals of Emergency Medicine, 30*(4):463–472.

Lamberg, L. (2001). Stalking disrupts lives, leaves emotional scars. *Journal of the American Medical Association, 286*(5):519, 522–523.

Minino, A. M., & Smith, B. L. (2001). Deaths: Preliminary data for 2000. *National Vital Statistics Report, 49*(12):1–40.

Muscari, M. (2002). Media violence: Advice for parents. *Pediatric Nursing, 28*(6):585–591.

Pears, K. C., & Capaldi, D. M. (2001). Intergenerational transmission of abuse: A two-generational prospective study of an at-risk sample. *Child Abuse and Neglect, 25*(11):1439–1461.

Rennison, C. M., & Rand, M. R. (2003). *Criminal Victimization, 2002.* Bureau of Justice Statistics (NCJ=19994). Retrieved from http://www.ojp.usdoji.gov/bjs/pub/press/cv02pr.htm.

Ristock, J. L. (2003). Exploring dynamics of abusive lesbian relationships: Preliminary analysis of a multisite, qualitative study. *American Journal of Community Psychology, 31*(3–4):329–341.

Schafer, J., Caetano, R., & Clark, C. L. (1998). Rates of intimate partner violence in the United States. *American Journal of Public Health, 88*(11):1702–1704.

Schuster, M. A., Stein, B. D., Jaycox, L. H., Collins, R. L., Marshall, G. N., Elliot, M. N., Zhiu, A. J., Kanouse, D. E., Morrison, J. L., & Berry, S. H. (2001). A national survey of stress reactions after the September 11, 2001, terrorist attacks. *New England Journal of Medicine, 345*:1507–1512.

Sygnatur, E. F., & Toscano, G. A. (2000). Work-related homicides: The facts. *Compensation and Working Conditions Online, 5*(1). Washington, DC: U.S. Department of Labor. Retrieved from http://www.bls.gov/opub/cwc/2000/Spring/art1full.pdf.

Tjaden, P., & Thoennes, N. (1998). *Prevalence, incidence, and consequences of violence against women: Findings from the National Violence Against Women Survey*. Atlanta: National Institute of Justice and the Centers for Disease Control and Prevention.

Tjaden, P., & Thoennes, N. (2000). *Extent, nature, and consequences of intimate partner violence: Findings from the National Violence Against Women Survey* (Publication NCJ 181867). Washington, DC: U.S. Department of Justice, Office of Justice Programs.

U.S. Department of Health and Human Services, Public Health Service. (1999). *Healthy People 2000 review 1998–99* (DHHS Publication No. 99-1256). Hyattsville, MD: Public Health Service.

U.S. Department of Health and Human Services, Administration for Children and Families, The Children's Bureau. (2004). *Child maltreatment 2002: Summary of key findings*. Washington, DC: U.S. Government Printing Office.

U.S. Department of Justice, Bureau of Justice Statistics. (1998). *Crime in the United States, 1998: Uniform crime reports*. Retrieved from http://www.fbi.gov/ucr/Cius_98/98crime/98cius29.pdf.

U.S. Department of Justice, Bureau of Justice Statistics. (2003). *Crime in the United States, 2002: Uniform crime reports*. Retrieved from http://fbi.gov/ucr/cius_02/html/web/index.html.

U.S. Department of Justice, Bureau of Justice Statistics. (2004). *Key crime and justice facts at a glance*. Retrieved July 1, 2004, from http://www.ojp.usdoj.gov/bjs/glance.htm.

Wathen, C. N., & MacMillan, H. L. (2003). Interventions for violence against women: Scientific review. *Journal of the American Medical Association, 289*(5):589–600.

Weiss, E. L., Longhurst, J. G., & Mazure, C. M. (1999). Childhood sexual abuse as a risk factor for depression in women: Psychosocial and neurobiological correlates. *American Journal of Psychiatry, 156*:816–828.

Willis, E., & Strasburger, V. C. (1998). Media violence. *Pediatric Clinics of North America, 45*(2):319–331.

What You'll Learn

http://healthyliving.jbpub.com

The Web site for this book offers many useful tools and is a great source for supplementary health information for both students and instructors. Visit the site at http://healthyliving.jbpub.com for information on these topics:

Pregnancy and Human Development
Managing Your Health: Genetic Counseling and Prenatal Diagnosis
Contraception
Across the Lifespan: Sexual Development

Chapter Overview

The functions and structures of the male and female reproductive systems

What happens throughout the menstrual cycle

How a woman can prepare her body for pregnancy

How a fetus develops

The changes in a pregnant woman from conception through the postpartum period

The causes of and treatments for infertility

The benefits and drawbacks of contraceptive methods

 Diversity in Health
Menopause

 Consumer Health
Home Pregnancy Tests

 Managing Your Health
*Genetic Counseling and Prenatal Diagnosis |
Enlargement of the Prostate*

Across
■ THE LIFESPAN ■

Sexual Development

Student Workbook

Self-Assessment: Contraceptive Comfort and Confidence Scale | Attitudes Toward Timing of Parenthood Scale

Changing Health Habits: Do You Want to Improve Your Reproductive Health?

Do You Know?

· *How well your contraceptive method works compared to others?*

· *What causes birth defects?*

· *When a woman is most likely to get pregnant?*

Reproductive Health

This striking photograph depicts the essence of **sexual reproduction**: the fertilization of an egg (ovum) by a sperm, a process also called conception. The photograph is color enhanced; the outside of the egg is shown as orange and the sperm as blue. A layer of cells that extend from the egg cover its surface. During the maturation of the egg, these outer cells secrete a thick gel-like material that covers the egg beneath. Together, the gel and the outer cells form a protective covering, which sperm must penetrate by means of digestive enzymes in their heads. Although it is difficult to see in this photograph, the head of only one sperm is making its way through these outer layers to ultimately fertilize this egg.

When the sperm enters the egg, it triggers the egg's final maturation. Following this process, the hereditary material from the sperm and the mature egg unite, forming a new cell—the zygote. This single cell has the potential to develop into a new individual.

Fertility, the ability to conceive a child, has been important to couples since the ancient civilizations. Fertility rites were practiced then and are still practiced in some parts of the world today. You may have seen fertility statues, with characteristically large breasts, pregnant bellies, or exaggerated penises, which are used in these ancient rites. Researchers have found that many ancient rites and customs have scientific merit. For example, if each partner of an infertile couple believes in the value of certain fertility practices, each may develop a positive emotional state, a factor that promotes fertility. In other examples, Hungarian peasant women bite their placenta after its delivery, and women in certain regions of China eat dried placenta. They believe these practices help the women remain fertile. Scientists know that the placenta contains large amounts of a hormone that is used to treat ovulatory failure. (The placenta is discussed on page 101.) This tradition, then, may be chemically beneficial to the women who practice it.

> **This striking photograph depicts the essence of sexual reproduction: the fertilization of an egg (ovum) by a sperm . . .**

Infertility is the inability of a couple to conceive a child after 1 year of unprotected sex. Couples may have reduced fertility for a variety of reasons; it is not necessarily due to "a problem" with one partner or the other. Factors that slightly impair the fertility of both sexual partners may interact to render a couple infertile. These factors include a low sperm count, a high percentage of abnormally shaped sperm, scarring in the female genital tract, structural defects of the uterus, and hormonal imbalances. Treatments for infertility are specific to the causes and include surgical procedures, hormone therapy, medication, and lifestyle changes. In addition to these therapies, physicians can harvest eggs and sperm to assist fertilization and implantation.

Whether physician-assisted, accompanied by ancient rites and customs, or accomplished with no intervention at all, fertilization is preceded by a variety of physiological processes that make it all possible, and that is where we begin this chapter.

sexual reproduction the fertilization of an egg (ovum; plural, ova) by a sperm.

testes (TES-tease) the male reproductive organs that produce sperm (the male sex cells) and testosterone (a male sex hormone).

scrotum (SKRO-tum) the sac of skin in which the testes are enclosed and hang outside the body.

epididymis (EP-ih-DID-ih-mis) a coiled tube that lies on the back of each testis and in which sperm mature.

vas deferens (VAZ DEF-er-enz) a tube that links the epididymis and the urethra, the passageway through which sperm exit the body.

■ The Male Reproductive System

The male reproductive system is structured for the development and maturation of sperm and for delivering sperm to the vagina. **Figure 5-1** is a diagram of a posterior view (a) and a lengthwise section of the male reproductive tract (b).

The Internal Organs of Sexual Reproduction

Sperm Development Sperm are produced in the **testes** (singular, testis), which hang outside the body (in the angle formed between the legs) encased in a sac of skin called the **scrotum**. The testes have two major functions: production of the sex hormone testosterone and production of sperm cells. The testes are packed with hundreds of feet of tubes (called *seminiferous tubules*) in which sperm are made.

Each day, the testes of an adult male produce hundreds of millions of sperm. Various conditions are necessary for proper sperm production. The testes must be cooler than body temperature to produce normal sperm; the position of the scrotum keeps the temperature of the testes below that of the rest of the body. It was formerly thought that wearing tight pants or tight undergarments held the testes so close to the body that the temperature within the tubules was raised. Research results show that there are no significant differences in the scrotal temperatures of men who wear tight underwear or pants and those

Figure 5-1 **The Male Reproductive System.** (a) Posterior view of the internal organs, and (b) lengthwise section (side view) of the internal organs.

POSTERIOR VIEW

SIDE VIEW

Ureter
Urinary bladder
Vas deferens
Seminal vesicle
Prostate gland
Rectum
Bulbourethral gland
Urethra
Epididymis
Anus
Testis
Penis
Glans penis
Pubis
Prostate gland
Urethra
Scrotum

(a)

(b)

who wear loose garments (Munkelwitz & Gilbert, 1998). Scientists think that blood flow near the surface of the scrotum increases when the groin temperature rises, dissipating the heat and lowering scrotal temperature.

Semen Formation After sperm are manufactured in the seminiferous tubules, they are gently moved along by the fluid in which they are suspended. The sperm move through a network of ducts to the **epididymis** (plural, epididymides). The epididymis is a coiled tube that lies on the back of each testis. Here is where the sperm mature, developing the ability to swim and to fertilize an egg.

Rhythmic contractions of the muscular walls of the epididymis slowly move the sperm to the **vas deferens** when maturation is complete. The vas deferens is a tube that links the epididymis and the urethra, the passageway through which sperm exit the body. Sperm are stored in the vas deferens until they are released from the body during **ejaculation**, their emission from the penis during **orgasm**, the peak of sexual excitement. Sperm can be stored for a few days in these ducts. If not ejaculated within that time, the sperm die and are ingested by the body's white blood cells. Newly synthesized sperm take their place. For this reason, men who have had vasectomies should not be concerned that sperm are accumulating in their bodies.

The sperm are suspended in relatively little fluid while stored in the vas deferens. A variety of organs referred to as accessory sex glands add fluid to the sperm as they exit the body during ejaculation. This fluid contains nutrients to fuel the sperm as they journey up the female reproductive tract, alkaline substances to neutralize the acidity of the vagina, and other chemicals to aid sperm movement. The secretions of the accessory sex glands (called seminal fluid) and the sperm make up the **semen**, or *ejaculate*.

During ejaculation, sperm are swiftly propelled through the vas deferens by the rhythmic contractions of its muscular walls. Just prior to the merging of the two vasa deferentia where they meet the urethra, the secretions of the paired **seminal vesicles** flow into the ejaculate. The thick secretions of the seminal vesicles add much of the volume to the ejaculate (approximately 60%) and contain the sugar fructose, which provides nutrition for the sperm.

As the ejaculate continues traveling through the male reproductive tract, the **prostate gland** adds its secretion. This single, walnut-sized gland lies just below the bladder. It surrounds the urethra and produces a milky fluid that protects sperm from the acidic environment of the woman's vagina.

During sexual arousal, the bulbourethral glands produce a mucus-like fluid that precedes the ejaculate. The *bulbourethral glands* (also called Cowper's glands), paired glands about the size of peas, are located on either side of the urethra just below the prostate. The secretions of these glands help neutralize the acidity of the male urethra and the vagina. These glands also contribute a small amount of lubrication for sexual intercourse. However, this fluid may contain sperm. For this reason (and others), the withdrawal method of birth control is not highly reliable.

The External Organs of Sexual Reproduction

The scrotum and the **penis** are the external organs of sexual reproduction (external genitals) in males (see Figure 5-1). Three columns of spongy tissue in the inner structure of the penis (Figure 5-2) become filled with blood during sexual arousal, which causes the penis to enlarge and become firm so that it can be

ejaculation the emission of semen from the penis during orgasm.

orgasm the peak of sexual excitement.

semen the ejaculate; the secretions of the accessory sex glands (called seminal fluid) and sperm.

seminal vesicles (SEM-ih-nal VES-ih-klz) paired male sex organs located near the junction of the two vasa deferentia, which produce thick fructose-containing secretions that are added to the ejaculate.

prostate gland a single, walnut-sized gland that lies just below the bladder, surrounding the urethra. The prostate produces a milky alkaline fluid that is added to the ejaculate.

penis a cylindrical external organ of sexual reproduction in males, which hangs in front of the scrotum.

Veins (constricted)
Artery (dilated)
Connective tissue
Spongy erectile tissue engorged with blood
Urethra
Spongy erectile tissue engorged with blood

(a) Section of erect penis

Veins (dilated)
Artery (constricted)
Connective tissue
Spongy erectile tissue
Urethra
Spongy erectile tissue

(b) Section of flaccid penis

Figure 5-2 **The Erect and Flaccid Penis.** (a) During an erection, blood fills the spongy erectile tissue of the penis. (b) When the blood drains from this tissue, as it does after orgasm, the penis becomes flaccid.

inserted into the vagina. During sexual intercourse the penis can become stimulated enough to result in orgasm, during which ejaculation occurs.

The Female Reproductive System

The female reproductive system is structured for the development and maturation of ova, for receiving sperm, for providing an environment in which a fertilized ovum can develop and mature, and for giving birth to the developed fetus. Figure 5-3 is a diagram of a lengthwise section of the female reproductive tract (a) and a posterior view (b).

The Internal Organs of Sexual Reproduction

Egg Development Ova are produced in the **ovaries**, which are two oval organs suspended by ligaments (a type of connective tissue) in the pelvic cavity. The almond-

Figure 5-3 The Female Reproductive System. (a) Side view (lengthwise section) of the internal organs, and (b) posterior view of the internal organs.

ovaries internal organs of female sexual reproduction within which eggs (ova) develop.

(a)

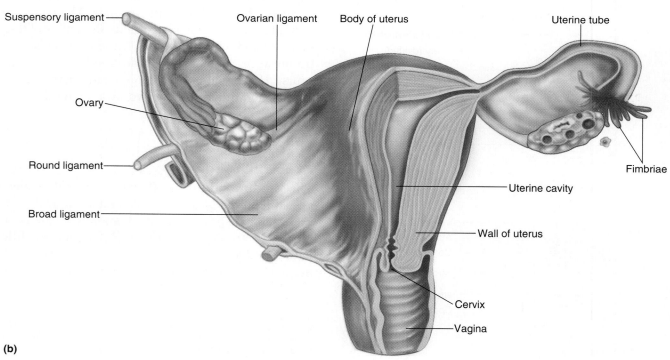

(b)

sized ovaries contain **follicles**, which are masses of cells that contain immature ova in various stages of development (Figure 5-4). Each follicle contains one ovum.

Unlike male sex cells, *all* female sex cells begin to develop before birth. This process stops before birth, and the potential eggs remain dormant throughout childhood. Each month after the onset of sexual maturity, or *puberty*, but prior to menopause, a few ova continue their development. Most of the time one ovum matures and bursts from an ovary each month; this process is **ovulation**. The ovulation of two ova can lead to the development of fraternal twins, if both are fertilized. Identical twins result when the two cells formed from the fertilized ovum's first division continue development as independent organisms. A woman's reproductive life span lasts from puberty to age 50 (on average), so only about 400 ova mature during this period.

Where Eggs Are Fertilized and Then Develop During ovulation, the egg is released into the pelvic cavity. Lying close to the ovaries are the *fimbriae*, the fringed edges of the **uterine tubes** (see Figure 5-3), also called *fallopian tubes* or *oviducts*. The uterine tubes are shaped somewhat like trumpets, with their wider ends near the ovaries and their narrower ends connected to the uterus. As the fimbriae move, they create a current of fluid that gently sweeps the ovum into the tube. If sperm are present, the uterine tube is also the site of fertilization. The fertilized ovum moves through the uterine tube as it journeys to the uterus.

The **uterus** is a hollow, muscular, pear-shaped organ that protects and nourishes the developing organism. The fertilized egg implants in the wall of the uterus and grows and develops during pregnancy, which will be discussed shortly.

The uterus opens into the vagina at the **cervix**, the narrow neck of the uterus. The cervix produces mucus.

At certain times of the month the consistency of the cervical mucus changes, facilitating sperm movement into the uterus around the time of ovulation and hindering it at other times. The **vagina** is a tube about 10 cm (approximately 4 in.) long. It receives the penis during intercourse, allows the passage of the menstrual flow, and is a birth canal.

The External Organs of Sexual Reproduction

The female external genitals (see Figure 5-3a) collectively are called the **vulva**. The vulva surrounds the vaginal opening. The urethra, the tube that carries urine from the bladder to the outside, lies anterior to the vagina.

Although the urethra is shared by the urinary and reproductive systems in men, it has no reproductive or sexual function in women. Because it is close to the anal area, the urethra can become infected by digestive tract microorganisms during sexual intercourse if these bacteria become lodged in this tube. If microorganisms are not washed from the urethra by urine, they may multiply and cause urethritis (also commonly known as cystitis, a urinary tract infection, or a bladder infection). Health care providers recommend that women who often develop such infections urinate after sexual intercourse and drink plenty of fluids to keep the urethra washed free of bacteria.

Located under a protective hood of tissue, the **clitoris** lies anterior to the urethra. This tiny structure has spongy tissue like that of the penis and becomes engorged with blood during sexual arousal. Like the penis, it has numerous nerve endings that send messages to the brain, which are interpreted as sensations of sexual pleasure when this organ is stimulated indirectly during sexual activity. (Rubbing the clitoris directly may result in discomfort.)

Extending from over the clitoris to an area behind the vagina, two thin hairless folds of skin called the **labia minora** (meaning "small lips") cover and protect the vaginal opening and urethra. Within the area bounded by the labia minora, lying near the vaginal and urethral openings and the

follicles masses of cells in the ovaries that contain immature ova (eggs) in various stages of development. Each follicle contains one ovum.

ovulation the maturation and release of an egg from an ovary, usually each month from puberty to menopause.

uterine tubes passageways that extend from each ovary to the uterus.

uterus a hollow, muscular, pear-shaped organ that protects and nourishes the embryo/fetus during development.

cervix the narrow neck of the uterus.

vagina a tube about 10 cm (approximately 4 in.) long that receives the penis during intercourse, allows the passage of the menstrual flow, and is a birth canal.

vulva the collective term for the external female genitals. The vulva surrounds the vaginal opening.

clitoris (KLIT-oh-ris) a female organ of sexual arousal. Located under a protective hood of tissue, the clitoris lies in front of the urethra.

labia minora (LAY-bee-ah my-NOR-ah) two thin, hairless folds of skin that extend from over the clitoris to an area behind the vagina. The labia minora cover and protect the vaginal opening and urethra.

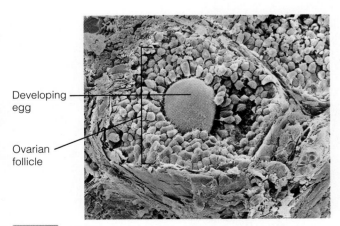

Developing egg

Ovarian follicle

Figure 5-4 A highly magnified, colorized photograph of a developing ovarian follicle with developing egg (ovum).

clitoris, are various glands that secrete lubricating substances during sexual activity. Next to these skin folds are the hairy, more rounded, and thicker **labia majora** ("large lips"). The labia majora extend forward to unite in a mound of fatty tissue called the **mons pubis**. The mons pubis provides a cushion over the pubic bone, a portion of the pelvic bones that is in front of the genitals.

The breasts are also external organs of sex and reproduction in women. Breasts primarily consist of fat and glandular tissue (Figure 5-5). Exercise will not increase breast size; it can develop only the underlying pectoral muscles. Although their major purpose is the production of milk to sustain an infant after birth, the breasts are also sensitive to sexual stimulation. The nipples contain nerve endings that are sensitive to touch;

smooth muscles in the nipples contract during sexual arousal, causing the nipples to become erect.

■ The Menstrual Cycle

Women, unlike men, experience a cyclic waxing and waning of their sex hormones each month. These hormonal changes orchestrate physiological changes in the ovaries and uterus. These changes are collectively called the **menstrual cycle**, which literally means "monthly cycle." The average length of a cycle is 28 days.

The menstrual cycle is usually described as beginning on the first day of the **menses** (menstrual period; Figure 5-6). The menses are the sloughing of the inner lining of the uterus, which is the **endometrium**. This lining develops gradually during the month, preparing for the implantation of a fertilized egg. If fertilization and implantation do not occur, the ovum dissolves and

labia majora (LAY-bee-ah mah-JOR-ah) hairy, rounded, and thick folds of skin that lie adjacent to the labia minora and extend forward to unite at the mons pubis.

mons pubis a mound of fatty tissue that lies over the pubic bone, cushioning it.

menstrual cycle (MEN-stroo-al) the monthly changes in the levels of the female sex hormones that orchestrate physiological changes in the ovaries and uterus.

menses (MEN-seez) the menstrual period; the sloughing of the endometrium.

endometrium (EN-doe-ME-tree-um) the inner lining of the uterus.

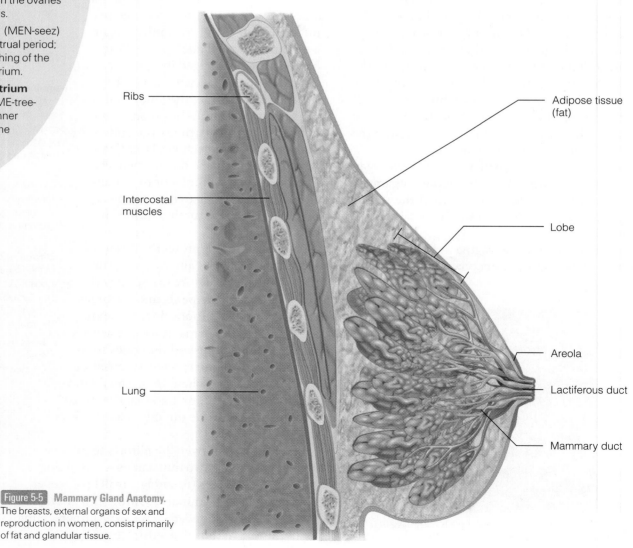

Ribs

Intercostal muscles

Lung

Adipose tissue (fat)

Lobe

Areola

Lactiferous duct

Mammary duct

Figure 5-5 **Mammary Gland Anatomy.** The breasts, external organs of sex and reproduction in women, consist primarily of fat and glandular tissue.

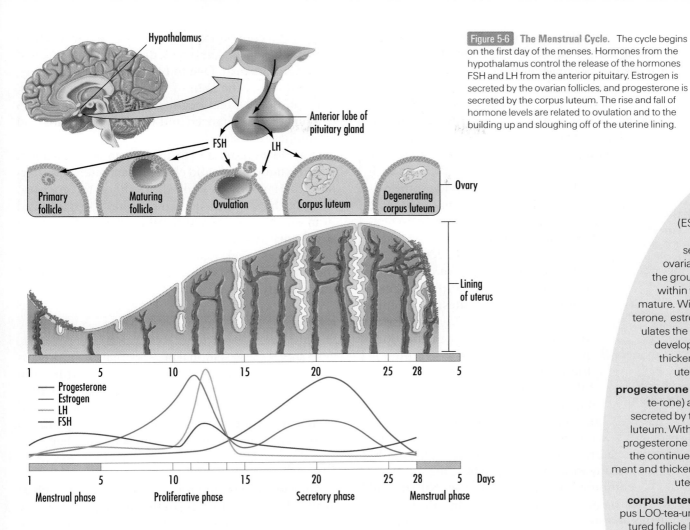

hormonal changes result in the lining being cast from the body. Each month a new lining develops.

What happens to the uterine lining is controlled by the hormones estrogen and progesterone. **Estrogen** is a hormone secreted by ovarian follicles, the groups of cells within which ova mature (see Figure 5-4); **progesterone** is secreted by the **corpus luteum**, the remnant of a follicle that has released its ovum.

Each month during her childbearing years, a woman's body prepares for a pregnancy. Usually only one ovarian follicle reaches the final stage of development in any particular cycle. About mid-cycle, hormonal changes trigger ovulation, the release of the egg from the ovary. The corpus luteum (meaning "yellow body") secretes high amounts of progesterone and lesser amounts of estrogen, which cause the uterine lining to grow, thicken, and develop a rich blood supply in preparation for the implantation of a fertilized ovum. If fertilization does not occur, the corpus luteum degenerates and stops producing hormones. Without hormonal stimulation, the uterine lining degenerates and is passed out of the body through the vagina during the menses.

If fertilization occurs, the corpus luteum does not degenerate. It produces estrogen and progesterone throughout pregnancy, maintaining the lining of the uterus. As the pregnancy develops, so does the **placenta**, a structure consisting of maternal and fetal tissues that also secretes hormones that help maintain the pregnancy. In addition, oxygen, nutrients, and wastes are exchanged between mother and fetus via the placenta (and umbilical cord).

Premenstrual Syndrome

Approximately 95% of American women in their reproductive years report mild to moderate discomfort during the week prior to menstruation as their hormonal levels drop. Up to 40% report that premenstrual symptoms such as depression, anxiety, irritability, mood swings, headaches, and bloating interfere with their relationships and their daily activities. This condition, originally termed *premenstrual tension syndrome* because

estrogen (ES-tro-jen) a hormone secreted by ovarian follicles, the groups of cells within which ova mature. With progesterone, estrogen stimulates the continued development and thickening of the uterine lining.

progesterone (pro-JES-te-rone) a hormone secreted by the corpus luteum. With estrogen, progesterone stimulates the continued development and thickening of the uterine lining.

corpus luteum (KOR-pus LOO-tea-um) the ruptured follicle left behind after ovulation.

placenta (plah-SEN-tah) a structure that develops after implantation of a fertilized ovum in the uterine wall and consists of maternal and fetal tissues that secrete hormones that help maintain the pregnancy.

most women experiencing it reported tension and anxiety among their symptoms, is now simply referred to as **premenstrual syndrome**, or **PMS**.

Approximately 5% of women report severe impairment (Daugherty, 1998; Ugarriza et al., 1998). This debilitating condition is called *premenstrual dysphoric disorder (PMDD)*. Symptoms of PMDD include clinical depression, anxiety, and irritability so severe that these problems interfere significantly with daily life. Research results provide some evidence that PMDD may be partly due to changing hormone levels of the brain neurotransmitter gamma-aminobutyric acid (GABA) (Epperson et al., 2002).

Most women with PMS are helped by one or more of the following treatments: counseling, lifestyle modification such as including exercise in their daily regimen, or medications prescribed for specific symptoms. Fluoxetine (Prozac) has shown usefulness in the treatment of PMS, acting to reduce symptoms of depression and anxiety that are linked to problems with the proper regulation of serotonin, a brain neurotransmitter. Additionally, many women are helped by using low-dose, combined oral contraceptives. Nutritional treatments include a diet low in salt, fat, caffeine, and sugar (Ugarriza et al., 1998). Taking calcium supplements has been shown to reduce the physical and psychological symptoms of PMS by almost 50% (Thys-Jacobs et al., 1998).

premenstrual syndrome (PMS) symptoms such as depression and anxiety that occur prior to the menses and that significantly interfere with daily life.

pregnancy the gestational process; the process of development of a new individual from fertilization until birth.

teratogens various environmental influences such as drugs, alcohol, viruses, and dietary deficiencies that can damage the embryo or fetus early in pregnancy.

Toxic Shock Syndrome

A disease called *toxic shock syndrome (TSS)* is associated with the menses. This disease became well known in the 1980s, when hundreds of women who used certain high-absorbency tampons during their menstrual periods were stricken. In TSS, staphylococcal (STAFF-ih-low-KAH-kul) bacteria grow in the blood-soaked tampon and in vaginal tissues, producing toxins that can enter the woman's bloodstream. Although TSS is associated with a wide variety of surgical conditions unrelated to the menses (such as skin, bone, and soft tissue infections), about two-thirds of all cases are related to tampon use during the menses. Additionally, TSS can occur from use of contraceptive diaphragms and sponges, but such occurrences are rare. Although TSS is an uncommon disease, women from 15 to 34 years old are at the highest risk. Approximately 3% of women who contract TSS die from its effects (Rivlin, 2000).

The most common symptoms of TSS are fever, muscle pain, headache, dizziness, diarrhea, vomiting, and a sunburnlike rash. One to two weeks after the onset of the disease, the skin of the palms, fingers, toes, and soles of the feet begins to peel. Generally TSS patients are hospitalized and treated with fluids and antibiotics.

To avoid contracting TSS from tampon use, women who use tampons should change them often and alternate their use with pads throughout the menses. Although high-absorbency tampons have been removed from the market, women should use only the level of absorbency they require. If during tampon use, a woman experiences fever, rash, dizziness, or diarrhea, she should remove the tampon and seek medical attention immediately.

Pregnancy and Human Development

Pregnancy is the gestational process, that is, the process of development of a new individual from fertilization until birth. What can a woman do to prepare her body for pregnancy? What can she do during the *prenatal* period, the time during which she is pregnant, to increase her chances of delivering a healthy baby?

Prepregnancy and Prenatal Care

Various **teratogens**, environmental influences such as drugs, alcohol, viruses, cigarette smoking, and dietary deficiencies, can damage the embryo or fetus. The highly sensitive periods of the developing structures of the embryo and fetus to teratogens occur primarily during the first 8 weeks after conception, possibly before a woman knows that she's pregnant. Therefore, if you are trying to become pregnant, to avoid birth defects you should take care of your body as if you were pregnant. The Analyzing Health-Related Information feature on page 127 discusses folic acid (folate), a B vitamin critical to proper neural tube development of the embryo. Table 5-1 lists various teratogens and their detrimental effects on the embryo/fetus.

A woman preparing for pregnancy should have a medical checkup to determine if her level of antibodies against rubella (German measles) is sufficient. She should also be screened for sexually transmitted infections (STIs), especially AIDS, and should avoid changing the cat's litter box to protect herself from contracting toxoplasmosis (infection with a microscopic parasite found in cat feces). Additionally, a woman preparing for pregnancy should seek her health care provider's advice regarding the use of medications.

It is important that a woman contemplating pregnancy eat a well-balanced and nutritious diet to enter

Table 5-1 Selected Teratogens Known to Cause Birth Defects

Teratogen	Explanation
Maternal Infectious or Noninfectious Disease	
Cytomegalovirus	A herpes-type virus that can cross the placenta and infect the embryo. Found in about 1% of newborns. Most defects affect the nervous system. Risk of brain damage is 50% after infection early in pregnancy. One in 10 affected fetuses die.
Diabetes mellitus	Risk of major malformations is about 18%. Heart malformations and neural tube defects are most frequent. Risk is greatest in uncontrolled or poorly controlled diabetes.
Phenylketonuria (PKU) untreated	Excess phenylalanine, not the defective gene, causes birth defects such as mental retardation and malformations of the heart.
Rubella	The German measles virus can cross the placenta and infect the embryo. Infection during the first 3 months of pregnancy is likely to result in abnormalities such as deafness, heart defects, and mental retardation.
Drugs, Other Chemicals, and Radiation	
Alcohol (chronic alcoholism—6 oz. or more per day—constitutes high risk)	Main characteristics of the birth defects caused by maternal chronic alcoholism are growth deficiency, hyperactivity, distractibility, small head, underdevelopment of the brain, and mental retardation. Moderate maternal drinking can affect the IQ and learning ability of offspring.
Anticonvulsant medication	Probability of birth defects varies with medications, dosage, and stage of pregnancy.
Chemotherapeutic agents	Drugs used to treat cancer can also harm the embryo or fetus.
Cocaine	Some possible birth defects from cocaine use during pregnancy are bleeding in the brain, death of part of the brain tissue, underdeveloped head and brain, prematurity, and seizures.
Diethylstilbestrol (DES)	A drug formerly prescribed for women who were in danger of having a miscarriage. This drug affected some of their female offspring, causing unusual vaginal, cervical, and uterine changes beginning in adolescence. Increased risk for developing a certain type of vaginal and cervical cancer.
Ionizing radiation	Extremely high exposure to x rays or exposure to radiation used in cancer therapy can affect the embryo or fetus and result in an underdeveloped head and brain.
Accutane	This synthetic form of vitamin A is used to treat certain types of acne. Birth defects that may result from use during pregnancy (when taken by mouth) include malformations of the ear, brain, and heart. Health care providers also suggest avoiding megadoses (more than 10,000 I.U.) of vitamin A during pregnancy.
Thalidomide	A drug taken for morning sickness in the 1960s. Taking this drug between 20 days and 36 days after conception resulted in major anatomical deformities of the limbs and heart.

this critical period with sufficient nutrient stores and blood levels to meet the needs of the pre-embryo and embryo before the placenta is established. (The body has both short-term and long-term nutrient storage capabilities.) Chapter 9 describes some nutritional guidelines for a prepregnancy diet; a woman should also consult her health care practitioner regarding proper nutrition during pregnancy. A pregnant woman should not assume that she is "eating for two" in the sense that she should double her food intake. Her need for calories, protein, and calcium are only somewhat greater than her prepregnancy needs. Excessive weight gain during pregnancy may mean excess body fat retained long after pregnancy. Although certain nutrients are extremely important (such as folate, which helps prevent neural tube defects), a pregnant woman

should take only the vitamin supplements that her health care provider prescribes. Some nutrients, such as vitamin A, are teratogens in certain quantities.

It is critical that a woman avoid drinking alcohol, smoking cigarettes, and taking any drugs (unless they have been prescribed) when preparing for pregnancy and during pregnancy. Chronic alcohol consumption can cause fetal alcohol syndrome, which can result in a variety of birth defects, including mental retardation, growth deficiency, and hyperactivity. Smoking a pack or more of cigarettes per day can result in a low-birth-weight baby who is weak, has a reduced brain size, and is vulnerable to illness. If a pregnant woman is addicted to drugs, her baby will be born addicted as well. In addition, she is more likely to experience complications during pregnancy and have a baby with severe

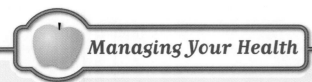

Genetic Counseling and Prenatal Diagnosis

You and your spouse have decided it's time to have a baby. You are both worried that a genetic disease may run in one of your families. (A genetic disease is caused by problems with the hereditary, or genetic, material.) Also, you're worried about the risk of birth defects because "mom" will be far past age 35 when she gives birth, and the likelihood of genetic diseases is higher than at younger ages. What can you both do to ensure the genetic health of your baby?

Your first step might be to discuss your concerns with an obstetrician/gynecologist. Your health care practitioner may send both of you to a genetic counselor to explore the incidence of genetic disease in your families and to determine the probability of you and your spouse having a child with a genetic disorder.

There are many reasons to seek genetic counseling. Parents with a child who has a genetic disease often choose genetic counseling to determine the probability that future children will be affected. In populations at high risk for certain genetic diseases, such as African Americans and sickle cell anemia, or Ashkenazi Jews and Tay-Sachs disease, families or prospective parents may visit genetics centers to undergo screening tests. Once screening has been done and the carriers and noncarriers of the disease have been identified, the genetic counselor can advise them of their probability of passing on problem genes to children.

After the baby is conceived and prior to birth, various techniques are available to tell for sure if the baby is affected with a wide variety of disorders. Tests performed on the fetus (or related tissues) to determine its health are called prenatal diagnoses. Methods that are frequently used are ultrasound, amniocentesis, and chorionic villus sampling (CVS). These methods can detect many, but not all, fetal abnormalities.

Ultrasound scanning, or sonography, is a common, painless, safe, and relatively inexpensive procedure for prenatal diagnosis that has been used since the 1960s. Ultrasound uses high-frequency sound waves to visualize the fetus, which can be seen as early as 7 weeks of development. The ultrasound probe is moved over the woman's abdomen. Sound waves enter the uterus and bounce off fetal structures in ways that reflect their density and makeup. The reflected waves are projected on a monitor screen (Figure 5-A), and their patterns are interpreted by a health care provider. Using this technique, a health care provider can detect many structural abnormalities, estimate the age of the fetus, confirm if multiple fetuses are present, and confirm fetal position. In addition, ultrasound is often used to help guide needle placement in amniocentesis, fetal blood sampling, and chorionic villus sampling.

Figure 5-A **Ultrasound in Pregnancy.** The ultrasound probe produces sound waves that bounce off fetal tissues. As the probe is moved across a pregnant woman's abdomen, images are visualized on a screen that provide information about the position, size, and physical condition of the fetus.

Another common type of prenatal diagnosis is **amniocentesis,** which was developed in the 1960s and was widely used by the 1970s. Amniocentesis involves the removal of some of the amniotic fluid that surrounds the fetus. This watery fluid protects the baby from jarring movements and contains waste products and some cells from the fetus. Geneticists observe these cells to determine whether the fetus will be born with a genetic abnormality. In addition, medical technicians can perform tests on the fluid to determine the presence of substances that are indicators of various conditions, such as certain neural tube defects and Rh disease (a blood incompatibility problem between mother and fetus).

To extract some amniotic fluid and cells from around the fetus, the physician inserts a thin, long needle through the abdominal and uterine walls of the mother until the needle pierces the amniotic sac (Figure 5-B). (The physician guides the needle using ultrasound so that it will not injure the fetus, and anesthetizes the abdominal wall with a local anesthetic.) After the fluid is withdrawn, the cells must be grown, or cultured, which takes approximately 4 weeks. This technique is now performed as early as 11 weeks of gestation, but is routinely performed between 15 and 18 weeks, so diagnosis is generally completed by the 19th to 22nd week. Physicians are studying even earlier amniocentesis testing. This procedure is considered safe; the risk of miscarriage due to amniocentesis is 0.25% to 0.5% (1 in 200 to 400).

Fetal blood sampling was developed in the 1970s. Extracting blood from the fetus is risky; however, blood can be withdrawn safely from the umbilical vein. With this technique, physicians can screen infants for various blood disorders such as sickle cell anemia and hemophilia. The risk of miscarriage with this technique is approximately 2% (2 in 100). This technique is least risky when performed between weeks 18 and 21 of pregnancy.

Amniocentesis

Uterus
Amniotic sac
Placenta

Centrifuge

Amniotic fluid withdrawn from cavity

Cells from amniotic fluid

Cell culture
- Analyzed for biochemical or chromosomal defects

Figure 5-B   Amniocentesis. In the amniocentesis procedure, a long, thin needle is used to pierce the mother's abdominal wall and uterus and withdraw amniotic fluid. Free fetal cells are found in this fluid and can be analyzed for the fetus's gender, age, and indications of chromosomal abnormalities.

Chorionic villus sampling was also developed around 1970 but came into wide use in the 1980s. The chorion is the outermost of the fetal membranes (Figure 5-C) that facilitate the exchange of nutrients, gases, and other materials such as waste products between the fetus and the mother.

Bladder   Chorionic villi   Placenta   Amniotic sac   Abdominal wall

Thin tube   Cervix   Fetus at 9-11 weeks

Figure 5-C   Chorionic Villus Sampling. A tube, or catheter, is inserted into the vagina, up through the cervix, and into the uterus. This tube is used to collect pieces of chorionic villi, which are part of the outer fetal tissue called the chorion (not part of the fetus). These cells are analyzed for chromosomal abnormalities.

The umbilical cord extends from the fetus to the chorion. Fingerlike projections called villi (singular, villus) extend from the chorion into maternal tissues at the placenta, the pancake-shaped part of the chorion that joins mother and fetus. In this way the blood of the fetus, circulating through blood vessels in the chorion and its villi, comes into close contact (but does not mix) with maternal blood vessels. To perform CVS, a physician inserts a thin tube or a needle into the vagina and up into the uterus. The instrument vacuums up a tiny sample of villi. Although this technique has the advantages of early testing (weeks 9 to 11) and quick analysis of cells (no culturing is needed), the risk of miscarriage is 2% to 4% (2 to 4 in 100). Additionally, in the early 1990s medical researchers discovered that CVS can cause birth defects of the limbs. If this procedure is conducted prior to 10 weeks of pregnancy, the risk is 20%, but drops to 7% at 10 weeks or more of gestation. The defects when CVS is performed at 10 weeks or later involve only the fingers or toes.

Today, using ultrasound to guide them, physicians are able to sample fetal skin and certain other tissues. In addition, some conditions can be treated before birth. Amazingly, the fetus can be given a blood transfusion while in the uterus. Open fetal surgery, a highly risky but potentially life-saving procedure, is new and experimental at this time. The choices that remain are terminating the pregnancy or carrying the fetus to term. If the second choice is made, prenatal diagnosis is extremely helpful to ensure that the baby receives the best possible medical care for its condition, beginning from its first breath.

amnio-centesis a prenatal test performed generally between the 15th and 18th weeks of gestation, in which some of the amniotic fluid that surrounds the fetus is removed and studied to determine whether the fetus has a genetic abnormality.

chorionic villus sampling a prenatal test performed generally between the 9th and 11th weeks of gestation, in which some of the fetal extra-embryonic tissue is removed and analyzed to determine whether the fetus has a genetic abnormality.

birth defects. Taking drugs and drinking alcohol occasionally can also damage the embryo or fetus. No safe level of these teratogens has been determined.

Women older than 35 years of age have a higher risk of having babies with Down syndrome (a genetic abnormality resulting in mental retardation) than younger women. Older women may choose to have diagnostic tests such as amniocentesis and chorionic villus sampling during pregnancy to detect possible genetic disease or other abnormalities in the fetus. In addition, couples often seek genetic counseling before becoming pregnant. If anyone in a couple's family has a genetic disease, seeking genetic counseling may be prudent. (The Managing Your Health essay "Genetic Counseling and Prenatal Diagnosis" discusses prenatal tests and counseling.)

pre-embryo the first 2 weeks of gestational development.

embryo the third through the eighth weeks of gestational development.

fetus the 9th through 38th weeks of gestational development.

Many women want to know if exercising during pregnancy will hurt the fetus. Generally, if a woman was exercising before she became pregnant, she can continue exercising while she is pregnant. However, a health care provider may suggest modifications in a pregnant woman's workout regimen. Also, some health care providers recommend that their previously sedentary patients start a mild exercise program to help them become stronger and develop stamina for the birth process. Chapter 11 discusses exercising and pregnancy in more detail in its Across the Lifespan section.

Healthy Living Practices

- Women preparing for pregnancy should have a medical checkup, eat a well-balanced and nutritious diet, and avoid drinking alcohol, smoking cigarettes, or using other drugs.
- Women and men concerned about the possibility of passing a genetic condition on to their offspring can seek genetic counseling when considering pregnancy.

Determining If You or Your Partner Is Pregnant

How do you know if you or your partner is pregnant? By noticing certain physical signs, you may become aware of this condition. A pregnant woman will not menstruate, so a missed menstrual period may be the first sign. However, a pregnant woman may experience *implantation bleeding* about a week before the expected time of the menstrual period. This small amount of blood flow from the uterus occurs when the fertilized ovum nestles into the uterine wall. Additionally, the breasts may feel sore, she may feel nauseated at certain times during the day or all day, and she may feel tired, moody, or both. These signs are bodily reactions to changes in hormone levels during pregnancy.

If a woman suspects that she is pregnant, she may choose to conduct a home pregnancy test or visit her gynecologist/obstetrician for such a test. The Consumer Health feature "Home Pregnancy Tests" on page 110 discusses how pregnancy tests work and provides guidelines for conducting such a test.

If a woman has missed more than one menstrual period and is certain that she is not pregnant, she should see her health care provider. *Amenorrhea* (ah-MEN-oh-REE-ah), or abnormal stoppage of the menses, is most often caused by stress, weight loss, or strenuous exercise regimens. However, it can have more serious causes, such as hormonal imbalances or tumorous growths.

Pregnancy and Fetal Development

Pregnancy usually lasts 38 weeks, or approximately 9 months. The delivery date is calculated to be 40 weeks from a woman's last menstrual period because *conception* (fertilization) usually occurs in the middle of the cycle. Typically pregnancy is described in terms of trimesters, or 3-month periods, during which certain developmental events take place. (Because months are more than 4 weeks, the month-to-week correlations given here are approximate.)

The first trimester is a crucial time of development when all the organ systems of the body are forming and becoming functional. Cells in the embryo migrate to key developmental positions, shaping the individual as it takes on a human form. In contrast, the second and third trimesters are periods of growth and refinement of the organ systems. Figure 5-7 through Figure 5-11 depict the development of the **pre-embryo** (the first 2 weeks of development), the **embryo** (weeks 3 through 8), and the **fetus** (weeks 9 through 38). Figure 5-7 also describes ectopic pregnancy, implantation of the embryo outside of the uterus.

While the fetus is developing, changing, and growing over 9 months, changes also take place in the mother's body. Figure 5-12 summarizes these changes. In addition, the pregnant woman may experience nausea, vomiting, frequent urination, leg cramps, vaginal discharge, fatigue, and constipation during the first trimester. Nausea, vomiting, and leg cramps (if present) usually subside by the second trimester.

Four-cell stage

Blastocyst

Uterus

FERTILIZATION

Uterine
(fallopian)
tube

Corpus luteum

IMPLANTATION
OF BLASTOCYST

OVULATION

Ovary

Endometrial
wall

Figure 5-7 **Fertilization and Implantation.** The first event in human development is fertilization, which takes place in the uterine (fallopian) tube. The fertilized ovum begins to divide as it moves along the tube to the uterus, and is now referred to as a pre-embryo. At 4 days after fertilization, the developing ball of cells begins to fill with fluid, a stage of pre-embryonic development termed the *blastocyst*. Approximately 6 days after fertilization, the blastocyst implants in the back wall of the uterus. During implantation, the embryo attaches firmly to the inner lining of the uterus. This illustration shows the journey of the fertilized ovum from the fallopian tube to the uterus. Occasionally implantation takes place outside of the uterus, a condition known as ectopic pregnancy. Pre-embryos may implant on an ovary, on the intestine, or in a fallopian tube. All ectopic pregnancies endanger the mother's life.

Figure 5-8 **Human Embryo between 4 and 5 Weeks of Development.** As the pregnancy moves into the third week, the pre-embryo is only one-tenth of an inch long. The flattened pre-embryo develops into a cylindrical embryo. Some of the organs, such as the heart, begin to develop. This 4.5-week-old embryo has established the beginnings of most of the major organ systems of the body. Its C-shaped body has a featureless head, a middle with the heart and liver bulging from the body, and a tail. During the fifth week, the embryo doubles in length from 4 mm (3/16″) to 8 mm (3/8″). The brain grows rapidly. Wrists, fingers, and ears begin to form during the sixth week of development. Although development has been rapid, growth has not. By the end of the sixth week, the embryo is a mere half-inch long.

Figure 5-9 **Human Fetus about 11 to 12 Weeks of Development.** During the seventh week, eyelids begin to cover the eyes, and the face begins to look somewhat human. By the eighth week, the last week in the embryonic period, the embryo grows to about an inch. Most of the body systems are functional by this time. The fetal period begins at week 9, lasts throughout the rest of the pregnancy, and is characterized by growth and functional maturation of the organs. During weeks 9 through 13 (the third month), facial features become more well developed, with eyelids completely covering the eyes and then fusing shut. (The eyes can be seen through the thin eyelids.) The genitals begin to develop, and the heart is now a four-chambered structure.

Figure 5-10 **Human Fetus about 5 Months (20 Weeks) of Development.** The second trimester comprises the fourth, fifth, and sixth months of development, or weeks 14 through 26. The organs that developed during the first trimester mature and grow during this trimester. As the fourth month passes, the genitals become fully formed. The sensory organs nearly finish their development and refinements of body structures occur. The mother becomes aware of fetal movements around the fifth month of pregnancy, the stage of development of the fetus in the photo. By the end of the fifth month, as fat deposits are laid down, the fetus begins to look more like a baby. Only 12 inches long and weighing 1 pound, it probably could not survive on its own. However, if born by the end of the sixth month, the fetus has a chance of surviving with special medical care.

Figure 5-11 **Human Fetus Nearly Full Term—8 to 9 Months.** During the third trimester, months seven through nine or weeks 27 through 38, the fetus primarily gains weight. Its lungs develop more fully, eyelids open, and the nervous system undergoes further development. However, the nervous system is not fully developed and its maturation continues after birth. At the end of the third trimester, the average fetus weighs about 7 ½ pounds and is 20 inches long.

Anterior pituitary enlarges (increases secretory activity)

Patches of pigment appear on face (brown-pink)

Thyroid gland enlarges (increases metabolism)

Breathing becomes more frequent

Heart enlarges slightly

Cortex of adrenal glands enlarges

Pigmented streaks appear on breasts (brown-pink)

Breasts enlarge

Nipples darken, enlarge, become erectile

Areolas darken (brown) and enlarge

Skin darkens (brown) around areolas

Diaphragm rises

Pigmented (brown-pink) streaks appear on skin of abdomen

Uterus enlarges 50 to 60 times original size

Brown line appears in center of abdomen

Brown pigment appears around vulva and striations on thighs

Figure 5-12 **A Summary of the Physical Changes That Take Place during Pregnancy.** (*Left*) The unpregnant female body; (*right*) changes that appear by 30 weeks of fetal development.

Table 5-2   Pregnancy Problems and Symptoms

Name of Condition (Alternative or former names)	Definition	Cause	Symptoms	Treatment
Ectopic pregnancy	Fertilized egg implants outside the uterus. Majority occur in the uterine tube.	Problems with anatomy of uterine tubes, possibly due to pelvic inflammatory disease or uterine surgery. Use of IUD.	Loss of menses, pelvic or abdominal pain, abnormal vaginal bleeding.	Surgery to remove embryo. Nonsurgical treatments may be used in certain situations.
Pregnancy-induced hypertension [PIH] (Preeclampsia) (Toxemia of pregnancy)	A group of metabolic disturbances.	Unknown.	High blood pressure, water retention, and an excess of protein in the urine, occurring in the third trimester. Primarily a disease of first pregnancy. Occurs with higher frequency in adolescent women and those older than 35 years.	Bed rest. Medication to reduce blood pressure and prevent seizures. Delivery usually cures the condition.
Eclampsia	An extension of PIH to the point of seizure, coma, or both.	Unknown.	Increase in blood pressure from that in PIH, abdominal pain, blurry vision, headache, shakiness. May occur in third trimester or postpartum.	Convulsions and high blood pressure are treated with medication. Delivery takes place as soon as patient is stabilized.
Diabetes mellitus associated with pregnancy (Gestational diabetes mellitus [GDM])	A metabolic disorder that leads to high glucose levels in the blood (see Chapter 9). In pregnancy, poor control of blood glucose levels can lead to fetal abnormalities.	Hormonal changes of pregnancy often result in a display of diabetes in women with risk factors for the disease.	See Table 9-3. Women with risk factors for diabetes (obesity and family history) should be screened prior to and during pregnancy for this disease.	Control of blood sugar level with diet and/or insulin injections.

Sources: Rivlin, M. E., & Martin, R. W. (Eds.). (2000). *Manual of clinical problems in obstetrics and gynecology* (5th ed). Philadelphia, PA: Lippincott, Williams & Wilkins. Zuspan, F. P., & Quilligan, E. J. (1998). *Handbook of obstetrics, gynecology, and primary care.* St. Louis, MO: Mosby.

At that time, additional changes may take place. In her last two trimesters, a pregnant woman may experience swelling of the legs and feet, varicose veins, backache, heartburn, and shortness of breath, in addition to continuing vaginal discharge, frequent urination, fatigue, and constipation. Table 5-2 lists various problem conditions that may occur during pregnancy.

The Birth Process

No one is certain what events signal the beginning of labor, the process of childbirth. Labor is also called parturition and takes place in three stages: cervical dilation, fetal delivery, and placental delivery. The birth process normally takes about 13 hours for the woman who is giving birth for the first time. In women who have previously given birth, the time shortens considerably and is about 8 hours.

Two main events occur during dilation: rhythmic contractions of the uterine muscles cause the cervix (the opening of the uterus) to dilate (widen) and to efface (thin out). In the nonpregnant state, the cervix is hard and tubelike with an extremely narrow opening. During the first stage of labor, the cervix becomes soft. The opening widens and the tissue stretches so that by the end of the first stage of labor the cervical opening is $3\frac{1}{2}$ in. to 4 in. wide and the tubular cervix no longer exists as such—it flattens and becomes continuous with the lower portion of the uterus (Figure 5-13). During this time (or prior to labor in some cases) the amniotic sac ruptures

labor (parturition) (PAR-too-RISH-un) the process of childbirth.

Home Pregnancy Tests

Most pregnancy tests rely on the detection of the hormone **human chorionic gonadotropin (hCG)**. This hormone is produced by embryonic tissues destined to become the placenta, the organ that allows the exchange of nutrients, gases, and wastes between the fetus and a pregnant woman. Pregnancy tests to detect hCG can be conducted on either blood or urine. Urine tests are most frequently used to detect hCG because urine is easier to collect than blood. This is the type of test in home test kits.

The way pregnancy tests work is that hCG binds with specific antibodies in the test. If a woman is *not* pregnant, hCG will not be present in her urine, binding will not occur, and the test will be negative. If a woman *is* pregnant, hCG will be present in her urine, binding will occur, and the test will be positive.

Home pregnancy tests are easy to use. These tests contain either a plastic stick with an absorbent part that is placed in the urine flow, or a plastic device with an opening containing absorbent material into which drops of urine are placed. While a woman waits, the urine moves through the absorbent material inside either type of device, and the

hCG (if present) attaches to an antibody that has a color label such as blue or red. The hCG-antibody complex then moves to another window where it binds to a second antibody attached to the absorbent material in either a line or a circle. Therefore, if hCG is present in a woman's urine, a colored line or circle appears, indicating that both antibodies have attached to the hCG and that the woman is pregnant.

It is important to follow the directions of a home test carefully and wait the prescribed length of time to "read" the result. Testing the first urine of the day is best because hCG is most concentrated in the first urine. However, today's home pregnancy testing kits are quite sensitive and you can use any urine of the day. You may conduct a home test on the day of a missed period or after that time; the results are 99% accurate. Be sure to check the expiration date on the package and only use tests that have not expired. Virtually all tests marketed today in the United States are reliable, but ask your pharmacist for help if you are unsure which test to choose. A woman who has a positive test should see her health care provider immediately for a confirmatory test (false positives occur rarely) and appropriate prenatal care.

---

human chorionic gonadotropin (hCG) in a pregnant woman, a hormone produced by embryonic tissues destined to become the placenta. Pregnancy tests rely on the detection of this hormone in the blood.

Braxton-Hicks contractions false labor; preparatory contractions that are not a part of labor.

breech birth a delivery in which the baby presents feet or buttocks first instead of the usual head-first position.

episiotomy (eh-PIZ-ee-OT-oh-me) a cut in the tissue surrounding the vaginal opening to widen it during a vaginal delivery so that the surrounding skin and tissues will be less likely to tear.

(the water breaks), releasing the amniotic fluid. (This fluid cushions the fetus during development.) The baby must be born within 24 hours of the rupture, or serious infection could occur.

In the beginning of her labor, a woman's uterine contractions may last for 30 seconds and be 15 to 20 minutes apart. As labor progresses, the contractions become stronger, longer, and more closely spaced. By the end of the first stage of labor, during a period called *transition*, contractions occur every 1 to 2 minutes and last up to a minute each.

Some women experience preparatory contractions that are not a part of labor, which are called **Braxton-Hicks contractions**, or *false labor*. False labor contractions can be distinguished from the contractions of true labor in that they occur irregularly, the intervals between contractions do not shorten, and the contractions do not increase in strength.

A woman experiencing these contractions should consult her physician to confirm that she is not in labor.

During the second stage of labor, the baby is born. The average time for this stage is 30 to 60 minutes. Uterine contractions continue and move the baby into the birth canal (vagina). The woman pushes and bears down, aiding this process. The head usually appears first, but some babies are born in the breech position, feet or buttocks first. A **breech birth** is a more complicated delivery than a head-first delivery and may require surgical removal of the baby through the abdominal wall—a cesarean section. During a vaginal delivery, the physician may perform an **episiotomy**, making a cut in the tissue surrounding the vaginal opening to widen the opening. (This cut is usually made in the direction of the anus.) Without this procedure, the skin and surrounding tissues may sustain more damage and heal with more difficulty than surgically cut tissue.

After the baby is born, its nose and mouth are cleared of mucus by suctioning. The umbilical cord is clamped in two places and cut between the clamps to prevent bleeding. Health care practitioners assess the baby's

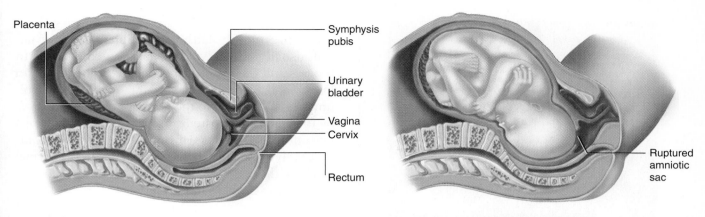

Placenta

Symphysis pubis

Urinary bladder

Vagina
Cervix

Rectum

(a) Early first-stage labor

Ruptured amniotic sac

(b) Later first-stage labor: the transition

Placenta

(c) Early second-stage labor

Placenta

Uterus

Umbilical cord

(d) Third-stage labor: delivery of placenta

Figure 5-13   The Stages of Labor.   (a) The position of the fetus at the beginning of labor. (b) Dilation, the cervix (the opening to the uterus) widens and thins. (c) Expulsion, the baby is born. (d) Placental delivery.

ability to adjust to life outside the uterus at 1 minute and then 5 minutes after birth.

Within 15 and 30 minutes after delivery of the baby, the uterus continues to contract, separating the fetal placental tissues from maternal tissues. During this third stage of labor, the placenta is expelled from the uterus. Figure 5-13 summarizes the birth process, showing the three stages of labor (a–d).

Circumcision

Although few data are available, they show that from about 45% to 70% of male newborns are circumcised in the United States (American Academy of Pediatrics, 1999). In some groups, such as followers of the Jewish and Islamic faiths, circumcision rates approximate 100% because the procedure is practiced for religious and cultural reasons. *Circumcision* is a surgical procedure to remove the foreskin of the penis, which is a fold of skin covering the end of the penis. The photos in Figure 5-14 show both an uncircumcised and a circumcised penis.

Existing scientific evidence demonstrates potential medical benefits of newborn male circumcision, such as lowered risk of urinary tract infections, especially in infants younger than 1 year of age, lowered risk of penile cancer, and lowered risk of STIs, especially syphilis and HIV infection. Circumcision may also reduce the prevalence and transmission of human papillomavirus, which is linked to the development of cervical cancer (Adami & Trichopoulos, 2002). However, the policy statement of the American Academy of Pediatrics notes that, in general, the differences in risk are small and the data are not sufficient to recommend routine circumcision of male newborns at this time. Additionally, circumcision has some risks as does any surgical procedure, though complications are rare and usually minor. Therefore, the AAP suggests that parents, in conjunction with their pediatricians, decide what is in the best interest of the child. If the decision is made for circumcision, the Academy strongly recommends giving the infant pain relief medication (AAP, 1999).

(a)

(b)

Figure 5-14 | **Circumcision.** (a) Uncircumcised penis. (b) Circumcised penis.

The Postpartum Period

The *postpartum period* is the 6 weeks after childbirth during which a mother's body returns to its prepregnant state. One of the areas of the body affected greatly, of course, is the reproductive system. The uterus returns nearly to its original size. Within 2 weeks, the cervical opening closes to a slit, and tissue damage that occurred to it during the birth process heals. The vagina, bruised and swollen from the newborn traveling through it, returns to normal after about 3 weeks. The episiotomy and any torn tissues surrounding the vaginal opening heal within 1 week.

A variety of other organ systems and tissues in the mother's body change during pregnancy and return to their prepregnant state during the postpartum period and beyond. For example, muscles in the pelvic region gradually regain their original tone, but this process may take up to 6 months. During the first few days after delivery, a woman may have trouble urinating due to bruising of the bladder, the effects of anesthetics, and swelling of the ureters, tubes that lead from the

kidneys to the bladder. The ureters may remain swollen for up to 3 months, although problems with urination usually last only a few days. During the birth process and the expulsion of the placenta, a woman loses blood. Her blood plasma and red blood cell volumes usually return to the normal nonpregnant state by the end of the postpartum period, but may take a few additional weeks. Hormonal changes are comparatively rapid after delivery; some return to normal levels by the end of the first postpartum day, but others take 1 to 2 weeks to normalize.

Many women experience *postpartum depression*, especially in the week after delivery. Approximately 40% to 85% of women experience mild depression, often referred to as "the baby blues." This mild form of depression, often accompanied by mood swings, is thought to be a result of the physical and mental stresses of childbirth, as well as the variety of physical (including hormonal) changes that take place during that time. Symptoms include periods of crying, sleep disturbances, loss of appetite, and confusion. The blues usually subside during the second postpartum week. Severe depression is rare (Glass & Bruner, 2000). Physicians usually recommend that a woman consult her health care provider to discuss treatment with a mild sedative if she is experiencing sleep problems, since a lack of sleep may contribute to her depression.

At the beginning of the postpartum period, many women also start breastfeeding their infants. The benefits of breastfeeding are discussed in the Across the Lifespan section of Chapter 9.

Healthy Living Practices

- If you are female and have missed a period, are nauseated at times, feel tired often, and are experiencing moodiness, check with a health care practitioner; you may be pregnant.
- A home pregnancy test can be used on the day of a missed period or thereafter to determine pregnancy. A health care practitioner can provide laboratory testing to confirm pregnancy.

■ Infertility

Infertility is the inability of a couple to conceive a child after 1 year of unprotected sex and affects approximately 10% of the U.S. population (Mitchell, 2002). Some infertility experts suggest that couples wait for 2 years before seeking help for infertility. Infertility is not necessarily due to "a problem" with one partner or the other. Factors that slightly impair the fertility of both sexual partners may interact to render a couple infertile.

One reason for male infertility is faulty sperm production. In normal sperm production, the semen contains approximately 80 to 120 million sperm per milliliter (ml). Since the ejaculate volume ranges from 2 to 8 ml, slightly less than a teaspoon to nearly 2 teaspoons, the total sperm ejaculated ranges from about 200 million to 800 million. A sperm count lower than 20 million sperm per ml, 40 million to 160 million total in the ejaculate, may impair fertility.

In addition to a low sperm count, a high percentage (usually more than 40%) of abnormally shaped sperm can affect male fertility. Abnormally shaped sperm such as those with two heads or abnormally shaped heads or tails (Figure 5-15) may not be able to swim well. These defects may reduce their chances of reaching the egg.

Male infertility is often related to a variety of environmental factors or diseases. Cigarette smoking, chronic alcoholism, various medications, and prolonged illnesses with accompanying fever all affect sperm production. Infection with the mumps virus can render a man sterile.

A man can also have a problem with sperm transport, which can cause infertility even if the sperm count is adequate for conception. Infections caused by certain STIs can block the vas deferens and injure these tubes. Erectile dysfunction is also a common cause of infertility if a man is unable to ejaculate.

There are a variety of causes of infertility in women. In some instances, the vagina cannot be penetrated due to an intact hymen or to vaginismus. Some abnormalities in the structure of the vagina, which may be present at birth or caused by scarring from STIs or trauma, allow only partial penetration. Unknowingly complicating the problem, couples having trouble with penetration often use lubricants that kill sperm. For example, one type of the popular K-Y jelly has spermicidal properties.

Once sperm travel up the vagina, they must pass through the cervix to reach the uterus and the fallopian tubes. Secretion of mucus by the cervix is important to sperm motility. Infection can damage the glands that secrete mucus or result in the presence of white blood cells. The properties of this mucus also change if a woman has an estrogen deficiency. Such changes in the quality and quantity of mucus can impair the sperm's ability to reach an egg.

Structural defects of the uterus do not usually cause infertility; usually such problems result in repeated miscarriage. However, the uterine (fallopian) tubes can be another fertility trouble spot. Infection with *N. gonorrhoeae* or *C. trachomatis* (see Chapter 14) can result in severe tissue destruction, completely blocking the tubes and causing sterility. Infections of other origins, such as from appendicitis or IUD complications, may result in less severe blockage. Pregnancy may occur, but the risk is increased for ectopic pregnancy. Endometriosis, the growth of abnormal tissue in the abdomen, is another cause of sterility, ectopic pregnancy, or both.

The ovaries can be the source of impaired fertility. Hormonal imbalances can interfere with ovulation, and a mumps infection, radiation, and chemotherapy can damage the ovaries. Additionally, function of the ovaries declines as a woman ages, reducing her ability to conceive. Dietary deficiencies and strenuous exercise, such as jogging 10 or more miles per week, have also been shown to affect ovary function.

infertility
inability to conceive a child after 1 year of unprotected sex.

To treat infertility, a physician skilled in this practice begins with extensive histories of the couple's health. This may be followed by a series of relatively simple tests such as a sperm count to rule out common causes of infertility. Other, more extensive, physical examinations may be necessary to determine the cause. In some instances, the cause cannot be determined. Treatments are specific to the known causes of the infertility and include surgical procedures, hormone therapy, medication, and lifestyle changes. In addition, nutritional treatment is currently being investigated. Research results reveal that the total normal sperm count rose in men after treatment with the nutritional supplements zinc sulfate and folic acid (Wong et al., 2002).

In addition to these therapies, physicians can harvest ova and obtain semen to assist fertilization and implantation. For example, if a couple has problems with sperm reaching the cervix, cervical conditions

Figure 5-15 **Abnormal Sperm.** Abnormal sperm exhibit various types of malformations. A normal sperm is shown at the top.

Normal sperm

that are hostile to sperm, or the health of the sperm themselves, a physician may suggest artificial insemination, which has been practiced in the United States for more than 50 years. During this procedure, semen is placed in the cervical opening during the time of ovulation. With intrauterine insemination, concentrated sperm are placed in the uterus.

Women who have no uterine tubes or blocked tubes that do not respond to surgery often choose in vitro fertilization (IVF) to conceive. "In vitro" means "in a test tube" or "in the laboratory." In vitro fertilization involves fertilization of ova with sperm in laboratory glassware, with subsequent implantation of zygotes (fertilized eggs) in the woman's uterus. The birth of the first baby conceived through in vitro fertilization took place in 1978.

In 1992 a new IVF technique called intracytoplasmic sperm injection, or ICSI, was developed to fertilize eggs directly. Early IVF techniques involved putting eggs and sperm together and allowing sperm to swim to and fertilize the eggs. In the late 1980s, a technique was developed in which a few sperm were injected into the space between the egg and its barrier, increasing the chance of fertilization. The new ICSI technique involves injecting a single sperm directly into the egg. It is used when men have a very low sperm count, nonmotile sperm, or sperm unable to penetrate the chemical barrier that protects the egg.

Any treatment of infertility in which the sperm and eggs are both handled outside of the body is called assisted reproductive technology. Although assisted reproductive technology has been helpful, new studies urge some caution. The use of assisted reproductive technology accounts for a disproportionate number of infants born with low birth weights (under 5.5 pounds) for both multiple births and single births (Schieve et al., 2002). Low-birth-weight infants are more likely to experience both physical and developmental problems than infants who weigh more than 5.5 pounds at birth. Additionally, infants conceived with assisted reproductive technology are twice as likely as naturally conceived infants to have a major birth defect (Hansen et al., 2002).

■ Contraception

Most of the time, people engage in sexual intercourse for nonreproductive reasons. The timing may not be right for a pregnancy, or their family may be complete. Therefore, couples usually use some form of **birth con-**

birth control (contraception) methods to avoid pregnancy.

abstinence a method of birth control that involves refraining from vaginal intercourse.

trol, or **contraception**, which are methods to avoid pregnancy. You can assess your attitude toward the timing of parenthood by using the self-assessment scale in the student workbook.

Couples and individuals have many factors to consider when choosing a birth control method. They might consider its cost, effectiveness, reversibility, side effects, ease of use, convenience, and effectiveness against STIs. They must also consider their age and whether they need contraception on a regular basis or if they have only infrequent contraceptive needs. Many people are also concerned about the ways in which a contraceptive interferes with or fits in with their lovemaking. Some people have religious considerations to think about when making this choice.

Because a woman has a long reproductive life lasting some 30 to 35 years (from her teenage years until age 50 on average), the form of contraception she chooses may vary to meet her needs throughout the stages of her life. A variety of contraceptive methods are available, each with its own risks, benefits, and level of effectiveness. Most methods are based on the female reproductive cycle and rely on a woman's taking action. However, many methods can rely on the action of both partners and be incorporated into lovemaking.

The effectiveness of a contraceptive method is an important factor to consider. The *theoretical effectiveness* of a contraceptive refers to the number of women who will not become pregnant out of 100 couples using a method consistently and properly as their only means of birth control for 1 year. For example, if a method is 80% effective, 80 of 100 women using this method will not become pregnant over a year; 20 women will become pregnant. *Actual effectiveness* refers to the number of women who will not become pregnant of 100 couples using a method under usual conditions. Many people forget to use the method or use it improperly, lowering its effectiveness. (Unprotected sex has an effectiveness rate of 15%. Put simply, having unprotected sex is not an effective means of birth control.) Table 5-3 lists the effectiveness of the various forms of birth control.

The "Contraceptive Comfort and Confidence Scale" in the student workbook will help you assess whether the method of contraception that you are using or considering is or will be effective for you.

Abstinence and Natural Methods

With respect to contraception, **abstinence** means refraining from vaginal intercourse. Without this act, a woman cannot get pregnant (unless sperm are introduced artificially into her reproductive tract by a physician). Abstinence is 100% effective and is an excellent alternative for young men and women who feel they are not ready to have sex. Also, people choose to abstain from sex during various periods of their lives for varied reasons.

Natural family planning, or **fertility awareness** (formerly called the *rhythm method*), is a group of birth control techniques in which a couple abstains from sexual intercourse during the time of the month when a woman is most likely to conceive. The actual effectiveness of these methods is about 80% because it is often difficult to determine when ovulation has occurred and fertilization can take place.

Table 5-3	Effectiveness of Various Birth Control Methods	
Method	**Actual Effectiveness (%)**	**Theoretical Effectiveness (%)**
Abstinence	—	100
Fertility awareness	75	91–99
Coitus interruptus (withdrawal)	73	96
Spermicides	79	85
Diaphragm	84	94
Contraceptive sponge (women who have not given birth)	80	91
Contraceptive sponge (women who have given birth)	60	80
Cervical cap (women who have not given birth)	84	91
Cervical cap (women who have given birth)	68	74
Male condom	85	98
Female condom	79	95
Combined oral contraceptives (the pill)	92	99.7
Progestin-only pill (the mini-pill)	97	99.5
Contraceptive patch	92	97.7
Contraceptive vaginal ring	92	97.7
Monthly contraceptive injection	97	99.95
Depo-Provera	97	99.7
IUDs (across types)	99.2–99.9	99.4–99.9
Female sterilization	99.5	99.5
Male sterilization	99.85	99.9

Ovulation usually takes place in the middle of a woman's reproductive cycle. If she has sex up to 72 hours before ovulation, she can become pregnant because sperm live approximately this long. The egg survives for 24 hours, so fertilization can occur for 1 day after ovulation also. In summary, fertilization can take place up to 3 days before and 1 day after ovulation.

The time of ovulation varies with the length of a woman's cycle and may vary within cycles of a consistent length. In fact, a woman can ovulate anytime during her cycle and can even become pregnant during her menstrual period. There are four ways to determine (but without 100% certainty) when ovulation takes place: the temperature method, the calendar method, mucus inspection, and the mucothermal method. All but the calendar method are based on changes that take place in a woman's body around the time of ovulation.

To use the *temperature method*, a woman takes her temperature with a special basal thermometer before she gets out of bed every day for a few months. Since the body temperature dips just before and rises just after ovulation (Figure 5-16), charting body temperature for a few months can help a woman determine when she ovulates and if ovulation is regular.

To use *mucus inspection*, a woman notes when her cervical mucus changes consistency. Four days before ovulation, cervical mucus (which flows to the vagina) becomes clearer and thinner. She should avoid intercourse from this time until the mucus changes back to its cloudier, thicker appearance. The *mucothermal method* combines this method with the temperature method described in the previous paragraph.

To use the *calendar method*, the woman records the length of her menstrual cycles for a year, beginning on day 1 of menstrual bleeding. After determining the length of her shortest and longest cycles, she uses a chart or formula to determine which days of the month she could become pregnant (Table 5-4). This method works best when a woman has cycles that are consistently the same length. If a woman's cycle varies greatly, "safe" times within her cycle will be shorter than if her cycles are more regular.

Coitus interruptus, or **withdrawal**, is another natural form of birth control. To use this method, the man senses when he is close to ejaculation, then removes his penis from his partner's vagina and genital area, interrupting intercourse. There are many problems

natural family planning (fertility awareness) formerly called the rhythm method; a group of birth control techniques in which a couple abstains from sexual intercourse during the time of the month when a woman is most likely to conceive.

coitus interruptus (withdrawal) (KO-ih-tus in-ter-RUP-tus) a form of birth control in which the man removes his penis from his partner's vagina and genital area, interrupting intercourse before ejaculation.

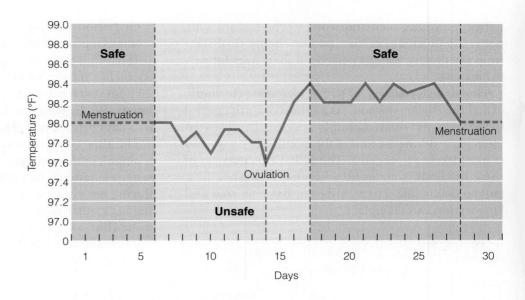

Figure 5-16 Basal Body Temperature Variations during the Menstrual Cycle. In this graph, basal body temperature is shown to vary during this "model" menstrual cycle. The time of ovulation is determined by noting the fall in temperature just before ovulation and the rise over 3 days just after. Remember, most menstrual cycles are not as regular as this "model" cycle. Safe days vary widely among women and may vary widely among an individual's cycles. The days prior to ovulation are considered "unsafe" because a woman does not yet know whether ovulation has occurred.

Table 5-4	How to Calculate Your Fertile Period		
If Your Shortest Cycle Has Been (no. of days)	Your First Fertile (Unsafe) Day Is	If Your Longest Cycle Has Been (no. of days)	Your Last Fertile (Unsafe) Day Is
21*	3rd Day	21*	10th Day
22	4th	22	11th
23	5th	23	12th
24	6th	24	13th
25	7th	25	14th
26	8th	26	15th
27	9th	27	16th
28	10th	28	17th
29	11th	29	18th
30	12th	30	19th
31	13th	31	20th
32	14th	32	21st
33	15th	33	22nd
34	16th	34	23rd
35	17th	35	24th

*Day 1 = First day of menstrual bleeding

with this method, however. A man must exercise a great deal of self-control, removing his penis from the vagina at a time when his desire may be to thrust more deeply. Also, he must be able to sense when he has enough time to remove himself before ejaculation. Additionally, sperm from a recent ejaculation may be present in the urethra and may be carried to the tip of the penis with drops of pre-ejaculatory fluid and result in pregnancy. To reduce the possibility of sperm in the pre-ejaculate, a man should urinate after ejaculation and carefully clean all semen from the penis. With perfect use, coitus interruptus is 96% effective. However, during actual use this form of contraception is only 81% effective. None of the natural methods of birth control protects against the transmission of STIs.

Chemical and Barrier Methods

Spermicides are chemicals that kill sperm. The most common active ingredient in spermicides marketed in the United States is nonoxynol-9. The inactive ingredients make up the carrier, or base, of the spermicides, which are sold as foams, creams, jellies, films, suppositories, and tablets. (Spermicides are also added to many brands of condoms.) The carrier distributes the spermicide in the vaginal canal. Shortly before vaginal sex, foams, creams, and jellies are placed high in the vagina near the cervix using an applicator, as shown in Figure 5-17A . Spermicidal films are placed near the cervix. Suppositories and tablets are placed in the vagina and given time to dissolve. Correct placement of the spermicide and timing of insertion are critical to the spermicide's effectiveness, which is 94% if these products are used correctly and consistently.

Advantages to using spermicides are that the side effects (such as allergy and vaginal irritation or infection) are minimal, they are used only when birth control is needed, and they are easy products to obtain over the counter. Disadvantages are a low rate of effectiveness and an increase in the frequency of genital lesions caused by nonoxynol-9. The presence of genital lesions increases the risk of contracting a sexually transmitted infection such as HIV during intercourse with an infected partner (Wilkinson et al., 2004; Lech, 2002).

Figure 5-17 **Contraceptive Foam and Jelly, Diaphragm, and Cervical Cap.**
(a) Contraceptive foam or jelly is placed high up in the vagina, covering the cervix, using a plunger-type applicator. This applicator and these contraceptive products are shown in the accompanying photo. (b) The diaphragm, which is shown in the photo, is ringed with contraceptive spermicide prior to insertion. The diaphragm is then pinched to narrow it and is then placed high in the vagina, covering the cervix. (c) The cervical cap, which is shown in the photo, is filled one-third full with spermicide prior to insertion. It is then inserted to cover the cervix.

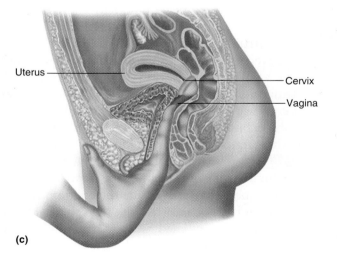

Barrier methods of contraception block the path that sperm must take to reach the ovum. These forms of contraception include male condoms, female condoms, diaphragms, and cervical caps (see Figure 5-17B and C). The Today Vaginal Contraceptive Sponge, an over-the-counter **sponge** that contains spermicide and is used like a diaphragm, was taken off the market in the United States in 1995. The Food and Drug Administration (FDA) discovered that the water system used in the manufacture of the product was contaminated with bacteria that cause diarrhea, although the sponges were never shown to be contaminated with this pathogen. A New Jersey pharmaceutical company purchased the Today Sponge from its original manufacturer in 1999. The FDA approved U.S. sales of the Today sponge in April, 2005.

Male condoms, the only form of birth control presently available for men other than vasectomy, are one of the most popular forms of birth control in the United States. The use of male condoms is also described in Chapter 14. Used for the prevention of pregnancy, condoms are 86% effective with actual use and 97%

spermicides chemicals that kill sperm.

barrier methods types of birth control that block the path that sperm must take to reach the ovum; these forms of contraception include male condoms, female condoms, diaphragms, and cervical caps.

sponge an over-the-counter product containing spermicide that is used like a diaphragm.

male condom a sheath used to cover the penis during sexual intercourse to help prevent pregnancy or sexually transmitted infections.

Figure 5-18 **How to Put on a Male Condom.**
The text explains each step.

(a)　　　　　**(b)**

(c)　　　　　**(d)**

effective with consistent and proper use. Scientists are currently developing new methods of birth control for men, including hormonal contraceptives that would stop sperm production (Swerdloff et al., 1998) and an antifertility drug called triptolide, which has been isolated from the plant *Tripterygium wilfordii* used in traditional Chinese medicine to treat inflammation (Lue, 1998).

Figure 5-18 illustrates the correct procedure for putting on a male condom: Put the condom on after the penis has become erect but before there is genital contact with a partner. Hold the top half-inch of the condom, squeezing the air out. This space will form a reservoir for semen. If air is not removed from this space, the semen cannot collect at the condom tip. Place the rolled-up condom over the head of the penis (Figure 5-18a). While still holding the tip, unroll the condom to cover the penis to its base (Figure 5-18b and c). Gently smooth out any air that may

female condom a polyurethane sheath with a ring at each end used to line the vagina during sexual intercourse to help prevent pregnancy or sexually transmitted infections.

have been trapped between the condom and the penis. After ejaculation, hold the condom firmly at its base to prevent slippage while you withdraw the still-erect penis from your partner's body. Remove the condom from the penis (Figure 5-18d), being careful not to spill semen on your partner and not to touch the exterior of the condom to your genital area. The outside of the condom may have become contaminated from an infected partner. Discard the used condom.

Approved by the FDA in 1993 the Reality **female condom**, a polyurethane sheath with a ring at each end, lines the vagina. Its use is also described in Chapter 14. Female condoms, used consistently and properly as a form of birth control, are approximately 95% effective. Their actual effectiveness, however, is 79%.

Figure 5-19 shows a female condom and the correct procedure for inserting one: Holding the closed end of the condom, squeeze the ring inside the condom so that it flattens and can be inserted into the vagina (Figure 5-19a). Insert the flattened ring and condom into the vagina (Figure 5-19b), gently pushing it up to the cervix

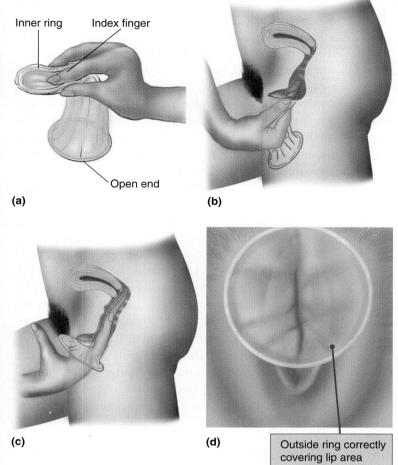

Inner ring   Index finger

Open end

(a)

(b)

(c)

(d)

Outside ring correctly covering lip area

assume its dome shape and to be held firmly in place over the cervix.

After insertion, a diaphragm is effective for 6 hours, so that a woman could insert the diaphragm well before sexual intercourse. However, spermicide must be added before each additional act of intercourse. After the last intercourse, the diaphragm must be left in place for at least 6 hours but must not be worn for more than 24 hours because of risk of infection. Used properly and consistently, the diaphragm is 94% effective. Currently under development are disposable, single-use diaphragms.

The **cervical cap** (Figure 5-17c) works much the same way as the diaphragm, but it is smaller and covers only the cervix. The cervical cap has not been in use in the United States until relatively recently; the Prentif cavity-rim cervical cap was approved by the FDA in 1988.

Before inserting a cervical cap, fill it one-third full with spermicide. When in place, it fits snugly around the base of the cervix and provides protection for 48 hours. Additional spermicide is not necessary with repeated intercourse, unlike the diaphragm. The cervical cap is 91% effective; however, its effectiveness is lowered to 74% in women who have given birth. In the future, silicone rubber cervical caps that release spermicide will become available.

Some women use **douching** as a contraceptive method. Douching is the use of specially prepared solutions to cleanse the vagina. *Douching is not effective for contraception.* By the time a woman can douche after sexual intercourse, sperm have already reached the cervix and uterus and cannot be washed away. Additionally, if a woman has used a contraceptive product containing spermicide, or has used spermicide alone as a contraceptive, douching may wash away the chemical and render it inactive.

as shown in Figure 5-19c. You should be able to feel the ring positioned past the pubic bone. Straighten out the part of the condom lining the vagina if it is twisted. The outside ring should cover the labia, as shown in Figure 5-19d. After intercourse, first twist the condom to close it at the vaginal opening, which will prevent sperm and pathogens from touching your genital area. Remove the condom with gentle pulling and discard. Female and male condoms are intended for one-time use.

The diaphragm has been in use in the United States longer than 60 years. Shown in Figure 5-17b, a **diaphragm** is a dome-shaped rubber cup bordered by a flexible spring that is designed to cover the cervix and surrounding area. This prescription item must be fitted by a health care practitioner.

Before inserting a diaphragm, place spermicide on both its sides and around its rim. Compress the spring, collapsing the diaphragm so that it can be inserted into the vagina. When the diaphragm reaches the cervical area, its spring pops open, causing the diaphragm to

diaphragm a dome-shaped rubber cup bordered by a flexible spring that covers the cervix and surrounding area during sexual intercourse to help prevent pregnancy.

cervical cap a dome-shaped rubber cup, smaller than a diaphragm, that covers the cervix during sexual intercourse to help prevent pregnancy.

douching (DOOSH-ing) the use of specially prepared solutions to cleanse the vagina; not an effective birth control method.

Hormonal Methods

Hormonal methods of birth control prevent pregnancy by suppressing ovulation. There are six types of hormonal contraceptive products: combined oral contraceptives (the pill), the contraceptive patch, the contraceptive vaginal ring, Implanon, Depo-Provera, and progestin-only pills (mini-pills).

Combined oral contraceptives suppress ovulation through the combined actions of estrogen and progestin (a synthetic form of progesterone). During the month there is a pill-free time when menstruation occurs.

The pill has numerous advantages. It is highly effective, decreases menstrual cramps, decreases the length of the menses and the amount of blood lost, has a protective effect against pelvic inflammatory disease, reduces the risk for ovarian and endometrial cancer (cancer of the uterine lining), reduces the risk for benign (noncancerous) breast disease, and helps prevent osteoporosis (thinning of the bones). The pill is a readily reversible form of contraception and, since 1965, has consistently been the contraceptive choice of approximately 25% of U.S. women who use contraceptives (Jones, 1999).

The pill has been available for nearly 45 years and is one of the best-studied prescription medications. The amount of estrogen and progestin in pills has decreased over the years, so today's pills are much safer than pills of the past. Cardiovascular disease is the most serious complication of the pill. Women at high risk for developing this complication of combined oral contraceptive use are those who are older than 50 years of age or who are older than 35 years of age and smoke cigarettes. Women who are sedentary, overweight, and have high blood pressure, diabetes mellitus, or an elevated serum cholesterol level are also at high risk.

A review of studies on the risk of cervical cancer in women taking oral contraceptives revealed that risk increases with increasing duration of use (Smith et al., 2003). The studies included women on combined oral contraceptives and progestin-only preparations, which are discussed shortly. Although the study results suggest that the risk may decrease after hormonal contraceptive use ceases, the authors of the review suggest that more data are needed to make this determination.

Four products have been developed recently that use the combined actions of estrogen and progestin: a new pill, a patch, a vaginal ring, and a monthly birth control shot. The new pill, which is called Seasonale, was approved by the FDA in 2003. This oral contraceptive has lower doses of hormones than conventional birth control pills. It is taken for 84 days instead of the usual 21 before the 7-day pill-free time and menstruation. With this new pill, a woman would have only four menstrual periods per year, one each season, instead of the usual thirteen. In addition to suppressing ovulation, this pill prevents buildup of the lining of the uterus. Therefore, the menses are light.

The contraceptive patch (Ortho Evra) was approved by the FDA in 2001 and became available in late April, 2002. The patch delivers hormones through the skin for 1 week. A woman uses three patches over 3 weeks, and then "goes off" the patch, during which time menstruation occurs. A primary advantage of the patch over conventional birth control pills is convenience: A woman needs to remember to change the patch only once a week rather than remembering to take a pill every day. Results of research show that women are more likely to use the contraceptive patch as directed as compared to contraceptive pills (Dittrich, 2002).

In 2001, the FDA approved the contraceptive vaginal ring (NuvaRing), which became available in mid-2002. This doughnut-shaped device fits in the vagina much like a diaphragm but works by releasing progestin and estrogen. Instead of taking a pill every day, a woman keeps the ring in place for 3 weeks, then removes it for 1 week, during which time she menstruates. Like the patch, the vaginal ring offers convenience: A woman only needs to remember to remove the ring after 3 weeks and insert a new one after a week without it.

Lunelle is a monthly birth control injection, which was approved by the FDA in 2000. This method of birth control contains both estrogen and progestin, works similarly to oral contraceptives, and carries similar risks. In addition, women gain, on average, 4 pounds per year while on this hormone regimen. Lunelle requires no home medications or visible skin patches, so it is considered a private form of birth control. Nevertheless, using Lunelle requires monthly visits to a clinic or, in Washington State, to a pharmacy to receive the injections.

Implanon, Depo-Provera, and mini-pills are all forms of progestin-only contraceptives. Progestin works to suppress ovulation in much the same way as combined oral contraceptives.

---

combined oral contraceptives "the pill"; suppress ovulation through the combined actions of estrogen and progestin.

Depo-Provera an injection of progestin that inhibits ovulation for 3 months.

mini-pills progestin-only contraceptive pills that are taken continually; menstruation does not occur.

intrauterine device (IUD) a small contraceptive device that either is covered with copper or contains a reservoir of progestin and is inserted into the uterus.

sterilization a permanent form of birth control that requires a surgical procedure.

tubal ligation female sterilization that is performed by cutting and tying off the uterine tubes so that the sperm and egg cannot unite.

vasectomy male sterilization that is performed by cutting and tying off the vas deferens to prevent sperm from becoming part of the ejaculate.

Uterus

Applicator

Cervix

Vagina

Figure 5-20 The intrauterine device (IUD) is a small apparatus that is inserted into the uterus. The active ingredient of an IUD is either copper or progestin.

■ IUD in place

Implanon is a matchstick-sized contraceptive implant. It is surgically inserted under the skin of the upper arm. While there, it releases progestin slowly and can inhibit ovulation for 3 years or longer. This implant is widely used in Europe, Britain, and Australia, but it is not yet available in the United States.

Depo-Provera, which has been used in the United States since 1992, is an injection of progestin that inhibits ovulation for 3 months. **Mini-pills** are progestin-only pills that are taken continually; menstruation does not occur. They have been in use in the United States for approximately 25 years.

Although highly effective, progestin-only contraceptives have a few serious disadvantages. These contraceptives change a woman's menstrual cycle. In addition to amenorrhea, these changes can include opposite effects: an increased number of days of menstruation with light bleeding or an increased number of days with heavy bleeding. Women find some of these changes unacceptable. Another disadvantage is that long-term use of progestin-only contraceptives may cause thinning of the bones due to low estrogen.

Intrauterine Devices

An **intrauterine device (IUD)** is a small apparatus that a health care practitioner inserts into the uterus (**Figure 5-20**). A string hangs from the base of the IUD and extends into the vagina; the presence of the string is an indication that the IUD is still in place. The active ingredient of the IUD is either copper, which covers the IUD, or progestin, which is contained in a reservoir within the IUD.

Although IUDs have a high rate of effectiveness (98% to 99.9%), the way in which they work has been a source of controversy. Results of several studies suggest that IUDs interfere with the movement of sperm through a woman's reproductive tract. There is little evidence to suggest that IUDs make it difficult for a fertilized ovum to implant, thereby aborting it (Dardano & Burkman, 1999).

Copper-containing IUDs have long been thought to cause pelvic inflammatory disease, or PID, which can lead to infertility. (PID is also discussed in Chapter 14.) However, evidence suggests that the risk of PID is highest during the time of insertion, if the uterine lining becomes contaminated with bacteria. After the first month of use, the risk of PID is the same as in women without IUDs. Research results (Hubacher et al., 2001) reveal that the use of copper IUDs is much safer than previously thought. The authors of the study suggest that women who are not at risk for sexually transmitted infections can use the copper IUD safely. They also note that this form of contraception is one of the safest, most effective, and least expensive reversible contraceptives available. Once an IUD is inserted, it does not need to be changed for 1 to 8 years, depending on the IUD used.

Sterilization

Sterilization is a permanent form of birth control. In the past, sterilization was only available as a surgical procedure, but in 2002 the FDA approved a nonsurgical, irreversible method of female sterilization called *Essure*. Using a local anesthetic, a physician inserts a tiny spring into each fallopian tube by passing it through the vagina and then the uterus. Over 3 months, the spring irritates the tube, causing it to produce scar tissue that blocks the tube. After the 3-month period, a physician injects dye into the uterus and up into the tubes. An x ray of the dye-injected area shows whether the tubes are fully blocked.

The surgical form of female sterilization is a **tubal ligation** and involves cutting and tying off the uterine tubes by means of clips, rings, or burning so that the sperm and egg cannot unite. Male sterilization is a **vasectomy** and involves cutting and tying off the

Uterine
(fallopian)
tube

Ovary

Uterus

(b)

(a)

vas deferens to prevent sperm from becoming part of the ejaculate. Tubal ligation is a medically more complicated and more costly procedure than vasectomy, but both are highly effective. Failure is most often due to surgical error or to the spontaneous rejoining of the tubes. **Figure 5-21** illustrates tubal ligation and vasectomy.

The surgical forms of sterilization can be reversed, but pregnancy rates vary depending on factors such as the type of procedure that was performed, the health of the tubes being rejoined, and the health and age of the patient. Microsurgical techniques provide excellent success rates.

Healthy Living Practices

- The most effective means to prevent an unwanted pregnancy are sexual abstinence and sterilization, followed closely by hormonal methods and IUDs.
- To reduce the risk of contracting or transmitting sexually transmitted infections, use a condom during sexual intercourse. The best way to protect yourself against STIs is to practice sexual abstinence.

■ Abortion

Sometimes contraceptive methods fail and an unplanned pregnancy occurs that a woman or a couple chooses to terminate. Sometimes pregnancy seriously jeopardizes a woman's health and ending the pregnancy is the only means of saving her life. There

are numerous other reasons why women and couples choose to terminate a pregnancy.

A controversial 1973 United States Supreme Court decision (*Roe v. Wade*) ruled that induced abortion is a legal medical procedure. States may regulate abortions in the second trimester to protect the health of the pregnant woman, but the decision to end a pregnancy during the first trimester is the private concern of a woman and her health care practitioner.

An **abortion** is the removal of the embryo or fetus from the uterus before it is able to survive on its own. During a *spontaneous abortion*, the body expels the embryo, usually because of serious genetic defects, although there may be other causes. Spontaneous abortions (miscarriages) generally occur during the first trimester. Ten to twenty percent of pregnancies end in spontaneous abortion.

During an *induced abortion*, a physician performs medical procedures that remove the embryo or fetus from the uterus. There are three principal ways to perform an induced abortion: vacuum aspiration, dilation and evacuation (D&E), and induction; the choice of method depends on the stage of development of the embryo or fetus.

The safest time to have an abortion is between 7 and 10 weeks of gestation. If an abortion is performed before 6 to 7 weeks or after 10 weeks, there is an increased risk of complications. Nevertheless, elective abortion in the United States is safe; less than 1% of women who have abortions experience serious complications.

The abortion procedure used when the embryo is at less than 8 weeks of development is **vacuum aspiration**, or *suction curettage*. (*Curettage* means clearing material from a surface.) It can be performed in the physician's office in approximately 10 to 20 minutes with the use of a local anesthetic. To perform a vac-

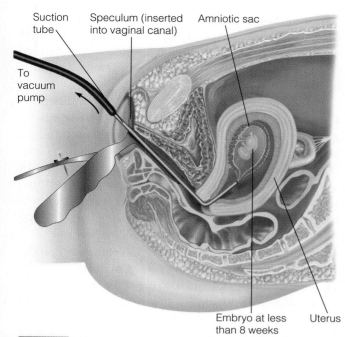

Suction tube

Speculum (inserted into vaginal canal)

Amniotic sac

To vacuum pump

Embryo at less than 8 weeks

Uterus

Figure 5-22 **Suction Curettage.** During this procedure, a thin, hollow tube is inserted through the vagina and cervix to the uterus. A suction aspirator (vacuum pump) draws tissue out of the uterus and into a container.

uum aspiration, the physician inserts a slender, hollow plastic tube through the vagina and cervix into the uterus. The tube is connected to a suction aspirator, which draws the tissue out of the uterus and into a container (**Figure 5-22**). After this procedure is completed, a narrow metal rod is inserted through the tube, and the uterine wall is scraped to be certain that all the tissue has been removed. Vacuum aspiration is used for 50% of abortions; the embryo is less than an inch long at this time.

Mifepristone (formerly known as **RU486** or the French abortion pill) is also a method to terminate early first-trimester pregnancies. In July of 1996, the FDA Advisory Committee on Reproductive Health Drugs determined that mifepristone is safe and effective. The FDA approved the drug for the termination of early pregnancy in late 2000. This drug, taken within 3 weeks of a missed period, induces abortion in 95% of pregnant women by blocking progesterone, which is necessary for the adequate development of the uterine lining. Without the buildup of this lining, implantation does not occur, and therefore, pregnancy is not established. Results of recent research suggest that the use of mifepristone to induce early abortion does not adversely affect subsequent pregnancies (Chen et al., 2004).

Abortions that are performed during 8 to 12 weeks of development use vacuum aspiration (suction curettage), but the cervix is also dilated (widened) to reduce the risk of damage to the uterus. This variation of suction curettage is called *dilation and curettage,* or *D&C.* Occasionally, general anesthesia is used for this procedure. Forty percent of all abortions are performed this way. In summary, 90% of abortions are performed in the first trimester by suction curettage or by dilation and curettage.

Early second-trimester abortions (13 to 16 weeks) are performed by **dilation and evacuation (D&E)**, also referred to as a *surgical abortion.* A D&E is performed somewhat like a D&C, except that there is greater dilation of the cervix and a larger suction device is used. In addition, the physician uses a special forceps to remove fetal parts.

Induction is used between 16 and 24 weeks of development, although D&E procedures are replacing induction as a safer, faster, and less expensive method of abortion at this stage of gestation. Induction means that labor is artificially induced (started). *Saline abortions* are one method of induction: A physician inserts a long needle through the abdominal wall and into the amniotic sac. A salt solution is injected into the sac, which causes the quick death of the fetus. The uterus begins contractions within 12 and 24 hours, and the woman delivers a dead fetus. This procedure is performed using a local anesthetic. Other types of solutions and prostaglandins (hormonelike substances that cause the uterus to contract) are also used for induction.

A special type of D&E procedure (the so-called partial birth abortion) is used to abort fetuses after 24 weeks. Only 1% of abortions are performed this late in a pregnancy. President George W. Bush signed the Partial-Birth Abortion Ban Act in November 2003, which criminalizes the procedure. Physicians from many states challenged the constitutionality of the law. Three federal judges from California, New York, and Nebraska ruled that the legislation had many constitutional defects and rejected the ban. Legal experts suggest that the law will eventually be brought to the U.S. Supreme Court for a ruling on its constitutionality.

abortion removal of the embryo or fetus from the uterus before it is able to survive on its own.

vacuum aspiration a method of early first-trimester induced abortion in which embryonic tissue is drawn out of the uterus by a suction device.

mifepristone (RU486) (MIFF-ih-PRIS-tone) a drug that induces early first-trimester abortions; this drug blocks progesterone, which is necessary for the adequate development of the uterine lining and implantation.

dilation and evacuation (D&E) surgical abortion; a technique used for early second-trimester abortion in which the cervix is dilated (widened) and the fetal tissues are suctioned from the uterus.

induction an abortion technique used between 16 and 24 weeks of gestation in which labor is artificially started.

Sexual Development

The gender of an individual is set at the time of fertilization and is determined by the type of sex chromosomes (genes) it receives from its parents. Females have two X chromosomes; males have an X and a Y.

During the 7th week of development, the embryo with a Y chromosome begins to develop testes. The developing testes secrete male hormones collectively called *androgens*. These hormones direct the development of a male reproductive system. Embryos and fetuses without a Y chromosome begin to develop ovaries during the 9th week. The absence of androgens results in the development of a female reproductive system.

After birth, the secretion of the androgen testosterone in male babies nearly ceases and does not resume until puberty, the time of sexual maturation. The female reproductive system does not become active until that time as well.

Puberty is a stage of development during which the endocrine (hormone) and reproductive systems mature. Puberty begins at approximately 10 to 11 years of age and concludes about 5 or 6 years later. Girls usually enter puberty about 2 years earlier than boys. Scientists do not know what triggers this developmental process.

During childhood, the production of a hormone that stimulates the release of male and female sex hormones is suppressed. At the onset of puberty, the suppression ceases and the brain begins releasing the hormone that regulates the production of testosterone in males and estrogen in females. As puberty proceeds, the brain secretes greater and greater amounts of this hormone; thus more and more testosterone or estrogen is secreted. It is these hormones that stimulate the physical changes of puberty. These changes include growth spurts due to the growth of the skeleton (especially the long bones), the development of pubic and underarm hair, and the growth and maturation of the reproductive tract.

In males, building levels of testosterone result in an enlarging of the testes and penis, deepening of the voice due to an enlargement of the voice box, development of facial hair, broadening of the shoulders, and enlargement of the arm, chest, and leg muscles. Under the direction of testosterone, the seminiferous tubules begin manufacturing sperm. A significant developmental event in pubertal boys is semen emission during sleep, called nocturnal emissions or wet dreams. Initially, sperm are not present in the semen.

In females, estrogen results in the development of the breasts and the rounding of the hips. Females experience **menarche**, the first menstruation, at around 12 years of age. The normal range for menarche is 8 to 15 years of age. A delay of the menarche may occur in girls with chronic diseases, such as diabetes mellitus, those with disorders that affect their nutritional status, such as anorexia nervosa, and those undergoing strenuous training, such as Olympic hopefuls.

When a woman reaches 45 to 55 years of age, most of her ovarian follicles (eggs) have matured, and the remaining follicles are old. During some months, these aging follicles do not reach maturity and ovulation does not take place. Without mature egg follicles, the normal cyclic secretion of estrogen and progesterone does not occur, and the menses become irregular. Eventually, all follicles stop maturing, estrogen and progesterone are no longer secreted, and the menses cease. The cessation of the menses is called **menopause**. This term means the final menstrual period, but it is widely used to refer to the few years of transition when a woman passes from her reproductive years to her nonreproductive years. The Diversity in Health essay discusses menopausal symptoms and attitudes across cultures.

As the hormonal changes of menopause take place, women usually experience symptoms such as hot flashes and physiological changes such as thinning of the vaginal walls and vaginal dryness. In addition, the loss of estrogen results in an increased risk of osteoporosis and heart disease. Therefore, some health care practitioners suggest hormone replacement therapy (HRT) for their patients on a short-term basis to help alleviate these symptoms. The hormones prescribed are either estrogen alone or estrogen in combination with progestin. Estrogen with progestin increases the risk of breast cancer and cardiovascular disease, and may increase the risk of ovarian cancer (Writing Group for the Women's Health Initiative Investigators, 2002; Beral et al., 2002; Anderson et al., 2003). Estrogen alone or with progestin does not protect and may have an adverse effect on cognitive function in women 65 years of age or older (Espeland et al., 2004; Shumaker et al., 2004). Low-dose estrogen alone, however, has been shown to increase bone density in postmenopausal women with minimal adverse effects (Prestwood et al., 2003). The addition of progestin in HRT reduces the risk of endometrial cancer.

puberty (PEW-ber-tea) a stage of sexual development during which the endocrine (hormone) and reproductive systems mature.

menarche (meh-NAR-key) the first menstruation.

menopause (MEN-oh-pawz) the cessation of the menses; a term widely used to refer to the few years of transition during which a woman passes from her reproductive years to her nonreproductive years.

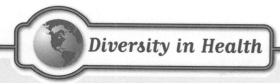

Menopause

Menopause is a time of transition for every woman who reaches her 50s, but transition is about the only thing women universally experience during this time. The symptoms of menopause and attitudes regarding this process vary extensively among women across cultures. Why do these differences exist?

One hypothesis is that if a society regards the menopause as a positive time, then the symptoms of menopause reported by its women will decrease in number and severity. Certain evidence seems to support this hypothesis. For example, during their childbearing years, the Rajput women of Northern India are socially constrained and cannot move about freely in their villages. Those who no longer menstruate are freed of this constraint. Interestingly, these women report no symptoms of menopause. Similarly, Mayan women look upon the menopause as a lifting of the burden of childbearing. They, too, report no symptoms of hot flashes or cold sweats such as are typically reported by North American women. Additionally, Yanomamo women (forest-dwellers who live near the border between Brazil and Venezuela) eagerly await menopause, which is considered the time of "older age," for this time of life brings increased status and decision-making power in their society.

Many researchers point out that it is difficult to form conclusions concerning symptoms and behaviors across cultures because the definition of terms such as *menopause* varies from culture to culture. In some cultures, there are no words in the language to identify particular menopausal symptoms or the menopause itself. Additionally, some symptoms are not recognized in Western medical literature as signs of menopause, but they are reported frequently by menopausal women in non-Western cultures. For example, Japanese women commonly report menopausal symptoms of shoulder stiffness and dizziness; Nigerian women frequently report having menopausal joint pains.

The diversity of the symptoms and experiences of women of various cultures regarding menopause cannot be attributed solely to differences in cultural beliefs. Their menopausal symptoms and experiences must also be evaluated in the context of their differences with respect to risk factors for death and disease. People of different cultures have different lifestyles that affect their health, which may account for some of the differences in the symptoms and perceptions of menopause across cultures.

Menopause is a significant time in a woman's life, and her attitude about and bodily response to "the change" is crucial to her susceptibility to disease, quality of life, and aging process. Currently, medical researchers are debating the significance of menopause to healthy aging. The experts disagree about the extent to which the decline in ovarian function contributes to physiological and psychological symptoms of menopause. Researchers are unanimous in their opinion that more research is needed to answer many of the questions we are just beginning to ask about this middle-life transition.

Sources: Mercer, C. (1999). Cross-cultural attitudes to the menopause and the aging female. *Age and Ageing, 28*(S2):12–17.
Lock, M. (1994). Menopause in cultural context. *Experimental Gerontology, 29*:307–317.
Woods, N. F. (1994). Menopause—challenges for future research. *Experimental Gerontology, 29*:237–243.

Men also undergo changes in their reproductive systems during middle age. Men are fertile throughout their lives, although the number of healthy, active sperm they produce decreases as they grow older. Middle-aged men experience a decline in testosterone, ejaculate with less force and less volume, and take longer to regain an erection after orgasm. In addition, the prostate gland usually enlarges. See the Managing Your Health essay "Enlargement of the Prostate."

Although both men and women undergo changes in their reproductive systems beginning at middle age, these changes do not have to impair their ability to have a healthy, enjoyable sex life extending into their elderly years.

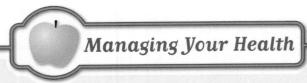
Enlargement of the Prostate

If you are male and over 45, your prostate may be enlarging slowly. If you are not yet 45, prostate enlargement may be in your future. This process of enlargement is common for middle-aged and older men; it is part of the aging process and may never be a cause for concern. However, about 50% of men in their 60s and about 90% of men in their 70s and 80s complain of problems caused by an enlarged prostate gland, also known as prostatic hyperplasia, or benign prostatic hypertrophy (BPH).

How can an enlarged prostate affect your health? Notice in Figure 5-1 that the prostate gland surrounds the urethra beneath the urinary bladder. As the prostate enlarges, it may squeeze the urethra, hampering the flow of urine through this tube. Therefore, the symptoms that may appear first as a result of BPH are difficulty in beginning to urinate, a decrease in the force of the urine stream, a dribbling of urine after urinating, a sensation of a full bladder after urinating, and a need to urinate 5 or 10 minutes after urinating.

As the prostate squeezes the urethra more and more, the muscles of the bladder wall respond by thickening as they forcefully push urine through the constricted urethra. This thickened bladder is irritated easily, however, and contracts more readily. Therefore, the following symptoms develop: an urgency to urinate and/or leaking of urine, more frequent urination, especially at night, and painful urination. Eventually, urine flow can be blocked to the point that emergency treatment is necessary.

There are several treatments for BPH. Surgery is usually undertaken when symptoms are severe. During the surgery, the portion of the prostate squeezing the urethra is removed.

One treatment is balloon dilatation. During this procedure, an inflatable device is inserted into the urethra through the opening at the tip of the penis. The device is inflated at the area of constriction and is then removed. This procedure widens the urethra to alleviate symptoms. Various medications also ease the symptoms of BPH.

Enlargement of the prostate may also be caused by prostate cancer. This cancer is the second most common cause of cancer deaths in men (lung cancer being the first). However, it usually does not appear in men younger than 55, and it is generally a slow-growing form of cancer. Its symptoms overlap with those of BPH and include difficult, frequent, and painful urination, and blood in the urine.

The symptoms of BPH and prostate cancer are more than just a nuisance. The restriction or blockage of urine flow can damage the kidneys; prostate cancer can spread, resulting in death. To avoid the discomforts and possible serious consequences of these conditions, therefore, the prostate should be examined regularly. The American Cancer Society recommends that men older than 50 have a digital rectal examination every year. During this examination, the physician inserts a gloved, lubricated finger into the rectum. Because the prostate lies next to the rectum (Figure 5-D), the physician can palpate (feel by pressing lightly) the size of the prostate.

Newer diagnostic techniques include transrectal ultrasound, in which the physician inserts an ultrasound probe into the rectum that results in an image of the prostate on a monitor.

A blood test has been developed to help detect prostate cancer. This test is known as prostate specific antigen (PSA) and helps find many prostate cancers years before they would otherwise be detected. See Chapter 13 for a discussion of prostate cancer and the PSA test.

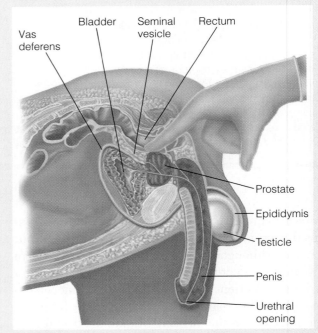

Figure 5-D **Digital Examination of the Prostate.** The physician can feel an enlargement of the prostate gland by inserting a gloved finger into the rectum.

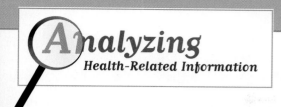

Analyzing
Health-Related Information

Explain why you think this Web site about folic acid is a reliable or an unreliable source of information. Use the model for analyzing health-related information to guide your thinking; the main points of the model are noted below. The model is fully explained on pages 13–15. If you wish to visit this site, the Web address is http://www.cdc.gov/node.do/id/0900f3ec80010af9.

1. Which statements are verifiable facts, and which are unverified statements or value claims?

2. What are the credentials of the agency that created the Web site? If this information is available, is the agency qualified as an expert in the topic area?

3. What might be the motives and biases of the agency that created the Web site? State reasons for your answer.

4. Which information in the Web site is relevant to the topic? Which information is irrelevant?

5. Is the source reliable? Does it have a reputation for publishing misinformation?

6. Does the Web site attack the credibility of conventional scientists or medical authorities?

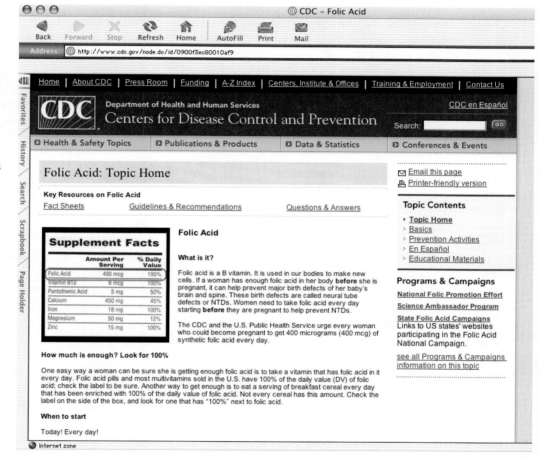

Based on your analysis, do you think that this Web site is a reliable source of health-related information? Summarize your reasons for coming to this conclusion.

CHAPTER REVIEW

Summary

Sexual reproduction involves the fertilization of an egg by a sperm, forming the first cell of a new individual. The male reproductive system produces sperm (male sex cells) and delivers them to the vagina of the female. Sperm are produced in the testes and are moved along the male reproductive tract with the seminal fluid secreted by accessory sex glands during ejaculation.

Eggs (ova; female sex cells) develop and mature in the female reproductive system, which also receives sperm and provides an environment in which a fertilized ovum can develop. Eggs mature in the ovaries, are fertilized in the uterine tubes, and develop in the uterus during pregnancy.

Women experience cyclic monthly hormonal changes that orchestrate physiological changes that take place in the ovaries and uterus. The changes are collectively called the menstrual cycle. During the menstrual cycle an ovum matures and is released from the ovary while the lining of the uterus thickens in preparation for the implantation of a fertilized ovum. If pregnancy does not occur, the uterine lining sloughs off during the menses.

If fertilization takes place, the embryo/fetus develops in the uterus of the female. This developmental process is termed *pregnancy,* or *gestation.* Various environmental influences (teratogens) such as drugs, alcohol, viruses, and dietary deficiencies can damage the embryo or fetus early in pregnancy. A woman preparing for pregnancy should have a medical checkup; eat a well-balanced and nutritious diet; avoid drinking alcohol, smoking cigarettes, and taking drugs; and possibly seek genetic counseling.

Women who become pregnant may notice physical signs of this condition such as a missed period, nausea, fatigue, and moodiness. A woman can conduct a home pregnancy test after a missed period or have a laboratory test performed to determine if she is pregnant.

Pregnancy lasts about 38 weeks and is typically described in terms of trimesters, or 3-month periods. During the first trimester, all the organ systems of the body form and become functional. The second and third trimesters are periods of growth and refinement of the organ systems.

The process of childbirth (labor) takes place in three stages: dilation, expulsion, and placental delivery. During dilation, the uterine muscles contract, causing the cervix to widen (dilate) and thin out (efface). During the second stage of labor the baby is born. Within 15 to 30 minutes after delivery of the baby, the placenta is expelled from the uterus.

Couples often want to avoid pregnancy for various reasons, so they choose some form of birth control, or contraception. Contraceptive methods are varied and can be grouped into five categories: abstinence and natural methods, chemical and barrier methods, hormonal methods, intrauterine devices, and sterilization. Each method has different advantages, disadvantages, and levels of effectiveness. Abstinence and sterilization are the most effective means of contraception, followed closely in effectiveness by hormonal methods and IUDs. Using condoms or practicing abstinence are the best ways to prevent the transmission of sexually transmitted infections while at the same time preventing pregnancy.

Sometimes contraceptive methods fail and an unplanned pregnancy occurs that a woman or a couple chooses to terminate. There are other reasons why women and couples choose to terminate a pregnancy, including health concerns of the mother. Terminating a pregnancy involves the removal of the embryo or fetus from the uterus before it is able to survive on its own. This process is called an induced abortion. In the United States today, there is great controversy over a woman's right to choose induced abortion. Ninety percent of abortions are performed during the first trimester using a procedure called suction curettage. The drug RU486, which is also effective in inducing abortion during the first trimester, was approved by the FDA in 2000.

The sex of an individual is set at the time of fertilization and is determined by the type of sex chromosomes (genes) that it receives from its parents. The male and female reproductive tracts develop during gestation. Further maturation does not continue until puberty, the time of sexual maturation, which begins at approximately 10 to 11 years of age and concludes about 5 or 6 years later. Men and women both undergo changes to their reproductive function during middle age. Women have a cessation of the menses as a result of physiological and hormonal changes and can no longer reproduce. Men can reproduce throughout their lives but at middle age experience a decline in testosterone and sexual functioning.

Applying What You Have Learned

1. A woman is 42 years old, unmarried, and has sex regularly with a single sexual partner. She has been using an intrauterine device but has developed an infection with the insertion of her most recent IUD. She must change to another method of birth control. If you were this woman, which method would you choose? Provide evidence that your choice is prudent. **Application**

2. In this chapter, much attention is given to the theoretical and actual effectiveness of various types of birth control. When you look at Table 5-3, which column should carry more weight in your decision making—the theoretical or the actual effectiveness? Give reasons for your answer. **Analysis**

3. You have been asked to lead a discussion in your health class about the pros and cons of legalized abortion. You may discuss any information in this chapter relevant to this issue. (You may add topics not mentioned in this chapter as well.) List the topics you will discuss and briefly describe the importance of each to the issue of abortion. **Synthesis**

4. Devise an assessment that will help people evaluate their attitudes toward abortion. Explain why you think that your assessment tool will accurately evaluate these attitudes. **Evaluation**

Key

Application	using information in a new situation.
Analysis	breaking down information into component parts.
Synthesis	putting together information from different sources.
Evaluation	making informed decisions.

Reflecting on Your Health

1. Contracting sexually transmitted infections can endanger your health and your ability to have children. What is the relationship between responsible sexual behavior and reproductive health in your life?

2. If you are a man, what did you learn in this chapter about female reproductive health that was new to you? If you are a woman, what did you learn in this chapter about male reproductive health that was new to you? How will this new knowledge affect your behavior toward the opposite sex? How might it affect your attitudes?

3. Most contraceptive methods focus on the female reproductive system. Because of this focus, should women have the primary responsibility for contraception? Why or why not?

4. In the United States, a woman's right to choose to have an abortion (other than a "partial birth" abortion) is protected by law. Do you think that the law should be changed to criminalize abortion in general? If so, why? Should abortion be legal only in certain circumstances? If so, when?

5. Table 5-1 lists selected teratogens. If a woman knowingly exposes her embryo or fetus to teratogenic drugs such as alcohol, should she be prosecuted in the criminal justice system? Why or why not?

References

Adami, H.-O., & Trichopoulos, D. (2002). Cervical cancer and the elusive male factor. *New England Journal of Medicine, 346*:1160–1161.

American Academy of Pediatrics (AAP). (1999). Circumcision policy statement. *Pediatrics, 103*:686–693.

Anderson, G. L., Judd, H. L., Kaunitz, A. M., Barad, D. H., Beresford, S. A., Pettinger, M., Liu, J., McNeeley, S. G., & Lopez, A. M., for the Women's Health Initiative Investigators. (2003). Effects of estrogen plus progestin on gynecologic cancers and associated diagnostic procedures: The Women's Health Initiative randomized trial. *Journal of the American Medical Association, 290*(13):1739–1748.

Beral, V., Banks, E., & Reeves, G. (2002). Evidence from randomized trials on the long-term effects of hormone replacement therapy. *Lancet, 360*(9337):942–944.

Chen, A., Yuan, W., Meirik, O., Wang, X., Wu, S., Zhou, L., Luo, L., Gao, E., & Cheng, Y. (2004). Mifepristone-induced early abortion and outcome of subsequent wanted pregnancy. *American Journal of Epidemiology, 160*:110–117.

Dardano, K. L., & Burkman, R. T. (1999). The intrauterine contraceptive device: An often-forgotten and maligned method of contraception. *American Journal of Obstetrics and Gynecology, 181*:1–5.

Daugherty, J. E. (1998). Treatment strategies for premenstrual syndrome. *American Family Physician, 58*:183–192, 197–198.

Dittrich, R., Parker, L., Rosen, J. B., Shangold, G., Creasy, G. W., & Fisher, A. C. (2002). Transdermal contraception: Evaluation of three transdermal norelgestromin/ethinyl estradiol doses in a randomized, multicenter, dose-response study. *American Journal of Obstetrics and Gynecology, 186*:15–20.

Epperson, C. N., Haga, K., Mason, G. F., Sellers, E., Gueorguieva, R., Zhang, W., Weiss, E., Rothman, D. L., & Krystal, J. H. (2002). Cortical γ-aminobutyric acid levels across the menstrual cycle in healthy women and those with premenstrual dysphoric disorder: A proton magnetic resonance spectroscopy study. *Archives of General Psychiatry, 59*:851–858.

Espeland, M. A., Rapp, S. R., Shumaker, S. A., Brunner, R., Manson, J. E., Sherwin, B. B., Hsia, J., Margolis, K. L., Hogan, P. E., Wallace, R., Dailey, M., Freeman, R., & Hays, J., for the Women's Health Initiative Memory Study Investigators. (2004). Conjugated equine estrogens and global cognitive function in postmenopausal women: Women's Health Initiative memory study. *Journal of the American Medical Association, 291*(24):2959–2968.

Glass, C. A., & Bruner, J. P. (2000). Postpartum depression. In M. E. Rivlin & R. W. Martin (Eds.), *Manual of clinical problems in obstetrics and gynecology*, 5th ed, pp. 204–208.

Hansen, M., Kurinczuk, J. J., Bower, C., & Webb, S. (2002). The risk of major birth defects after intracytoplasmic sperm injection and in vitro fertilization. *New England Journal of Medicine, 346*:725–730.

Hubacher, D., Lara-Ricalde, R., Taylor, D. J., Guerra-Infante, F., & Guzmán-Rodrígues, R. (2001). Use of copper intrauterine devices and the risk of tubal infertility among nulligravid women. *New England Journal of Medicine, 345*:561–567.

Jones, K. P. (1999). Oral contraception: Current use and attitudes. *Contraception, 59*(1 Suppl):17S–20S.

Lech, M. M. (2002). Spermicides 2002: An overview. *European Journal of Contraception & Reproductive Health Care, 7*(3):173–177.

Mitchell, A. A. (2002). Infertility treatment—more risks and challenges. *New England Journal of Medicine, 346*:769–770.

Munkelwitz, R., & Gilbert, B. R. (1998). Are boxer shorts really better? A critical analysis of the role of underwear type in male subfertility. *Journal of Urology, 160*:1329–1333.

Prestwood, K. M., Kenny, A. M., Kleppinger, A., & Kulldorff, M. (2003). Ultralow-dose micronized 17[beta]-estradiol and bone density and bone metabolism in older women: A randomized controlled trial. *Journal of the American Medical Association, 290*(8):1042–1048.

Rivlin, M. E. (2000). Toxic shock syndrome. In M. E. Rivlin & R. W. Martin (Eds.), *Manual of clinical problems in obstetrics and gynecology*, 5th ed, pp. 306–310.

Schieve, L.A., Meikle, S. F., Ferre, C., Peterson, H. B., Jeng, G., & Wilcox, L. S. (2002). Low and very low birth weight in infants conceived with use of assisted reproductive technology. *New England Journal of Medicine, 346*:731–737.

Shumaker, S. A., Legault, C., Kuller, L., Rapp, S. R., Thal, L., Lane, D. S., Fillit, H., Stefanick, M. L., Hendrix, S. L., Lewis, C. E., Masaki, K., & Coker, L. H. (2004). Conjugated equine estrogens and incidence of probable dementia and mild cognitive impairment in post-menopausal women: Women's Health Initiative memory study. *Journal of the American Medical Association, 291*(24):2947–2958.

Smith, J. S., Green, J., Berrington de Gonzales, A., Appleby, P., Peto, J., Plummer, M., Franceschi, S., & Beral, V. (2003). Cervical cancer and use of hormonal contraceptives: A systematic review. *Lancet, 361*:1159–1167.

Swerdloff, R. S., Bagatell, C. J., Wang, C., Anawalt, B. D., Berman, N., Steiner, B., & Bremner, W. J. (1998). Suppression of spermatogenesis in man induced by Nal-Glu gonadotropin releasing hormone anatagonist and testosterone enanthate (TE) is maintained by TE alone. *Journal of Clinical Endocrinology and Metabolism, 83*:3527–3533.

Thys-Jacobs, S., Starkey, P., Bernstein, D., & Tian, J. (1998). Calcium carbonate and the premenstrual syndrome: Effects on premenstrual and menstrual symptoms. Premenstrual Syndrome Study Group. *American Journal of Obstetrics and Gynecology, 179*:444–452.

Ugarriza, D. N., Klingner, S., & O'Brien, S. (1998). Premenstrual syndrome: Diagnosis and intervention. *Nurse Practitioner, 23*(9):40–45, 49–52.

Wilkinson, D., Ramjee, G., Tholandi, M., & Rutherford, G. (2002). Nonoxynol-9 for preventing vaginal acquisition of HIV infection by women from men. *The Cochrane Database of Systematic Reviews,* issue 4. Article No. CD003936. Chichester, UK: John Wiley & Sons.

Wong, W. Y., Merkus, H. M. W. M., Thomas, C. M. G., Menkveld, R., Zielhuis, G. A., & Steegers-Theunissen, R. P. M. (2002). Effects of folic acid and zinc sulfate on male factor subfertility: A double-blind, randomized, placebo-controlled trial. *Fertility and Sterility, 77*:491–498.

Writing Group for the Women's Health Initiative. (2002). Risks and benefits of combined estrogen and progestin in healthy, postmenopausal women: Principal results from the Women's Health Initiative randomized controlled trial. *Journal of the American Medical Association, 288*:321–333.

What You'll Learn

http://healthyliving.jbpub.com

The Web site for this book offers many useful tools and is a great source for supplementary health information for both students and instructors. Visit the site at http://healthyliving.jbpub.com for information on these topics:

Human Sexual Behavior
Sexual Dysfunctions
Sexual Orientation
Romantic Relationships
Across the Lifespan: Sexuality

Chapter Overview

How biological and psychological factors influence sexual behavior

The phases of the sexual response cycle

Symptoms of and treatments for sexual dysfunctions

How culture affects sexuality

The nature versus nurture debate and sexual orientation

The diversity of sexual behavior

Definitions and theories of love and commitment

 Diversity in Health
The Virtue of Virginity

 Consumer Health
Ginseng and Sexual Prowess

 Managing Your Health
Minding Your Sexual Manners | Tips for Better Sex

ACROSS
THE LIFESPAN

Sexuality

Student Workbook

Self-Assessment: The Love Attitudes Scales | Communication Patterns Questionnaire

Changing Health Habits: Would a Behavior Change Improve Your Relationships?

Do You Know?

· *What are common sexual practices?*
· *How living together affects future marriage?*
· *How to communicate effectively?*

Relationships and Sexuality

Sex is everywhere in our society. You can find sexually explicit images and information in movies, books, and TV shows, on the Web, and in the lyrics of popular music. If you browse through magazines or scan billboards, you are likely to see pictures of attractive young men and women in advertisements for clothes, perfumes, and cars. Whether their product is a movie or pair of jeans, promoters and advertisers know that "sex sells." What does sex mean to you?

The term *sex* refers to one's gender, male or female, as well as to sexual intercourse and other intimate physical activities that involve the genitals. Sexuality, however, is more than gender or reproductive organs. **Sexuality** is the aspect of personality that encompasses an individual's sexual thoughts, feelings, attitudes, and actions. Each person has a unique collection of private and public sexual experiences that shapes his or her sexuality.

Numerous biological, psychological, social, and cultural forces interact to influence a person's sexual development, sexual health, and interpersonal relationships (Figure 6-1). Sexuality is woven into every aspect of human life; sex affects a person's identity, self-esteem, emotions, personality, relationships, lifestyle, and overall health.

Being knowledgeable about sexuality is important for maintaining good health and optimal well-being. Misinformation can lead to serious consequences, such as unintentional pregnancies or sexually transmitted infections. Additionally, people who are well informed about sexuality can communicate effectively with their medical practitioners and sexual partners regarding reproductive or sexual concerns.

Throughout life, you make various sexually related decisions, for example, deciding with whom to have an intimate sexual relationship. Such decisions can have serious effects on your health and well-being, as well as those of others. By considering how your actions may affect yourself and your sexual partners, you can become a more sexually responsible person.

> "... promoters and advertisers know that 'sex sells.'"

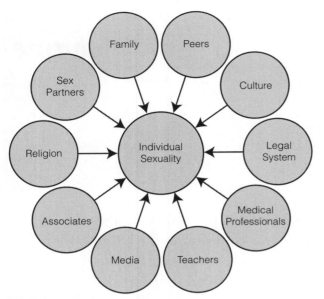

Figure 6-1 **Sexuality Model.** Numerous biological, psychological, social, and cultural forces interact to influence sexual development, sexual health, and interpersonal relationships.

Human Sexual Behavior

The reproductive activity of most complex animals includes behaviors commonly referred to as courtship and mating. Unlike other animals, humans exhibit a variety of complex sexual behaviors that do not necessarily result in reproduction. People often engage in sexual activity for pleasure and relaxation or to help maintain the emotional bonds of their intimate relationships. Some individuals, however, use their sexuality to dominate, exploit, or harm others. What factors influence human sexual behavior?

The Biology of Sexual Behavior

The motivation to pursue sexual activity, the sex drive, or *libido,* is an instinctual behavior moderated by the sex hormones. The ovaries and the testes, glands that make up part of the hormonal (endocrine) system, secrete these chemical messengers. The endocrine system is so named because of the endocrine glands, such as the ovaries and the testes, which secrete the hormones. Glands are individual cells or groups of cells that secrete substances. They are called *endocrine* because they release substances within (endo-) the body, rather than secreting substances that exit the body, such as sweat.

The endocrine system plays an important role in sexual functioning. The pituitary, located in the brain, and the ovaries and testes produce hormones that affect sexual functioning (Figure 6-2). Additionally, the hypothalamus, located above the pituitary, produces hor-

mones that trigger the secretion of pituitary hormones. During puberty in males, pituitary hormones activate the maturation of the male reproductive structures and the release of increased levels of the male sex hormone, testosterone. Testosterone plays a role in the maturation of the male reproductive structures, stimulates the development of sperm, and triggers and maintains the development of the secondary sexual characteristics such as the growth of a beard and the deepening of the voice. During puberty in females, pituitary hormones cause maturation of the ovaries, which then begin secreting the female sex hormones estrogen and progesterone. Estrogen stimulates maturation of the uterus and vagina, development of the female secondary sexual characteristics such as the development of breasts, and a change in the distribution of body fat.

During middle age, the production of sex hormones declines. After 40 years of age, men produce less testosterone and fewer sperm (Feldman et al., 2002). Despite this reduction, elderly men can still father children. When women reach menopause, usually between 45 and 55 years of age, their estrogen and progesterone levels decrease dramatically. As a result, menopausal women are no longer fertile. However, most healthy elderly men and women continue to have an interest in sex, and they engage in sexual activity. In a study

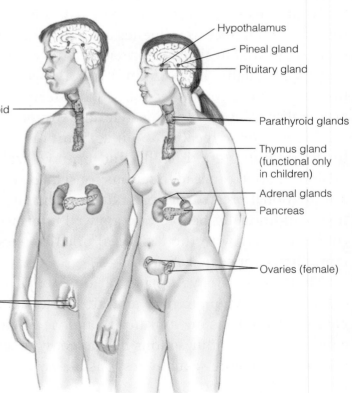

Figure 6-2 **Endocrine Glands.** The pituitary, ovaries, and testes produce hormones that affect sexual functioning. The hypothalamus produces hormones that trigger the secretion of pituitary hormones.

conducted for the American Association for Retired Persons, about 50% of those aged 45 through 59 reported having sex at least once a week. Among those aged 60 through 74, 30% of men and 24% of women reported having sex at least once a week (Jacoby, 1999). Research conducted for the 2003 General Social Survey (Smith, 2003) revealed that among those over 70 years of age, 39% were currently sexually active.

The Psychology of Sexual Behavior

Certain thoughts, sensations, and emotions modulate sexual behavior, as do the sex hormones. Included in this psychological mix are factors that can influence sex-

ual behavior positively, such as satisfaction with one's body, good physical and emotional health, absence of beliefs that can hinder sexual responsiveness or enjoyment, previous positive sexual experiences, and high self-esteem.

Many **sexologists**, scientists who study human sexuality, think that people who have high self-esteem are more likely to have positive attitudes concerning their sexuality than persons with poor self-concepts. However, people frequently judge their bodies and sexual prowess against unrealistic standards of physical attractiveness

sexuality the aspect of personality that encompasses a person's sexual thoughts, feelings, attitudes, and actions.

sexologists scientists who study human sexuality.

Consumer Health

Ginseng and Sexual Prowess

You've probably seen ads for ginseng in magazines, on television, or on the Web. The ads often make claims such as "Ginseng will boost your energy and sexual stamina," or "Ginseng has been used for centuries in maintaining overall health and vitality," or "Ginseng will reduce stress and the effects of aging." "Can it do that?" you wonder. "Heck," you think, "may as well try it. What can I lose?"

Ginseng is an herb that grows wild or is cultivated in eastern Asia and North America. For hundreds of years, the root of the plant has been used in Asia for medicinal purposes and as an aphrodisiac because it often looks like a human body. But what do we know about ginseng? Will it make you more sexually "potent"? Can it harm you or, alternatively, enhance your health?

On the positive side, studies in Taiwan show that sperm motility is enhanced after sperm are incubated with extracts of ginseng. Is sperm motility enhanced in men who take ginseng? There is still no answer to that question. Does ginseng affect sexual arousal or performance? Ginseng has been shown to significantly enhance libido and copulatory behavior in male rats and mice. This herb appears to have a direct effect on penile tissue, which could be responsible for its copulatory performance-enhancing actions. Nevertheless, these effects have not been studied in humans, and scientists agree that much needs to be learned regarding the ability of ginseng to facilitate libido in males.

On the negative side, medical researchers know that drug interactions occur with many herbals. Ginseng, in particular, may alter bleeding (or clotting) time, the time it takes for blood to stop flowing from a tiny wound. Ginseng also interacts with anticoagulant drugs, which "thin" the blood; that is, they decrease the ability of the blood to clot. Therefore,

anticoagulants and ginseng should not be taken together. Ginseng also may interfere with the heart medication digoxin (digitalis), which affects the force and rate at which the heart beats.

In addition to its interaction with anticoagulants and digoxin, ginseng should not be used if a person is taking estrogens or corticosteroid drugs such as cortisone because of possible additive effects. Ginseng may also affect blood glucose levels, so it should not be taken by persons with diabetes mellitus. For those on the antidepressant drug phenelzine sulfate (Nardil), ginseng could provoke a manic episode (an extreme excited state). Its general side effects may include headache and involuntary muscular contractions.

Should you take ginseng to boost your sexual prowess? This herb is commonly used in Asia to treat sexual dysfunction in humans. In addition, animal studies provide evidence that ginseng may be useful in such treatment, and it may enhance libido and copulatory behavior in males. However, clinical tests of the effects of ginseng on human sexual behavior have not been conducted, and the possibility of drug interactions exists. Therefore, you might not want to rely on ginseng for better bedroom calisthenics just yet.

Sources: Chen, J. C., Xu, M. X., Chen, L. D., Chen, Y. N., & Chiu, T. H. (1999). Effect of *Panax notoginseng* extracts on inferior sperm motility in vitro. *American Journal of Chinese Medicine, 27*:123–128.

Ernst, E. (2002). The risk-benefit profile of commonly used herbal therapies: Ginkgo, St. John's wort, ginseng, echinacea, saw palmetto, and kava. *Annals of Internal Medicine, 136*:42–53.

Miller, L. G. (1998). Herbal medicinals: Selected clinical considerations focusing on known or potential drug-herb interactions. *Archives of Internal Medicine, 158*:2200–2211.

Murphy, L. L., & Jer-Fu Lee, T. (2002). Ginseng, sex behavior, and nitric oxide. *Annals of the New York Academy of Sciences, 962*:372–377.

and sexual ability that are presented in the media. As a result, some individuals develop feelings of sexual inadequacy and low self-esteem because they feel sexually unattractive or inept. People who have these feelings may be unable to enjoy their sexuality and may be unable to form fulfilling intimate relationships.

The Sexual Response

The sexual response in both males and females is governed primarily by the nervous system rather than by hormones. Hormones are chemicals secreted in one part of the body that have an effect in another. **Testosterone**, the "male" hormone (women also secrete testosterone), helps maintain the sex drive, or libido.

The two major physical changes that occur during sexual arousal are vasocongestion and myotonia. **Vasocongestion** occurs as blood flow away from the sexual organs is reduced. The spongy tissue of the penis and clitoris expands with blood and these structures become erect. **Myotonia**, an increase in muscle tension, occurs throughout the body.

Both sexes have broader responses than just these events. This pattern of responses is termed the *sexual response cycle*. First defined by Masters and Johnson, it is usually thought of as having four phases: excitement, plateau, orgasm, and resolution (Figure 6-3).

During the *excitement phase* of the sexual response cycle, both men and women have a heightened sexual awareness. Certain thoughts, sights, touches, and even sounds or odors lead to a rush of blood to the clitoris and vaginal opening in women and to the penis in men.

In men, the penis expands as blood fills spaces in its columns of spongy tissue. As a result, the penis becomes erect, and the expansion of the tissue compresses the veins that take blood away from this organ (see Figure 5-2). Consequently, as blood flow into the penis increases, blood flow out of the penis decreases. This decrease in outward blood flow maintains the erection.

In women, glands in the vulvar area secrete mucuslike fluid. The congestion of blood in the vulvar area and in the vagina swells the labia and pushes fluid through the vaginal wall. These fluids are lubricants for sexual intercourse. Blood also rushes to the breasts.

testosterone a male sex hormone (androgen) that plays a role in the development of functionally mature sperm and is responsible for the development and maintenance of male secondary sexual characteristics such as the deepening of the voice and the growth of facial hair.

vasocongestion a condition in which the spongy tissue of the penis and clitoris expands with blood during sexual arousal.

myotonia an increase in muscle tension throughout the body during sexual arousal.

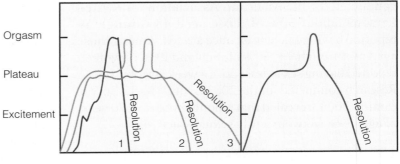

Female response   Male response

Figure 6-3 **The Female and Male Human Orgasmic Responses.** The female response is much more variable than is the male response, as shown by the three female patterns and one male pattern illustrated here.

In response, the breasts swell. The nipples become erect as smooth muscles contract. Many women also exhibit a *sex flush* at this time, a reddening of the skin as blood flow through it increases.

As sexual excitement continues, the *plateau phase* begins. The heart rate, blood pressure, respiration rate, and level of muscle tension all increase. During the plateau phase, the erection of the male intensifies as the penis is massaged rhythmically by intercourse (anal or vaginal), manual stimulation, or oral stimulation. Sensory impulses from tactile sensations in both sexes reinforce their sexual sensations. In women, the lower third of the vagina constricts around the penis. The upper two-thirds of the vagina widens as the uterus and cervix lift up, creating a space for the semen. Continued stimulation of the clitoris and penis leads to the next phase of the sexual response—the orgasmic phase.

In men, ejaculation occurs during the *orgasmic phase*. This involuntary response (over which men can exert some voluntary control) results when the nervous system sends messages to muscles in the walls of the vas deferens and urethra to contract. At the same time, the seminal vesicles and prostate receive messages to release their secretions. The pelvic muscles also rhythmically contract. Orgasm in women is characterized by rhythmic contractions of the pelvic muscles and vaginal walls. Both sexes experience a peak of sexual pleasure at orgasm. Erection and ejaculation are the two primary components of the male sex act. The clitoris of the female becomes erect during sexual activity and she achieves orgasm, but women do not ejaculate like men.

During the *resolution phase* the body returns to its pre-arousal state. The heart rate, blood pressure, and respiration slow; the muscles relax. In males, the erection subsides (the penis becomes flaccid) and sometimes fatigue sets in. Depending on the man and his age, he will not be able to develop another erection for a few minutes to a few hours. This time is the *refractory period*. Unlike men, women have the capacity to reach the orgasmic phase again (have multiple orgasms) in sequence or rather quickly after dropping to the plateau phase.

Sexual Dysfunctions

A *dysfunction* is an impaired bodily process or a behavior that hinders the development or maintenance of healthy relationships. *Sexual dysfunctions* relate to the psychological and physical conditions that interfere with the sexual response.

Erectile Dysfunction (Impotence)

A common problem with the sexual response that occurs in men, particularly middle-aged and older men, is *impotence*. More properly called **erectile dysfunction (ED)**, impotence is the inability of a man to develop and/or sustain an erection firm enough for penetration. The incidence of ED rises as men age, from 7% in men aged 18 to 29 to 18% in men aged 50 to 59 (Laumann et al., 1999). Some men with various degrees of erectile dysfunction are able, with proper stimulation, to reach orgasm and ejaculate.

Until the last decade, impotence was thought to be primarily a psychological problem, a conclusion based on research studies conducted by well-known sex therapists Masters and Johnson. However, medical researchers have discovered that approximately 70% to 80% of cases of impotence are due to physical problems. The most common cause of physically based impotence is blood vessel disease.

In order to develop and maintain an erection, blood must fill the spongy tissue of the penis and compress the veins that bring blood away from the penis. If a man has fatty deposits clogging his penile arteries, blood flow to the penis may be insufficient to develop and maintain an erection. The drugs Viagra (sildenafil), Levitra (vardenafil), and Cialis (tadalafil) work by widening blood vessels in the penis, thus increasing blood flow. A rub-on cream (Alprox-TD) also widens penile blood vessels, but this product is not yet available in the United States. To maintain sexual potency throughout mid-life and old age, men are encouraged to eat a low-fat diet, exercise regularly, and stop smoking (Esposito et al., 2004).

Erectile dysfunction can also be caused by a variety of other conditions, such as diabetes mellitus; damage to the spinal nerves or other nerves involved in erection; damage to the arteries that bring blood to the penis; certain medications used to control high blood pressure, anxiety, or depression; illness or injury that damages the penis; and hormonal imbalances. Results of recent research (Kunelius et al., 2002) show that use of a testosterone patch improves sexual function in men aged 50 to 70 years who exhibit symptoms of hormonal imbalance.

Alcohol and illegal drugs such as marijuana, heroin, and cocaine have also been shown to affect penile function negatively. In addition, stress can be a cause of impotence. Epinephrine (adrenaline), a chemical released by the body during the stress reaction, impedes a man's ability to have an erection.

Physicians warn that minor physical problems can cause problems with erection that can worry a man and lead to psychological problems with erection. A significant finding to help distinguish between a physical and psychological cause for impotence is whether the man has a normal pattern of erections while asleep but not while engaged in sex with his partner. Men are encouraged to seek medical help for impotence immediately so that underlying, and possibly serious, physical problems can be diagnosed and treated promptly. If physical problems are not the cause, the psychological health of the patient as well as the health of his relationships should be explored.

erectile dysfunction (ED) a sexual dysfunction in which a man is unable to develop and/or sustain an erection firm enough for penetration of the vagina. Also called impotence.

premature (rapid) ejaculation a common male sexual dysfunction in which a man consistently attains orgasm shortly after intercourse and before he wishes it to occur.

Premature (Rapid) Ejaculation

Premature ejaculation, also called **rapid ejaculation**, is another common male sexual dysfunction. The phrase "premature ejaculation" means that a man consistently attains orgasm shortly after intercourse begins (in less than 2 minutes more than 50% of the time) and before he wishes it to occur. The prevalence of this dysfunction is difficult to determine, but survey data show that premature ejaculation affects approximately one-quarter to one-third of men (Grenier & Byers, 2001; Laumann et al., 1999).

The cause of premature ejaculation is a controversial topic among medical researchers and psychologists who study sex-related disorders. One hypothesis suggests that premature ejaculation is related to anxiety. Another hypothesis is that men who exhibit premature ejaculation may be physically more sensitive to sexual stimulation. However, other research results refute this claim (Paick et al., 1998).

Whatever its cause, premature ejaculation usually can be overcome with proper treatment, which may include medication (Evanoff & Newton, 1998). The most common treatment is the "squeeze" technique, which helps a man learn to delay orgasm. To employ this technique, the man's partner uses her fingers to squeeze the front and back (not sides) of the penis where the glans meets the shaft (see Figure 5-1) or the base of the penis when the man feels as though he will ejaculate. After a few seconds, she releases her fingers. The couple waits 30 seconds and then resumes sexual activity until his orgasm is once again imminent. The squeeze is once again applied. This process is repeated as often as the couple desires. After a few sessions of using this technique, the male usually is able to delay ejaculation without help (Greenberg et al., 2004); however, the squeeze technique shows poor long-term success (Evanoff & Newton, 1998). In some cases, a couple may need to seek counseling from a qualified sex therapist to help them adjust their sexual techniques or to address other issues that may relate to the problem. Although premature ejaculation adversely affects sexual satisfaction, it does not appear to affect overall relationship and personal functioning (Byers & Grenier, 2003).

Hypoactive Sexual Desire Disorder

Hypoactive sexual desire disorder (HSDD) refers to a low interest in sex. This disorder affects both men and women, although HSDD occurs more often in women. (The term *frigid* was formerly used to refer to women with HSDD, but this term is no longer used because of its negative connotations.)

It is difficult to estimate accurately the prevalence of HSDD because no criteria have been established that define abnormal (or normal) levels of sexual desire. Additionally, desire varies among individuals and between partners, and decreases as people age. However, when interviewed for the National Health and Social Life Survey (NHSLS), approximately 30% of women and 15% of men between the ages of 18 and 59 reported that they lacked interest in sex over the prior year (Laumann et al., 1999; Warnock, 2002).

Hypoactive sexual desire disorder has a variety of psychological and physical causes, such as restrictive views regarding sex, a history of sexual abuse, relationship problems, certain chronic diseases such as rheumatoid arthritis, fatigue, stress, illness, and abnormal hormone levels. Treatment includes the identification and elimination of the cause. Problems within the relationship or those rooted in long-held, deep-seated feelings and beliefs require counseling and therapy for resolution. Other treatments include rest,

vaginismus
(VAJ-in-NIZ-mus) a sexual dysfunction of women in which the lower portion of the vagina contracts involuntarily at the anticipation of penetration, preventing it.

relaxation, hormone treatments, and changes in medications that a patient may be taking (Warnock, 2002). Additionally, many therapists suggest that couples practice *sensate focus,* a type of sex therapy developed by Masters and Johnson. This technique involves lovers caressing, touching, and exploring the sensual areas of each other's bodies in ways that produce pleasure, promote trust and communication, and reduce anxiety. Neither partner pressures the other for sex.

Female Sexual Arousal Disorder

Female sexual arousal disorder (FSAD) is a condition in which a woman receives no erotic pleasure from sexually oriented stimulation and is continually unable to attain or maintain arousal and lubrication during intercourse. The disorder primarily affects postmenopausal women due to hormonal changes, although infections, medical conditions, medications, surgeries, stress, depression, alcohol, drugs, and cigarette smoking may affect arousal as well. Nonmedical treatment strategies include the use of erotic materials, sensual massage, position changes, and the use of lubricants. Medical and drug treatments include psychological therapy, estrogen replacement therapy, testosterone therapy, and the EROS clitoral therapy device, which is a small vacuum pump designed to increase blood flow to the area. In addition, results of studies conducted by Berman and colleagues (2001) show that sildenafil (Viagra) is useful in treating FSAD and improves the female sexual response.

Vaginismus

Vaginismus is a sexual dysfunction of women in which the muscles of the lower third of the vaginal canal contract involuntarily (and often painfully) at the anticipation of sexual intercourse, the insertion of tampons, or a pelvic examination. The muscular contractions are strong enough to prevent penetration. Women with vaginismus do not usually have other sexual dysfunctions and can achieve orgasm by stimulating the clitoris. Vaginismus appears to have both physical and psychological causes. A review of the literature (Reissing et al., 1999) suggests that vaginismus is a neglected health problem of women, and that this sexual dysfunction has not been studied adequately since its name was coined in 1861.

A variety of physical conditions can cause pain during intercourse (*dyspareunia*) and result in vaginismus. Causes of dyspareunia include a poorly healed episiotomy (an incision made to widen the vaginal opening during the birth process); infections, sores, or lesions of the vagina or vulva; sexually transmitted infections (STIs); or inadequate lubrication during intercourse. If a woman experiences pain during intercourse because of one or more of these conditions, involuntary vaginal contractions may occur as the body attempts to protect itself from penetration and subsequent pain. If the cause of the pain eventually subsides, the contractions may still occur as a conditioned response.

Psychogenic vaginismus usually begins without a physical cause. The results of studies show that this type of vaginismus occurs as a protective response to perceived pain or violation of the body, with the most common cause being child sexual abuse (Greenberg et al., 2004).

Treatments for vaginismus have high success rates and include desensitization through exercises with dilators (Schnyder et al., 1998). Treating physical causes may resolve the condition. If a psychological cause exists, treatment usually includes behavioral therapy and counseling.

Culture and Sexuality

Society strongly influences the sexual attitudes and behaviors of a population by identifying acceptable sexual activities and placing restrictions on others. For example, some cultures value sexual abstinence before marriage; others value sexual experimentation during childhood. A **value** is a belief that an idea, object, or action has worth. The Diversity in Health essay "The Virtue of Virginity" provides a cross-cultural perspective concerning the value of sexual abstinence before marriage.

An individual usually formulates a personal value system before adulthood. A *value system* is a collection of beliefs that helps a person identify and classify things as being good or bad, or neither good nor bad. This value system guides the reasoning and behavior of the individual, especially in sexual decision making.

Many Americans derive their sexual values from Judeo-Christian religious teachings. However, people in the culturally diverse U.S. population adhere to a variety of sexual values, some of which conflict with traditional Judeo-Christian teachings. No universally accepted set of sexual values applies to Americans.

Widely accepted values can help people determine behavioral norms, but these norms often change over time and across cultures. Before World War I, for example, it was socially unacceptable for "proper" American men or women to expose much of their bodies in public. Today, most Americans think that it is acceptable for people to wear clothing that exposes much of their

Figure 6-4 **Culturally Appropriate Clothing.** In most Islamic countries, the only socially acceptable style of clothing for women covers their entire bodies except eyes and hands.

bodies, especially in warm weather. However, in some cultures, persons are punished severely if they appear in public dressed in revealing outfits; the only socially acceptable style of clothing is that which has been worn for centuries (Figure 6-4).

Gender Identity and Roles

Gender is the classification of a person's sex based on many criteria, among them anatomic and chromosomal characteristics. **Gender identity** is an individual's perception of himself or herself as male or female. Various biological, social, and environmental forces mold a child's gender identity.

Before birth, genetic and hormonal factors influence the sexual development of the embryonic brain. After birth, social factors have a major impact on gender identity. As children interact with people, they observe and learn gender roles and sexual stereotypes. A **gender role** refers to patterns of behavior, attitudes, and personality attributes that are traditionally considered in a particular culture to be feminine or masculine. A **sexual stereotype** is the widespread association of certain perceptions with one gender. Examples of sexual stereotypes are associating the

value the belief that an idea, object, or action has worth.

gender the classification of a person's sex based on many criteria, among them anatomic and chromosomal characteristics.

gender identity an individual's perception of himself or herself as male or female.

gender role patterns of behavior, attitudes, and personality attributes that are traditionally considered in a particular culture to be feminine or masculine.

sexual stereotype the widespread association of certain perceptions with one gender.

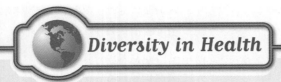
The Virtue of Virginity

Some American parents teach their children to consider virginity a gift that is given to spouses on their wedding night. Since the majority of American youth have sexual intercourse before leaving their teens, the importance of virginity before marriage appears headed for extinction. For many people, however, virginity continues to be highly valued.

Since ancient times, people from various cultures have used the condition of a bride's hymen to document her sexual history. In these cultures, an intact hymen is considered a sign of virginity. Although the hymen has no known biological function, this thin membranous tissue usually covers part of the outer entrance to the vagina. Most hymens have at least one opening that is wide enough to permit the discharge of menstrual blood. In many instances, this opening is too narrow for a penis to penetrate without tearing the hymen.

According to the Old Testament of the Bible, a man who thought that his bride was not a virgin on their wedding night was entitled to have his townspeople stone her to death. In some ancient societies, a newly wed woman who could not prove her virginity might be banished from her hometown, tortured, or killed. Her lover, if known, often received the same treatment. Today, virginity is still an important criterion for selecting a mate, especially in India, Indonesia, China, Taiwan, Iran, Turkey, and Arab nations. In most of these places, however, a new bride with sexual experience usually receives less harsh treatment than in the past. She may be rejected by her husband and returned to her family as "used goods." Facing embarrassment and ridicule from neighbors, the woman's family may disown her.

According to Islamic tradition, a woman's virginity is the basis for her honor and that of her family, her future groom, and his family. Muslims, followers of Islam, would arrange early marriages for their female children to ensure that these girls entered puberty as virgin brides. Fatima Mernissi (1987), a sociologist in the African country of Morocco, thinks that Muslim men maintain their respect and pride by controlling the sexuality of their wives, daughters, and sisters. In many Muslim communities, young women are required to be heavily veiled in the presence of strange men and in public (see Figure 6-4). If they do not wear veils, young women may be punished severely or labeled as prostitutes because their appearance is sexually tempting to men. Older Muslim women often appear unveiled in public because it is assumed that they are no longer sexually attractive.

Marriage customs in rural parts of Africa, Asia, and the Mediterranean often include some ritual that "proves" the bride has lost her virginity on her wedding night. In parts of Greece, the groom's friends gather outside the window of the newly married couple on the morning after the wedding to receive the news that the bride is no longer a virgin. After the groom makes the expected announcement, the gathering of friends celebrates by firing guns into the air. In many Middle Eastern villages that are populated with followers of Islam, it is customary for the groom to display his bride's underpants or their bloodstained sheets as evidence.

The social value of virginity is so powerful that plastic surgeons in Japan and Italy routinely reconstruct hymens so that their unmarried female patients who have been sexually active can give the impression that they are virgins. In some societies, new brides keep a small amount of chicken blood handy to smear on sheets during the wedding night, or they make a small cut near the vaginal opening that will bleed during sexual intercourse.

Economic factors also play a major role in perpetuating the value of premarital virginity. In many cultures, property is handed down from fathers to sons. Therefore, families strive to protect their financial interests and lines of inheritance by seeking virgin brides for male relatives. An unmarried woman who is not a virgin could be pregnant with a male child whose father is from another family. Without DNA testing to confirm a child's paternity, rural people in underdeveloped regions rely on an intact hymen as a sign of virginity. Along with this view of women as property, cultural norms of sexual chastity, female virginity, pure bloodlines, and family honor may also serve to control women's behavior.

In some societies, physicians perform virginity examinations to document premarital virginity. Even though cultural, historical, economic, and other factors perpetuate virginity examinations, the Turkish Medical Association has deemed these exams a form of gender-based violence. In 1999 Turkey banned virginity tests after five teenaged girls committed suicide by ingesting rat poison, rather than face the tests. Another drowned herself. In 2001, however, Turkey's health minister authorized virginity tests for nursing students. Those found to have lost their virginity were to be expelled from school. There was a public outcry against the testing, and in February 2002, the Turkish government closed a loophole in its law, removing wording that allowed school administrators to determine whether girls were virgins.

Source: Mernissi, F. (1987). *Beyond the veil: Male-female dynamics in modern Muslim society.* Bloomington, IN: Indiana University Press.

color blue with boys and pink with girls, or associating passiveness with females and aggressiveness with males.

Throughout the world, obvious biological differences between the sexes form the basis for traditional gender roles. In many cultures, for example, women are responsible for routine child-rearing and household management. This traditional gender role assignment likely developed for a variety of reasons, such as a woman's biological role in giving birth and nursing infants. It is also likely that because men, in general, are physically stronger than women, their customary roles have been protecting and providing for their families, especially in hunter-gatherer or agrarian societies.

In addition to biological factors, culture (often determined by race and ethnicity) and religion heavily influence sexual attitudes and behaviors. In many cultures, men learn to be sexually aggressive and women learn to be sexually passive. According to these sexual stereotypes, men are always eager for sex, and they are expected to demonstrate their interest and aggressiveness by initiating sexual encounters. Women are expected to be less interested in sex than men and to show their passiveness by accepting the sexual advances of men willingly.

In the United States, parents, friends, teachers, and the media influence children's perceptions of gender roles. For example, mothers appear to be a primary socializing agent for their daughters. The results of studies of mothers' and daughters' attitudes over time toward children, marriage, and careers reveal that mother/daughter attitudes are similar when the girls are adolescents and young teens. When daughters become adults, their gender role attitudes still appear to be significantly similar to those of their mothers; the attitudes of both groups change over time in similar patterns.

How do students' perceptions of gender roles change while they are in college? Bryant (2003) found that in general, students attending colleges and universities across the United States perceived male and female roles in a less traditional manner when they left college than when they entered. Nevertheless, at college entry and four years later, women held more egalitarian gender role attitudes (equality of the sexes) than did men. Experiences that appear to be relevant in shaping students' perceptions of gender roles are academic engagement, peers, and women's studies courses.

Some Americans reject traditional gender stereotypes because these attitudes and practices can create and foster sexism. **Sexism**, discrimination and bias against one sex, is common in many societies. For many women in the United States and other countries, sexist prac-

tices affect their status and health at work, school, and home. Sexual harassment and violence against women are forms of sexism. Men can experience sexism as well; White American males often feel the object of sexist practices in the workplace when hiring guidelines favor females.

Over the past two decades, societal norms in the United States have moved to a more liberal interpretation of appropriate role behaviors for women. Women are now more comfortable asking men out on dates. Men and women may feel free to initiate or refuse sexual activity. Additionally, a growing number of Americans feel free to choose nontraditional careers and adopt flexible gender roles. In a few families, traditional sex roles are reversed. For example, a woman may decide to work outside of the home while her male partner chooses to stay at home to care for their children and manage household tasks.

Transsexualism

In some instances, a person's gender identity conflicts with his or her biological sex, a condition known as *gender dysphoria*. An individual with this disorder feels trapped in the body of the opposite sex, and is a **transsexual**. To satisfy their self-concepts, transsexuals often dress and act like members of the opposite sex. According to the International Foundation for Gender Education, from 1 in 1,000 to 1 in 10,000 people are transsexuals. These recent estimates suggest that about half are male-to-female and half female-to-male transsexuals (Greenberg et al., 2004).

Transsexuals frequently undergo psychotherapy and hormonal treatments to help them deal with their gender identity conflicts; others choose to have sex reassignment surgery to change their sexual appearances. Physicians who perform sex reassignment surgeries usually remove certain reproductive organs and reconstruct the genitals of the patient to make them resemble those of the opposite sex. After transsexual surgery, however, the newly fashioned reproductive organs do not function like the organs of people who were born with them.

sexism discrimination and bias against one sex.

transsexual a person who is dissatisfied with his or her biological gender.

Healthy Living Practices

- To help you make responsible decisions concerning your sexuality, consider how your sexual behavior affects yourself and others.

Sexual Orientation

One of the most emotionally charged aspects of human sexuality is **sexual orientation**, that is, the direction of a person's romantic thoughts, feelings, and attractions. Survey data from European and American studies indicate that about 90% to 95% of people identify themselves as **heterosexual**, sexually attracted to members of the opposite sex (Sell et al., 1995; Smith, 2003; Greenberg et al., 2004). The remainder identify themselves as **homosexual** or **bisexual**. Homosexuals are sexually attracted to members of their own sex; bisexuals engage in sexual activity with both sexes.

Of the homosexual population, about 65% to 75% are males, and the remaining are females, although this figure is often debated (Greenberg et al., 2004). Homosexual men and women are commonly referred to as *gay* people; homosexual women are also called *lesbians*. Sexologist Alfred Kinsey proposed that sexual orientation is a continuum with exclusively heterosexual and homosexual designations at opposite ends, and degrees of bisexuality within this continuum (Kinsey et al., 1953) (Figure 6-5). Sexual orientation does not vary much across sociodemographic groups (Smith, 2003).

Nature or Nurture?

Do people, particularly homosexuals, choose their sexual orientation? Until recently, it was generally believed that homosexuality was learned behavior, and that children became homosexual by having early social and sexual experiences with gay individuals. At present, researchers cannot find a common childhood characteristic that predicts adult sexual orientation. Children may have same-sex experiences with other children, but most of them develop heterosexual orientations as they mature. Some gays and lesbians report that they knew they were different at an early age, but they did not recognize their homosexuality until they were in their teens or early 20s. Today, mental health experts generally agree that homosexuals do not decide their sexual orientation, nor can gay people alter their sexual preferences easily, if at all.

Researchers have also been studying the biological basis of homosexuality. Results of studies of the early 1990s show physical differences in small groups of cells in the hypothalamus of the brains of heterosexual and homosexual men (LeVay, 1991). In 1993 molecular geneticist Dean Hamer and his colleagues (1993) announced that a particular region of the X chromosome in homosexual males was involved in male sexual orientation in some, but not all, gay men. Males inherit this sex chromosome (condensed piece of hereditary material) from their mothers. The particular region of the X chromosome was dubbed the "gay gene." However, the results of more recent research do not support the presence of a gene that influences sexual orientation (Rice et al., 1999; Wickelgren, 1999).

Many scientists hypothesize that exposure of the fetal brain to male hormones is linked to homosexuality. They also think that handedness (whether a person is right- or left-handed) may be linked to such exposure. Research results associate handedness with sexual orientation in transsexuals and homosexuals. That is, both groups are disproportionately left-handed compared to the proportion of lefties in the heterosexual population (Green & Young, 2001; Lalumiere et al., 2000). Although these findings and other research results point to the brain as key in the development of sexual orientation, researchers concur that there is no consistent theory for sexual orientation and gender identity development at this time, and suspect that a combination of factors is involved.

Homosexuality and Society

Since ancient times, homosexuality has existed in most societies. Homosexuals are members of every racial, ethnic, socioeconomic, religious, and occupational group. While many homosexuals choose to conceal their sexual orientation, especially from their coworkers and neighbors, others have decided to "come out," expressing their sexual preferences openly.

Homophobia is an intense fear of or hostility toward homosexuals. However, not every person who objects

---

sexual orientation the direction of a person's romantic thoughts, feelings, and attractions toward people of the same or different sex.

heterosexual a person who is sexually attracted to members of the opposite sex.

homosexual a person who is sexually attracted to members of his or her own sex.

bisexual a person who engages in sexual activity with both sexes.

homophobia an intense fear of or hostility toward homosexuals.

100% Heterosexual	A few homosexual fantasies or experiences	More heterosexual than homosexual	Bisexual	More homosexual than heterosexual	A few heterosexual fantasies or experiences	100% Homosexual

Figure 6-5 **Kinsey's Continuum of Sexual Orientation.** Sexuality researcher Alfred Kinsey thought that sexual orientation is a continuum with exclusively heterosexual and homosexual designations on the ends and degrees of bisexuality between them.

to homosexuality is afraid of gay people or is hostile toward them. Therefore, *antihomosexual* may be a more descriptive term than *homophobic* to describe people who harbor such fears and hostilities.

Many heterosexuals do not accept homosexuality because they think gay sexual behavior is unnatural or it contradicts their religious beliefs. Other people are afraid of contact with gays because they associate acquired immune deficiency syndrome (AIDS) with homosexuality. Results of research studies show that in general, women hold fewer negative attitudes and beliefs toward homosexuals than men do, and exhibit fewer antihomosexual behaviors (Johnson et al., 1997; Whitley & Kite, 1995).

Homosexuals may feel isolated and have low self-esteem as a result of hostility and rejection from their families and other members of society. Family counseling can improve relations between homosexual children and their parents. Additionally, gay people may enhance their self-concepts by forming social networks with other homosexuals.

In 1996 U.S. President Bill Clinton signed the "Defense of Marriage" bill, which does not recognize marriages between homosexuals and allows states to ignore same-sex marriages that have been performed in other states (Carney, 1996). Gay couples, however, often cohabit and form lifetime commitments, commonly called domestic partnerships. Since domestic partners often contribute to the economic survival of their households, share property, and raise children, they want the same legal rights and protections that heterosexual married couples have, such as the right to claim insurance benefits when their partners die.

As of July 1, 2000, Vermont recognized civil unions between gays in that state. Some cities, such as San Francisco and Seattle, and a few states now recognize certain legal aspects of homosexual partnerships, such as the right to adopt children from one of their previous marriages. Massachusetts legalized gay marriage on May 17, 2004. In early 2004, San Francisco Mayor Gavin Newsom issued 4,000 marriage licenses to gay couples even though California only recognized marriage between a man and a woman. In August 2004, however, the California Supreme Court ruled unanimously that San Francisco's mayor overstepped his authority and declared the marriages of gay and lesbian couples that had been sanctioned by the city "void from their inception and a legal nullity." Then in March 2005, a San Francisco Superior Court judge overturned California's ban on gay marriage. As of this writing, opponents of gay marriage, led by President George W. Bush, were trying to amend the U.S. Constitution to outlaw gay and lesbian marriages.

Diversity in Sexual Behavior

Common Sexual Practices between Partners

Most heterosexuals are familiar with the notion of "having sex" or **sexual intercourse** as vaginal sex, the insertion of a penis into a vagina. Vaginal sex, or **coitus**, is the most common and popular form of intimate sexual activity among heterosexual adults. On average, adult Americans report that they engage in coitus about once a week. Married individuals report having vaginal sex more frequently than never-married, divorced, or widowed persons. The results of various surveys indicate that the longer a couple has been married, the less frequently they engage in coitus (Smith, 2003).

Couples often engage in **petting** as a pleasurable substitute for or a prelude to coitus. Petting activities include a variety of sex acts that range from kissing and fondling breasts to performing oral sex. Additionally, a heterosexual couple may rub their genital areas together, without allowing the penis to penetrate the vagina. For people who want to reduce their risk of pregnancy or sexually transmitted infections, petting can be a safe alternative to vaginal sex.

Although not as popular as vaginal sex, oral sex is becoming a common sexual activity. **Cunnilingus** is the use of the mouth and tongue to stimulate a woman's genitals; **fellatio** refers to oral stimulation of a male's genitals. In the early part of this century, heterosexuals, even those who were married, rarely practiced oral sex. By the 1970s, sex manuals and sexuality textbooks had begun to suggest that couples incorporate oral sex into their sexual routines. More than 75% of American men and nearly as many American women report that they have either received or given oral sex (Michael et al., 1994). Women who are unable to have orgasms during coitus are often able to have them while receiving oral sex.

sexual intercourse penetration of the vagina by a penis.

coitus (KO-ih-tus) the act of a penis penetrating a vagina, often referred to as vaginal intercourse.

petting sexual activities that may be a substitute for or prelude to coitus.

cunnilingus (KUN-ih-LING-gus) use of the mouth and tongue to stimulate a woman's genitals.

fellatio (feh-LA-she-oh) use of the mouth and tongue to stimulate a male's genitals.

Some couples find anal sex, the practice of stimulating the anal area with the penis, mouth, or fingers, to be pleasurable. Although anal intercourse is a common sexual practice of gay males, a growing number of heterosexual couples are experimenting with the activity; 10% to 20% of heterosexuals report having had anal sex at least once (Michael et al., 1994). When women, however, are asked to rate how much they enjoy various sexual activities, they usually rank anal sex among the least liked.

Many women find anal intercourse unappealing because the practice can be painful. The muscles surrounding the anal opening normally tighten when stimulated. As a result of this tightening, large hard objects have difficulty entering the anus. Forcing the object into the anus can tear its delicate tissues and produce pain.

Anal sex also can spread infection. If anal sex is followed by coitus, bacteria can be spread from the rectum into the vagina or the *urethra,* the tube that carries urine from the bladder. These bacteria may cause troublesome vaginal and bladder infections. After anal sex, one should wash the fingers or penis thoroughly before inserting them into a vagina or another rectum to reduce the risk of spreading harmful bacteria. Women should urinate after vaginal sex to help remove some of the bacteria that have entered the urethra, reducing the risk of a bladder infection. Anal sex also increases the risk of contracting HIV and other sexually transmitted infections from an infected partner. Using latex condoms during anal sex reduces but does not eliminate this risk.

celibacy (sexual abstinence) refrainment from sexual intercourse, usually by choice.

Solitary Sexual Behavior

Sex does not necessarily require a partner for it to be a pleasurable experience. People who practice masturbation, or solitary sex, can achieve orgasms by stroking or rubbing their own sexually sensitive body parts, especially the genitals. Although people may feel guilty or ashamed because they masturbate, the practice is common. In the National Health and Social Life Survey (NHSLS), nearly 60% of the male and about 40% of female respondents between 18 and 59 years of age reported that they had masturbated at least once during the past year (Michael et al., 1994). Data from other studies generally indicate that nearly all men engage in solitary sex at some point in their lives.

People often think that only adolescent boys and single men masturbate, but women and married or cohabiting individuals also practice solitary sex, especially when their partners are unavailable. Some women masturbate because they do not have orgasms during vaginal intercourse. These women may be reluctant to communicate with their partners about their most sexually sensitive body parts or about sexual practices that they think are stimulating. Whatever their reasons for masturbating, people can relieve sexual tension safely with this practice. No physiological harm comes from masturbating, nor is there evidence that it leads to an inability to establish sexual relationships (Greenberg et al., 2004).

Celibacy

Celibacy, or **sexual abstinence**, is refrainment from sexual intercourse, usually by choice. Celibacy can be a way of life; the clergy of some religions practice sexual abstinence. Some celibate individuals engage in alternative sexual practices such as petting and masturbation. Temporary sexual abstinence during the woman's peak period of fertility is a feature of natural family planning methods (see Chapter 5). Late in pregnancy, couples may decide to avoid vaginal intercourse, especially if the activity is too awkward and uncomfortable.

Celibacy is not known to be harmful; indeed, it is the most effective measure for preventing pregnancies and sexually transmitted infections. Therefore, most health experts recommend that teenagers practice sexual abstinence before marriage.

Healthy Living Practices

- Wash after touching the anal area so as not to spread bacteria that live in the rectum to other parts of the body.
- To reduce the risk of transmitting the virus that causes AIDS, use latex condoms during vaginal or anal intercourse.
- Practicing sexual abstinence is the most reliable way to avoid pregnancy and sexually transmitted infections.

■ Romantic Relationships

Defining Love

Giving and receiving love are so important to a person's well-being that social scientists have speculated about it and studied its origins, characteristics, and stages. What is love? Why do people fall in love?

Love is difficult to define because the term has different meanings for different people. One definition is that *love* is a collection of behaviors, thoughts, and emotions that are associated with a psychological attraction toward other individuals. There are numerous kinds or degrees of love and a variety of feelings associated with love. Liking, fondness, affection, attraction, infatuation, and lust are feelings related to love. Also, the love of two friends can be quite different from the feelings between parent and child or husband and wife. According to sexologists William H. Masters and Virginia E. Johnson, all forms of love involve the element of **caring**, the expression of concern for someone's well-being.

Zick Rubin, one of the first psychologists to develop a questionnaire to measure the meanings of love, attempted to differentiate between loving and liking. He found that loving had characteristics of intimacy, attachment, caring, and commitment while liking had characteristics of affection and respect (Rubin, 1973). **Intimacy** is the disclosure of one's most personal thoughts and emotions to a trusted individual. **Attachment** is the desire to spend time with someone to give and receive emotional support. **Commitment** is the determination to maintain the relationship even when times are difficult. **Affection** is a feeling of fondness toward another. **Respect** is the feeling that another has value and deserves attention.

Most humans seek loving relationships with other individuals to meet their emotional needs. Love that is fulfilling is reciprocal; that is, when one loves another, he or she is loved in return. Individuals who are in love feel free to achieve self-actualization (see Chapter 2) because their relationship fosters mutual independence as well as emotional, social, and spiritual growth.

Psychologists' Theories about Love

Beginning with Sigmund Freud in 1922, psychologists have tried to explain the phenomenon of love. Early "love theorists" such as Freud were clinical psychologists, professionals who diagnose, treat, and study mental or emotional problems and disabilities. Most of their theories relied on ideas that people loved others as a remedy for their own problems or deficiencies, rather than loving others for themselves.

In recent decades, social psychologists have formulated theories on love. These professionals explore questions by examining the individual in a social context while taking into account personality, which is the distinctive pattern of behavior, thoughts, motives, and emotions that characterizes an individual.

In 1956 Eric Fromm presented his ideas about love in *The Art of Loving*. A basic idea in Fromm's book, as noted in its title, is that loving is an art and, as such, must be learned and practiced. Fromm also distinguished between types of love, such as motherly love and erotic love.

In 1973 John Alan Lee theorized that six styles of loving exist. His ideas have since been upheld by results of studies of other researchers. Table 6-1 lists these styles with their names (derived from the Greek), meanings, and characteristics. To see with which of Lee's style you most closely align, take "The Love Attitudes Scale" provided in the student workbook.

In 1986 Robert Sternberg developed a triangular theory of love that incorporates three components—intimacy, commitment, and passion—as symbolized by

caring the expression of concern for someone's well-being.

intimacy disclosure of one's most personal thoughts and emotions to a trusted individual.

attachment the desire to spend time with someone to give and receive emotional support.

commitment the determination to maintain a relationship even when times are difficult.

affection fondness.

respect the feeling that another has value and deserves attention.

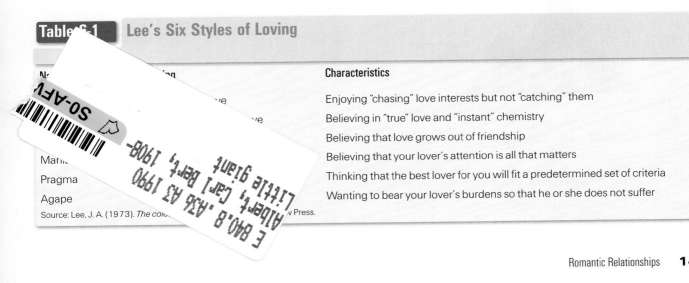

Table 6-1	Lee's Six Styles of Loving	
Name	Meaning	Characteristics
		Enjoying "chasing" love interests but not "catching" them
		Believing in "true" love and "instant" chemistry
		Believing that love grows out of friendship
		Believing that your lover's attention is all that matters
Pragma		Thinking that the best lover for you will fit a predetermined set of criteria
Agape		Wanting to bear your lover's burdens so that he or she does not suffer

Source: Lee, J. A. (1973). *The colors of love.* New Press.

the points of a triangle, as Figure 6-6a shows. His intimacy component includes behaviors that foster a feeling of warmth, while the commitment component refers to the decision to love as well as to make a relationship last. Passion, in the love triangle, refers not only to sexual passion but also to the fulfillment of needs that elicit a passionate response. The balance of these three components affects the shape of the triangle. Amount of love affects the area of the triangle.

People in a love relationship often have feelings of intimacy, commitment, and passion that differ from those of their partners. Although two people may be in love with each other, their "love triangles" will not match if one loves the other more than is reciprocated, and if one differs from the other in the balances of the three kinds of love. According to Sternberg, couples with similar love triangles are more likely to

be satisfied with their relationships because they share more love-related feelings and attitudes, as Figure 6-6b shows, than couples with mismatched triangles, as in Figure 6-6c . Sternberg has developed a questionnaire to measure love according to his love triangles theory (Sternberg, 1997, 1998).

Finally, Sternberg asserts that although there are only three components of love, these three components combine in various ways to produce seven kinds of love (Sternberg, 1998). For example, an absence of all three components (intimacy, commitment, and passion) results in nonlove. The presence of all three components results in consummate love. Table 6-2 lists Sternberg's kinds of love and their components.

Love Attachments

The early bonds, or attachments, that develop between parents and their offspring may influence the ability of the children to form close, secure relationships when they are adults. *Attachment* is a biological drive in which a child seeks nearness to or contact with a specific person, such as a parent, when he or she is frightened, tired, hungry, or ill. A child will exhibit attachment behavior, such as eye contact, smiling, crying, and clinging, to obtain or maintain desired proximity to this person. How the person responds to the child largely determines the type of attachment the child will form: secure, ambivalent, or avoidant.

For example, when an infant is hungry, he or she will exhibit attachment behavior, such as crying, to evoke a nurturing response from the attachment figure (e.g., mom or dad). A nurturing response to this need usually includes touching, eye contact, smiling, and providing milk. When the infant receives this nurturing

Figure 6-6 **Sternberg's Love Triangle.** Psychologist Robert Sternberg created a model that incorporates three components of love—intimacy, commitment, and passion—at the points of a triangle. Couples with identical "love triangles" (a) are more likely to be satisfied with their relationships because they share more sexual feelings and attitudes than couples with similar (b) or highly mismatched triangles (c).

Table 6-2	Sternberg's Seven Kinds of Love		
	Components of Love		
Kind of Love	Intimacy	Passion	Commitment
Nonlove	−	−	−
Liking	+	−	−
Infatuated love	−	+	−
Empty love	−	−	+
Romantic love	+	+	−
Companionate love	+	−	+
Fatuous love	−	+	+
Consummate love	+	+	+

Source: Sternberg, R. J. (1998). *Cupid's arrow: The course of love through time.* Cambridge, UK: Cambridge University Press, p. 17. Reprinted by permission of the author.

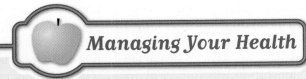

Minding Your Sexual Manners

The following guidelines can help you make socially responsible decisions regarding your sexual behavior.

1. Never force sex on another person, regardless of the situation.
2. Understand that at any time in a relationship, when a person says no, that means no, not yes or maybe.
3. Avoid situations that can impair your ability to make responsible sexual decisions, especially situations that involve alcohol and other drug use.
4. Be prepared to prevent pregnancies or sexually transmitted infections. Do not engage in risky sexual behaviors. Protect yourself and your partner by using a new latex condom with each act of sexual intercourse.
5. Communicate your concerns about the risks of pregnancy and sexually transmitted infections to your partner.
6. Share the responsibility of preventing pregnancies and sexually transmitted infections with your partner.
7. Respect the sexual privacy of your partner and your relationship.
8. Consider the feelings of others. Public displays of intimate behavior can offend or embarrass people.
9. Do not sexually harass others.
10. Treat your partner with care and respect.

Adapted from Hatcher, R. A., Sanderson, C. A., & Smith, K. L. (1990). Sexual etiquette 101. *SIECUS Report, 18*:9.

response consistently, trust is built. When the infant does not receive this response consistently, the child may develop mistrust and may stop his or her attachment behavior. Over time, symptoms may emerge such as lack of eye contact, destructive behavior, and poor peer relationships. Some children who have poor attachments to their parents may avoid becoming emotionally close to people in adulthood.

Experts think that children who have emotionally distant and neglectful parents may mature into *anxious lovers*. Anxious lovers often have considerable doubts about the quality of their sexual relationships, are unable to trust their partners, and may be unable to form long-term commitments. However, if parents meet the emotional needs of their children and frequently display affection toward them, the children are likely to mature into secure lovers. Secure lovers are more likely to form trusting and committed relationships with other adults than are anxious lovers.

Love Changes over Time

Early in a relationship, when physical attraction is greatest and partners know very little about one another, their passion is high. Preoccupied with their sexual desire for each other, passionate lovers think about their partners and want to be with them constantly.

Some people experience *infatuation*, a passionate but unrealistic attraction to someone. Infatuated individuals often exaggerate the positive characteristics of their partners while ignoring their faults. A relationship that is based on infatuation may not survive, especially when one or both lovers become aware of their partners' weaknesses and find these faults unacceptable.

Eventually, the intense sexual attraction that characterizes the initial stage of a romantic relationship subsides. The couple, if sexually active, usually engages in sex less frequently than in the earlier phase of their relationship. They enjoy being together, but they can endure separations. Other aspects of their relationship, such as companionship, often deepen. Although couples in this stage of love have conflicts, committed partners usually try to resolve their problems.

Not every couple experiences the stages of love in this order. Sometimes passionate love affairs evolve from romantic companionate relationships, such as when friends become lovers. Whatever the course of a romantic relationship, however, it will have phases of growth and change. If you are involved in an intimate relationship, the Managing Your Health features "Minding Your Sexual Manners" above and "Tips for Better Sex" on page 150 provide suggestions that may help you maintain the intimacy of this partnership.

Establishing Romantic Commitments

Have you ever been in love? Why did you fall in love with that person? Studies have shown that physical attraction is the most important factor that determines whether two individuals become romantically interested in one another. People often use other criteria as well, such as social status, occupation, and wealth, to select their sexual partners. Not surprisingly,

Americans spend millions of dollars annually to enhance their "sex appeal" by purchasing make-up, jewelry, clothing, and expensive cars.

Initially, two people who are physically attracted to each other usually make and hold eye contact. Couples may describe this behavior as "falling in love at first sight." After two people find each other physically appealing, they need to determine if they are **compatible**; that is, if they are capable of existing together in harmony.

Which characteristics are important for establishing long-term satisfying and compatible relationships? Individuals in such relationships are usually close in age, and they usually share similar racial, ethnic, religious, and educational backgrounds (Figure 6-7). Members of couples who have extremely different backgrounds or dissimilar characteristics can certainly form satisfying and lasting relationships, but these situations are less common than those described previously.

compatible capable of existing together in harmony.

cohabitation unmarried persons living together.

extrarelational sex sexual relationships with individuals who are not one's spouse or primary sex partner.

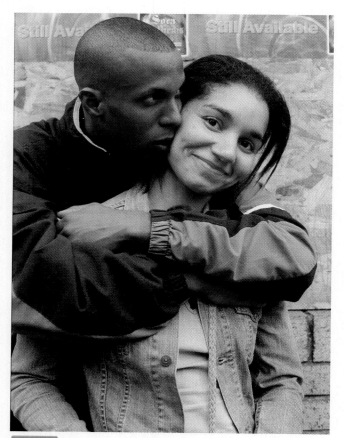

Figure 6-7 **Many Personal Characteristics Contribute to Compatibility.** Although this man and woman do not share the same racial background, they are similar in age and may have other similarities that foster their compatibility as a couple.

Sexual satisfaction is another characteristic related to the establishment of long-term satisfying and compatible relationships. Several studies have shown an association between sexual satisfaction and overall relationship satisfaction in marriage. One study focused on the association between sexual satisfaction and relationship quality in premarital heterosexual couples (Sprecher, 2002). Research results showed that over time, sexual satisfaction was positively associated with relationship satisfaction, love, and commitment for both men and women. When change occurred in sexual satisfaction over time, change also occurred in relationship satisfaction, love, and commitment. Overall, sexual satisfaction had stronger links with relationship quality for men than for women.

Types of Romantic Commitments

Cohabitation In the second half of the twentieth century, a growing number of unmarried people decided to live with their heterosexual partners. In 1960, 439,000 adult heterosexual couples lived together; in 2000, the number rose to nearly 4.6 million (U.S. Bureau of the Census, 2000). The practice of unmarried couples living together is called **cohabitation**.

Why do people live together rather than get married? Among young people, the widespread belief is that cohabitation is a way to find out if they and their partners really get along. Cohabitation is viewed as a way to avoid a bad marriage and eventual divorce (National Marriage Project, 2004). However, results of studies show that people who cohabit before marriage (with the exception of those who are engaged and have set a wedding date) are *not* more likely to enjoy longer and happier marriages than individuals who do not live together before marrying. Studies conducted in the United States, Sweden, and Canada document higher divorce rates among couples who cohabited before marriage than among those who did not. Research results suggest that this increased risk of divorce may be due to self-selection; that is, persons who are less able to sustain long-term relationships may choose to cohabit prior to marriage, rather than to marry without first living with their partners (Lillard et al., 1995). Additionally, research data show that multiple cohabiting experiences do *not* help people learn to have better relationships. In fact, persons with multiple cohabiting experiences are more likely to have failed future relationships than persons who do not cohabit. Although this negative correlation of cohabitation on later marriage stability is not totally understood, no positive contribution of cohabitation to marriage has been found (Popenoe & Whitehead, 2002).

In spite of a negative correlation between cohabitation and marriage stability, cohabitation is emerging as a significant experience for young adults and is replacing marriage as the first living-together union. Researchers estimate that 25% of unmarried women in the United States between the ages of 25 and 39 are currently living with a heterosexual partner. Approximately 50% are estimated to have cohabited at one time.

Marriage In the United States and in most other countries, marriage is a legally binding commitment between an adult man and an adult woman. (Massachusetts allows marriage and Vermont allows civil unions between persons of the same sex.) Most Americans desire marriage as a lifelong and loving partnership, and expect sexual faithfulness, emotional support, mutual trust, and lasting commitment (Popenoe & Whitehead, 1999). However, research results show a moderate decline in marital quality since the 1970s (Figure 6-8).

Along with being less satisfied with their marriages, Americans are also marrying a bit later in life today than in recent decades. In 1960 the median age at first marriage was 20 years for women and 23 years for men. (The median is the point below which 50% of the scores fall.) By 2004, the median age of first marriage had increased to 25 years for women and 27 years for men. Americans have also become less likely to marry; from 1970 to 2002 the annual number of marriages per 1,000 unmarried women aged 15 and older has declined by about 40% (National Marriage Project, 2004).

What factors help make a marriage successful? Partners in successful marriages often demonstrate positive problem-solving and communication skills. When conflicts arise, couples with these skills can openly discuss their feelings, and they are willing to negotiate and compromise to find solutions. Additionally, partners in successful marriages share basic values, have mutual concerns, and exhibit high degrees of physical intimacy.

Extrarelational Sex Some people have sexual relationships with individuals who are not their spouses or primary sex partners. Although most Americans disapprove of such **extrarelational** sexual activity, particularly when married couples are involved, results of a recent survey show that persons aged 40 to 59 are more likely to have extramarital sex than are older people or younger people (Smith, 2003). (Having sex with someone other than one's spouse is commonly referred to as *extramarital sex* or *adultery.*) The majority of married Americans report that they are faithful to their spouses. Experts, however, have difficulty obtaining an accurate estimate of the number of Americans who have had extramarital sex because people may be unwilling to reveal this information. Nevertheless, results from recent national surveys suggest that approximately 20% of spouses in the United States have been unfaithful (Atkins et al., 2001; Smith, 2003).

Separation and Divorce In spite of having high hopes for happiness and success during their wedding celebrations, many couples see their marriages end in separation or divorce. Nearly half of recent first marriages may end in divorce; the divorce rate for younger per-

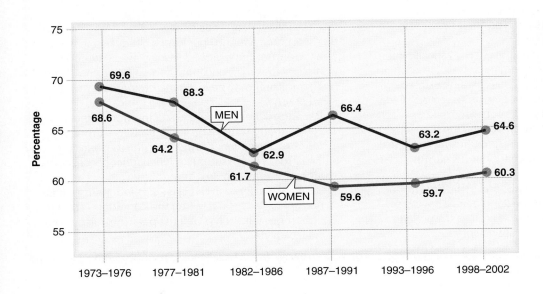

Figure 6-8 Percentage of Married Persons Age 18 and Older Who Said Their Marriages Were "Very Happy," by Period, United States. Source: General Social Survey, conducted by the National Opinion Research Center of the University of Chicago.

sons has risen in recent years (Kreider & Fields, 2002). Accurate data concerning the number of married persons who separate permanently are unavailable. Teenage marriages are especially vulnerable to dissolution. Women who marry when they are younger than 20 years of age are much more likely to be in a failed marriage as women who marry when they are at least 20 years of age (Bramlett & Mosher, 2001).

Early in the twentieth century, divorce was uncommon in this country. In 1940 the U.S. divorce rate was 2 divorces per 1,000 persons. The divorce rate rose during World War II and peaked at more than 4 divorces per 1,000 at the war's end. The rate fell during the 1950s to nearly prewar rates, and rose again in the 1960s and 1970s. From 1979 through 1981, the U.S. divorce rate was at its highest level of the twentieth century, slightly more than 5 divorces per 1,000. The decline in the divorce rate has been relatively steady since that time, and in 2003 was at 3.8 for every 1,000 persons (Figure 6-9). Currently in the United States, more than 1 million divorces occur annually.

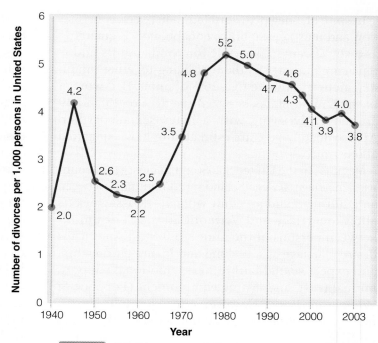

Figure 6-9 **U.S. Divorce Rates: 1940 to 2003.** Since 1981 the divorce rate has declined in the United States. Sources: U.S. Bureau of the Census, National Center for Health Statistics.

 Managing Your Health

Tips for Better Sex

1. Develop the nonsexual sides of your relationship; sharing common interests such as music, camping, and sports can help maintain the partnership outside the bedroom.
2. Communicate with your partner. Convey specific information to each other concerning the sexual activities that are the most pleasurable as well as the least desirable. If you like having your breasts kissed or you do not like having your buttocks squeezed, say so.
3. Make sex more interesting by varying the situations in which it occurs. Be creative; find unusual locations, wear provocative sleepwear or undergarments, or try new positions for sex.
4. Allow enough time for sex. Spend some time talking, touching, caressing, and kissing before having sexual intercourse. These activities can be the prelude to a more satisfying sexual relationship.

5. Avoid worrying about orgasms or sexual performances. You may find that it is not essential to have orgasms or accomplish penetration during every sexual encounter to feel sexually satisfied.
6. Think about fulfilling your lover's needs before yours. If you are not interested in receiving sexual stimulation at the same time, concentrate on satisfying your lover. Your partner may be willing to reciprocate at some other time.
7. Recognize that there are no recipes for perfect sex. Focus on the sensations and emotions surrounding the sexual experience rather than the mechanics.
8. Avoid making an issue out of your partner's occasional lack of interest in sex or inability to have sexual intercourse. Even in the best of relationships, it is normal to have times when the conditions are not right for sex. If such problems persist, seek professional advice.

Marriages fail for numerous reasons. People frequently cite reasons for dissolving their marriages that involve problems with their spouses, particularly extramarital sexual activity, emotional immaturity, and alcoholism. Other factors that contribute to marital separation and divorce include the failure to communicate with or to understand one's spouse; gender role disagreements; personality, interest, and value differences; and the desire for more personal freedom. In most instances, more than one factor contributes to the breakup of a marriage.

After their divorces are final, many people begin to search for new partners, and they eventually remarry—men at a higher rate than women. Remarriages do not have better success rates than first marriages. Divorced people who remarry have a greater probability of subsequent divorce than do persons marrying for the first time (Ceglian & Gardner, 1999).

Healthy Living Practices

- To increase your child's chances of being able to form secure and trusting relationships as an adult, consider ways to be more attentive to his or her emotional needs; display your affection frequently.
- To increase your likelihood of having a happy and long-term marriage, avoid cohabitation prior to making this commitment and communicate as effectively as possible with your spouse.

■ Communication in Relationships

Effective communication is a cornerstone of interpersonal and sexual relationships. In order to communicate effectively, people must express themselves as accurately and as clearly as possible but also must listen with attentiveness, openness, and patience. To express yourself accurately and clearly, first say exactly what you mean. If you avoid being straightforward so that you will not hurt someone's feelings, for example, the person with whom you're communicating may not understand your message. Second, your statements must be specific, not vague. For example, telling your partner that you would like him to be more spontaneous will probably make him question what you really mean. Do you always want him to act in a spontaneous manner? Has he never been spontaneous? Or do you really mean that you had wanted him to accept yesterday's last-minute party invitation, and wished that he could have just dropped what he was doing, changed his clothes, and dashed out the door with you? Third, avoid sending mixed messages. For example, don't tell your partner that everything is fine when she can tell from your behavior and expression that you are really feeling "down." Or, don't say, "I don't want to worry you, but I think I have a sexually transmitted infection."

Another mechanism to foster effective communication is to express your feelings using "I" statements when discussing issues with a partner. Then go on to say what you need to try to maintain (or change) the feeling. Statements that begin with "You" can hinder open communication between partners, particularly if the speaker is criticizing the listener's behavior or blaming this person for something. For example, instead of saying "You always spend too much time with your friends," you could say "I feel lonely and miss you terribly when you are out with your friends. (Express the feeling.) Could I join you on those occasions so that we could spend more time together?" (State the remedy.) Try not to fall into the trap of "false" I statements. "I feel like you spend too much time with your friends" is really a "you" statement.

Besides being able to express oneself clearly, an effective communicator has good listening skills. Failure to hear information accurately or completely can create misunderstandings that result in conflicts. In discussions, good listeners restate or paraphrase what they have heard their partners say. This practice allows speakers, if necessary, to correct or clarify what they have said. For example, if your partner says, "When we get together with your friends or your family, you always ignore me," you could respond by saying, "I didn't realize that you feel neglected in those situations. What can I do to make you feel more included?" To evaluate your communication patterns, use the "Communication Patterns Questionnaire" in the student workbook.

In addition to words, people use nonverbal forms of communication, such as body positioning (body language) and facial gestures, to express their thoughts (Figure 6-10). Touching is a form of nonverbal communication that can convey important information about intimate sexual feelings. Many people report that being held, kissed, massaged, or fondled by their partners is as sexually gratifying as sexual intercourse. Sensual touching does not have to involve the genitals; gently massaging your partner's back, for example, can convey your feelings of love to this individual.

Nonverbal Communication. Nonverbal forms of communication, such as body postures and facial gestures, can convey thoughts. What do this couple's nonverbal signals communicate?

Healthy Living Practices

- To encourage discussions between you and your partner about issues that concern the relationship, use "I" statements to express your feelings and avoid using "You" statements. "You" statements can anger or belittle your partner.

- Listen carefully to your partner during your discussions. Repeat what your partner says to avoid misunderstandings. If your partner gives unclear responses to your questions, ask for additional information.

Across
THE LIFESPAN

Sexuality

Most preschoolers masturbate. Parents who think masturbation is a healthy and normal aspect of sexuality usually let their children know that the behavior is inappropriate in public but do not attempt to stop this behavior in private. Preschool children typically play games in which they act out adult gender roles. By this age, children have learned that there are differences between the sexes. Children are curious about sexuality; they may "play doctor" by examining each others' genitals. Additionally, young children often ask questions such as "Where did I come from?" If parents are uncertain how to answer this or other questions about sexual matters, they can usually find a collection of age-appropriate sexuality books that they can read with their children at their libraries. Of course, parents should read these books themselves before they read them with their children.

It is not unusual for elementary school-age children to engage in mutual sex play, activities that may include rehearsing adult sexual behaviors. Sex experts consider such sex play normal behavior when it is playful, occurs infrequently, and does not involve coercion.

The ability to reproduce begins during puberty. Many teens avoid sexual activity because they fear becoming pregnant, contracting sexually transmitted infections, and losing self-esteem or parental trust. The media, however, expose American youth to sexually explicit images that may conflict with parental values and encourage sexual experimentation. Additionally, peers or older persons can exert considerable pressure on teens to engage in sex. To help youth maintain their abstinence, parents and educators can teach teens how to use sexual assertiveness skills.

In spite of efforts to promote teenage abstinence, only slightly more than 1 in 4 American teenagers refrains from having sex. By grade 10, about 44% of young girls in the United States have had sexual intercourse. By grade 12, about 62% have engaged in coitus (Centers for Disease Control and Prevention [CDC], 2004).

Michael Benson from Northwestern University Medical School and Edward Torpy from Loyola University in Chicago conducted an anonymous survey of almost 1,000 urban students in grades 6 to 8. After analyzing the results of their survey, Benson and Torpy (1995) concluded that, among other things, gender, age of puberty, and ethnic group are associated with virginity loss. Sex education, religious affiliation, grade average, and self-esteem were among the variables that were not associated, either positively or negatively, with virginity.

Results of a 2003 study conducted by the Centers for Disease Control and Prevention (CDC) across genders and races revealed that by approximately age 13, more boys reported sexual activity than girls. About 32% of male black students indicated that they were sexu-

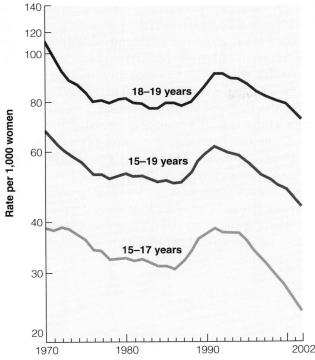

NOTE: Rates are plotted on a log scale.

Figure 6-11 Birth Rates for Teenagers by Age: United States, 1970–2002.
Source: Martin, J. A., et al. (2003). Births, final data for 2002. *National Vital Statistics Reports, 52*(10). Hyattsville, MD: National Center for Health Statistics.

ally active; this percentage was nearly three times that of their Hispanic peers and over six times that of their white peers. Overall, 19% of black students, about 8.3% of Hispanic students, and 4.2% of white students initiated sexual intercourse before 13 years of age (CDC, 2004).

In comparing behavior trends in youth from 1991 through 2003, the CDC has found that the percentage of high school students who have ever had sexual intercourse has decreased from about 54% in 1991 to about 47% in 2003. More students are using condoms; in 1991 about 46% of sexually active students used a condom at their last sexual intercourse, while in 2003, 63% reported having done so (CDC, 2004).

The teenage birth rate has declined from 1991 to 2002 (Figure 6-11). Compared with women in their 20s, pregnant teenagers have a greater risk of experiencing serious complications during pregnancy and delivery as well as of giving birth to premature, underweight babies. Premature infants are born before the 37th week of pregnancy. The risk of giving

birth to a premature, low-birth-weight infant is especially high for pregnant adolescents between 10 and 14 years of age. Underweight premature newborns have a greater risk of serious health and developmental problems than normal-weight newborns who are born at term, that is, between the 37th and 41st weeks of pregnancy.

Most unmarried teenage girls who give birth to live infants keep their babies rather than give them up for adoption. Adolescent mothers are more likely to be unmarried, poor, and have less education than mothers who give birth when they are older. Many teenage mothers have difficulty improving their educational and socioeconomic levels when they become adults.

Some unwed teenage fathers choose to fulfill their parental responsibilities by providing financial and emotional support for their children. Many of them live with or marry the mother of their children. The long-term outlook for these cohabitations or marriages is not good. Data from one study of teenage fathers indicate that only about 16% of these individuals continue to live with their child and its mother 15 months after the baby's birth (Hardy et al., 1989).

With respect to the elderly, sex has enduring importance. Sexuality does not end because a person is older (Pfizer, 2002) (Figure 6-12). According to a 1998 survey conducted by the National Council on Aging (NCOA), nearly half of Americans age 60 or older engage in sexual activity at least once a month (NCOA, 1998). Results of this study reveal that sexual inactivity in the later years of life usually is due to medical disabilities or lack of a sexual partner rather than to lack of desire.

Figure 6-12 Sexuality Has No Age Limit.

Older adults experience a gradual decline in sexual functioning. Therefore, elderly individuals should recognize that their sexual responses are likely to be different from when they were young adults. For example, it usually takes longer for the older adult to become adequately sexually stimulated before sex, and orgasms are less intense. Chronic diseases such as diabetes and heart disease can further limit an aged person's sexual responses or interest in sex. Certain antihypertensive and antidepressant medications can produce side effects that impair sexual functioning; affected individuals should discuss their sexual problems with their physicians. Frequently, changing medications can be helpful. In some cases, medical treatments are available that can improve sexual functioning. Elderly individuals who have sexual impairments that do not respond to treatment can rely on noncoital forms of sexual expression such as kissing, caressing, cuddling, and oral sex to obtain pleasure and fulfillment. In fact, the results of one study of 200 older married couples reveal that affectionate behavior is more crucial to their happiness than sex (Mathias-Riegel, 1999).

Besides physical factors, significant social changes such as the loss of a spouse or moving into a nursing home can have negative impacts on the sexuality of aged individuals. Widows and widowers may have difficulty meeting sexual partners. Elderly nursing home residents may not feel free to express their sexuality because they lack privacy. As the number of elderly Americans rises, addressing sexual needs in this age group will become an increasingly important issue.

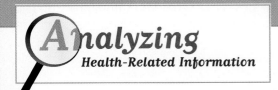

Analyzing
Health-Related Information

Explain why you think the Web site reproduced below is a reliable or an unreliable source of information. Use the model for analyzing health-related information to guide your thinking; the main points of the model are noted to the right. The model is fully explained on pages 13–15. If you wish to visit this site, the Web address is http://www.vigorelle.com.

1. Which statements are verifiable facts, and which are unverified statements or value claims?
2. What are the credentials of the person who wrote the information posted on the Web site? If this information is available, do the author's background and education qualify him or her as an expert in the topic area?
3. What might be the motives and biases of the person who wrote information on the Web site? State reasons for your answer.
4. Which information on the Web site is relevant to the topic? Which information is irrelevant?
5. Is the source reliable? Does it have a reputation for publishing misinformation?
6. Does the Web site attack the credibility of conventional scientists or medical authorities?

Based on your analysis, do you think that this Web site is a reliable source of health-related information? Summarize your reasons for coming to this conclusion.

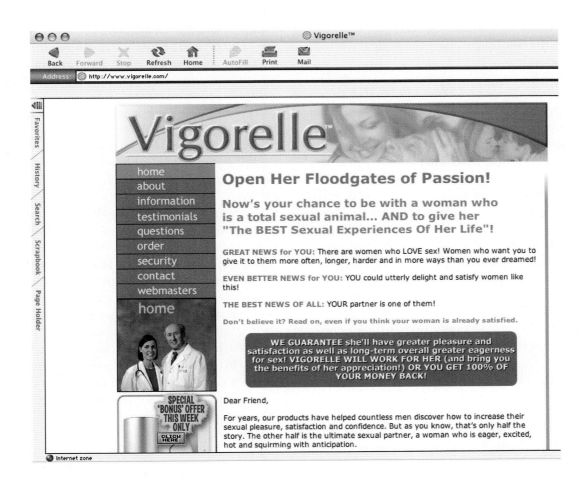

CHAPTER REVIEW

Summary

Human sexuality is a complex set of thoughts, feelings, attitudes, and behaviors that are related to reproduction as well as to being male or female. Numerous biological, psychological, social, and cultural forces interact to influence sexuality. Sexuality influences all aspects of an individual's life, including identity, self-esteem, emotions, personality, relationships, lifestyle, and health. Being knowledgeable about sexuality is important for maintaining good health and optimal well-being.

The sexual response of individuals engaging in sexual activity is usually described in phases. During the excitement phase, both men and women have a heightened sexual awareness. During the plateau phase, the heart rate, blood pressure, respiration rate, and level of muscle tension all increase and the erection of the male intensifies. During the orgasmic phase, men ejaculate, while women's vaginal walls contract rhythmically. During the resolution phase the body returns to its prearousal state.

Some people have sexual dysfunctions that interfere with their sexual response. Common sexual dysfunctions include erectile dysfunction, the inability of a man to develop and/or sustain an erection firm enough for penetration; premature ejaculation, consistently attaining orgasm shortly after intercourse begins and before a man wishes it to occur; hypoactive sexual desire, a low interest in sex, which occurs in both sexes but is more prevalent in women; and vaginismus, a sexual dysfunction of women in which the muscles of the lower third of the vaginal canal contract involuntarily at the anticipation of vaginal penetration.

Instincts, sensations, and hormones drive reproductive behavior, but social, cultural, and religious factors heavily influence a person's sexual attitudes, values, and behaviors. Sexually responsible people consider how their sexual behavior affects themselves and others.

Gender is the classification of the sex of a person based on many criteria, among them anatomic and chromosomal characteristics. Gender identity is an individual's perception of himself or herself as male or female. Various biological, social, and environmental forces mold a child's gender identity. A gender role refers to patterns of behavior, attitudes, and personality attributes that, in a particular culture, are traditionally considered feminine or masculine. In the United States today, gender roles are undergoing dramatic changes and are becoming more flexible than in the past.

Sexual orientation, the direction of one's romantic thoughts, feelings, and attractions, can be toward the same sex, the opposite sex, or both sexes. Biological factors, such as genetics, and environmental influences, such as childhood experiences, probably contribute to the formation of one's adult sexual orientation.

Sexual partners may engage in a variety of intimate activities, including petting as well as vaginal, oral, and anal sex. However, sex does not require a partner for it to be a pleasurable experience—most people masturbate at some point during their lives. Some people choose to refrain from sexual activity for a variety of reasons, such as health concerns or religious beliefs. Abstaining from sexual activity is not known to be harmful, and it is an effective measure for preventing pregnancies and sexually transmitted infections.

People need to establish and maintain satisfying attachments to others for optimal health and well-being. People who have high self-esteem, are satisfied with their bodies, are in good health, and have positive feelings about their sexuality are likely to form fulfilling intimate relationships. Although love is difficult to define, people in loving relationships share feelings of caring, respect, attachment, commitment, and intimacy.

Various psychologists have developed theories about love. However, experts generally agree that love changes over time. Early in a relationship, when physical attraction is greatest and partners know very little about one another, their passion is high. Eventually, the intense sexual attraction that characterizes a romantic relationship in its initial stages subsides. Other aspects of the relationship, such as companionship, often deepen. Compatibility, the ability to exist in harmony, is crucial in the development of a healthy emotional attraction between partners. Usually important for establishing a compatible relationship is the sharing of similar interests, attitudes, and values.

More couples are choosing to cohabit before marriage, but this practice results in a higher risk of divorce than not living together prior to marriage. Those who are married are less satisfied with their marriages and are marrying later in life than in recent decades. Effective communication is an essential ingredient for main-

From:

ACCEPTANCE POST OFFICE
COMPUTE POSTAGE DUE

MEDIA MAIL

TOTAL POSTAGE DUE $_____

POSTAGE_____

MERCHANDISE RETURN LABEL

PERMIT NO. 1   FITCHBURG MA 01420
JONES & BARTLETT PUB.   231 INDUSTRIAL PARK

POSTAGE DUE UNIT
US POSTAL SERVICE
881 MAIN STREET
FITCHBURG MA 01420-9998

NO POSTAGE
NECESSARY
IF MAILED
IN THE
UNITED STATES

We value your opinion of our book.
Please fill in and mail the attached card.
No postage is required.
If you prefer to submit this information via the World Wide Web, please visit us at http://www.jbpub.com/comcard.htm.

Detailed course information will help us update our records.

Name of course coordinator, if other than yourself, will permit sending new information or supplementary material, such as answer books, new problems, etc., to the proper person.

Thank you.

Jones and Bartlett Publishers, Inc.
40 Tall Pine Drive
Sudbury, MA 01776
Phone 978 443 5000 / 800 832 0034
Fax 978 443 8000
E-mail info@jbpub.com

Please detach this stub before mailing.

Date _____

I have received a copy of _____
_____
(Please enter title and author of book here)

This book is / is not appropriate for my course because: _____

May we quote you in our advertising? ☐ yes ☐ no

Course name _____ Enrollment _____
Author of text now in use _____ Professor(s) in charge of course _____
Likelihood of change _____ Decision date _____
Do you expect to adopt our book? _____ When? _____

Name _____ **Title** _____

School _____ **Dept.** _____

Address _____

City _____ **State** _____ **Zip** _____

Telephone _____ **Office Hours** _____

E-mail _____ ☐ **Please send me updates on J&B products via e-mail**

Are you interested in reviewing texts in this field? ☐ yes ☐ no
Do you have plans to write any textbooks, software, etc.? ☐ yes ☐ no
If yes, in what area? _____
Which multimedia products to you use when teaching? _____
Are you using ☐ IBM or ☐ Macintosh computers? _____

We appreciate
acknowledgement of your
receipt of our book

We also value your
opinion of the materials received.

Please detach and mail
this postage-paid card.

Thank you.

Visit our website at
http://www.jbpub.com

NO POSTAGE
NECESSARY
IF MAILED
IN THE
UNITED STATES

BUSINESS REPLY MAIL
FIRST CLASS MAIL   PERMIT NO. 40   SUDBURY, MA

POSTAGE WILL BE PAID BY ADDRESSEE

Jones and Bartlett Publishers Inc.
40 Tall Pine Drive
Sudbury, MA 01776-9848

taining satisfying and successful marriages and intimate relationships.

Children are curious about sex; they frequently play sex games with other children and ask their parents questions about sex. Children's sex play is normal behavior when it is playful, occurs infrequently, and does not involve coercion.

Today, teens are becoming sexually active at an earlier age and have more sex partners than those of previous generations. Although the teenage birth rate has declined, it is still high. Compared with women in their 20s, pregnant teenagers have a greater risk of serious complications during pregnancy and delivery, as well as of giving birth to premature and underweight new-

borns. Additionally, adolescent mothers are more likely to be unmarried, poor, and have less education than mothers who give birth when they are older. Many teenage mothers have difficulty improving their educational and socioeconomic levels when they become adults.

Sexuality does not end at a particular age. Most healthy elderly men and women continue to be interested and participate in sexual activity. However, sexual functioning declines with aging; sexual responses in older persons are different from when they were young adults. As the number of elderly Americans rises, addressing sexuality needs in this age group will become an increasingly important issue.

Applying What You Have Learned

1. Develop a plan to improve the way you convey your feelings in relationships. Application
2. Analyze your present intimate relationship or a past one. Explain why you think it will be (or was) a short-term or long-term relationship. Analysis
3. Propose a checklist of characteristics that you could use to select a suitable partner. Explain why these characteristics are important. Synthesis
4. Develop a position concerning the promotion of masturbation as a safe sex alternative. How would you defend your position? Evaluation

Key

Application	using information in a new situation.
Analysis	breaking down information into component parts.
Synthesis	putting together information from different sources.
Evaluation	making informed decisions.

Reflecting on Your Health

1. What is the source of your sexual values (e.g., your parents, your religious upbringing, etc.)? Do you feel comfortable with those values? Why or why not? Do you feel as though your peers share some or all of your values, or do you feel intimidated or pressured to change your values?
2. Do you think that "traditional" gender roles are appropriate in American society today? If you think that some are appropriate and some are not, pick one example from each category and explain your feelings about their appropriateness or inappropriateness.
3. Do you agree with former Surgeon General Jocelyn Elders' opinion that sex education in America's

schools should include instruction about masturbation? Why or why not?
4. Think about a current or former intimate relationship you had. Do you think that your love relationship fits one of Lee's six styles of loving or one of Sternberg's kinds of love? How does it fit or not fit?
5. Think about the nature of your verbal interactions with someone important to you—a parent or spouse, for example. How could you communicate more effectively with that person using suggestions in this chapter?

References

Atkins, D. C., Baucom, D. H., & Jacobson, N. S. (2001). Understanding infidelity: Correlates in a national random sample. *Journal of Family Psychiatry, 15*:735–749.

Benson, M. D., & Torpy, E. J. (1995). Sexual behavior in junior high school students. *Obstetrics and Gynecology, 85*:279–284.

Berman, J. R., Berman, L. A., Lin, H., Flaherty, E., Lahey, N., Goldstein, I., & Cantey-Kiser, J. (2001). Effect of sildenafil on subjective and physiologic parameters of the female sexual arousal response in women with sexual arousal disorder. *Journal of Sex and Marital Therapy, 27*(5):411–420.

Bramlett, M. D., & Mosher, W. D. (2001). *First marriage dissolution, divorce, and remarriage: United States.* Advance data from *Vital and Health Statistics* No. 323. Hyattsville, MD: National Center for Health Statistics.

Bryant, A. N. (2003). Changes in attitudes toward women's roles: Predicting gender-role traditionalism among college students. *Sex Roles, 48*(3/4):131–142.

Byers, S. E., & Grenier, G. (2003). Premature or rapid ejaculation: Heterosexual couples' perceptions of men's ejaculatory behavior. *Archives of Sexual Behavior, 32*(3):261–270.

Carney, D. (1996). GOP bill restricting gay unions clears . . . but does not yield political dividends. *Congressional Quarterly Weekly Report, 54*(36):2598–2599.

Ceglian, C. P., & Gardner, S. (1999). Attachment style: A risk for multiple marriages? *Journal of Divorce and Remarriage, 31*:125–139.

Centers for Disease Control and Prevention. (2004). Youth Risk Behavior Surveillance—United States, 2003. *Morbidity and Mortality Weekly Report, 53*(SS-2).

Esposito, K., Giugliano, F., Di Palo, C., Giugliano, G., Marfella, R., D'Andrea, F., D'Armiento, M., & Giugliano, D. (2004). Effect of lifestyle changes on erectile dysfunction in obese men: A randomized controlled trial. *Journal of the American Medical Association, 291*(24):2978–2984.

Evanoff, A., & Newton, W. P. (1998). Treatment of premature ejaculation. *Journal of Family Practice, 46*:280–281.

Feldman, H. A., Longcope, C., Derby, C. A., Johannes, C. B., Arauho, A. B., Coviello, A. D., Brenner, W. J., & McKinlay, J. B. (2002). Age trends in the level of serum testosterone and other hormones in middle-aged men: Longitudinal results from the Massachusetts male aging study. *Journal of Clinical Endocrinology and Metabolism, 87*:589–598.

Fromm, E. (1956). *The art of loving.* New York: Harper.

Green, R., & Young, R. (2001). Hand preference, sexual preference, and transsexuals. *Archives of Sexual Behavior, 30*:565–574.

Greenberg, J. S., Bruess, C. E., & Haffner, D. W. (2004). *Exploring the dimensions of human sexuality* (2nd ed.). Sudbury, MA: Jones & Bartlett.

Grenier, G., & Byers, E. S. (2001). Operationalizing premature or rapid ejaculation. *Journal of Sex Research, 38*:369–378.

Hamer, D. H., Hu, S., Magnuson, V. L., Hu, N., & Pattatucci, A. M. (1993). A linkage between DNA markers on the X chromosome and male sexual orientation. *Science, 26*:321–327.

Hardy, J. B., Duggan, A. K., Masnyk, K., & Pearson, C. (1989). Fathers of children born to young urban mothers. *Family Planning Perspectives, 21*:159–163.

Jacoby, S. (1999). Great sex: What's age got to do with it? *Modern Maturity, 42*(5):40.

Johnson, M. E., Brems, C., & Alford-Keating, P. (1997). Personality correlates of homophobia. *Journal of Homosexuality, 34*:57–69.

Kinsey, A. C., Pomeroy, W. B., Martin, C. E., & Gebhard, P. H. (1953). *Sexual behavior in the human female.* Philadelphia: Saunders.

Kreider, R. M., & Fields, J. M. (2002, February). *Number, timing, and duration of marriages and divorces: 1996* (Current Population Reports P70-80). Washington, DC: U.S. Census Bureau.

Kunelius, P., Lukkarinen, O., Hannuksela, M. L., Itkonen, O., & Tapanainen, J. S. (2002). The effects of transdermal dihydrotestosterone in the aging male: A prospective, randomized, double blind study. *Journal of Clinical Endocrinology and Metabolism, 87*:1467–1472.

Lalumiere, M., Blanchard, R., & Zucker, K. (2000). Sexual orientation and handedness in men and women: A meta-analysis. *Psychological Bulletin, 126*:575–592.

Laumann, E. O., Paik, A., & Rosen, R. C. (1999). Sexual dysfunction in the United States: Prevalence and predictors. *Journal of the American Medical Association, 281*:1537–1544.

Lee, J. A. (1973). *The colours of love*. Ontario, Canada: New Press.

LeVay, S. (1991). A difference in hypothalamic structure between heterosexual and homosexual men. *Science, 253*:1034–1037.

Lillard, L. A., Brien, M. J., & Waite, L. J. (1995). Premarital cohabitation and subsequent marital dissolution: A matter of self-selection? *Demography, 32*:437–457.

Mathias-Riegel, B. (1999). Intimacy 101: A refresher course in the language of love. *Modern Maturity, 42*(5):46.

Michael, R. T., Gagnon, J. H., Laumann, E. O., & Kolata, G. (1994). *Sex in America*. Boston: Little, Brown.

National Council on Aging. (1998). *Healthy sexuality and vital aging* [Executive summary]. Washington, DC: Author.

National Marriage Project. (2004). *The state of our unions: The social health of marriage in America*. Piscataway, NJ: Rutgers University.

Paick, J. S., Jeong, H., & Park, M. S. (1998). Penile insensitivity in men with premature ejaculation. *International Journal of Impotence Research, 10*:247–250.

Popenoe, D., & Whitehead, B. D. (1999). *The state of our unions*. New Brunswick, NJ: National Marriage Project.

Popenoe, D., & Whitehead, B. D. (2002). *Should we live together? What young adults need to know about cohabitation before marriage. A comprehensive review of recent research*. Piscataway, NJ: Rutgers University and The National Marriage Project.

Reissing, E. D., Binik, Y. M., & Khalife, S. (1999). Does vaginismus exist? A critical review of the literature. *Journal of Nervous and Mental Disease, 187*:261–274.

Rice, G., Anderson, C., Risch, N., & Ebers, G. (1999). Male homosexuality: Absence of linkage to microsatellite markers at Xq28. *Science, 284*:665–667.

Rubin, Z. (1973). *Liking and loving*. New York: Holt, Rinehart, & Winston.

Schnyder, U., Schnyder-Luthi, C., Ballinari, P., & Blaser, A. (1998). Therapy for vaginismus: In vivo versus in vitro desensitization. *Canadian Journal of Psychiatry, 43*:941–944.

Sell, R. L., Wells, J. A., & Wypij, D. (1995). The prevalence of homosexual behavior and attraction in the United States, the United Kingdom, and France: Results of a national population-based sample. *Archives of Sexual Behavior, 24*:235–248.

Smith, T. W. (2003). *American sexual behavior: Trends, socio-demographic differences, and risk behavior*. Chicago, IL: National Opinion Research Center.

Sprecher, S. (2002). Sexual satisfaction in premarital relationships: Associations with satisfaction, love, commitment, and stability. *The Journal of Sex Research, 39*(3):190–196.

Sternberg, R. J. (1986). A triangular theory of love. *Psychological Review, 93*:119–135.

Sternberg, R. J. (1997). Construct validation of a triangular love scale. *European Journal of Social Psychology, 27*:313–335.

Sternberg, R. J. (1998). *Cupid's arrow: The course of love through time*. Cambridge, UK: Cambridge University Press.

U.S. Bureau of the Census. (2000). *Marital status by sex, unmarried partner households, and grandparents as caregivers: 2000*. Retrieved from http://www.census.gov.

Warnock, J. K. (2002). Female hypoactive sexual desire disorder: Epidemiology, diagnosis and treatment. *CNS Drugs, 16*(11):745–753.

Whitley, B. E. Jr., & Kite, M. E. (1995). Sex differences in attitudes toward homosexuality: A comment on Oliver and Hyde (1993). *Psychological Bulletin, 117*:46–154, discussion 155–158.

Wickelgren, I. (1999). Discovery of "gay gene" questioned. *Science, 284*:571.

What You'll Learn

Drug Use and Abuse

Drugs. For many people, this word produces thoughts of shadowy characters secretively injecting illegal and dangerous compounds into their veins. This word may also evoke images of boarded-up crack houses, young people "zoned out" like this boy after injecting heroin, and women being assaulted while under the influence of date-rape drugs. To others, the word *drugs* brings positive thoughts, such as physicians prescribing medicines to relieve the signs and symptoms of illness. Other images might include your sitting comfortably in the dentist's chair while drugs block the pain of the drill, or a person with cancer being treated with powerful chemical therapies to eliminate deadly abnormal cells. What are drugs? Why do drugs elicit both negative and positive images?

Drugs are nonfood chemicals that alter the way a person thinks, feels, functions, or behaves. For thousands of years, people have taken naturally occurring drugs that produce medicinal benefits or **psychoactive** (mood-altering or mind-altering) effects. Nearly everyone uses drugs, for a variety of reasons. Most people have taken aspirin or other pain relievers to treat headaches, sipped cups of coffee or caffeinated soft drinks to stay awake, or drunk alcoholic beverages to celebrate special occasions or to complement meals. Each of these familiar products contains drugs that have beneficial uses, but they can have serious negative effects on the health and well-being of individuals when used improperly. Additionally, inappropriate drug use contributes to numerous social problems that plague our society, such as crime, unemployment, and family violence and dissolution.

This chapter examines the effects of certain drugs on the functioning of the brain, the general nature of drug use and abuse, and the various problems associated with the use of these chemicals. Table 7-1 lists the major types of drugs that affect brain functioning and provides examples of each. Since many Americans use alcoholic beverages and tobacco, Chapter 8 focuses on the effects of these products on health. Some people take steroid hormones to improve their appearance; see p. 296 in Chapter 11 for more information concerning the effects of steroids on health.

> *Drugs . . . can have serious negative effects on the health and well-being of individuals when used improperly.*

Table 7-1 Psychoactive Drugs: Effects on the Body

Drug Category	Trade or Other Names	Physical Dependence	Psycho- logical Dependence	Tolerance	Possible Side Effects	Overdose Effects	Withdrawal Effects
Stimulants	Caffeine, cocaine (snow, Big C), methamphetamine, crystal meth (crystals), Preludin, Ritalin, Dexadrine or "dex," black beauties, black hollies	Possible	High	Yes	Alertness, euphoria, increased pulse rate and blood pressure, sleeplessness, lack of appetite	Fever, hallucinations, convulsions, death	Prolonged sleep, irritability, depression, anxiety, moodiness, headaches
Depressants	Alcohol,* barbiturates (Goofballs), Valium, Halcion, Quaalude, GHB, GBL, "roofies" (Rohypnol)	Varies	Varies	Yes	Slurred speech, drunken behavior	Depressed breathing, dilated pupils, coma, death	Depression, anxiety, sleeplessness, convulsions, death
Opiates	Heroin (China white), morphine, codeine-containing products, methadone, Demerol, OxyContin, Vicodin, Darvon, Percodan	Moderate to high	Moderate to high	Yes	Euphoria, sleepiness, depressed breathing, nausea	Slowed breathing, convulsions, coma, death	Teary eyes, watery nose, yawning, tremors, anxiety, abdominal cramps
Marijuana (cannabis)	Pot, hash, hashish oil, Acapulco gold, blunts, buds, Colombo, weed	Unknown	Moderate	Possible	Euphoria, relaxation, increased appetite, distorted time perception	Anxiety, paranoia	Anxiety, depression
Hallucinogens	LSD blotters, mescaline, STP, psilocybin, high doses of PCP, peyote, psychedelic mushrooms, ketamine	None (LSD and mescaline) Others: unknown	Unknown	Yes	Euphoria, hallucinations, poor time perception	Anxiety, psychotic behavior	None reported
Inhalants	Gasoline, paint thinners and removers, freon, aerosols, butyl nitrate	None	Possible	No	Euphoria, sleepiness, confusion, slurred speech	Brain, kidney, or liver damage; headaches; death	Anxiety
Drugs with mixed effects	Nicotine,* PCP, MDMA (Ecstasy)	Unknown	High (PCP) Unknown (MDMA)	Yes	Hallucinations and altered per-	Psychosis, possible death (PCP)	Unknown

*See Chapter 8.
Sources: *Drugs of abuse* (1996). Washington, DC: U.S. Department of Justice, Drug Enforcement Administration; Goldberg, R. (1997). *Drugs across the spectrum.* Englewood, CO: Morton Publishing Co.; and Hanson et al. (2004). *Drugs and society.* Sudbury, MA: Jones & Bartlett Publishers.

■ Drug Use, Misuse, and Abuse

The typical American household has a supply of pain relievers, cold remedies, cough syrups, and other medications. *Medications* are drugs that have beneficial uses such as treating diseases or correcting physiological abnormalities. Medicinal drugs are frequently misused. **Drug misuse** is the temporary and improper use of a legal drug. Table 7-2 lists some typical misuses of drugs.

A prescription is necessary to legitimately purchase the most powerful and potentially hazardous medications. Most of the active compounds in prescription drugs have been tested scientifically for safety and effectiveness. However, people can buy thousands of medicines without prescriptions, commonly called over-the-counter, or OTC, drugs. Many over-the-counter remedies contain chemicals that have not been evaluated scientifically. Although people often think that OTC drugs are completely safe, any substance that has druglike effects can be dangerous if used improperly. Aspirin and antihistamines, for example, are toxic (poisonous) when ingested in high doses. A later section of this chapter examines problems associated with the use of certain OTC drugs.

Foods are not considered drugs, but many foods contain substances such as caffeine that affect the body. Furthermore, when some vitamins and minerals are consumed in large doses, they have druglike activity in the body. For example, physicians occasionally prescribe large doses of niacin (a B vitamin) to lower the blood cholesterol levels of certain patients. Many people, however, take massive doses of vitamins and minerals without consulting physicians because they think these nutrients are always safe to ingest. However, many vitamins and minerals are toxic when taken in such high doses. Chapters 9 and 16 discuss hazards associated with consuming large amounts of nutritional supplements.

In some instances, drug use becomes **drug abuse**, the intentional improper or nonmedical use of any drug. Drug abuse occurs whenever the use of a substance negatively affects the health and well-being of the user, his or her family, or society. People are more likely to abuse psychoactive drugs than other drugs because of their effects on the mind.

The government controls the use of most psychoactive drugs because of their potential for abuse. Title II of the Comprehensive Drug Abuse Prevention and Control Act of 1970, usually referred to as the Controlled Substances Act, is the legal foundation of narcotics enforcement in the United States. It classifies many psychoactive substances into five drug schedules according to their potential for abuse and medical usefulness (Table 7-3). Schedule I drugs are commonly abused and have little medicinal value. In the

drugs nonfood chemicals that alter the way a person thinks, feels, functions, or behaves.

psychoactive having mind-altering or mood-altering effects.

drug misuse the temporary and improper use of a legal drug.

drug abuse the intentional improper or nonmedical use of any drug.

Table 7-2 — Typical Drug Misuse Behaviors

Behavior	Example
Discontinuing the use of prescribed medications prematurely even though you have been instructed to take it for a longer period	Taking an antibiotic only until symptoms disappear
Mixing drugs	Taking barbiturates and drinking alcohol at a party (combining these depressant drugs can be fatal)
Taking more than the recommended dosage	Consuming ten multiple vitamin and mineral supplements instead of one daily
Saving and using medications past their expiration date	Taking a pain reliever that was prescribed 5 years ago
Sharing medicines	Giving your prescribed allergy medicine to a friend

---

Table 7-3 — Drug Schedules

Schedule	Examples of Drugs	Description
I	Heroin, LSD, mescaline, methaqualone, peyote, psilocybin, THC, hashish, marijuana, Rohypnol ("roofies" or the "date-rape drug")	No current accepted medical use; high potential for abuse
II	Ritalin, PCP, Percodan, Dilaudid, cocaine, methadone, Marinol, Demerol, morphine, amphetamines, barbiturates (fast-acting)	Current accepted medical use; high potential for abuse
III	Paregoric, anabolic steroids, Tylenol with codeine, Vicodan, opium	Current accepted medical use; medium potential for abuse
IV	Valium, Librium, Serax, Halcion, Darvon, Placidyl, phenobarbital, Miltown	Current accepted medical use; low potential for abuse
V	APC with codeine, Robitussin A–C, Lomotil, Phenergan	Current accepted medical use; lowest potential for abuse

Sources: *Physicians' desk reference*. (1996). Oradell, NJ: Medical Economics Company, Inc.; and *Drugs of abuse*. (1996). Washington, DC: U.S. Department of Justice, Drug Enforcement Administration.

euphoria
(you-FOR-ee-a)
an intense feeling
of well-being com-
monly called a "high."

detoxification the
process of converting
harmful substances into
less dangerous com-
pounds.

intoxication the state of
being poisoned by a drug
or other poisonous sub-
stance.

polyabuse abusing
more than one drug at a
time.

synergism (SIH-ner-
jism) the multiplied
effects produced by
taking combina-
tions of certain
drugs.

United States, it is illegal to use, possess, or sell Schedule I drugs. Schedule V drugs are infrequently abused and have important medicinal uses. Schedule II, III, IV, and V drugs are available by prescription.

Officials with the Drug Enforcement Administration (DEA) evaluate medical and scientific information from the U.S. Department of Health and Human Services (HHS) before classifying a drug as a controlled substance. The placement of a drug into one of the five schedules does not necessarily reflect its potential for being abused or producing harmful effects. Heroin, PCP, and marijuana are Schedule I drugs, but the effects of abusing heroin or PCP are more serious than those of abusing marijuana. Alcohol and nicotine are not scheduled drugs, yet the widespread abuse of these addictive substances is responsible for disabling and killing more people each year than the combined use of all controlled drugs.

People abuse illegal drugs such as cocaine, legally available psychoactive substances such as alcohol, some prescription drugs, and OTC remedies. Many individuals abuse a combination of legal and illegal drugs. Regardless of its legal status, no drug is completely safe. The risk that a drug will cause serious side effects largely depends on the type of drug, the amount taken over time, and the health of the person using the drug.

Healthy Living Practices

- Since no drug is completely safe, consider the effects a drug can have on your health and well-being before using it.

Psychoactive Drugs: Effects on the Mind and Body

How Psychoactive Drugs Affect the Brain

Psychoactive drugs affect the nervous system, the communications network of the body, by changing the way the brain perceives and processes information received from the environment. Chapter 2 describes the nervous system, which includes the brain and spinal cord (central nervous system, or CNS) and the sensory and motor nerves that transmit messages to and from the central nervous system.

Psychoactive drugs interact with nerve cells in the brain, altering the activity of chemical transmitters that carry messages from one nerve to another. As a result, these drugs influence perceptions, thought processes, feelings, and behaviors. Many commonly abused drugs affect specific regions of the brain, referred to as reward centers because they have a positive influence on mood and alertness. As a result, when used initially, these drugs often produce **euphoria**, an intense feeling of well-being commonly called a "high." Although altering the normal internal chemical environment of the brain affects a person's mood and behavior, external conditions can modify these responses.

What Happens to Drugs in the Body?

After being taken, psychoactive drugs enter the bloodstream and eventually reach the brain, where they produce their characteristic effects. As drugs circulate, the body may eliminate small amounts of these substances in urine, feces, or exhaled breath. In most instances, the remaining drugs undergo **detoxification**, the process of converting harmful substances into less dangerous compounds that can be excreted. Detoxification usually occurs in the liver. The body stores some drugs, primarily in fat, for days and possibly weeks after exposure, particularly when detoxification occurs slowly. Until the body completely eliminates a drug, small amounts of the substance may be detectable in blood or urine.

A state of **intoxication** occurs when the amount of a substance reaches poisonous levels in the body. This level varies among individuals, but genetic factors, body size, physical health, and prior drug exposure influence a person's ability to metabolize, or process, a drug. The signs and symptoms of intoxication include slurred speech, poor muscular coordination, and mental confusion.

An *overdose* occurs when an excessive amount of a drug circulates in the bloodstream and overwhelms the ability of the body to detoxify or eliminate the substance rapidly. Overdoses of OTC, prescription, and illegal drugs can damage or destroy tissues. In some instances, drug overdoses can be fatal. Table 7-1 (page 162) describes some signs and symptoms of overdoses of various psychoactive drugs.

Polyabuse, abusing more than one drug at a time, is a common practice. For example, individuals often drink alcoholic beverages while they use heroin, barbiturates, cocaine, or other drugs. When people take different drugs that have similar actions, the effects of each drug may be greatly multiplied. This phenomenon, called **synergism**, can be deadly. Alcohol and barbiturates, for example, are depressant drugs that slow the functioning of the central nervous system. If a person drinks a few alcoholic beverages while taking barbiturates, the combined effects of these substances can depress respiration severely, producing coma or death. Polyabuse can cause drug interactions in addition to synergism that can have serious and even fatal outcomes. Many people are not aware that drinking alcohol while taking acetaminophen, a compound contained in popular over-the-counter pain relievers such as Tylenol, can cause liver failure and death.

Healthy Living Practices

- To avoid the effects of drug synergism or interactions, do not combine drugs, including alcohol and OTC medicines, without consulting a physician or registered pharmacist.

■ Illegal Drug Use in the United States

The Prevalence of Illegal Drug Use

Researchers conduct surveys and interviews to estimate the prevalence of illegal (*illicit*) drug use in the United States. For example, the 2003 National Survey on Drug Use and Health sampled 67,784 Americans 12 years of age or older. From the data they collected, researchers concluded that in 2003 an estimated 19.5 million Americans were illicit drug users, meaning they had used an illicit drug in the month prior to the interview (Substance Abuse and Mental Health Services Administration [SAMHSA], 2004). The 2003 figure represents no change in the number of illicit drug users between 2002 and 2003. Nevertheless, far fewer Americans were using these substances than in the late 1970s. In 1979 researchers estimated that 25 million people in the United States used illegal drugs.

According to the 2003 National Survey on Drug Use and Health, more men than women take drugs, 10% and 6.5%, respectively, and certain segments of the American population use illicit drugs more than do other groups. Slightly over 18% of unemployed adults were current users of illicit drugs in 2003; nearly 8% of full-time employed adults took these substances. Among people aged 18 and older in 2003, those who lacked high school diplomas had higher rates of illicit drug use (9%), and college graduates had the lowest rate of use (5.2%) (SAMHSA, 2004).

Rates of illegal drug use are especially high among teenagers and young adults (Figure 7-1). Since 1975 researchers at the University of Michigan's Institute for Social Research have conducted Monitoring the Future, an annual survey of American high school and college students, to ascertain their use of drugs. Data from the 2003 survey indicate that approximately 37% of full-time college students took one or more illegal drugs during 2000, up from 30.6% in 1992. In 2003, 34% of college students used marijuana, up from nearly 28% in 1992. Additionally, the use of LSD ("acid") rose in

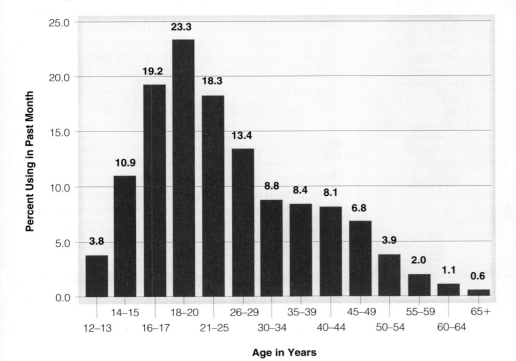

Figure 7-1 **Percentage of People by Age in the United States Who Were Illicit Drug Users in 2003.** Source: Substance Abuse and Mental Health Services Administration (2004). *Results from the 2003 National Survey on Drug Use and Health* (DHHS Publication No. SMA 04-3964). Rockville, MD; National Clearinghouse for Alcohol and Drug Information.

the mid-90s from 1989, and has since begun to fall. In 2003, 1.4% of college students reported taking LSD during the previous 12 months. In 1994 this figure was about 5%; in 1989 it was 3.4% (Johnston et al., 2004b).

Why Do People Use Psychoactive Drugs?

Drug users often provide numerous reasons to explain why they began taking psychoactive substances. Most people begin taking mood-altering drugs for non-medical purposes. Some individuals use alcohol or other drugs simply as a pleasurable experience. Others use drugs to cope with their psychological problems, reduce stress, or escape from unpleasant aspects of their lives. Curiosity often motivates many teenagers and young adults to experiment with drugs. Movies and advertisements may stimulate this curiosity by showing, for example, sophisticated and attractive people smoking cigars or drinking alcoholic beverages while engaging in enjoyable activities (Figure 7-2).

Figure 7-2 **Former Basketball Star Michael Jordan Smoking a Cigar While Playing Golf.** The media frequently portray sophisticated and attractive people using drugs while engaging in enjoyable activities. As a result, some young people copy these unhealthy behaviors.

Additionally, teenagers may use drugs to experience new behaviors, relieve peer pressure, or enhance social interactions (Hanson et al., 2004).

Patterns of Psychoactive Drug Use

Drug experimentation and illicit use often occur during the teen years and peak between the ages of 18 and 20 (see Figure 7-1). Most drug abusers in this age group begin by smoking cigarettes, then they consume alcoholic beverages like beer or wine. Some youth inhale chemicals such as those in aerosols and plastic cements to obtain their mind-altering effects. Alcohol, nicotine, marijuana, and inhalants are often referred to as "gateway" drugs because adolescents use these substances before moving on to other psychoactive drugs (Hanson et al., 2004).

Many adolescents stop experimenting with new drugs after using alcohol or nicotine. If they continue trying drugs, teenagers are likely to use marijuana next. Marijuana use declined about 2% among eighth, tenth, and twelfth graders in the United States in 2003. About 13% of eighth graders, 28% of tenth graders, and nearly 35% of twelfth graders surveyed in the Monitoring the Future study reported that they had tried marijuana in 2003 (Johnston et al., 2004a).

Any combination of stimulants, depressants, or hallucinogens may follow marijuana use. After trying these drugs, some young people move on to use opiates. However, not every youthful drug user follows this stepping-stone pattern of drug experimentation. For example, many teenagers who experiment with alcohol or marijuana do not try other psychoactive drugs.

The recreational use of illegal drugs generally declines with increasing age beyond age 20 as traditional adult roles, including marriage, parenthood, and careers, are adopted. As they age, many individuals recognize that abusing illicit drugs can be self-destructive. Nevertheless, older adults are at greater risk of abusing prescription drugs than are adolescents and young adults (Simoni-Wastila & Strickler, 2004).

■ Drug Dependence

Most people who use psychoactive drugs such as alcohol or marijuana take them for pleasure, to relax, or to feel comfortable in social settings, which is termed *recreational drug use*. To assess your use of drugs, complete the questionnaire in the student workbook entitled "Are You Dependent on Drugs?"

Drug dependence or **addiction** occurs when users develop a habitual pattern of taking drugs that produces a compulsive need, which is both physical and psychological. The terms *dependency* and *addiction* are often used interchangeably to describe any compulsive behavior that interferes with one's health, work, and relationships.

Dependent individuals are unable to avoid using drugs; most have a history of unsuccessful attempts to stop. Over time, these people escalate their intake of drugs even as they recognize that their actions are harmful to themselves and others. People who are dependent on drugs are so preoccupied with the need to obtain and use these substances that other aspects of their lives, such as handling the responsibilities of family and work, become less important.

Physiological and Psychological Dependence

When people take certain psychoactive drugs repeatedly over an extended period, their bodies make various physiological adjustments to function as normally as possible. For example, dramatic chemical changes occur in the brains of chronic drug users that influence their thought processes and behaviors. As a result, these individuals display the characteristic signs and symptoms of *physical dependence* or *physical addiction:* drug tolerance and withdrawal.

After chronic exposure to certain drugs, the body develops **tolerance**, the ability to endure larger amounts of these substances while the adverse effects decrease. When this occurs, users discover that their usual dose of drugs no longer produces the desired degree of physical or psychological effects. To get the desired effects, people must take larger quantities, which results in increased tolerance. This upward spiral is more difficult to break at each successive level, increasing the risk of overdose.

Withdrawal is a temporary physical and psychological state that occurs when certain drugs are discontinued. The signs and symptoms of withdrawal include trembling, anxiety, and pain. In cases of barbiturate addiction, withdrawal symptoms are so severe they can cause death. Table 7-1 indicates psychoactive drugs' potentials for producing tolerance, withdrawal, and addiction.

Psychological dependence is a person's need to use certain psychoactive drugs regularly to obtain their pleasurable effects and to relieve boredom, anxiety, or stress. Psychologically dependent people experience powerful cravings for these substances, which motivates drug-seeking behavior. However, it may be difficult to distinguish psychological dependence from physical dependence. As mentioned earlier, psychoactive drugs produce physiological changes in the brain that influence behavior. Thus, these changes may affect a person's emotional responses, including feelings about the need to take psychoactive substances.

Not everyone who habitually uses or abuses psychoactive substances becomes dependent on their use. For example, individuals who drive after becoming drunk at bars or parties are abusing alcohol, but they are not necessarily alcoholics. It is difficult to determine when the habitual use of a psychoactive substance becomes a dependency. Scientists are interested in determining why some people seem to be more susceptible to drug dependency and addiction than others.

Risk Factors for Drug Dependency

Like many other health problems, there is no single risk factor for drug dependency. Substance addiction results from complex interactions among biological, personal, social, and environmental factors. Results of research conducted by the National Institute on Drug Abuse (NIDA) (2003) suggest that certain conditions in the home are probably the most crucial risk factors for children becoming drug abusers. Such factors include home environments in which parents abuse drugs or suffer from mental illness; ineffective parenting, particularly with children who have difficult temperaments or conduct disorders; and a lack of mutual child–parent attachments and parental nurturing. Risk factors for drug abuse that relate to a child's behavior outside of the home include inappropriately shy or aggressive behavior in the classroom; poor school performance; poor social skills; friendships with peers who use drugs; and a belief that parents, the school, peers, and the community approve of drug use. Conversely, *protective factors*, those associated with reduced potential for drug abuse, include strong family and school ties; parental monitoring of behavior with clear rules of conduct; involvement of parents in the lives of children; academic success in school; and the belief that parents, the school, peers, and the community do not approve of drug use.

drug dependence or addiction a state in which one develops a habitual pattern of taking drugs that usually produces a compulsive need to use these substances, tolerance, and withdrawal.

tolerance an adaptation to drugs in which the usual dose no longer produces the anticipated degree of physical or psychological effects.

withdrawal a temporary physical and psychological state that occurs when certain drugs are discontinued.

Healthy Living Practices

- To avoid the destructive effects of a drug dependency or addiction, do not use psychoactive substances unless you are under a physician's care.

Stimulants

Throughout the world, people have used various stimulant drugs for thousands of years to relieve fatigue, suppress appetite, and improve mood. (See the Diversity in Health essay "Khat.") Stimulants enhance chemical activity in parts of the brain that influence emotions, sleep, attention, and learning. Within minutes after taking stimulants, users are more alert, excitable, and restless. Additionally, these drugs increase blood pressure levels and heart rates.

Amphetamines and Methamphetamines

Synthetic stimulants are amphetamines, methamphetamines, and nonamphetamines (see Table 7-1). Amphetamines such as Dexedrine increase energy and alertness, lessen the need to sleep, produce euphoria, and suppress appetite. In the early 1980s, 21% to 22% of college students reported using amphetamines within the past year. Their use dropped significantly each year from 1983 to 1992, when only 3.6% of college students reported using this drug. From 1993 to 2000, its use rose again, ranging from 4.2% in 1993 to 7.2% in 2001. In 2003, 7.1% of college students reported using amphetamines, and 2.6% reported using methamphetamines (Johnston et al., 2004c).

Methamphetamines ("speed") are more powerful forms of amphetamines that have few medically approved uses. Methamphetamine is taken orally (usually as a pill) or the powder is snorted. It can also be injected or smoked. In small doses, methamphetamines produce euphoria, appetite loss, excessive perspiration, and pounding heartbeats. The effects of taking larger doses can be frightening: chest pains, irregular heartbeat, fever, hallucinations, and convulsions. People who drive while on methamphetamines exhibit erratic driving patterns such as weaving and drifting off the road. They are also prone to exceeding the speed limit and being involved in high-speed collisions. Nevertheless, results from a University of Washington study revealed that stimulants such as methamphetamines were the most frequently used drugs by commercial tractor-trailer drivers while operating their vehicles (Couper et al., 2002).

Overdoses of methamphetamines can be deadly by resulting in cardiovascular collapse or strokes. When taken by pregnant women, the drug can result in birth defects such as cleft lip and palate, and heart defects. Fetal growth is also stunted (Plessinger, 1998). Withdrawal from methamphetamines often results in anxiety, fatigue, sleeplessness, paranoia, delusions, and severe depression.

In the 1980s drug suppliers from Korea, Taiwan, and the Philippines introduced an illegal crystalline form of methamphetamine called *crystal meth* (also referred to as *meth, crank, ice,* and *glass*). Using crystal meth can produce violent behavior and damage the liver, kidneys, and lungs. To meet the rapidly growing demand for the substance in the United States, amateur chemists are producing crystal meth in crude laboratories in their homes. The use of such "homemade" drugs is extremely dangerous.

Club Drugs Amphetamines and methamphetamines are two drugs in a group called *club drugs* or *party drugs*. Club drugs also include alcohol, GHB, GBL, and Rohypnol (depressants); LSD (acid) and ketamine (special K) (both are hallucinogens); and MDMA (Ecstasy, a drug with mixed effects). Adolescents, teenagers, and young adults use these drugs at raves (all-night parties) and in other social situations to reduce anxiety, induce euphoria, or build energy to keep on dancing or partying. However, these drugs are not harmless "fun" drugs because they can have long-lasting negative effects on the brain. (We discuss these drugs in this chapter, with the exception of alcohol, which is discussed in Chapter 8.)

Recent research results show that chronic methamphetamine abuse damages certain areas of the brain more than others. Figure 7-3 shows this damage: The red

Areas of Greatest Loss
— Emotion, reward (limbic system)
— Memory (Hippocampus)

0%	3%	5%
Loss	Loss	Loss

Average difference in brain tissue volume of methamphetamine users, as compared with nonusers

Figure 7-3 **Brain Decay Caused by Methamphetamine Use.** This MRI image of one hemisphere of the brain shows areas of brain-volume loss in a methamphetamine user.

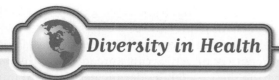

Khat

Which psychoactive drug is associated with weddings and weekends? If your answer is alcohol, you may be wrong. In the East African countries of Somalia and Ethiopia, people chew *khat,* the leaf buds and leaves of the native bush *Catha edulis,* to celebrate weddings and other special events. For centuries, people from these cultures have chewed or smoked khat or drunk tea brewed from its leaves as a socially acceptable and enjoyable pastime. Many homes in Somalia have a special room in which family members and their friends gather to munch khat and chat. Like alcohol and other psychoactive substances that are more familiar to Americans, khat contains chemicals that are known to produce both pleasurable and harmful side effects.

Khat contains cathionine and cathine, compounds that are chemically similar to amphetamines. Not surprisingly, khat produces psychological and physiological responses that resemble those produced by amphetamines and other stimulants. After using khat, people report feeling euphoric and alert; they have little desire to eat, sleep, or engage in sex. Additionally, khat users experience elevated blood pressures and heart rates. After the stimulating and mood-elevating effects of the drug subside, khat users feel anxious and irritable.

Khat impairs thought processes such as mental concentration and judgment; therefore, driving while under its influence can be hazardous. Men who use khat regularly may develop permanent impotence; women who use khat during pregnancy are at risk of giving birth to underweight newborns. Over time, chewing khat damages teeth, contributing to dental decay. During Somalia's civil war, reports appeared in the Western press that khat-chewing members of the country's warring militia displayed aggressive, paranoid, and psychotic behavior. These responses usually result from overdoses of khat.

In the early 1990s thousands of Somalians and Ethiopians fled the civil unrest raging in their homelands and sought refuge in Western countries, including England and the United States. After settling in the West, many of these immigrants maintained their habit of using khat. To satisfy their demand, the immigrants purchase khat leaves that have been flown into North America or the United Kingdom from East Africa.

Concerned about the drug's effects on the central nervous system, officials at the U.S. Drug Enforcement Administration added cathine to its list of controlled substances in 1988. In 1993 the Food and Drug Administration issued an import alert that recommended detention of khat by customs officials to prevent its entry into the United States. Currently, khat use does not pose a major drug enforcement problem. However, the problem of illegal khat use may become more widespread in the United States as more East African immigrants settle in this country.

Sources: Belew, M., Kebede, D., Kassaye, M., & Enquoselassie, F. (2000). The magnitude of khat use and its association with health, nutrition and socioeconomic status. *Ethiopian Medical Journal, 38*(1):11–26; Hassan, N. A., Gunaid, A. A., El-Khally, F. M., & Murray-Lyon, I. M. (2002). The effect of chewing khat leaves on human mood. *Saudi Medical Journal, 23*:850–853; and Mwenda, J. M., Arimi, M. M., Kyama, M. C., & Langat, D. K. (2003). Effects of khat (*Catha edulis*) consumption on reproductive functions: A review. *East African Medical Journal, 80*:318–323.

areas are those with the greatest tissue loss. The limbic region, which is involved in drug craving, reward, mood, and emotion, lost 11% of its tissue. The hippocampus, which is involved in memory making, lost 8% of its tissue. The persons examined in the study were in their 30s and had used methamphetamine for 10 years (primarily by smoking it approximately every other day, using 4 grams a week) (Thompson et al., 2004).

Ritalin and Other Medically Useful Stimulants Amphetamines and chemically related stimulants have few medicinal uses. One medicinally useful stimulant is Ritalin, prescribed for people with attention disorders. Ritalin abuse increased among high school seniors from an annual prevalence of 0.1% in 1992 to 2.8% in 1997. Abuse levels remained somewhat steady for the next six years and were at 2.3% in 2003. Among college students, the Ritalin abuse level was 4.7%, considerably higher than for young adults of similar ages not enrolled in college (3%) (Johnston et al., 2004b, 2004c). Physicians may also prescribe stimulants to treat narcolepsy, an uncommon condition characterized by episodes of falling asleep during the day. Although the practice is controversial, some physicians prescribe amphetamines to suppress the appetites of people who are trying to lose weight. Stimulants suppress appetite, but the effects are usually short-lived.

Cocaine

Cocaine is a white powdery substance extracted from the leaves of the coca bush, which is not the same plant as the cacao tree from which cocoa and chocolate are derived. Crack is a rock crystal form of cocaine that can be heated and its vapors smoked (inhaled); its name comes from the cracking sound that is heard during the heating process. The powdered form of cocaine can be snorted (inhaled through the nose) or dissolved in water and injected. Most people snort, rather than inject, cocaine.

This potent stimulant has some medical uses, particularly as an **anesthetic**, a substance that interferes with normal sensations. However, cocaine was the most widely used illegal stimulant in the United States during the late 1970s and early 1980s, a time during which the public was misinformed about the drug and its dangers. Additionally, many health care practitioners did not understand the dangers of cocaine use or its addictive nature, and, as a consequence, cocaine was viewed as glamorous and was used by many celebrities as well as millions of other Americans. The popularity of cocaine declined dramatically between 1985 and 1992, most likely from public understanding that accompanied increased knowledge about this drug and its dangerous effects (Hanson et al., 2004). The level of cocaine use has not changed significantly since 1992. Nevertheless, experts estimate that approximately 2.3 million Americans were current cocaine users in 2003 (SAMHSA, 2004).

anesthetics
drugs that interfere with normal sensations.

Cocaine is highly addictive. In laboratory studies of the drug's effects, animals prefer to self-administer cocaine rather than engage in reproductive behavior or obtain food. Many people who are dependent on cocaine demonstrate similar responses. Cocaine abusers often dissociate themselves from their families, friends, and associates.

Chronic cocaine abuse produces serious health problems (see Table 7-1). People who snort cocaine regularly often suffer from chronic irritation of their nasal passages. This irritation causes nosebleeds, and it can destroy the septum, the cartilaginous tissue that divides the area between the two nostrils. Additionally, snorting cocaine and smoking crack damage lung tissue and increase susceptibility to respiratory tract infections.

Long-term use of cocaine may interfere with normal sexual functioning. Men who use cocaine regularly often experience an inability to achieve erections and a reduced sexual drive. Women who are chronic users may experience difficulty achieving orgasms, infertility, and menstrual problems.

Cocaine use can have deadly consequences. People with hepatitis or AIDS can spread these diseases by sharing their used hypodermic needles with uninfected drug users. Additionally, cocaine use increases the risk of dying suddenly from life-threatening disorders of the circulatory system such as irregular and rapid heartbeat, high blood pressure, stroke, and heart attacks. Death is especially likely when people take cocaine with other psychoactive substances such as alcohol and heroin. During the past two decades, several well-known individuals have died as a result of using cocaine (Figure 7-4).

While under the influence of cocaine, some individuals experience severe psychotic reactions, including paranoia, that may result in violent behavior. It is not uncommon for cocaine abusers to report having delusions such as the sensation that bugs are crawling beneath their skin. The psychological symptoms of cocaine intoxication also lead some users to attempt suicide, and a number of them succeed.

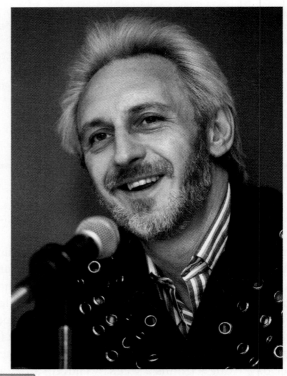

Figure 7-4 **Celebrities Who Have Died as a Result of Using Cocaine.** Cocaine use increases the risk of dying suddenly from life-threatening disorders of the circulatory system, such as irregular and rapid heartbeat, stroke, and even heart attacks. During the past two decades, several well-known individuals have died as a result of using cocaine, including comedian/actor John Belushi, actor River Phoenix, comic Chris Farley, and bassist John Entwistle of the rock band The Who (shown above).

Caffeine

Worldwide, caffeine is the most widely used psychoactive substance (Nehlig, 1999). Caffeine and its related chemical compounds occur naturally in several varieties of plants that we use to make foods and beverages, including coffee, tea, and cocoa. People may ingest caffeine when they consume caffeinated soft drinks or they take certain over-the-counter medications. Table 7-4 lists the amounts of caffeine contained in certain beverages, foods, and over-the-counter products.

Caffeine has been generally recognized as a stimulant that causes limited dependence. People often benefit from taking small amounts of caffeine (less than 250 milligrams per day) because the stimulant improves work capacity, level of alertness, and mood. However, after abstaining from caffeine for about half a day, a person who is accustomed to taking the drug typically experiences withdrawal symptoms that include headache, tiredness, irritability, and depression.

The average American consumes about 200 mg of caffeine daily—the equivalent of about two cups of coffee or five cola beverages. People who drink a few cups of caffeine-containing beverages daily usually do not suffer ill effects. However, individuals who consume more than 600 mg per day often experience psychological as well as physical problems known as *caffeinism*. The manifestations of caffeinism include nervousness, trembling, irritation of the stomach lining, insomnia, increased urine production, diarrhea, sweating, and rapid heart rate. People who do not regularly consume caffeine or who are sensitive to it may develop caffeinism after taking as little as 250 mg of the drug daily.

Most research data indicate that typical patterns of moderate caffeine consumption are not harmful to healthy persons (Hanson et al., 2004). Recent data also show that pregnant women can consume caffeine in moderate amounts without affecting the birth weight of their babies (Clausson et al., 2002).

Table 7-4 Caffeine Content of Popular Beverages, Foods, and Products

Food, Beverage, or Product	Typical Amount/ Range (mg)
Coffee	
Cappuccino (2 oz)	100
Espresso (2 oz)	100
Brewed, drip method (5 oz)	60–180
Brewed, percolator (5 oz)	40–170
Instant (5 oz)	30–120
Decaffeinated, brewed (5 oz)	2–5
Decaffeinated, instant (5 oz)	1–5
Tea	
Brewed, U.S. brands (5 oz)	20–90
Brewed, imported brands (5 oz)	25–110
Instant (5 oz)	25–50
Iced (5 oz)	28–32
Cocoa-Containing Products	
Cocoa (5 oz)	2–20
Chocolate milk (5 oz)	1–4
Milk chocolate (1 oz)	1–15
Dark chocolate, semi-sweet (1 oz)	5–35
Chocolate flavored syrup (1 oz)	4
Soft Drinks (12 oz)	
Dr. Pepper	40
Cola-type beverages	
Regular	30–46
Diet	2–58
Caffeine-free	0
Mountain Dew, Mello Yello	52
Jolt	75–100
Over-the-Counter Medications	
Vivarin (1 pill)	200
Nōdōz (1 pill)	100
Anacin, Empirin, or Midol (2 pills)	64
Excedrin (2 pills)	130

Sources: Based on Caffeine: Grounds for concern? (1994). *University of California at Berkeley Wellness Letter, 10*(6):5; Goldberg, R. (1997). *Drugs across the spectrum.* Englewood, CO: Morton Publishing Co.; and Sizer, F., & Whitney, E. (1997). *Nutrition, concepts and controversies.* Belmont, CA: Wadsworth Publishing Co.

Healthy Living Practices

- If you have ill effects such as anxiety or sleep disturbances from consuming too much caffeine, gradually wean yourself from the drug to avoid its withdrawal symptoms, especially headaches.

◼ Depressants

Depressants produce **sedative** (calming) and **hypnotic** (trancelike) effects as well as drowsiness. These drugs slow the activity of the cerebral cortex, the part of the brain that is responsible for thought processes. Depressant drugs include alcohol, barbiturates such as

sedatives
drugs that produce calming effects.

hypnotics
drugs that produce trancelike effects.

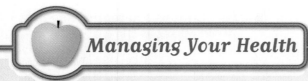
phenobarbital (Luminal), and minor tranquilizers such as diazepam (Valium).

Dangerous side effects can result when people misuse depressants. All of these drugs slow the heart and respiratory rate, which increases the risk of dying from respiratory failure after taking an overdose. Combining depressants—for example, drinking alcohol while taking Valium—produces synergistic effects. Such synergism of depressants can be life threatening.

Tolerance and dependency occur with regular use of depressants. Withdrawal from these drugs can cause *delirium* (mental confusion and disorientation) and *seizures* (abnormal brain activity that results in uncontrollable muscular movements). Some addicted people die while undergoing withdrawal from depressants.

Sedatives and Tranquilizers

Physicians frequently prescribe sedatives and minor tranquilizers, especially for people suffering from insomnia or mild anxiety. In many instances, people can treat their mild anxiety or insomnia without powerful depressants. Anxious individuals can try to reduce their feelings of stress by practicing the relaxation techniques described in Chapter 3. The Managing Your Health feature "Falling Asleep without Prescriptions" provides suggestions that may induce sleep without the use of depressants or other drugs. Prescription medications used to treat anxiety and sleep disorders are often abused. In 2003, 1.8 million people abused tranquilizers and 225,000 abused sedatives (SAMHSA, 2004).

Rohypnol

Rohypnol (row-HIP-nole), commonly called roofies (along with a variety of other street names), is one of a few "date-rape drugs." (See "GHB and GBL.") While under the influence of Rohypnol, women are unable to resist rapists, and they cannot recall, for various lengths of time, what happened to them while under the influence. Because of concern about Rohypnol and other similarly abused sedative-hypnotics, Congress passed the "Drug-Induced Rape Prevention and Punishment Act of 1996" to increase federal penalties for use of any controlled substance to aid in sexual assault.

After 1996, Rohypnol use declined. It was used by approximately 1.3% of high school seniors in 2003 and only 0.4% of college students (Johnston et al., 2004b).

Although not approved for use in the United States, this drug is widely available in Mexico, Colombia, and Europe, where it is used for the treatment of insomnia. Like other depressants, its effects include sedation, muscle relaxation, and anxiety reduction. It also causes dizziness, loss of motor control, lack of coordination, slurred speech, confusion, and gastrointestinal disturbances, all of which can last 12 hours or more.

GHB and GBL

Gamma hydroxybutyrate, better known as *GHB*, was formerly sold in health food stores as a dietary supplement to induce sleep and build muscle. Its over-the-counter sale was banned by the FDA in 1990. The longer periods of sleep it induced were supposed to allow release of human growth hormone, which has been linked with increased muscle mass. However, GHB users reported unpleasant side effects such as nausea and shaking. More dangerously, this drug has induced seizures and coma in some users (Kam & Yoong, 1998). With legislation passed in February 2000, GHB became a Schedule I drug.

In January 1999 the FDA warned consumers about a drug related to GHB: gamma butyrolactone, or *GBL*. After ingestion, the body converts GBL to GHB. Some products labeled as dietary supplements contain GBL, and claim to build muscles, improve physical performance, enhance sex, reduce stress, and induce sleep. However, GBL-related products have been associated with reports of at least 55 adverse health effects, including seizures, vomiting, slowed breathing, slowed heartbeat rate, and coma. One death had been reported from GBL at the time of the FDA warning. The FDA considers GBL an unapproved drug. After the FDA warning, all but one manufacturer of GBL-related products agreed to recall these drugs and to stop their manufacture and distribution.

Healthy Living Practices

- Do not accept drinks from casual acquaintances or strangers; they may contain dangerous drugs.
- Do not drive or operate machinery while under the influence of depressant drugs because these substances can impair your thought processes and muscular coordination.
- Do not drink alcohol while taking other depressants. The synergistic effect of combining these compounds can be deadly.

■ Opiates

Opiates include *opium,* the dried sap extracted from seedpods of opium poppies shown in Figure 7-5 , and drugs such as codeine, morphine, heroin, and Percodan that are derived from opium. Synthetic opiates include Darvon and Demerol. These compounds have important medical uses as sedatives, analgesics, and narcotics. **Analgesics** alleviate pain; **narcotics** alter the

Figure 7-5 Longitudinal Section through a Seedpod of the Opium Poppy. The dried sap extracted from opium poppy seedpods is used to make the narcotic opium. Some white sap can be seen on the cut edge of this seedpod.

perception of pain and induce euphoria and sleep. (Many people incorrectly use the term *narcotic* to describe any illegal drug.)

In addition to relieving pain, opiates slow the activity of the intestinal tract, so they are useful in treating severe diarrhea. Physicians frequently prescribe codeine-containing syrups to subdue severe coughing. Despite their medicinal value, opiates are extremely dangerous when taken in an uncontrolled manner. These drugs are highly addictive; people who use opiates daily develop dependence and tolerance within a few weeks.

Using opiates, especially heroin, can cause a variety of serious health problems as well as death. Excessive doses of opiates depress the CNS, slowing respiration and reducing mental functioning. Such overdoses require immediate medical attention. Sharing needles that are used to inject heroin intravenously can cause life-threatening bacterial infections and viral diseases, such as AIDS and hepatitis.

analgesics (an-al-GEEZ-iks) drugs that alleviate pain.

narcotics drugs that induce euphoria and sleep as well as alter the perception of pain.

Opium and Heroin

After it enters this country, opium is chemically converted to heroin by drug dealers. They also add various materials, such as quinine or cornstarch, to dilute the drug's concentration. Substances that dilute the concentration of a drug are called *adulterants.* Since heroin abusers lack information concerning the potency of their drug purchases after chemical conversion by drug dealers, they risk taking overdoses or having allergic reactions to the adulterants.

Heroin is one of the most widely abused illegal drugs worldwide (Hanson et al., 2004). Since heroin imported from Colombia and Mexico is cheaper than it used to be and is very potent, teenagers are able to snort heroin rather than inject it, making it easier for them to use this drug for the first time (Schwartz, 1998). Survey data indicate that approximately 0.8% of American high school seniors have used heroin in the year prior to the survey. This percentage is higher than from the 1980s through the early 1990s. After 1993, heroin use among high school students rose until 2000, but may be beginning to drop (Johnston et al., 2004b).

OxyContin and Vicodin

In 2001 news reports of abuse of the time-released opiate pain reliever OxyContin became common. OxyContin is a medication prescribed primarily for patients with terminal cancer and other illnesses that cause moderate to severe chronic pain. By 2002, hundreds of people had died from OxyContin abuse, and researchers began collecting data on the use of OxyContin by high school students, college students, and adults. In 2003, the percentages of eighth, tenth, and twelfth graders, college students, and adults aged 19 to 45 using OxyContin during the year prior to being surveyed (the annual prevalence) were 1.7%, 3.6%, 4.5%, 2.2%, and 2.6%, respectively. These figures were higher than those of 2002, and show that the highest use is among tenth and twelfth graders, not among college students (Johnston et al., 2004b).

OxyContin is a time-release medication with the synthetic opiate oxycodone as its active ingredient. Persons who abuse this prescription medication chew, crush, or dissolve the pills and then inject, inhale, or take them orally, which delivers the medication all at once rather than slowly over time. The result is a rapid and intense euphoria that does not occur when the drug is taken as prescribed, but such ingestion carries the dangers of opiates mentioned previously. Abusers also take OxyContin with other pills, marijuana, or alcohol, which can result in serious injury or death.

Vicodin is also a drug prescribed to reduce pain. Abuse of this drug is more prevalent than abuse of OxyContin. In 2003, the annual prevalence of abuse of Vicodin among eighth, tenth, and twelfth graders, college students, and adults aged 19 to 45 was 2.8%, 7.2%, 10.5%, 7.5%, and 8.6%, respectively. As with OxyContin, these figures were higher than those of 2002, and show that the highest use is among twelfth graders. Use among tenth graders and college students is about equal.

■ Marijuana

Marijuana is the most widely used illicit drug in the United States. An estimated 14.6 million Americans over 12 years of age used marijuana in 2003 (SAMHSA, 2004).

The marijuana plant (*Cannabis sativa*) contains the psychoactive compound delta-9-tetrahydrocannabinol, or THC. *Hashish* is a dried resin made from marijuana flowers, which contain a higher concentration of THC than the leaves of the plant. Also extracted from marijuana flowers, hashish oil contains a greater percentage of THC than hashish. A few drops of hashish oil added to a cigarette produce psychoactive effects that are the same as smoking a marijuana cigarette, or *joint*.

When people smoke marijuana or hashish, THC enters the brain rapidly. THC alters muscular coordination and normal thought processes such as mental concentration, problem solving, time perception, and short-term memory. Not only are these effects likely to decrease educational achievement in young people (Fergusson et al., 2004), but also they can have serious consequences for drivers. Results of a study on the effects of marijuana on driving abilities reveal that smoking one marijuana cigarette affects drivers' equilibrium and ability to brake quickly during the hour following ingestion of the drug (Liguori et al., 1998). Additionally, an analysis of the blood and urine from fatally injured drivers indicates that drug use (including alcohol) is a factor in 52% of motor vehicle fatalities. After alcohol, the most common drug found in the blood was marijuana, and marijuana was most prevalent in the 15- to 30-year age group (Logan & Schwilke, 1996).

Marijuana and hashish smoke contain numerous irritants that can damage the bronchial tubes and lungs. Some of these irritants are the same cancer-causing substances found in cigarette smoke (Fung et al., 1999). Compared to smoking filter-tipped cigarettes, smoking marijuana results in about a fivefold increase in the amount of carbon monoxide in the blood, about a threefold increase in the amount of tar inhaled, and retention in the respiratory tract of one-third more inhaled tar (Wu et al., 1988). Results of studies also show that smoking marijuana has effects on the respiratory system that may increase risk for the development of lung infections and lung cancer (Barsky et al., 1998; Baldwin et al., 1997).

Although many users think that marijuana enhances their sexual responsiveness, results of some studies have found that the drug interferes with reproductive functioning. Men who use marijuana may experience a temporary reduction of their normal testosterone levels. *Testosterone* is a sex hormone that maintains sex drive and sperm production. This effect decreases the sperm count and increases the proportion of abnormal sperm, qualities that are associated with reduced fertility and an increased probability of fetal abnormalities (Hanson et al., 2004).

Most Americans who smoke marijuana use the drug occasionally, particularly while they are in social settings. Although low-THC cannabis (the form generally available in the United States) rarely produces physical dependence when taken infrequently and in low doses, it can cause psychological dependence. Psychologically addicted persons mentally crave the euphoric effects of THC; experience a heightened sensitivity to and distortion of sight, smell, taste, and sound; have mood changes; and have a slowed reaction time (Hanson et al., 2004).

Among marijuana's medical uses is that it reduces the fluid pressure in the eyes of people with glaucoma. However, physicians usually prescribe other medications to treat this disorder. Marinol, a drug that contains synthetic THC, eases the side effects of nausea and vomiting that often accompany chemotherapy during cancer treatment. Other drugs are available to control these side effects. Marijuana is also used to ease the symptoms of wasting syndrome in AIDS patients, muscle spasms in patients with muscle disorders such as multiple sclerosis, and the pain of migraine headaches. It can also help control seizures (Taylor, 1998).

Marijuana has been approved for medical use in 11 states: California, Colorado, Oregon, Nevada, Maine, Washington, Alaska, Montana, Vermont, Arizona, and Hawaii. Laws in these states also remove state-level criminal penalties for cultivation, possession, and use of medical marijuana. However, in June 2005 the U.S. Supreme Court ruled that federal authorities may prosecute patients whose physicians prescribe marijuana for their medical use, and that state laws do not protect users from the federal ban on the drug.

Most opponents of using smoked marijuana for medical purposes are not against the medical use of synthetic THC as pills or injectable drugs. Since most supporters of the medical use of smoked marijuana are against using synthetic THC, many suggest that their motivation for support is not scientific or medical but rather a "back door" method of legalization (DuPont, 1999).

■ Hallucinogens

When taken internally, hallucinogens produce *hallucinations*, abnormal and unreal sensations such as seeing distorted and vividly colored images. Many people report feeling pleasantly detached from their bodies or united with their environment while using hallucinogens. Hallucinogens, however, can produce frightening psychological responses such as anxiety, depression, and the feeling of losing control over your mind. The physical side effects of hallucinogens include elevated blood pressure, dilated pupils, and increased body temperature. Although chronic users of these drugs may develop psychological dependence and tolerance, physical addiction and withdrawal do not occur.

In the United States, the most potent and commonly abused hallucinogens are LSD, mescaline, psilocybin (SIGH-low-SIGH-bin), PCP, and ketamine. These drugs have no approved medical uses, and their recreational use is illegal. Native Americans, however, are permitted to use *peyote*, a cactus that contains mescaline, in certain religious rites.

LSD

LSD (lysergic acid diethylamide) is a colorless, odorless, flavorless compound that is manufactured in pill, solution, and powder form. It is an extremely potent drug; taking very small amounts produces vivid hallucinations that can last up to 12 hours. While taking LSD, some people have severe psychotic reactions, such as paranoid delusions. Additionally, for days or weeks after taking LSD, users may have "flashbacks" in which they experience mild hallucinations. Medical practitioners usually reassure these people that flashbacks are harmless and subside over time and that few, if any, long-term psychological problems result from hallucinogen use (Halpern & Pope, 1999). Although no scientific evidence links use of LSD with the development of fetal abnormalities, LSD can stimulate uterine contractions, so pregnant women should avoid it (Goldberg, 1994).

During the early 1980s, LSD use by college students declined dramatically, from 6.3% in 1982 to 2.2% in 1985. By 1992, however, LSD use among college students had climbed to 5.7% and peaked in 1995 at 6.9%. Use declined throughout the rest of the 1990s, dropping precipitously in 2002 and 2003. In 2003 only 1.4% of college students had used LSD in the year prior to their being asked about their use (Johnston et al., 2004b).

Mescaline

A small, round, spineless cactus that grows in Mexico and Texas produces the hallucinogen mescaline, or peyote (Figure 7-6). After eating peyote, people have hallucinations that last 1 to 2 hours. These "trips" are milder and easier to control than LSD trips. Since pure mescaline is difficult to produce for illicit sale, most mescaline sold on the streets contains LSD as the psychoactive agent.

Psilocybin

Many mushrooms, including several wild-growing varieties that are found throughout the United States, contain psilocybin. After eating these fungi, sometimes called *magic mushrooms,* people experience elevated blood pressure, body temperature, and pulse rate. Psilocybin produces euphoria and hallucinations, but these psychoactive effects are not as intense or long-lasting as those produced by LSD. Unpleasant responses to psilocybin ingestion include wide mood swings and uncontrollable movements of arms and legs. Although fatal overdoses from psilocybin have not been reported, users may die if they eat other wild mushrooms that are poisonous.

analogs
drugs that are chemically similar but have different effects in the body.

PCP

PCP (commonly called *angel dust* or *rocket fuel*) is difficult to classify because the drug produces hallucinogenic, depressant, stimulant, or anesthetic effects depending on the dose in which it is taken. Within a few minutes after taking PCP, users begin to experience its psychoactive effects, which can last up to 6 hours.

Unlike other hallucinogenic drugs, high doses of PCP can cause severe toxic reactions. Taking 1 mg to 5 mg of PCP produces confusion and loss of muscular coordination; users also feel warm, sweaty, relaxed, and euphoric. As the level of intake increases to about 10 mg, users become confused, paranoid, and agitated; they act drunk, have hallucinations, and report numb-

Figure 7-6 Peyote Cactus *(Lophophora williamsii).* This small, round, spineless cactus grows in Mexico and Texas and produces the hallucinogen mescaline, or peyote.

ness in their arms and legs. Taking 10 mg to 25 mg produces the signs and symptoms of PCP toxicity, including trancelike or psychotic behavior. Doses that exceed 25 mg to 50 mg can produce fever, convulsions, coma, elevated blood pressure, and death. People who survive the acute toxic effects of PCP often feel depressed and anxious. Additionally, they may show signs of brain damage such as confusion and disorientation that can take weeks to disappear.

Ketamine

In the 1960s drug researchers developed ketamine, a PCP analog that has fewer troublesome side effects than PCP. An **analog** is chemically similar to another drug and may or may not produce similar responses. Today, legally manufactured PCP analogs such as Ketalar (ketamine hydrochloride) have limited human and veterinary medical use as anesthetics.

Teens and young adults most commonly abuse ketamine by snorting the drug for its dreamlike or hallucinatory effects. In addition, the drug can be swallowed, smoked, drunk, or injected intramuscularly. Ketamine injection is highly risky because multiple injections typically occur during a single "session" in large groups, and the drug is drawn from shared bottles of liquid ketamine. These behaviors put ketamine injectors at risk of infectious diseases such as hepatitis C and HIV. At high doses, ketamine can cause delirium, amnesia, impaired motor function, high blood pressure, and potentially fatal respiratory problems. These effects are magnified when the drug is taken with sedatives or depressants, such as alcohol, which is a common practice.

- Do not eat wild mushrooms. Some are poisonous and can cause death.

- Use household products that release toxic fumes, such as paints, glues, and lighter fluids, in well-ventilated areas to avoid inhaling these chemicals.

■ Inhalants

Inhalants are gases that produce euphoria, dizziness, confusion, and drowsiness shortly after they are inhaled, or *huffed*. Numerous household products release such gases; these include paints and fingernail polishes that contain acetone, and lighter fluids that contain butane (Table 7-5). Freon, a refrigerant previously used in air conditioners, is a toxic gas also.

Inhalants irritate the mucous membranes lining the eyes, mouth, nose, throat, and lungs. Inhalant abusers often develop watery, reddened eyes and a persistent cough. Some users experience double vision, nausea, vomiting, fainting, and a ringing sensation in their ears. Many teenagers are unaware of the serious health effects of inhalant use: brain damage, irregular heartbeat, anemia, liver damage, kidney failure, coma, or death.

Inhalant use begins at young ages—sometimes in the fifth grade—and its use drops as students grow older. Inhalants are the second most widely used class of illicit drugs for eighth graders (after marijuana), and the fourth most widely used for tenth graders (after marijuana, amphetamines, and Vicodin). In 2003, the annual prevalence for inhalant use for eighth graders was 8.7%; for tenth graders, 5.4%; and for twelfth graders, 3.9%. Lowest use is by college students and young adults (Johnston et al., 2004b).

■ Designer Drugs: Drugs with Mixed Effects

People who have some knowledge of chemistry can alter the chemical structure of a controlled substance to make a new compound that is not classified as a controlled drug. The new compound, called a *designer drug,* usually produces psychoactive responses similar to the drug from which it was produced. Designer drugs are relatively easy and inexpensive to produce. Thus, people who make these drug analogs can reap considerable profits from selling them.

After officials with the DEA determine that a designer drug has the potential to be abused, they can classify the compound as a controlled substance. However, underground chemists often avoid prosecution by continuing to modify the substance, producing new generations of the drug that the DEA does not control. Table 7-6 lists some of the best-known designer drugs, their psychoactive effects, and potential health risks.

Designer drugs are often more toxic than the compounds from which they are derived. China white, for example, is 1,000 times more potent than its parent drug, fentanyl, a powerful synthetic opioid often used for general anesthesia or in the treatment of chronic pain. China white and other fentanyl analogs have been responsible for at least 100 deaths (Hanson et al., 2004).

Ecstasy

The illegal designer drug *Ecstasy,* or *MDMA* (3,4-methylenedioxymethamphetamine), became a controlled substance in 1985. Chemically similar to mescaline and methamphetamine, Ecstasy produces both hallucinogenic and stimulant effects. Ecstasy users report that the drug improves their self-esteem and increases their desire to have intimate contacts with other people. However, users may experience panic and anxiety, hallucinations, tremors, rapid heart rate, loss of coordination, and psychotic behavior. Some users report more serious side effects such as irregular heartbeat, hypertension, fever, memory loss, and seizures. Since

Table 7-5	Common Products That Contain Toxic Inhalants

Glues

Aerosols

Cleaning solutions

Fingernail polishes and fingernail polish removers

Fuels and lighter fluids

Paints and paint thinners

PVC cement

Hair spray

Typing correction fluid

Table 7-6 Popular Designer Drugs

Designer Drug	Original Drugs	Psychoactive Effects	Possible Health Risks
MPPP MPTP	Meperidine (Demerol)	Heroinlike euphoria (depressant)	Parkinsonian syndrome: drooling, uncontrollable skeletal muscle movements, muscle rigidity (permanent)
China white	Fentanyl (Sublimaze)	Euphoria, respiratory depression	Death from respiratory failure
Ecstasy, XTC, Adam, M & M, MDMA	Mescaline–methamphetamine	Euphoria, CNS stimulant, hallucinations	Panic, anxiety, paranoia, increased and irregular heart rate, fever, hypertension, brain damage, seizures, death
Love drug (MDA)	Mescaline–methamphetamine	Euphoria, talkativeness, increased need to make friends	Fever, rapid heart rate, hypertension, seizures, death

the 1980s several people have died after taking this drug.

The use of Ecstasy by high school students, college students, and young adults rose sharply between 1998 and 2001. In 2002 and again in 2003, use declined in all three groups. In 2003 annual prevalence rates for eighth, tenth, and twelfth graders were 2.1%, 3.0%, and 4.5% respectively. For college students, the prevalence rate was 4.4%, and for adults aged 19 to 45, it was 4.5% (Johnston et al., 2004b; Strote et al., 2002).

Over-the-Counter Drugs

If you walk down the aisles of a pharmacy or discount department store, you are likely to see a huge array of over-the-counter (OTC) medicines. Television advertisements promote a variety of OTC products that "shrink hemorrhoids," "promote regularity," or "kill germs." The demand for these products is growing as more Americans practice self health care to reduce their health care costs.

The FDA regulates the production and marketing of prescription and nonprescription medications in the United States. To be sold in this country, an OTC medicine must be effective and safe when people follow the product information that comes with it (in packages or on labels). Although the FDA does not evaluate the safety or effectiveness of every OTC product that is marketed, the agency requires that active ingredients in products be evaluated for safety and usefulness. *Active* ingredients have an effect on the body; *inert* ingredients do not affect the body. Products that contain unsafe or ineffective ingredients or that have dishonest labeling cannot be sold. Herbal products that are sold as food supplements in health food stores are not regulated by the FDA. Some of these products contain substances that produce druglike effects and are toxic (see the Consumer Health boxes in Chapter 1 and on page 179).

Misuse and abuse of OTC medicines is common. As mentioned in the beginning of this chapter, the improper use of these medications can be harmful. Furthermore, some OTC products contain substances such as alcohol that can produce serious psychoactive effects, especially when they are taken in large doses.

Look-Alike Drugs

The active ingredient in "stay-awake" pills is the stimulant caffeine. Some manufacturers produce caffeine-containing capsules or pills that look like prescription amphetamines or related prescribed stimulants. The production and sale of these look-alike drugs are difficult to regulate because they contain caffeine, an allowed substance. Frequently, people who sell street drugs misrepresent look-alike stimulants as amphetamines to unsuspecting users.

Weight Loss Aids

Nearly anyone who has tried to lose weight knows that it is frustrating and that hunger seems to be constant. Many overweight people have taken various pills, powders, beverages, and foods for years to promote weight loss and prevent hunger. The Consumer Health box in Chapter 10 describes the potential harmful effects of these products and the drugs they contain.

Over-the-Counter Medicines: Safety and the FDA

The FDA reports that Americans spend more than $18 billion annually on the estimated 300,000 drugs that are available without prescriptions. According to the American Pharmaceutical Association, people initially use self-care practices, such as OTC drugs, to treat 60% to 90% of all ailments. Painkillers and cold, sinus, and cough remedies are among the best-selling OTC products. The demand for these and other OTC products will continue to grow as more American consumers practice self health care to reduce their health care costs.

Some OTC drugs are useful, but others are ineffective. To protect consumers, the Food and Drug Administration (FDA) regulates the testing, production, marketing, and labeling of medical devices and medications; the safety of foods and truthfulness of information on their labels; and the safety of cosmetics. A medical device or OTC medicine that is sold in the United States must be effective for its intended use and safe when its instructions are followed.

The FDA also requires that the active ingredients in OTC products be evaluated for safety and usefulness.

Active ingredients have an impact on the body; inert ingredients do not affect the body. The FDA allows manufacturers of OTC products to use ingredients that are generally recognized as safe (GRAS), generally recognized as effective (GRAE), and generally recognized as honestly labeled (GRAHL). The FDA employs investigators who review information that appears on the labels of OTC products. Products that contain unsafe or ineffective ingredients, or that have labels displaying dishonest information, cannot be sold.

In 1998 the FDA proposed an easy-to-read and easy-to-understand labeling format for OTC drugs. Figure 7-A shows the information that must appear on the labels of an OTC medicinal product. Note that the label clearly displays warnings concerning the safe use of the product. Always follow instructions on the package or label concerning the use of any OTC medication.

Individuals, physicians, and staff of health care facilities can report cases of harm that result from using medicinal and nutritional products. If you have any problem with a medication, medical device, or dietary supplement, report the problem to the FDA's MedWatch hotline by calling 1-800-332-1088.

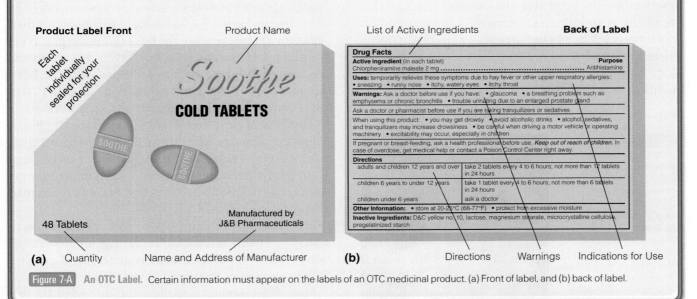

Product Label Front   Product Name   List of Active Ingredients   Back of Label

Each tablet individually sealed for your protection

Soothe
COLD TABLETS

SOOTHE

48 Tablets   Manufactured by J&B Pharmaceuticals

(a) Quantity   Name and Address of Manufacturer

Drug Facts

Active ingredient (in each tablet)   Purpose
Chlorpheniramine maleate 2 mg .... Antihistamine

Uses: temporarily relieves these symptoms due to hay fever or other upper respiratory allergies: • sneezing • runny nose • itchy, watery eyes • itchy throat

Warnings: Ask a doctor before use if you have: • glaucoma • a breathing problem such as emphysema or chronic bronchitis • trouble urinating due to an enlarged prostate gland

Ask a doctor or pharmacist before use if you are taking tranquilizers or sedatives

When using this product: • you may get drowsy • avoid alcoholic drinks • alcohol, sedatives, and tranquilizers may increase drowsiness • be careful when driving a motor vehicle or operating machinery • excitability may occur, especially in children

If pregnant or breast-feeding, ask a health professional before use. *Keep out of reach of children.* In case of overdose, get medical help or contact a Poison Control Center right away.

Directions

adults and children 12 years and over	take 2 tablets every 4 to 6 hours; not more than 12 tablets in 24 hours
children 6 years to under 12 years	take 1 tablet every 4 to 6 hours; not more than 6 tablets in 24 hours
children under 6 years	ask a doctor

Other Information: • store at 20-25°C (68-77°F) • protect from excessive moisture

Inactive Ingredients: D&C yellow no. 10, lactose, magnesium stearate, microcrystalline cellulose, pregelatinized starch

(b)   Directions   Warnings   Indications for Use

Figure 7-A   **An OTC Label.** Certain information must appear on the labels of an OTC medicinal product. (a) Front of label, and (b) back of label.

Ephedrine

During asthma attacks, affected people often use prescription or over-the-counter products that contain ephedrine or pseudoephedrine to dilate their bronchial tubes. Since ephedrine and pseudoephedrine act as mild stimulants, some individuals misuse medicines that contain these compounds as "pep pills." Ephedrine and pseudoephedrine can produce high blood pressure, sleeplessness, irregular and rapid heart rate, and restlessness; taking high doses of either substance may evoke psychotic symptoms.

In 2004, FDA officials banned the sale of ephedrine-containing dietary supplements because of their dangerous side effects. The ban targets ephedra supplements that have been advertised for weight loss, muscle building, and athletic performance, but an April 2005 court ruling prevents the FDA from enforcing its ban against products containing 10 milligrams of ephedrine or less. The Chinese herb *ephedra*, or *ma huang*, is a natural source of ephedrine and still may be used in traditional Asian medicine in the United States.

People who use ephedra as a stimulant think that it is safe and not addictive. However, the drug can cause heart attacks, seizures, and even death. Since 1997 the FDA has required warning and dosage restrictions on products that contain ephedrine. In addition to ephedra, numerous herbs or plant extracts—such as lobelia, comfrey, yohimbine, *Ginkgo biloba*, or sassafras—contain substances that can produce harmful side effects when ingested as supplements or teas (Figure 7-7).

Figure 7-7 **Hazardous Herbs.** Numerous plants can be toxic. Lobelia (shown here) induces vomiting; overdoses can result in convulsions, loss of consciousness, and death.

Drug Treatment and Prevention

Treating Drug Dependency

When some people recognize that they have a problem controlling their use of drugs, they voluntarily discontinue abusing drugs without the assistance of specialized treatment programs. Other people seek treatment after realizing that they cannot stop abusing substances on their own. Many of these individuals require medical supervision in special clinical settings to manage withdrawal signs and symptoms safely. In some instances, people do not want treatment for their substance abuse because the behavior is too gratifying for them or they deny that they have a drug problem. In cases involving criminal activities, legal authorities may require that addicted individuals either complete drug treatment or serve prison sentences.

The goal of drug treatment is to reduce the likelihood that abusers will return to their previous drug use behaviors. Currently, three major forms of long-term drug abuse treatment exist: methadone maintenance, outpatient drug-free programs, and residential therapeutic communities.

Methadone treatment is used to treat addiction to opiates; methadone reduces the cravings for these drugs. This controversial treatment is generally used after other attempts at treatment have failed.

Most abusers prefer *outpatient drug-free programs* that provide medical care and a wide variety of counseling and psychotherapy approaches while patients continue to live with their families and work in their communities. These programs do not include use of methadone.

Self-help groups are a popular and useful adjunct to professional outpatient drug treatment. Individuals recovering from drug dependency attend regular meetings to receive encouragement and social support from other former substance abusers. Alcoholics Anonymous (AA) is one of the oldest, most effective self-help programs (see Chapter 8). Many other community-based self-help programs that treat drug abuse, such as Narcotics Anonymous, are modeled after AA.

In severe cases, drug abusers may undergo detoxification and then live for several months in controlled environments called *residential therapeutic communities* or *group homes.* Living in these communities reduces the likelihood that patients will be exposed to drugs while they resocialize, or readjust to general society. While in group homes, patients also receive medical care, social services, and psychological counseling. After they leave residential therapeutic communities, individuals usually attend community- or hospital-based counseling sessions to prevent *relapse,* the return to drug abuse. For people who lack health insurance, the high cost of medical care is a major barrier to obtaining treatment in a therapeutic community.

Most drug treatment programs that last fewer than 90 days have limited long-term effectiveness (NIDA, 1999a). Results of studies show that length of time in drug treatment is the best single predictor of positive post-treatment outcomes (DesJarlais & Hubbard, 1999). Many drug-dependent people need more than 3 months of outpatient care or living in controlled environments to change their substance-related behaviors and attitudes. Additionally, recovering addicts often need to acquire job skills while they are in therapy to improve their chances of becoming drug-free, productive members of society.

A considerable number of patients finish treatment but relapse within a few weeks or months of abstinence. Former addicts are more likely to relapse if they have severe mental illness or polyabuse, and if they return to communities where illicit drugs are available and are widely used. Recovering drug addicts are more likely to abstain from using drugs if they are married or in stable relationships, supported by their families, and employed. In 2003, 1.8 million Americans received treatment for their drug use (SAMHSA, 2004).

Preventing Drug Misuse and Abuse

The U.S. government devotes much of its drug prevention efforts to reducing the supply of illicit drugs. These efforts include destroying crops such as marijuana and coca plants; stopping the flow of illegal substances through U.S. borders; and prosecuting individuals who manufacture, sell, and purchase drugs illegally. Such measures, however, are not effectively reducing the demand for illicit drugs in this country. Many people think that social and economic programs to reduce poverty and unemployment would decrease the demand for illegal drugs. Additionally, educational programs that promote drug-free lifestyles, especially among children and young adults, may help reduce the prevalence of drug abuse.

The National Institute on Drug Abuse conducted research for 20 years to determine which drug prevention programs have the highest degree of long-term effectiveness. They found that successful prevention programs

- enhance protective factors and reverse or reduce known risk factors,
- use interactive methods such as peer discussion groups,
- target all forms of drug use,
- teach skills to resist drugs when offered,
- strengthen personal commitments against drug use,
- increase social skills and assertiveness, and
- reinforce attitudes against drug use.

Additionally, drug education programs that involve parents, media, and the community are more successful than programs that limit educational activities to classrooms. The research-based programs for general populations of students that are effective include Project STAR, the Life Skills Training Program, and Project Family (NIDA, 1999b).

Healthy Living Practices

- If you or someone you know is abusing drugs, obtain help from local substance abuse programs or from your health care practitioner.

Across
THE LIFESPAN

Drug Use and Abuse

Pregnant drug users are at risk for miscarriage, *ectopic* ("tubal") pregnancy, and stillbirth (giving birth to a dead infant). Babies born to women who used cocaine, opiates, amphetamines, or marijuana regularly during pregnancy are more likely to be premature (born too soon) and smaller than infants who were not exposed to these drugs before birth. Compared with other infants, premature or underweight newborns are more likely to have serious health problems early in life. Drug-exposed newborns also tend to have smaller than normal head circumferences, a sign that brain growth

CRITICAL THINKING

The following ad promotes a book that describes how to eliminate addictive urges. Read the advertisement and evaluate it using the model for analyzing health-related information. The main points of the model are noted below; the model is fully explained on pages 13–15.

1. Which statements are verifiable facts, and which are unverified statements or value claims?
2. What are the credentials of the person who wrote the ad? If this information is available, does the author's background and education qualify him or her as an expert in the topic area?
3. What might be the motives and biases of the person who wrote the ad? State reasons for your answer.
4. Which information in the ad is relevant to the product? Which information is irrelevant?
5. Is the source reliable? Does it have a reputation for publishing misinformation?
6. Does the ad attack the credibility of conventional scientists or medical authorities?

Based on your analysis, do you think that this ad is a reliable source of health-related information? Explain why you would or would not buy the book. Summarize your reasons for coming to this conclusion.

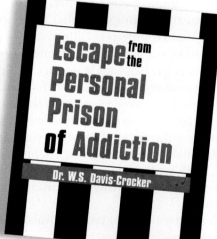

Escape from the Personal Prison of Addiction

Dr. W. S. Davis-Crocker

Is your life being ruined by chemical addictions? Wouldn't it be wonderful to say "no" to drugs and to stick to it? Now you can learn a simple technique to take control of your destructive behaviors.

After years of scientific research, Dr. W. S. Davis-Crocker has unlocked the neurobiochemical secrets of addiction. In her newest book, *Escape from the Personal Prison of Addiction,* Dr. Davis-Crocker, world-renowned author and founder of the Davis-Crocker Institute for the Study of Habituation, describes how to rid yourself of addictions painlessly.

Finally, there is hope for addicts. In just three days of practicing the advice in her book, your cravings for alcohol, cigarettes, heroin, and even chocolate will vanish! There is no need for you to use special medications or costly psychotherapy.

To order your copy of *Escape from the Personal Prison of Addiction,* call ▬▬▬. All major credit cards accepted.

Also register to attend Dr. Davis-Crocker's next seminar in your area. Enrollment is limited, so call the toll-free number now to reserve your seat, and we'll send you our informative pamphlet *Why Me?* at no charge.

has been negatively affected. Pregnant women should consult their physicians before taking any drug.

The news media have reported that many children who were exposed to drugs before birth experience various developmental problems, such as motor movement impairments and learning delays. Some researchers think that such problems are the result of the environment in which these children are raised. Children from low socioeconomic backgrounds are at risk of having developmental problems for a variety of reasons. Before they are born, their mothers are less likely to obtain adequate prenatal medical care. Lack of prenatal care increases a woman's risk of having problems during pregnancy that can affect her health and that of her infant. Additionally, low-income parents may not have the financial resources or parenting skills to provide effective intellectual stimulation for their preschool children.

Studies are needed to monitor the drug use of pregnant women and follow their children for several years. The results of such long-term research may clarify the extent to which prenatal drug exposure influences the mental and physical development of children (Eyler & Behnke, 1999; Tronick & Beeghly, 1999). Results of one recent study revealed that children exposed to cocaine before birth had significant cognitive deficits and were twice as likely as nonexposed children to have developmental delays (Singer et al., 2002).

Adolescents who have certain characteristics are more likely to use alcohol and other drugs than adolescents without these characteristics. These drug use risk factors include gender, family income, parents' use of drugs, latchkey status, and peer drug use. Adolescent males are more likely to use psychoactive drugs and in higher amounts than adolescent females. In general, teenagers from low-income families are more likely to use psychoactive substances than youth from high-income families. Adolescents whose parents use mind-altering drugs have a higher risk of using these substances than the children of non–drug users. Latchkey kids have a higher risk of using drugs than children who have adult supervision when they come home after school. Teenagers whose closest friends are drug users are more likely to take psychoactive substances than children without drug-using friends. **Table 7-7** lists risk factors associated with illicit drug among children and teenagers. Approximately 51% of high school students who were seniors in 2003 have used illegal drugs at some time in their lives (Johnston et al., 2004b).

In spite of living in situations that promote substance use and abuse, many young people abstain from taking psychoactive drugs. Teenagers who stay in high school, attend classes regularly, make good grades, and get along well with their parents generally avoid using

Table 7-7	Adolescents: Risk Factors for Drug Use

Experiences that increase risk of drug use
   Academic failure
   Early antisocial behavior
   Early drug experimentation

Personality characteristics that increase risk of drug use
   Rebelliousness
   Low self-esteem
   Sensation seeking

Environmental situations that increase risk of drug use
   Family disorganization
   Family history of drug use
   Drugs readily available
   Drug use among friends/peers
   Poor socioeconomic status of community

Source: Based on Gilchrist, L. D. (1991). Defining the intervention and target population. In C. G. Leukefeld & W. J. Bukoski (Eds.), *Drug abuse prevention intervention research: Methodological issues* (NIDA Research Monograph No. 107). Washington, DC: U.S. Government Printing Office.

drugs. These children have personality traits that are collectively referred to as *resiliency*. Resilient children accept responsibility, adapt to change, manage stress, solve problems, and are achievement- and success-oriented. Resilient young people have the ability to remain psychologically, socially, and spiritually healthy even though their families are dysfunctional or not supportive.

The abuse of illicit drugs is not a widespread problem among the elderly in the United States. However, many elderly take a variety of prescribed medications to treat problems such as insomnia, depression, hypertension, and heart disease. These aged individuals have a higher risk of becoming intoxicated from taking medications because their bodies do not detoxify and eliminate the substances as effectively as younger ones. More research is needed to determine medication levels that are safe and effective for elderly individuals.

The risk of serious drug interactions and drug synergism is high among aged people who take more than one prescribed drug. In many instances, elderly persons appear to have suffered a stroke, developed Alzheimer's disease, or become severely depressed when actually their confusion and weakness are the side effects of taking numerous prescribed medicines in bad combinations or the wrong amounts or schedules.

Healthy Living Practices

- Do not use drugs of any kind during pregnancy without the approval of your physician.

CHAPTER REVIEW

Summary

Drugs are nonfood chemicals that alter the way a person thinks, feels, functions, or behaves. Many drugs have beneficial uses as medicines, but these substances can have serious negative effects on the health and well-being of people who use them improperly. People often abuse psychoactive, or mood-altering, drugs. Drug abuse contributes to numerous social problems that plague our society, such as crime, unemployment, and family violence and dissolution.

By interacting with nerve cells in the brain, psychoactive drugs influence perceptions, thought processes, feelings, and behaviors. Additionally, environmental factors can affect how people act and feel while under the influence of psychoactive drugs.

In most instances, the liver converts drugs into less dangerous compounds that can be eliminated in urine, feces, or exhaled breath. When the body is unable to detoxify and eliminate excessive amounts of a drug rapidly, the characteristic signs and symptoms of intoxication occur. Drug overdoses and polyabuse may produce serious, even deadly, effects.

In 2003 an estimated 19.5 million Americans over 12 years of age were illegal drug users. Rates of illegal drug use are especially high among teenagers and young adults. Initially, these individuals typically use alcohol, nicotine, or inhalants; they then may move on to marijuana. Some persons experiment with or use other illegal drugs after marijuana. In general, illegal drug use declines after age 20.

Dependency and addiction describe any habitual behavior that interferes with a person's health, work, and relationships. Drug dependence or addiction occurs when users develop a pattern of taking drugs that usually produces a compulsive need to use these substances, a tolerance for them, and withdrawal when they are discontinued. The type of substance taken, the social environment of the person, his or her personality, and genetics influence an individual's chances of developing a drug dependency.

Depressants such as alcohol and barbiturates slow the activity of the cerebral cortex, producing sedative and hypnotic effects as well as drowsiness. Thus, people should not drive or operate machinery while under the influence of depressants. Misusing depressants can be deadly.

Stimulants enhance chemical activity in parts of the brain that influence emotions, sleep, attention, and learning. Caffeine is the most commonly consumed legal stimulant in this country. Stimulants such as Ritalin and cocaine have few medical uses. Cocaine is addictive and frequently abused. In the United States, the use of illegal methamphetamines is growing rapidly.

Opiates have important medical uses as sedatives, analgesics, and narcotics. When misused, opiates are highly addictive and extremely dangerous.

Marijuana, which contains THC as its major psychoactive compound, is the most widely used illicit drug in the United States. Although marijuana does not produce physiological dependence, some people become compulsive users. Marijuana smoke contains numerous irritants that can damage the bronchial tubes and lungs. Some of these compounds are the same cancer-causing substances found in cigarette smoke.

Hallucinogens alter the brain's ability to perceive sensory information, producing abnormal and unreal sensations. In the United States, the most potent and commonly abused hallucinogens are mescaline, psilocybin, LSD, ketamine, and PCP. High doses of PCP and ketamine can be deadly.

Many common household products release toxic fumes that can produce psychoactive effects when inhaled. Teenagers may use inhalants before they move on to other psychoactive drugs. Inhalants can depress respiration, resulting in coma or death.

Amateur chemists make designer drugs by altering the chemical structures of controlled substances. In some cases, these drug analogs are more toxic than the compounds from which they were derived.

The FDA regulates the production and marketing of all medications in the United States. Some health food and OTC products contain substances that are harmful or that produce psychoactive effects, especially when they are misused or abused.

The primary goal of drug treatment is to help abusers become drug-free. Drug treatment usually involves participation in outpatient treatment programs and self-help groups. Drug prevention programs that target school-age children typically provide information about drugs and teach drug resistance and refusal skills.

Drug use during pregnancy increases the risk of miscarriage, ectopic pregnancy, and stillbirth. Women who use cocaine, opiates, amphetamines, and marijuana regularly during pregnancy are more likely to give birth to premature and smaller infants than pregnant women who do not use these drugs. The extent to which prenatal drug exposure influences the long-term mental and physical development of children is unclear.

Approximately 51% of American high school seniors have experimented with illicit drugs. Although drug abuse is rare among the aged, these individuals may experience harmful effects from taking prescribed medicines because they do not detoxify and eliminate drugs as effectively as younger individuals or because they misuse or become confused by multiple prescriptions.

Applying What You Have Learned

1. Why do people abuse certain drugs such as cocaine and not others such as aspirin? **Application**
2. Have you ever used a medication improperly? If your answer is yes, describe your misuse of the drug. **Analysis**
3. Plan an educational program for fifth-grade students that discourages illicit drug use. **Synthesis**
4. One of your friends thinks that marijuana is safe and that its use should be decriminalized. Evaluate this person's position by considering the health effects on the population if marijuana were legalized. **Evaluation**

Key

Application	using information in a new situation.
Analysis	breaking down information into component parts.
Synthesis	putting together information from different sources.
Evaluation	making informed decisions.

Reflecting on Your Health

1. Do you use drugs responsibly? Explain why you do or do not.
2. Under what circumstances would you intervene to stop a friend from abusing drugs?
3. What are you currently doing or what would you do to encourage your children not to use illegal drugs?
4. What kinds of over-the-counter drugs do you use? Do you think that your use of these drugs is helpful or harmful to your health?

5. If you abuse drugs, do you think that your health or the health of others is adversely affected by your behavior? Why or why not? After reading this chapter and learning about the health effects of illegal drugs, are you motivated to stop your drug abuse? Why or why not?

References

Baldwin, G. C., Tashkin, D. P., Buckley, D. M., Park, A. N., Dubinett, S. M., & Roth, M. D. (1997). Marijuana and cocaine impair alveolar macrophage function and cytokine production. *American Journal of Respiratory & Critical Care Medicine, 156*:1606–1613.

Barsky, S. H., Roth, M. D., Kleerup, E. D., Simmons, M., & Tashkin, D. P. (1998). Histopathic and molecular alterations in bronchial epithelium in habitual smokers of marijuana, cocaine, and/or tobacco. *Journal of the National Cancer Institute, 90*:1198–1205.

Clausson, B., Granath, F., Ekbom A., Lundgren, S., Nordmark, A., Signorello, L. B., & Cnattingius, S. (2002). Effect of caffeine exposure during pregnancy on birth weight and gestational age. *American Journal of Epidemiology, 155*:429–436.

Couper, F. J., Pemberton, M., Hughes, M., & Logan, B. K. (2002). Prevalence of drug use in commercial tractor-trailer drivers. *Journal of Forensic Science, 47*:562–567.

DesJarlais, D. C., & Hubbard, R. (1999). Treatment for drug dependence. *Proceedings of the Association of American Physicians, 111*:126–130.

DuPont, R. L. (1999). Examining the debate on the use of medical marijuana. *Proceedings of the Association of American Physicians, 111*:166–172.

Eyler, F. D., & Behnke, M. (1999). Early development of infants exposed to drugs prenatally. *Clinics in Perinatology, 26*:107–150.

Fergusson, D. M., Horwood, L. J., & Beautrais, A. L. (2004). Cannabis and educational achievement. *Addiction, 99*:650–651.

Fung, M., Gallagher, C., & Machtay, M. (1999). Lung and aero-digestive cancers in young marijuana smokers. *Tumori, 85*:140–142.

Goldberg, R. (1994). *Drugs across the spectrum.* Minneapolis/St. Paul: West Publishing Company.

Halpern, J. H., & Pope, H. G. (1999). Do hallucinogens cause residual neuropsychological toxicity? *Drug & Alcohol Dependence, 53*:247–256.

Hanson, G., Venturelli, P. J., & Fleckenstein, A. E. (2004). *Drugs and society.* Sudbury, MA: Jones and Bartlett Publishers.

Johnston, L. D., O'Malley, P. M., Backman, J. G., & Schulenberg, J. E. (2004a). *Monitoring the Future national results on adolescent drug use: Overview of key findings 2003* (NIH Publication No. 04-5506). Bethesda, MD: National Institute on Drug Abuse.

Johnston, L. D., O'Malley, P. M., Backman, J. G., & Schulenberg, J. E. (2004b). *Monitoring the Future national survey results on drug use, 1975–2003: Volume 1, Secondary school students* (NIH Publication No. 04-5507). Bethesda, MD: National Institute on Drug Abuse.

Johnston, L. D., O'Malley, P. M., Backman, J. G., & Schulenberg, J. E. (2004c). *Monitoring the Future national survey results on drug use, 1975–2003: Volume 11, college students and adults ages 19–45* (NIH Publication No. 04-5508). Bethesda, MD: National Institute on Drug Abuse.

Kam, P. C., & Yoong, F. F. (1998). Gamma-hydroxybutyric acid: An emerging recreational drug. *Anaesthesia, 53*:1195–1198.

Liguori, A., Gatto, C. P., & Robinson, J. H. (1998). Effects of marijuana on equilibrium, psychomotor performance, and simulated driving. *Behavioral Pharmacology, 9*:599–609.

Logan, B. K., & Schwilke, E. W. (1996). Drug and alcohol use in fatally injured drivers in Washington State. *Journal of Forensic Sciences, 41*:505–510.

National Institute on Drug Abuse. (1999a). *Principles of drug addiction treatment: A research-based guide* (NIH Publication No. 99–4180). Washington, DC: National Institutes of Health, National Institute on Drug Abuse.

National Institute on Drug Abuse. (1999b). *The sixth triennial report to Congress from the secretary of Health and Human Services. Drug abuse & addiction research: 25 years of discovery to advance the health of the public.* Washington, DC: National Institutes of Health, National Institute on Drug Abuse.

National Institute on Drug Abuse. (2003). *Preventing drug use among children and adolescents: A research-based guide* (2nd ed.). Washington, DC: U.S. Government Printing Office.

Nehlig, A. (1999). Are we dependent upon coffee and caffeine? A review on human and animal data. *Neuroscience and Biobehavioral Reviews, 23*:563–576.

Plessinger, M. A. (1998). Prenatal exposure to amphetamines: Risks and adverse outcomes in pregnancy. *Obstetrics and Gynecology Clinics of North America, 25*:119–138.

Schwartz, R. H. (1998). Adolescent heroin use: A review. *Pediatrics, 102*:1461–1466.

Simoni-Wastila, L., & Strickler, G. (2004). Risk factors associated with problem use of prescription drugs. *American Journal of Public Health, 94*(2):266–268.

Singer, L. T., Arendt, R., Minnes, S., Farkas, K., Salvator, A., Kirchner, H. L., & Kliegman, R. (2002). Cognitive and motor outcomes of cocaine-exposed infants. *Journal of the American Medical Association, 287*:1952–1960.

Strote, J., Lee, J. E., & Wechsler, H. (2002). Increasing MDMA use among college students: Results of a national survey. *Journal of Adolescent Health, 30*:64–72.

Substance Abuse and Mental Health Services Administration. (2004). *Results from the 2003 National Survey on Drug Use and Health* (DHHS Publication No. SMA 04–3964). Rockville, MD: National Clearinghouse for Alcohol and Drug Information.

Taylor, H. G. (1998). Analysis of the medical use of marijuana and its societal implications. *Journal of the American Pharmaceutical Association, 38*:220–227.

Thompson, P. M., Kayashi, K. M., Simon, S. L., Geaga, J. S., Hong, M. S., Sui, Y., Lee, J. Y., Toga, A. W., Ling, W., & London, E. D. (2004). Structural abnormalities in the brains of human subjects who use methamphetamine. *Journal of Neuroscience, 24*:6028–6036.

Tronick, E. Z., & Beeghly, M. (1999). Prenatal cocaine exposure, child development, and the compromising effects of cumulative risk. *Clinics in Perinatology, 26*:151–171.

Wu, T. C., Tashkin, D. P., Djahed, B., & Rose, J. E. (1988). Pulmonary hazards of smoking marijuana as compared with tobacco. *New England Journal of Medicine, 318*:347–351.

WARNING
TOBACCO USE CAN MAKE YOU IMPOTENT

Cigarettes may cause sexual impotence due to decreased blood flow to the penis. This can prevent you from having an erection.

Health Canada

WARNING
CIGARETTES HURT BABIES

Tobacco use during pregnancy reduces the growth of babies during pregnancy. These smaller babies may not catch up in growth after birth and the risks of infant illness, disability and death are increased.

Health Canada

WARNING
YOU'RE NOT THE ONLY ONE SMOKING THIS CIGARETTE

The smoke from a cigarette is not just inhaled by the smoker. It becomes second-hand smoke, which contains more than 50 cancer-causing agents.

Health Canada

WARNING
CIGARETTES ARE HIGHLY ADDICTIVE

Studies have shown that tobacco can be harder to quit than heroin or cocaine.

Health Canada

What You'll Learn

Chapter Overview

Factors related to and consequences of alcohol abuse and dependence

Alcohol's effects on college students

How to control your alcohol consumption

How alcoholism is diagnosed and treated

Who uses tobacco products and why

The short- and long-term health effects of tobacco use

The benefits and process of quitting

 ### Diversity in Health
Tobacco Drinking?

 ### Consumer Health
Kretecks and Bidis: Unwrapping the Facts

 ### Managing Your Health
Drinking and Date-Rape Drugs | Guidelines for Safer Drinking | How to Say No to Secondhand Smoke | Tips for Quitters

Across THE LIFESPAN

The Effects of Alcohol and Tobacco Use

Student Workbook

Self-Assessment: Why Do You Smoke? | The CAGE Questionnaire

Changing Health Habits: Do You Want to Change a Smoking or Drinking Habit?

Do You Know?

· *Whether clove cigarettes are safer than regular cigarettes?*
· *The major reasons why college students drink?*
· *How smoking can affect your sex life?*

Alcohol and Tobacco

Canada has the distinction of being the first country in the world to implement strong visual warnings on tobacco product packaging, as shown in the photos. The regulations that allowed for these images became law in June 2000, and took effect in early 2001. These messages cover more than 50% of each cigarette pack, containing images and words that are larger and much more graphic than the four surgeon general's warnings currently printed on cigarette packs in the United States. They are difficult to ignore each time a smoker pulls out a pack to light up. Additionally, as part of Canada's comprehensive strategy to reduce serious disease and death caused by tobacco, the federal government requires the insertion of health information leaflets in cigarette packs with detailed toxic emission data printed along the outside. The Canadian government also increased taxes on tobacco products in late 2001, and many Canadian provinces concurrently raised their tobacco products taxes.

Smoking among all Canadians older than 15 years fell from 30% to 23% from 1991 to 2001 and continued to drop to 21% in 2003. Smoking among Canadian youths aged 15 to 19 years rose from 21% to 28% from 1991 to 1999 but declined to 23% by the first half of 2001 and to 18% by 2003. Twelve percent reported daily smoking (Health Canada, 2001, 2004). Smoking among American youths rose and declined in a similar manner. Cigarette use rose from 1991 to 1996 for eighth and tenth graders, and from 1991 to 1997 for twelfth graders. It has since declined steadily for all groups, with 4.5% of eighth graders, 8.9% of tenth graders, and 15.8% of twelfth graders smoking cigarettes daily in 2003 (Johnston et al., 2004a).

"These messages cover more than 50% of each cigarette pack . . ."

Smoking cigarettes and drinking alcohol are behaviors that often begin in adolescence. Most adolescents view these behaviors as acceptable because advertisements encourage such thinking, especially ads that target this age group, such as the Joe Camel advertisement shown in Figure 8-1a. Launched in 1987, the Joe Camel campaign was very attractive to young children as well as adolescents. Although a 12-year decline in adolescent smoking had occurred prior to the Joe Camel campaign, the decline stopped with its introduction, and the incidence of smoking in the 14- to 17-year-old age group increased (Pierce, 1998). Joe Camel ads were finally banned as part of the 1998 tobacco settlement with the states and five territories (Ebnet, 1998).

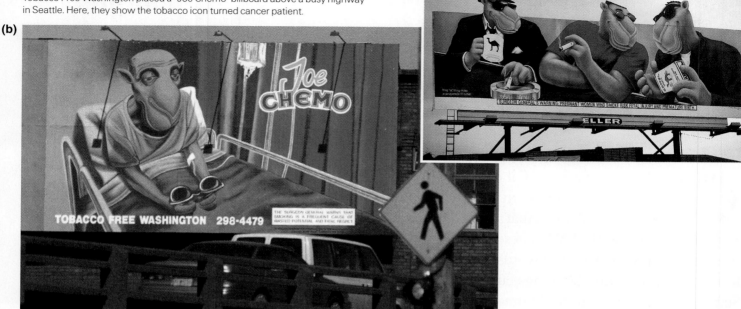

(a)

Figure 8-1 **Joe Camel.** (a) Such cigarette advertisements are criticized because they appear to target preteens and teens. (b) To counter Joe Camel advertising, Tobacco Free Washington placed a "Joe Chemo" billboard above a busy highway in Seattle. Here, they show the tobacco icon turned cancer patient.

The 1998 settlement prohibited tobacco companies from taking "any action, directly or indirectly, to target youth . . . in the advertising, promotion or marketing of tobacco products." Nonetheless, in 2004 tobacco companies began marketing "candy" cigarettes—those having fruit flavors, such as Twista Lime and Midnight Berry. Chewing tobacco was being promoted that had such flavors as apple, vanilla, and cherry. One brand of cigarettes was being advertised using hip-hop music. Such products and marketing strategies appear to target adolescents, teens, and young adults.

Many medical researchers and health care professionals think that advertising alcohol and other drug-related products such as cigarettes encourages the use of all drugs. The practice of promoting alcohol and tobacco use is particularly dangerous because they are two primary "gateway" drugs. That is, most people follow a pattern of progression in drug use from alcohol and/or tobacco to marijuana to "hard" drugs (Hanson et al., 2004).

Both tobacco and alcohol can have devastating effects on health. Before you read this chapter, consider taking one or both of the self-assessments for this chapter in the student workbook. Clinicians use the CAGE screening test to detect alcohol abuse or alcoholism. The National Cancer Institute's quiz "Why Do You Smoke?" will help you understand the roots of your smoking behavior. If you do not smoke cigarettes or drink alcoholic beverages, you probably know family members, coworkers, or friends who may benefit from these self-assessments. Taking these tests could be their first steps to healthier lifestyles.

Alcohol

Alcohol Use, Abuse, and Dependence

Alcohol use is quite prevalent in the United States, probably more prevalent than you might think. If every man, woman, and child over the age of 14 drank alcohol, each would have to consume approximately 600 12-ounce cans of beer per year to account for the annual consumption of alcohol in this country! Of course, not everyone over 14 years of age consumes alcoholic beverages; therefore, some who drink alcohol consume much more than this amount. Some consume less.

According to the 2003 National Survey on Drug Use and Health, 50.1% of Americans older than 12 years are current alcohol users, which means that they had at least one drink in the month before they took the survey. This group includes binge alcohol users and heavy alcohol users. For the purposes of the survey, *binge alcohol users* had five or more drinks on the same occasion at least once in the month prior to the survey. *Heavy alcohol users* had five or more drinks on the same occasion on at least five days in the month prior to the survey (Substance Abuse and Mental Health Services Administration [SAMHSA], 2004a). (All heavy

Table 8-1	Drinking Levels as Shown in Standard Drinks per Week

Drinking Level	Amount
Abstainer	Fewer than 12 drinks in lifetime or no drinks in the past year
Light	3 or fewer drinks/week
Moderate	More than 3 drinks but no more than 7 drinks/week for women and no more than 14 drinks/week for men
Heavier	More than 1 drink/day for women and more than 2 drinks/day for men

*One standard drink is 0.5 oz absolute alcohol, 12 oz beer, 5 oz wine, or 1.5 oz 80-proof liquor. (Amounts for beer and wine vary depending on their alcohol content.) Source: National Institute on Alcohol Abuse and Alcoholism.

Table 8-2	Alcohol Dependence Syndrome

Having three or more of the following symptoms over a year usually indicates alcohol dependence syndrome:

- A strong desire or compulsion to drink
- Difficulty in controlling the amount of alcohol consumed and when it is consumed
- Withdrawal symptoms when alcohol is not consumed, or consuming alcohol to avoid withdrawal symptoms
- Evidence of tolerance, that is, increased amounts of alcohol are needed to achieve the effects originally produced by lower amounts
- Progressive neglect of other interests because of drinking, while spending an increased amount of time obtaining and drinking alcohol, and recovering from its effects
- Continued use of alcohol despite clear evidence of its physical and/or psychological effects on the user

alcohol users are also binge alcohol users.) Table 8-1 lists the number of drinks consumed by light to heavier drinkers as measured in standard drinks per week.

Many people who consume alcoholic beverages use alcohol responsibly. Responsible drinkers do not allow drinking alcoholic beverages to threaten their physical or psychological health or interfere with their relationships or interactions with others. Additionally, their behavior while drinking does not threaten the health or well-being of others.

Alcohol use becomes **harmful use** when a person drinks alcoholic beverages while knowingly damaging his or her physical and/or psychological health. A person who sustains injuries from accidents while drinking or becomes depressed from drinking, for example, is engaging in harmful use.

Alcohol abuse encompasses the symptoms of harmful use but also includes a social dimension. When drinking, the alcohol abuser has problems interacting with people in his or her family, in social settings, or at work. Typically, the abuser uses alcohol in physically dangerous situations, such as when driving a car. However, he or she does not develop tolerance to the drug, exhibit withdrawal symptoms when not drinking (see Chapter 7), or compulsively use alcohol. Both harmful use and alcohol abuse are patterns of behavior, not just one-time occurrences, and are usually considered to be present if the behavior has occurred for at least one month or has occurred repeatedly over a longer period of time.

Alcohol abuse becomes **alcohol dependence**, or **alcoholism**, when certain other symptoms occur that are part of the *alcohol dependence syndrome*. Table 8-2 lists the symptoms of this syndrome. A diagnosis of dependence is usually made if a person exhibits three or more of these symptoms over a year's time. Approximately

10% of those who drink alcohol experience problems related to their alcohol use. These people account for 50% of all alcohol consumed in the United States. Currently, 14 million Americans are dependent on alcohol, and approximately 75,000 people die each year from harmful effects of excessive alcohol use, dying—on average—30 years prematurely (Centers for Disease Control and Prevention [CDC], 2004a).

Factors Related to Alcohol Abuse and Dependence

About 100 years ago, alcoholics were thought simply to have a "weak character" or to suffer from "moral weakness." Since that time, especially within the past 50 years or so, scientists have gathered evidence showing that alcoholism has a variety of origins, many of them biological. In addition, research results show the importance of the interactions among heredity, brain effects, and psychological, social, and developmental factors in the development of alcoholism. A cause of alcoholism is unknown, however.

Heredity For centuries, people have observed that alcoholism runs in families. Researchers have explored environmental and hereditary (genetic) factors of alcoholics to determine which are significant in the development of alcoholism.

harmful use drinking alcoholic beverages while knowingly damaging one's physical and/or psychological health.

alcohol abuse includes the symptoms of harmful use, but when drinking the abuser exhibits long-term social interaction problems and uses alcohol in physically dangerous situations.

alcohol dependence (alcoholism) a syndrome characterized by at least three of the following symptoms: a compulsion to drink, difficulty in controlling the amount of alcohol consumed, withdrawal symptoms when alcohol is not consumed, evidence of tolerance, progressive neglect of other interests because of drinking, and continuing to use alcohol despite its physical and psychological effects on the user.

By studying the family history of alcoholics, scientists determined that people who have a first-degree relative (parent, brother, or sister) with alcoholism have a higher risk of developing alcoholism than people in the general population. Scientists estimate this risk to be from 4 to 7 times higher. Sons of alcoholic fathers are at greatest risk. Additionally, data from adoption, twin, and animal studies indicate that there is a genetic component to alcoholism.

Scientists also study the reactions of people at risk for developing alcoholism (those who have a first-degree alcoholic relative) in comparison with those not at risk for alcoholism. In general, those at risk do not react to the consumption of alcohol with the same intensity as those not at risk. Some scientists think that persons at risk for alcoholism may not perceive that they are becoming intoxicated until they have had far more to drink than those not at risk for alcoholism.

Two other genetically linked factors are thought to influence the development of alcoholism: temperament and behavior. *Behavior* is the way people act—what they do. *Temperament* means disposition—the characteristic way in which people emotionally respond to the things and people around them. Temperament and behavior are thought to be inherited traits that are modified by interactions with the environment (see Chapter 2). Certain characteristics of temperament and behavior appear to be associated with enhanced risk for alcoholism: hyperactivity, impulsivity, aggression, short attention span, quickly changing emotions, slowed ability to calm oneself following stress, thrill-seeking behavior, and inability to delay gratification.

Brain Effects When a person drinks alcoholic beverages, various behavioral changes occur that are commonly called **intoxication**, impairment of the functioning of the central nervous system (the brain and spinal cord). Table 8-3 lists the changes that characteristically take place as a person consumes more and more alcohol. In this table, alcohol consumption and blood alcohol concentrations (BACs) are listed as ranges because the number of drinks as related to the body weight determines the concentration of alcohol in the blood. That is, in general, the larger the person, the greater the amount of alcohol that must be consumed for a specific blood alcohol concentration. Blood alcohol concentrations also rise more quickly in women than in men. One of the reasons for this occurrence is that women have proportionately more fat and less water in their bodies than do men. Alcohol is more sol-

intoxication impairment of the functioning of the central nervous system as a result of ingesting toxic substances like alcohol.

tolerance a physiological response in chronic users of drugs in which increased amounts of the drug are required to achieve effects previously produced by lower amounts.

Table 8-3	Effects of Various Levels of Alcohol Consumption on Inexperienced Drinkers	
Number of Standard Drinks	Blood Alcohol Concentration (BAC)*	Effects
1–2	0.02 to 0.06%	Euphoria; reduction in anxiety
3–5	0.08 to 0.15%	Impairment of judgment, motor coordination, and emotional control; involuntary rapid eye movements; double vision; speech disorders; may be accompanied by aggressive behavior as alcohol level rises
7–8	0.20 to 0.25%	Sedation; impairment of ability to learn and remember information
12–18	0.40 to 0.50%	Loss of adequate respiration; dangerously low blood pressure; dangerously low internal body temperature; coma or death may result

*Blood alcohol concentration is expressed in percentages: A BAC of 0.05% means an alcohol concentration of 5 milliliters (ml) for every 10,000 ml of blood.

uble in water than in fat; therefore, if a woman drinks the same amount as a man, her generally smaller size and lower water content result in a higher concentration of alcohol in watery body tissues such as the blood. Additionally, the stomach enzyme that breaks down alcohol before it reaches the bloodstream is less active in women than it is in men.

Why do certain changes take place in the body when a person consumes alcoholic beverages? The answer has to do with how alcohol affects interactions among nerve cells in the brain. As discussed in Chapter 7, psychoactive drugs (including alcohol) act at communication points among nerve cells. Psychoactive drugs interfere with the normal activity of the chemicals that carry nerve impulses from one nerve cell to another. The manner of this interference varies among drugs.

Alcohol acts on parts of the brain that are responsible for drives and emotions, as well as the part of the brain that coordinates skeletal muscle movements. It also affects the "thinking" part and reward centers in the brain.

Many people drink alcohol to "get drunk," but other factors often contribute to excessive alcohol consumption. Anxious people, for example, may use alcohol to relieve their anxieties. Researchers think that persons with a family history of alcoholism are more likely to be motivated to drink alcohol to get "high," while persons with no family history of alcoholism are more likely to be motivated by anxiety.

At high doses, alcohol also has effects that are aversive; that is, they are sufficiently unpleasant (such as nausea and vomiting) that people often lose their desire to drink. Severe aversive effects, such as unconsciousness, result in a person's inability to continue drinking. Therefore, aversive effects help curb excessive alcohol consumption.

Chronic drug users develop **tolerance** to the drug; that is, increased amounts of alcohol are required to achieve effects previously produced by lower amounts. Tolerance develops because the chronic use of the drug stimulates liver enzymes to break down the drug with increasing swiftness. Also, brain cells become less responsive to the drug over time. Tolerance develops for both the pleasant and unpleasant effects of alcohol consumption, so chronic drinkers do not experience the aversive effects as quickly as do occasional drinkers. Therefore, their alcohol consumption is not curbed as quickly.

Psychological, Social, and Developmental Factors People drink for reasons other than to experience the "brain effects" of feeling good or reducing anxiety. Similarly, people curb their drinking or abstain from drinking for reasons other than aversive brain effects that may stimulate nausea and vomiting. Many of these reasons are *psychological,* having to do with thoughts, feelings, attitudes, and expectations about alcohol. Some of the reasons are *social,* relating to interactions with friends, relatives, and coworkers. Still other reasons are *developmental,* relating to the psychological, social, and biological changes in individuals over time and as they mature.

People often consume alcoholic beverages because they expect positive psychological effects from their drinking, such as enhancing social interactions, feeling pleasurable effects, or producing sedation. People develop their expectations concerning alcohol from experience, observation, and what they are told. In fact, a person's beliefs about alcohol can be predictive of their future drinking habits: Heavy drinkers tend to view the positive effects of alcohol as arousing, while light drinkers tend to view the positive effects as sedating.

Individuals often consume alcohol to ease their social interactions or because it's the thing to do in a particular social setting. With adolescents and young adults, peers may pressure one another to drink alcohol. The section "Alcohol and College Students" explores the role of peer pressure in the drinking patterns of college students. Cultural factors are additional impor-

tant social reasons for drinking alcohol. In many cultures, people consume alcohol with meals or as a part of other traditional social activities.

Abusive and alcohol-dependent drinking patterns often begin in adolescence. A wide variety of factors affect children as they mature and influence the development of patterns of drinking alcoholic beverages. The biggest early risk factor for alcohol abuse and dependence is having a parent who is an alcoholic or who abuses alcohol. Children of alcoholics are two to four times more likely to become alcoholics than children of nonalcoholics (Hanson et al., 2004). Additionally, a child reared in an alcoholic family has a 50% greater risk of developing alcoholism than a child who is not reared in such an environment (Pullen, 1994).

Another way in which parents influence their children is by their parenting practices. Teenagers who report receiving high levels of nurturing and support from their parents also report fewer alcohol-related problems than teenagers who report little parental nurturing and support. Teenagers who report feeling close to their parents drink alcoholic beverages less frequently than teenagers who report that they do not feel close to their parents. Children are more likely to use alcohol if their parents are not involved in their activities, there is a lack of or inconsistent discipline, and the parents have low educational aspirations for the children. Positive family relationships, involvement, and attachment appear to discourage youths' initiation into alcohol use.

Psychological, social, and developmental factors all interact with genetic factors to result in behavior. These interactions explain why not all alcoholics have a family history of alcoholism, and why not all persons with a family history of alcoholism become alcoholics. These dynamic interactions occur throughout life, with varying contributions from genes and environment at different times.

Alcohol and College Students

Alcohol abuse is a serious problem that often appears to begin or accelerate during the college years. In fact, the most abused drug among college students is alcohol. Most studies of alcohol use by college students examine psychological and social issues; those issues are discussed here. However, researchers are calling for studies to examine economic, political, and ecological factors of college alcohol use, such as the alcohol environment on college campuses and their surrounding communities (Dowdall & Wechsler, 2002). Studies show that college students drink alcohol for a variety of reasons. Table 8-4 lists the primary reasons that stu-

Table 8-4	College Students: Major Reasons for Drinking

College students report that they drink alcohol because

- It helps them celebrate special occasions
- They enjoy the taste of alcohol
- They want to relieve tension
- It helps them relax
- It helps them feel more comfortable in social settings
- They want to get drunk
- It relieves boredom
- It just seems like the thing to do
- They want to forget about schoolwork

Source: Adapted from Klein, H. (1992). Self-reported reasons for why college students drink. *Journal of Alcohol and Drug Education, 37*(2):14–27.

Table 8-5	College Students: Major Reasons for Not Drinking

College students report that they abstain from drinking alcohol because

- Disapproval/Lack of interest (against religious/moral convictions)
- Risks and negative effects (hangovers/alcoholism/medication interactions)
- Social responsibility (might interfere with job/family/school/relationships)
- Loss of control (negatively affects mood/effects unpleasant)
- Lack of availability (expense/hard to obtain)
- Health concerns (in training/fattening/bad for health)

Source: Adapted from Johnson, T. J., & Chen, E. A. (2004). College students' reasons for not drinking and not playing drinking games. *Substance Use & Misuse, 39*:1139–1162.

dents give to explain why they drink. However, there are differences between moderate and heavy drinkers with regard to their reasons for drinking (Klein, 1992).

Moderate drinkers who do not abuse alcohol do not cite many reasons for their drinking. They drink to celebrate important occasions or because they enjoy the taste of alcohol. They do not drink with any goal in mind such as getting drunk.

Heavy drinkers who abuse alcohol, however, often state many reasons for their drinking, including the reasons listed in Table 8-4, but their drinking tends to be escapist and goal-oriented. College men are more likely to be in this category than women.

Certain student characteristics correlate with alcohol abuse. Although any student may abuse alcohol, abusers are more likely to be younger students with low self-esteem, high levels of anxiety, a mildly assertive personality, and at least one alcoholic parent. The freshman and sophomore years are the most likely times for students to exhibit alcohol abuse. Additionally, students who have a GPA lower than 2.0 are more likely than students with higher GPAs to abuse alcohol (Glindemann et al., 1999; Pullen, 1994).

Drinking alcohol during the college years poses many risks for students, including driving after drinking, getting behind in school work, and getting into trouble with campus or local police (Wechsler et al., 2000). In fact, many students who abstain from alcohol do so because they want to avoid such risks. Alcohol can also be a vehicle for date-rape drugs. The Managing Your Health box "Drinking and Date-Rape Drugs: Safety Tips for Women" provides guidelines to help women avoid ingesting these dangerous substances in alco-

holic beverages. Table 8-5 lists the primary reasons some students abstain from drinking alcohol.

Binge Drinking and Drinking Games College men who belong to fraternities, especially those who live in fraternity houses, make up a large proportion of students who drink heavily. Drinking in fraternities, as in other campus social groups including many sororities, is perceived as promoting a feeling of unity and cohesiveness among their members.

In 2001, about 75% of college students who lived in fraternities and sororities binge drank, versus about 55% of students who lived in off-campus housing alone or with a roommate, 45% who lived in residence halls, 30% who lived off-campus with parents, and 27% who lived off-campus with a spouse. Additionally, high proportions of nondrinking students who lived in fraternity or sorority housing experienced negative effects resulting from the behavior of bingeing students with whom they lived, such as having their study or sleep interrupted or having to take care of a drunken student. Nevertheless, attendance and heavy drinking at fraternity and sorority house parties declined significantly from 1993 to 2001 (Wechsler et al., 2002).

Students who live in fraternity or sorority houses are not the only college students who binge drink. In fact, age 21 is the peak of binge drinking behavior, with 50.2% of all persons in this age group reporting binge drinking (SAMHSA, 2004b).

Binge drinking is often accompanied by drinking games. There is a high prevalence of drinking games on college campuses, with approximately 76% of college men and 50% of college women reported to be engaging in these activities (Johnson & Sheets, 2004).

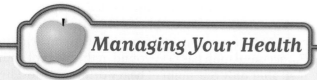

Table 8-6 lists specific motives for playing drinking games. Compare this table with Table 8-4 and you will see similarities. Although some motives for playing drinking games seem specific to the games (e.g., competition), current research has not conclusively established that the motives for playing drinking games are separate from the general motives for drinking (Johnson & Sheets, 2004).

In drinking games, participants follow rules that specify when and how much they must drink and that mandate certain verbal, physical, or memory skills. When players make mistakes, they are required to drink. The more game players drink, the more they make mistakes, and the amount of alcohol they consume increases. The danger of unconsciousness, coma, and death increases as alcohol consumption increases.

Table 8-6	College Students: Major Reasons for Playing Drinking Games

· Competition and thrills
· Conformity (to fit in)
· Novelty (to try something different)
· Fun and celebration
· Social lubrication
· Sexual manipulation (in order to have sex with someone or get a date)
· Boredom
· Coping (to forget about problems)

Source: Adapted from Johnson, T. J., & Sheets, V. L. (2004). Measuring college students' motives for playing drinking games. *Psychology of Addictive Behaviors, 18*(2):91–99.

What can you do to help an intoxicated person avoid serious medical consequences or death? A person who has slurred speech, a staggering gait, double vision, and is lethargic (but is able to be aroused by voice) should be stopped from drinking and taken away from the source of the alcohol. A person with signs of more severe intoxication, such as incoherence, incontinence, irregular breathing, repeated vomiting, and inability to be aroused with a strong stimulus like a slap, should be taken to an emergency room immediately.

How the Body Processes Alcohol

When an alcoholic beverage is consumed, the alcohol in the drink is absorbed into the bloodstream from the stomach and intestinal tract. The blood transports alcohol to the "detoxification center" of the body—the liver. The liver degrades harmful substances such as drugs by changing them into compounds that are safer or easier to excrete.

The liver can degrade only a certain amount of alcohol per hour, no matter how much has been consumed. That rate depends, in part, on the concentration of enzymes that degrade alcohol in the liver, and this enzyme concentration varies among individuals. Nevertheless, alcohol is absorbed into the bloodstream more quickly than it can be broken down by the liver, and the excess alcohol stays in the blood. Therefore, the consumption of alcohol needs to be controlled to prevent its accumulation in the blood, resulting in an increase in the blood alcohol level.

The stomach also degrades some alcohol. Eating food while drinking alcoholic beverages results in the alcohol being held in the stomach for a longer time with the food. Therefore, more of it gets broken down in the stomach, and less alcohol enters the bloodstream. A person who drinks while eating will have a slower rise in the blood alcohol level than will a person who drinks on an empty stomach. Conversely, aspirin and cimetidine (an ulcer drug) inhibit the breakdown of alcohol in the stomach. A person who takes either of these drugs along with alcohol will have a quicker rise in the blood alcohol level than will a person who does not take these drugs when drinking alcohol.

Consequences of Alcohol Abuse and Dependence

Diseases and Conditions The harmful use and abuse of alcohol result in multiple effects on the body that are serious threats to health. Alcohol consumption does not affect all individuals in the same way; various effects result from differences among abusers' genetic makeup, general health, and drinking patterns. In spite of these differences, however, excessive alcohol consumption exerts its most serious effects on the liver, cardiovascular system, immune system, reproductive system, and brain. It also affects how vitamins are used by the body and can result in vitamin deficiencies. In pregnant women, it has devastating effects on the fetus.

Diseases of the Liver Because the liver is the major detoxification site for alcohol, it is particularly prone to harm by chronic alcohol consumption. Years of drinking can result in three types of liver disease: fatty liver, alcoholic hepatitis, and cirrhosis of the liver. The symptoms of each may overlap, and a person can have more than one of these conditions simultaneously. Women tend to develop these conditions at lower levels of alcohol intake than men (see p. 192).

Nearly 90% of heavy drinkers develop a *fatty liver* because alcohol induces the accumulation of fat in liver cells. This process begins immediately upon drinking: Fat accumulation has been found in the livers of young men after only one night of heavy drinking. Most liver cells are not specialized for fat storage, and their ability to perform their normal functions declines when they store fat. These liver cells eventually die; the scar tissue that remains produces cirrhosis.

Approximately 15% to 30% of alcoholics develop *liver cirrhosis* (Figure 8-2). This disease develops as alcohol begins to kill liver cells. Liver cells have the ability to regenerate, much like skin heals from a small cut. However, if cell damage is extensive, the liver cannot produce new cells quickly enough to replace destroyed ones. Connective tissue cells fill the spaces left by the dead cells, similar to the way scar tissue may fill the gap of tissue caused by a severe cut. However, connective tissue is not functional liver tissue, and the liver's ability to perform its many important functions declines. Eventually the person must have a liver transplant or he or she will die.

Approximately 40% of chronic abusers develop *alcoholic hepatitis*. Hepatitis is an inflammation of the liver, which can be caused by hepatitis viruses or by toxic chemicals such as alcohol. A severe case of hepatitis can result in death.

The majority of individuals who develop cirrhosis of the liver have been drinking heavily for 10 to 20 years. Women, however, are more at risk than men for liver disease. Because women detoxify alcohol less efficiently than men, the concentration of alcohol in their blood rises more quickly than in men when both consume the same number of drinks. Therefore, serious forms of alcoholic liver disease occur more

(a)

(b)

Figure 8-2   **A Healthy and an Unhealthy Liver (with Cirrhosis).**   (a) Healthy liver tissue is smooth and dark red/brown.
(b) The liver with cirrhosis develops scar tissue and nodules (bumps) as it works to repair damage.

frequently in women than in men. Additionally, women are more likely than men to develop these conditions at lower levels of alcohol consumption and after shorter periods of alcohol dependence. Hereditary factors and body weight, as well as sex, appear to play a role in susceptibility to liver disease. Results of recent studies also show that obese alcoholics have a two to three times higher risk of having alcoholic liver disease than nonobese alcoholics (Bunout, 1999).

Cardiovascular Disease and Cancer There is considerable evidence that limiting alcohol consumption to 1 oz or less of ethanol per day (two drinks or less) decreases the risk of death from coronary artery disease and stroke (see Chapter 12). However, heavier drinking is associated with cardiovascular diseases such as cardiomyopathy (heart muscle disease), hypertension (high blood pressure), arrhythmias (disturbances in heart rhythm), and stroke. In fact, very heavy drinking (about five drinks per day) is associated with a fourfold increase in the risk of stroke (Hillbom et al., 1999).

Alcohol abuse is a risk factor for certain cancers. The heavy consumption of alcohol can cause cancers of the esophagus and liver. It is also associated with the development of stomach cancer and increases the likelihood of larynx and mouth cancer in smokers. People who smoke cigarettes and drink alcohol, even in moderate amounts, multiply their risk of cancer of the esophagus 12 to 19 times, because together these drugs have a multiplier effect. That is, when people take both drugs routinely, their risk of cancer is much higher than if the risk of each was added (Castellsague et al., 1999).

Even when not abused, alcohol can raise the risk of cancer. Consuming three or more drinks per week raises a woman's risk for developing breast cancer. Additionally, data suggest that women who drink alcohol while taking estrogen in postmenopausal estrogen replacement therapy may increase their breast cancer risk more than if they used either one alone (Ginsberg, 1999).

Immune System Suppression The immune system (see Chapter 14), which protects the body from invasion by pathogens, also suffers as a result of chronic alcohol abuse. This behavior impairs the functioning of the immune system, predisposing the drinker to infectious diseases such as colds, pneumonia, and tuberculosis. Chronic alcohol abuse even suppresses the activity of certain immune system cells that defend the body against the spread of cancer.

Detrimental Effects on the Reproductive System Alcohol affects the reproductive systems of both men and women. It affects the functioning of the testes, decreasing the amount of the sex hormone, testosterone, these

organs produce. Alcoholic men often experience shrinking of the testicles, impotence, and loss of libido, or sex drive. In women, alcohol affects the functioning of the ovaries. The menstrual periods of alcoholic women are often irregular or cease altogether. As a result, alcoholic women often have difficulty becoming pregnant. Alcoholic women also have a higher rate of early menopause than nonalcoholic women. During pregnancy, alcohol consumption can have devastating effects on the fetus. This topic is discussed in the Across the Lifespan section of this chapter (see pages 217–218).

Detrimental Effects on the Brain Alcohol consumption has multiple effects on the brain. Chronic alcoholics may experience brain disorders. One of the most serious is the Wernicke-Korsakoff syndrome. This syndrome includes mental confusion, abnormal eye movements, and an inability to coordinate skeletal muscles, which results in abnormal posture and a staggering gait. Scientists have discovered that this syndrome may be due to the alcoholic's inability to use the B vitamin thiamin properly. Some alcoholics are deficient in this vitamin (and many other nutrients) because their diets consist primarily of alcohol rather than food. In either case, if given thiamin, the abstinent alcoholic can be cured of the abnormal eye movements, posture, and gait. However, the person is left with anterograde amnesia—the inability to remember new information for more than a few seconds.

Another effect of alcohol on the brain is intoxication, the impairment of the central nervous system (see Table 8-3). *Withdrawal* is another brain effect of alcohol, but only in alcohol-dependent individuals who stop drinking or reduce their alcohol intake. Withdrawal symptoms usually occur about 24 to 36 hours after an alcoholic stops drinking. Typically, the alcoholic experiences mild agitation, shaking, anxiety, loss of appetite, restlessness, and insomnia. Five to 15% of alcoholics experience grand mal seizures (convulsions) during withdrawal. Additionally, a small percentage of alcoholics have severe withdrawal symptoms that include hyperactivity, hallucinations, disorientation, and confusion. This severe withdrawal syndrome is called *delirium tremens,* or *DTs.*

Some researchers suggest that a *hangover* is a mild form of withdrawal that can occur in anyone who consumes alcoholic beverages heavily during a session of drinking. The signs of a hangover can include headache, mental slowness, dry mouth, fatigue, diarrhea, anxiety, stomach pains, and tremors. If the "mild withdrawal" explanation is true, it explains why consuming additional alcohol temporarily relieves hangover effects.

The following news release appeared on the Web site of the National Institute on Alcohol Abuse and Alcoholism. It was posted on April 9, 2002. Read the news release and explain why you think it is a reliable or an unreliable source of information. Use the model for analyzing health information to guide your thinking; the main points of the model are noted below. A full explanation of the model can be found on pages 13–15.

1. Which statements are verifiable facts, and which are unverified statements or value claims?
2. What are the credentials of the person writing the article? If this information is available, does the author's background and education qualify him or her as an expert in the topic area?
3. What might be the motives and biases of the person writing the article? State reasons for your answer.
4. Which information is relevant to the issue or main point of the article; which information is irrelevant?
5. Is the source reliable? Does it have a reputation for publishing misinformation?
6. Does the article attack the credibility of conventional scientists or medical authorities?

Based on your analysis, do you think that this article is a reliable source of health-related information? Summarize your reasons for coming to this conclusion.

College Drinking Hazardous to Campus Communities

Task Force Calls for Research-Based Prevention Programs

by NIAAA Press Office

The consequences of college drinking are larger and more destructive than commonly realized, according to a new study supported by the National Institute on Alcohol Abuse and Alcoholism (NIAAA). Commissioned by the NIAAA Task Force on College Drinking, the study reveals that drinking by college students age 18–24 contributes to an estimated 1,400 student deaths, 500,000 injuries, and 70,000 cases of sexual assault or date rape each year. It also estimates that more than one-fourth of college students that age have driven in the past year while under the influence of alcohol.

"The harm that college students do to themselves and others as a result of excessive drinking exceeds what many would have expected," says lead author Ralph W. Hingson, Sc.D., Professor of Social Behavioral Sciences and Associate Dean for Research at Boston University School of Public Health. "Our data clearly point to the need for better interventions against high-risk drinking in this population." Dr. Hingson and colleagues from Boston University, the Harvard University School of Public Health, and the U.S. Substance Abuse and Mental Health Services Administration, derived their data by integrating a number of national databases containing information about drinking and its consequences. Their study appears in the March 2002 issue of the *Journal of Studies on Alcohol*.

"These numbers paint a picture of a deeply entrenched threat to the health and well-being of our young people," adds Raynard S. Kingston, M.D., Ph.D., Acting Director of NIAAA. "This study, and the NIH report released today by the Task Force on College Drinking, are an urgent call to action for educators, researchers, students and society in general. Today, NIAAA is sending the Task Force report to every college in the United States. The findings of the Task Force also serve as a timely reminder for students and others to assess their personal drinking habits on National Alcohol Screening Day, which takes place this week on April 11. The 2,500 screening locations across the country include sites at more than 550 colleges and universities."

A blue-ribbon panel of more than three dozen college presidents, scientists, and students, the Task Force was convened by NIAAA's National Advisory Council to conduct a comprehensive review of research on college drinking and the effectiveness of methods to prevent it. The Hingson study is one of two dozen studies commissioned by the Task Force as part of this review. Most of the commissioned papers have been published in a special supplement to the March 2002 issue of the *Journal of Studies on Alcohol*. The Task Force's report, titled "A Call to Action: Changing the Culture of Drinking at U.S. Colleges," outlines recommendations for college administrators and researchers to address high-risk college drinking.

"The consequences of excessive drinking are far too common on many college campuses nationwide, and efforts to reduce high-risk drinking and its related problems have largely failed," says Task Force co-chair Mark Goldman, Ph.D., Distinguished Research Professor of Psychology at the University of South Florida. "But we need not accept high-risk drinking on our campuses as inevitable. If colleges and communities work together, they can change these harmful drinking patterns. We hope this report will help them do that, by providing tools to help them make more informed decisions."

A Minority of Heavy Drinkers

Though common on many campuses, alcohol abuse does not run rampant among all college and university students. Previous studies have shown that most students drink moderately or abstain, with the proportion of nondrinkers increasing from 15 to 19% between 1993 and 1999. Other evidence, however, points to an increase in more extreme forms of college drinking. About 40% of students binge drink, defined as five or more drinks in a row for men and four or more drinks for women. In a recent survey, about 20% of students reported bingeing more than three times in the last two weeks. This group of frequent binge drinkers accounts for nearly 70% of all the alcohol consumed by college students.

"Although a minority of college students engage in high-risk drinking, all students, and their parents, faculty, and members of the surrounding community suffer the negative consequences of alcohol abuse, such as assault, vandalism, and traffic accidents," says Reverend Edward Malloy, President of the University of Notre Dame, and co-chair of the Task Force. "And I've lived in college dormitories for much of my adult life, so I know firsthand the impact irresponsible drinking has on the quality of residential life."

According to the Task Force research, drinking rates are highest among incoming freshmen, males, members of fraternities or sororities, and athletes. Students who attend two-year institutions, religious schools, commuter schools, or predominantly or historically black colleges and universities drink the least.

Recommended Strategies and Future Research

The Task Force studied research on alcohol prevention among college students to find out what works, what doesn't, and what research is needed to develop better prevention programs. They noted that research on prevention of college drinking is relatively new and the data are incomplete.

"The evidence supporting the alcohol abuse prevention strategies in the literature varies widely," explains Dr. Goldman, "often reflecting the fact that some strategies have not been as thoroughly studied as others or have not been evaluated in college settings."

However, the Task Force noted that alcohol research clearly indicates that multiple factors, from genetic and biological characteristics, to family and cultural backgrounds, to particular college environments interact to produce various drinking patterns. They called for the use of comprehensive, integrated programs with multiple complementary components to address the problem.

"Prevention strategies must simultaneously target three constituencies: the student population as a whole; the college and its surrounding environment; and the individual at-risk or alcohol-dependent drinker," says Dr. Goldman. "Research strongly supports strategies that target each of these factors."

The Task Force developed a *3-in-1 Framework* to help colleges and universities design prevention programs that target each of these constituencies. The framework identifies the target area(s) that each strategy addresses and uses the following four-tier system to rank the strength of the scientific evidence available to support or refute each strategy:

- **Effective and Targeted at College Students**—(examples: combining cognitive-behavioral skills with norms clarification; brief motivational interventions; altering students' expectations about the effects of alcohol)
- **Effective with General Populations and Could Be Applied to College Environments**—(examples: enforcement of minimum-drinking-age laws; restrictions on alcohol retail outlet density, responsible beverage service policies; formation of campus and community coalitions)
- **Promising**—(examples: reinstate Friday classes and exams and Saturday morning classes; expand alcohol-free dormitories; consistently enforced discipline for alcohol policy violations; awareness of personal liability issues; "Safe-Ride" programs; regulation of happy hours and sales)
- **Ineffective**—(examples: interventions that rely entirely on providing information about problems related to risks from drinking)

"Another dominant theme that emerged from our work," says Reverend Malloy, "is the importance of science-based research in establishing alcohol policies and prevention programs. Although research alone will not solve the problem, it will point the way to solutions."

The Task Force's report urges expanded funding for studies of underage and excessive college drinking and calls on NIAAA to assume primary responsibility for:

- Supporting the research community's efforts to address existing knowledge gaps and alter the culture of drinking on campus;
- Facilitating long-term campus-community research aimed at preventing hazardous student drinking; and
- Imparting what is known about the patterns of college drinking and the quality of current interventions to encourage college presidents, administrators, and other campus and community leaders to adopt policies and implement strategies based on research.

In addition to its main report, the Task Force's findings and recommendations are available in the following formats:

- Two Task Force panel reports—*High-Risk Drinking in College: What We Know and What We Need to Learn* and *How to Reduce High-Risk College Drinking: Use Proven Strategies, Fill Research Gaps;*

- A handbook for college planners on implementing and evaluating alcohol prevention programs; and
- Brochures for college and university presidents, student peer educators, and parents.

These materials are available on the Web at: www.collegedrinkingprevention.gov.

They also may be ordered by calling NIAAA at 301-443-3860.

NIAAA is a component of the National Institutes of Health (NIH). NIAAA conducts and supports a broad program of biomedical and behavioral research on the causes, treatment, and prevention of alcohol abuse and alcoholism and its medical consequences.

Source: National Institute on Alcohol Abuse and Alcoholism, National Institutes of Health. Available at www.niaaa.nih.gov/press/2002/college.htm. Accessed December 26, 2004.

Other physiological effects of drinking alcohol may cause hangovers, however. Alcoholic beverages contain certain acidic compounds that have toxic effects on the body. These compounds differ among types of alcoholic beverages and affect whether someone will experience a hangover. Another compound called formaldehyde (a preservative of dead animals) is produced by the body when it cannot keep up with the breakdown of alcohol being consumed. The buildup of formaldehyde contributes to a hangover. Additionally, alcohol causes the body to lose water. This dehydration occurs in brain cells as well as other body cells. Pain accompanies their rehydration.

Whatever the causes of a hangover, home remedies such as taking vitamins, getting in a cold shower, or drinking coffee will not cure the "morning-after" pain of drinking too much. Time alone will cure a hangover.

Effects on Behavior and Safety

Serious and Fatal Injuries Statistics show that alcohol use and abuse are related to serious and even fatal injuries. Alcohol frequently contributes to water-related accidents, motor vehicle accidents, general aviation crashes, domestic and nondomestic violence including sexual assault and rape, suicides, and homicides.

Data show that 40% of all fatal motor vehicle crashes in 2000 were alcohol-related (CDC, 2001). Approximately one-third of all victims of homicide and unintentional-injury death (excluding those in car crashes) are intoxicated at the time of their deaths. Additionally, about one-fifth of suicide victims are intoxicated when they take their own lives (Smith et al., 1999). In comparison, less than one-tenth of individuals in a London study who died of natural causes had alcohol in their blood at the time of death (Cox et al., 1997).

Automobile Accidents Drinking and driving are potentially deadly because alcohol impairs the perceptual, intellectual, and motor skills needed to operate motor vehicles safely. Traffic accidents are the leading cause of death among people aged 1 to 24 years and the third leading cause of death after cancer and heart disease in adults aged 25 to 44 years (Krochanek & Smith, 2004). In all states, the District of Columbia, and Puerto Rico, the legal blood alcohol concentration (BAC) limit for operating an automobile is 0.08%. All states have a lower unlawful BAC threshold for youth under 21, and in some cases, under 18 (U.S. Dept. of Transportation [DOT], 2004). Figure 8-3 shows approximate BAC by body weight and the time from the first drink. Note the number of drinks a person can have over a period of time before he or she is considered legally drunk. Also realize that some impairment occurs after a person consumes only one drink.

Alcohol-related fatal automobile accidents occur more frequently at certain times of the day and during certain days of the week than others. In 2003, approximately 49% of drivers and motorcycle operators killed during the weekend had BACs of at least 0.01% compared to 27% killed during weekdays. Similarly, 57% of drivers and motorcycle operators killed during nighttime hours had BACs of 0.01% or more compared to only 16% of drivers killed during daytime hours (U.S. DOT, 2004). Automobile fatalities are defined as alcohol-related when at least one automobile driver or nonoccupant of the car[s] involved in the crash, such as a pedestrian or cyclist, has a BAC of 0.01% or higher.

Alcohol Impairment Chart: Female

Drinks	Approximate Blood Alcohol Percentage									
	Body Weight in Pounds									
	90	100	120	140	160	180	200	220	240	
0	.00	.00	.00	.00	.00	.00	.00	.00	.00	Only safe driving limit
1	.05	.05	.04	.03	.03	.03	.02	.02	.02	Impairment begins
2	.10	.09	.08	.07	.06	.05	.05	.04	.04	Driving skills affected
3	.15	.14	.11	.10	.09	.08	.07	.06	.06	Possible criminal penalties
4	.20	.18	.15	.13	.11	.10	.09	.08	.08	
5	.25	.23	.19	.16	.14	.13	.11	.10	.09	
6	.30	.27	.23	.19	.17	.15	.14	.12	.11	Legally intoxicated
7	.35	.32	.27	.23	.20	.18	.16	.14	.13	Criminal penalties
8	.40	.36	.30	.26	.23	.20	.18	.17	.15	
9	.45	.41	.34	.29	.26	.23	.20	.19	.17	
10	.51	.45	.38	.32	.28	.25	.23	.21	.19	

Your body can get rid of one drink per hour
Each 11/2 oz. of 80 proof liquor, 12 oz. of beer or 5 oz. of table wine = 1 drink.

Alcohol Impairment Chart: Male

Drinks	Approximate Blood Alcohol Percentage								
	Body Weight in Pounds								
	100	120	140	160	180	200	220	240	
0	.00	.00	.00	.00	.00	.00	.00	.00	Only safe driving limit
1	.04	.03	.03	.02	.02	.02	.02	.02	Impairment begins
2	.08	.06	.05	.05	.04	.04	.03	.03	
3	.11	.09	.08	.07	.06	.06	.05	.05	Driving skills affected
4	.15	.12	.11	.09	.08	.08	.07	.06	Possible criminal penalties
5	.19	.16	.13	.12	.11	.09	.09	.08	
6	.23	.19	.16	.14	.13	.11	.10	.09	Legally intoxicated
7	.26	.22	.19	.16	.15	.13	.12	.11	Criminal penalties
8	.30	.25	.21	.19	.17	.15	.14	.13	
9	.34	.28	.24	.21	.19	.17	.15	.14	
10	.38	.31	.27	.23	.21	.19	.17	.16	

Your body can get rid of one drink per hour
Each 11/2 oz. of 80 proof liquor, 12 oz. of beer or 5 oz. of table wine 5 = 1 drink.

Pennsylvania Liquor Control Board
Alcohol Education PLCB

Figure 8-3 **Blood Alcohol Concentration (BAC) by Weight and Gender.** These graphs show the approximate BACs of men and women in various weight ranges. All states have set 0.08% as the legal BAC limit while driving. However, you may be convicted of driving under the influence (DUI) of alcohol if evidence exists that your driving is impaired. Commercial drivers may be convicted of a DUI at a BAC of 0.04%. Reprinted with permission from the Pennsylvania Liquor Control Board.

Figure 8-4 shows that alcohol-related fatal car crashes peak between midnight and 3 A.M. Comparatively few alcohol-related crashes occur between 6 A.M. and 3 P.M., but the percentage rises throughout the late afternoon and evening until the midnight-to-3 A.M. peak. A significant percentage occur from 3 A.M. to 6. A.M. as well. These statistics together show that a person driving at night and in the early morning hours, especially on a weekend, is more likely to be involved in a fatal alcohol-related motor vehicle accident than driving during the day and during the week. Taking public transportation or cabs on weekend nights is safer than driving for both drinkers and nondrinkers alike.

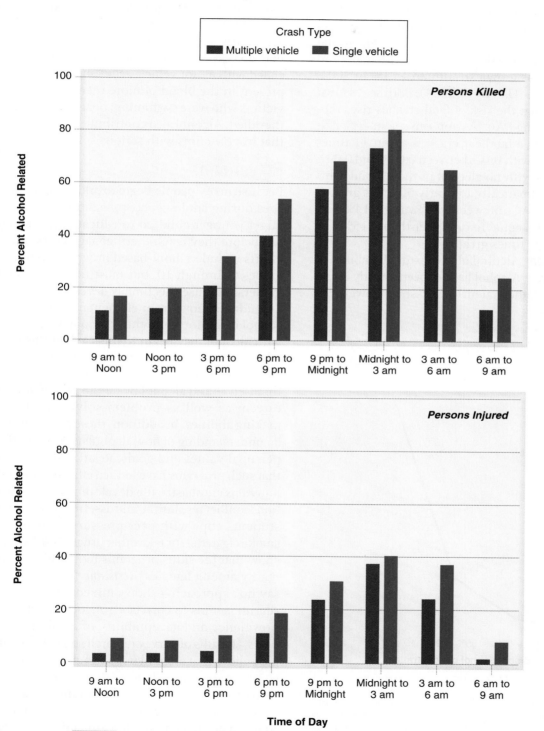

Figure 8-4 Percentage of Persons Killed or Injured in Alcohol-Related Crashes by Time of Day.
Source: U.S. Department of Transportation. (2004). *Traffic safety facts* (DOT HS 809 775).
Available at http://www.nrd.nhtsa.dot.gov/pdf/nrd-30/NCSA/TSFAnn/2003/TSF2003-Early.htm.

Alcohol-related automobile deaths dropped from 60% of total traffic fatalities in 1982 to about 40% in 2003. The drivers with the highest intoxication rates in fatal crashes were young adults aged 21 to 24 years (U.S. DOT, 2004).

Women who drink and drive must remember that their BACs rise more quickly than the BACs of males who consume the same number of drinks. Recent data indicate that females are increasingly involved in fatal automobile accidents. In 1982, 10.1% of drivers in fatal crashes with a BAC of 0.08% or more were female, and this percentage has grown steadily to 15.1% in 2004, an increase of 50% (U.S. DOT, 2004). Both sexes must also remember that the risk of fatal crashes rises rapidly with increasing BAC. As you can see in Figure 8-5, the risk of having a fatal car crash is about 11 times greater for drivers with BACs between 0.05% and 0.09% than for persons with no alcohol in their blood. This risk increases dramatically, to nearly 50 times greater, for drivers with BACs between 0.10% and 0.14%. For drivers with BACs equal to or higher than 0.15%, the risk is almost 400 times greater.

Airplane Accidents Alcohol also impairs the ability of pilots to fly aircraft. Alcohol has not been directly implicated in U.S. commercial airline crashes; however, it appears to play a more prominent role in general aviation crashes. Hangover effects (see page 197) may impair pilot performance for several hours even after alcohol has been eliminated from the blood (Yesavage & Leirer, 1986).

Water-Related Accidents Alcohol is also a significant factor in water-related accidents. Researchers estimate that alcohol consumption is associated with between 30% and 70% of adult drownings (Driscoll et al., 2004). The highest percentages are associated with males older than 25 years. Most alcohol-related drownings are associated with motor vehicle accidents, but alcohol is also present in the blood of more than half the drowning victims who were swimming, boating, or rafting when they died. Alcohol also contributes to diving accidents that leave victims with serious spinal cord injuries.

Prevention

Because many people begin drinking alcoholic beverages during adolescence, prevention programs often target younger children to educate them about alcohol before they reach their teenage years. Prevention efforts include school-based programs for children in grades 5 through 10, but most target fifth and sixth graders. Because this time is developmentally critical as students move from elementary school to middle school or junior high, those who have experimented with alcohol may begin to misuse it at this time.

There are a variety of school-based programs. *Affective education* seeks to influence students' feelings about themselves and alcohol by helping them develop self-esteem as well as problem-solving and decision-making abilities. In addition, these programs promote an understanding of how alcohol use can interfere with personal values and goals. Results of research show that such programs have limited effectiveness. *Life skills programs* emphasize the development of communication, conflict resolution, and assertiveness skills to help students cope with peer pressure to drink alcohol, smoke cigarettes, or take other drugs. Results of research show that life skills programs reduce alcohol use primarily among females. *Resistance training*—the "Just say no" approach—shows mixed results. *Normative education* aims to correct erroneous beliefs about the prevalence and acceptability of alcohol use among peers. (Results of survey research show that young people believe that alcohol use among their peers is more common than it really is.) Adding normative components to alcohol education programs for adolescents appears useful. In fact, normative education is a recent trend in adolescent alcohol education. Current normative programs include teaching students how to resist peer influence and often incorporate activities

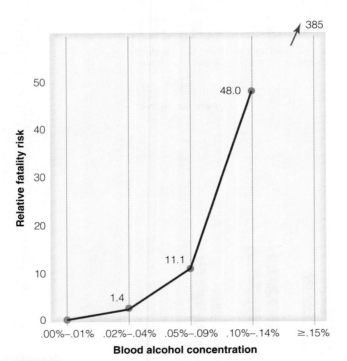

Figure 8-5 Fatality Risk at Various Levels of Blood Alcohol Concentration. This graph shows that as the BAC rises, the likelihood of being killed while driving a car increases. As the BAC approaches the legal limit for drunkenness (0.08% to 0.10%), the risk of being killed rises dramatically. Source: Zador, P. L. (1991). Alcohol-related relative risk of fatal driver injuries in relation to driver and age and sex. *Journal of Studies on Alcohol,* 52(4):302–310. Reprinted with permission. Copyright by Alcohol Research Documentation, Inc. Rutgers Center of Alcohol Studies, Piscataway, NJ 08854.

and events outside of the classroom (National Institute on Alcohol Abuse and Alcoholism [NIAAA], 2000).

Prevention efforts that focus on the entire population of drinkers are called *environmental approaches.* Such approaches are important because 50.1% of Americans are current alcohol users (SAMHSA, 2004a), and many drinkers experience moderate to severe alcohol-induced impairment at least occasionally. These drinkers are all at risk for alcohol-related injuries and health problems.

One prevention strategy for the general population was the requirement by the U.S. government to place warnings on alcoholic beverage containers beginning in 1989. However, survey data show that only about one-fourth of adults realize that the labels exist. Researchers have not found evidence that warning labels reduce alcohol consumption and its health-related effects. Another prevention strategy was the establishment of 21 as the minimum age for purchase and consumption of alcohol. Evidence suggests that this strategy significantly reduced youth drinking and related problems such as alcohol-related traffic accidents in those under the age of 21 (Wagenaar & Toomey, 2002).

A 5-year community alcohol trauma prevention trial conducted in California determined that coordinated community-based interventions can reduce high-risk alcohol consumption and alcohol-related injuries from car crashes and assaults. The types of interventions that were used included limiting the access of underage drinkers to alcohol, increasing the local enforcement of drinking and driving laws, and encouraging responsible alcoholic beverage service focused on reducing drunkenness and driving after drinking (Holder et al., 2000).

How to Control Your Alcohol Consumption

Studies show that light drinkers have certain behavior patterns that help them curb their drinking. These attributes are listed in the Managing Your Health box "Guidelines for Safer Drinking" and are effective rules for controlling alcohol consumption.

Diagnosis and Treatment of Alcoholism and Alcohol Abuse

According to the 2003 National Survey on Drug Use and Health (SAMHSA, 2004a), approximately 1.1 million Americans received treatment for alcohol abuse during the year prior to the survey. Various types of treatments are available for those who need help. Screening techniques help identify those persons who need treatment.

The CAGE screening test, printed in the student workbook, is considered one of the most effective screening devices for alcohol abuse or alcoholism. A variety of other screening instruments are available also.

Health care professionals who determine that their patients are alcohol dependent refer them to substance abuse specialists for evaluation and possible treatment. Patients that show nondependent problem drinking are often encouraged to participate in brief intervention programs.

Managing Your Health

Guidelines for Safer Drinking

1. Think about your alcohol drinking behaviors beforehand and plan how you will drink.
2. Drink slowly, and alternate alcoholic beverages with nonalcoholic beverages.
3. Eat before or while drinking.
4. Set a limit on the amount of alcohol you can drink at one time. Base this limit on the number of drinks someone with your body weight can drink and still remain below a BAC of 0.05% (see Figure 8-3); count drinks to stay within this limit.
5. Set a limit on how long you will drink; ideally, drink for an hour or less.
6. Drink only to enhance a good time and not to combat stress or to avoid dealing with problems.
7. Become skillful at assertively refusing drinks.
8. Don't drink daily (to avoid developing tolerance).
9. Cultivate alternatives to drinking that compete with its benefits (such as relaxing or socializing).
10. Practice social skills such as approaching people and engaging them in conversation while sober so you won't need alcohol to feel comfortable in social settings.

Source: Adapted from Vogler, R., Webber, N. E., Rasor, R., Bartz, W. R., & Levesque, J. (1994). *Journal of Alcohol and Drug Education, 39*(3):99–112.

In the past, physicians and substance abuse practitioners thought that an alcoholic could not be helped until he or she "hit bottom" and then asked for help. A person who did not ask for help was considered to be denying his or her alcoholism and lacking motivation to change. Current thinking regards motivation as a process of behavioral change rather than a trait that people have or do not have.

Before treatment, the role of clinical intervention is to help the patient understand the serious dangers inherent in his or her abusive or dependent drinking behavior. Once the alcoholic realizes the need to change his or her behavior, he or she tries to decide what course of action to take. The clinician helps the patient select a course of action or treatment program that best suits his or her needs.

Both inpatient and outpatient programs exist. *Inpatient treatment,* in which the alcoholic resides at a treatment facility, is sometimes used for the early phases of treatment, particularly acute detoxification. During this time, the patient abstains from alcohol and experiences withdrawal symptoms (see page 197). Approximately 10% to 13% of patients need medication during this time to help them reduce potentially life-threatening effects of withdrawal. During the detoxification period, patients participate in group therapy and alcohol education sessions for several hours daily. Recovering alcoholics usually live with patients to help them through the process. Such programs usually last 28 days. Near the end of this process the alcoholic's family is usually asked to participate in treatment.

Due to rising medical costs, acute detoxification, as well as further treatment, may take place in *outpatient programs.* Such programs, developed over the past 25 years, have been extremely successful. Approximately 90% of patients are now treated in outpatient facilities. In these programs, the patient spends a specific amount of time at the treatment facility but lives at home.

After a person has sought treatment for alcohol abuse or dependence, the next stage in behavior change is *maintenance.* For long-term maintenance treatment, recovering alcoholics take part in group meetings and attend individual counseling sessions once or twice a week at outpatient facilities, participate in self-help group meetings, and sometimes participate in family therapy. The maintenance period usually lasts one year.

Sometimes *relapse* occurs. During a relapse, a recovering alcoholic returns to his or her drinking habits. Relapse can be triggered by a variety of factors such as stress, depression, alcohol craving, negative life events, and interpersonal tensions. To recover once again, the patient goes through the stages of behavior change. Treatment to prevent an initial or repeated relapse often involves self-help groups.

Alcoholics Anonymous (AA) is the best known and most widely available of the self-help groups. Governed by its own members, the organization's philosophy is that alcoholism is a physical, emotional, and spiritual disease for which there is no cure. Recovery is a lifelong process that involves attention to AA's Twelve Steps, which are listed in Table 8-7. AA also has related support groups for family members and friends of alcoholics such as Alateen and Al-Anon.

Although not as well known, other self-help groups exist. The Secular Organization for Sobriety (SOS) is a group similar to AA, except its program does not include spiritual aspects. The Rational Recovery (RR) program is also a secular organization and emphasizes the importance of alcoholics becoming aware of their irrational beliefs, self-perceptions, and expectancies in

---

Table 8-7 **The Twelve Steps of Alcoholics Anonymous**

1. We admitted we were powerless over alcohol—that our lives had become unmanageable.
2. Came to believe that a Power greater than ourselves could restore us to sanity.
3. Made a decision to turn our will and our lives over to the care of God as we understood Him.
4. Made a searching and fearless moral inventory of ourselves.
5. Admitted to God, to ourselves, and to another human being the exact nature of our wrongs.
6. Were entirely ready to have God remove all these defects of character.
7. Humbly asked Him to remove our shortcomings.
8. Made a list of all persons we had harmed, and became willing to make amends to them all.
9. Made direct amends to such people wherever possible, except when to do so would injure them or others.
10. Continued to take personal inventory and when we were wrong promptly admitted it.
11. Sought through prayer and meditation to improve our conscious contact with God, as we understood Him, praying only for knowledge of His will for us and the power to carry that out.
12. Having had a spiritual awakening as the result of these Steps, we tried to carry this message to alcoholics, and to practice these principles in all our affairs.

Source: The Twelve Steps are reprinted with permission of Alcoholics Anonymous World Services, Inc. Permission to reprint the Twelve Steps does not mean that AA has reviewed or approved the contents of this publication, nor that AA agrees with the views expressed herein. AA is a program of recovery from alcoholism only—use of the Twelve Steps in connection with programs and activities which are patterned after AA, but which address other problems, or in any other non-AA context, does not imply otherwise.

order to be successful in changing their behavior. These groups suggest abstinence as a preferred drinking goal but emphasize personal choice. One self-help approach for women is Women for Sobriety. This group emphasizes women's issues such as assertiveness, self-confidence, and autonomy as part of the change process.

Healthy Living Practices

- To be a responsible drinker, do not allow your drinking to threaten your health, endanger the safety of others, or interfere with business or personal relationships.

- If drinking alcohol is damaging your physical and/or psychological health, you should seek medical help.

- If you use alcohol in physically dangerous situations, have developed a tolerance to alcohol, exhibit withdrawal symptoms when you are not drinking, and compulsively use alcohol, you are probably alcohol dependent and should seek medical help.

- Be sure to eat while drinking alcoholic beverages so that less alcohol will enter the bloodstream.

- If you consume alcohol, drink only 1 oz of ethanol per day or less to decrease the risk of coronary artery disease and stroke. Heavier alcohol consumption is associated with a variety of heart and blood vessel diseases.

- Do not drive after consuming alcoholic beverages. Alcohol impairs many of the skills needed to operate motor vehicles safely. As your blood alcohol concentration increases, your risk of having a car crash increases dramatically.

■ Tobacco

Types of Tobacco Products

Cigarettes are the most prevalent tobacco product in the United States. In 2003 an estimated 60.4 million Americans smoked cigarettes, representing 25.4% of the population age 12 and older. Smoking rates increase with age to 20 years, and then generally decline with age. In 2003, 12.2% of youths aged 12 to 17 were current cigarette smokers, 40.2% of young adults aged 18 to 25 years were current smokers, and 24.7% of adults aged 26 and older were current smokers (SAMHSA, 2004b).

Cigarette use has declined significantly since 1996/1997 in youth aged 12 to 17 (Johnston et al., 2004b), and modestly in adults 18 years and over (CDC, 2004c). Nevertheless, smoking increased significantly for college students during 1998 and 1999 while it was declining in these other groups. The year 2000 showed a decline in college student smoking, and that decline continued through 2003 (Johnston et al., 2004b). The Consumer Health box "Kreteks and Bidis: Unwrapping the Facts" on page 206 describes types of cigarettes that were becoming popular particularly with high school students, but whose popularity declined between 2001 and 2003 (Johnston et al., 2004b).

Smoking cigars and pipes is not as prevalent in the American population as smoking cigarettes. In 2003 approximately 9.4% of men smoked cigars, versus 1.7% of women. Most cigar or pipe smokers are 18 to 25 years old (SAMHSA, 2004b). Generally, women do not smoke pipes.

In 2003 6.4% of American men but only 0.4% of American women used *smokeless tobacco*, which includes *snuff* and *chewing tobacco* (SAMHSA, 2004b). Snuff, the most popular form of smokeless tobacco, is powdered or finely cut tobacco. It may be used loose or wrapped in a paper pouch. Although snuff can be inhaled, most users in the United States today place snuff between the cheek and gum. This practice is called *dipping.*

Chewing tobacco is loose leaf tobacco or a plug of compressed tobacco, which is sometimes called a *quid.* It is placed in the cheek. It can be chewed, as its name suggests, or, more often, it is sucked. During the time that snuff or chewing tobacco remains in the mouth, it forms a liquid that smokeless tobacco users usually spit out. For this reason smokeless tobacco is often called spitting tobacco.

Worldwide, a variety of other tobacco products exist besides those mentioned here. Additionally, methods of tobacco use vary among cultures. The Diversity in Health essay "Tobacco Drinking?" on page 208 describes a few tobacco-related practices of various South American cultures.

Who Uses Tobacco and Why?

As mentioned earlier, most people who smoke cigarettes began this habit when they were adolescents. Figure 8-6 shows the ages at which adults say they started smoking. Only 11% of adult smokers started this habit after age 18. Smokeless tobacco use usually begins in early adolescence or in childhood also.

Data show that during the early 1990s through 1996/1997 there was an increase in the percentage of high school students who smoked cigarettes daily. However, those percentages have declined steadily to 2003 (Figure 8-7). About 22% of high school students of all ages responded that they were current cigarette smokers on the National Youth Risk Behavior Survey in 2003 (CDC, 2004d). Despite all that is known today about the health consequences of cigarette smoking, about one-fourth of twelfth-grade students still do not believe that there is a great risk in smoking a pack or more of cigarettes per day (Johnston et al., 2004a). The *Healthy People 2010* objective is to reduce the number of new, young smokers to 12%.

The use of smokeless tobacco among adolescent boys rose dramatically from 1970 to the mid-1990s, but by 2003 was down by about one-half from its high. In 2003, 4.1% of eighth graders, 5.3% of tenth graders, and 6.7% of twelfth graders used smokeless tobacco (Johnston et al., 2004a). In general, females show little use of smokeless tobacco compared to males.

Psychosocial Reasons for Using Tobacco Products

Adolescents initially try tobacco products for a variety of reasons. Adolescents who have family members or friends who smoke cigarettes or use smokeless tobacco are more likely to begin these habits than teenagers who do not observe these behaviors in people close to them. Many adolescents try smoking, chewing, or

---

$ Consumer Health

Kreteks and Bidis: Unwrapping the Facts

Kreteks (clove cigarettes) and bidi cigarettes appeared to be popular with American youth in the late 1990s, but by 2001 their use was declining. Clove cigarettes, developed in Indonesia in the early 1900s and presently manufactured there, have been imported into the United States since 1968. Bidis, manufactured primarily in India and other Southeast Asian countries, were not widely used in the United States until the mid-1990s.

Clove cigarettes look much like tobacco cigarettes and are made with or without filter tips. Most are wrapped with white paper, but some have brown or black coverings. Clove cigarettes contain approximately 40% ground cloves and 60% tobacco, although the specific amount varies among manufacturers and brands. Clove oil is added as well, often discoloring the cigarette paper. As these cigarettes burn, the cloves make a crackling sound. (*Kretek* means "crackle" in Indonesia.)

Many users of clove cigarettes think that they are less dangerous to smoke than regular cigarettes because 40% of their content is cloves rather than tobacco. However, they are making an incorrect, and possibly deadly, assumption. Clove cigarettes are rolled tighter than regular cigarettes, resulting in a denser product. Put simply, there is less air in clove cigarettes than in regular cigarettes, so the tobacco content of kreteks is similar to that of regular cigarettes. Additionally, tests show that clove cigarettes deliver, on average, twice as much tar, nicotine, and carbon monoxide as do moderate tar-containing American cigarettes.

Clove cigarettes also contain an anesthetic called eugenol (a natural component of the cloves), which can cause allergic reactions in some. This anesthetic numbs the backs of smokers' throats and windpipes. Researchers think that this numbing effect is the reason that smokers inhale kretek smoke more deeply and retain it in their lungs longer than when smoking regular cigarettes. They also suspect that this numbing effect may encourage smoking by people who might otherwise find smoking cigarettes harsh and distasteful.

Bidis are small, strong-smelling brown cigarettes wrapped in leaves (much like cigars) and are tied with a string. They are smaller and thinner than regular cigarettes and come in flavors such as cherry, mango, chocolate, and strawberry. Results from a 1999 survey of students in grades 7 through 12 conducted in Massachusetts reveal that young people smoke bidis because they like the flavor and find bidis cheaper and easier to buy than regular cigarettes. Additionally, they perceived bidis to be safer than smoking regular cigarettes. However, as with clove cigarettes, this assumption is false. Tests show that bidis produce approximately 3 times the amount of carbon monoxide and nicotine as American cigarettes, and about 5 times the amount of tar. Additionally, smokers inhale more often and more deeply when smoking bidis than when smoking regular cigarettes because the leaf wrapper does not burn well.

So, are smoking kreteks and bidis safe alternatives to smoking regular cigarettes? The answer is an emphatic no! In fact, the data show that these alternative smoking products pose even greater health risks than regular cigarettes.

Sources: Centers for Disease Control and Prevention. (1999). Bidi use among urban youth—Massachusetts, March–April 1999. *Morbidity and Mortality Weekly Report, 48*:796–799.
Johnston, L. D., O'Malley, P. M., & Bachman, J. G. (2002). *Monitoring the future national results on adolescent drug use: Overview of key findings 2001.* Rockville, MD: NIH.

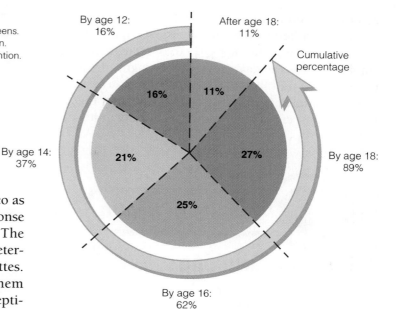

Figure 8-6 **Age at Which Adults Say They Started Smoking.**
Most smokers started this habit when they were in their teens or preteens.
Sources: Substance Abuse and Mental Health Services Administration.
Office on Smoking and Health, Centers for Disease Control and Prevention.

By age 12:
16%

After age 18:
11%

Cumulative
percentage

16%   11%

By age 14:
37%

21%   27%

By age 18:
89%

25%

By age 16:
62%

dipping simply to experiment. Others use tobacco as a way to feel older and more independent, as a response to advertising, or as a response to social pressure. The influence of peers is the most important factor in determining when and how adolescents first try cigarettes.

Certain characteristics of adolescents make them more likely to use tobacco: low self-esteem, susceptibility to peer pressure, a sensation-seeking nature, a rebellious personality, depression or anxiety, low academic achievement, and a low level of knowledge about the immediate health risks of smoking. Additionally, adolescents who think that their parents do not care about them or adolescents who are alone much of the time are more likely to try smoking. Girls are significantly less likely to begin smoking if they are involved in an organized sport. However, participation in sports does not affect boys' initiation into smoking.

Nicotine Addiction Why do teenagers and adults continue smoking and using smokeless tobacco? Most people continue because they are addicted to **nicotine**. Nicotine is a psychoactive drug that acts at communication points among nerve cells in the brain, as do other psychoactive drugs. It becomes addicting during the first few years of use.

The many reasons that people say they continue to smoke (other than craving or being addicted to cigarettes) include the following:

- It is arousing and gives them energy.
- It helps concentration.
- It lifts the mood.
- It reduces anger, tension, depression, and stress.
- It is a habit.
- It is a pleasurable activity.

However, some of the pleasure of smoking (as well as using smokeless tobacco) is really the relief of the symptoms of nicotine withdrawal. During the day, as a person smokes, he or she builds up tolerance to

nicotine an addictive psychoactive drug found in tobacco.

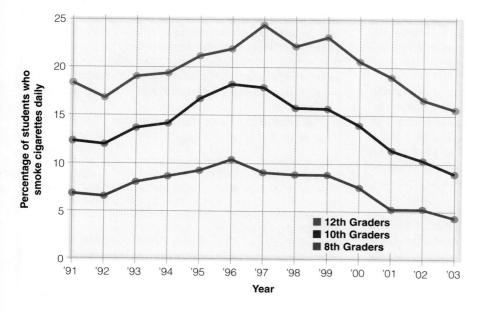

Figure 8-7 **Cigarettes: Trends in Daily Use by Eighth, Tenth, and Twelfth Graders.**
Source: Johnston, L. D., O'Malley, P. M., & Bachman, J.G. (2004). *Monitoring the future national survey results on drug use, 1975–2003: Vol. 1, Secondary school students.* Bethesda, MD: National Institute on Drug Abuse.

■ 12th Graders
■ 10th Graders
■ 8th Graders

Percentage of students who smoke cigarettes daily

Year

nicotine. Nicotine withdrawal symptoms become more pronounced between each successive cigarette. To relieve these symptoms (Table 8-8), most cigarette addicts smoke more as the day goes on. Overnight, the level of nicotine in the blood drops and tolerance decreases; thus, the smoker is resensitized to the effects of nicotine. The first cigarette of the day is usually quite satisfying to the smoker as the cycle of tolerance and then resensitization begins once again.

The Health Effects of Tobacco Use

In 1964, U.S. Surgeon General Luther Terry issued a landmark report that linked cigarette smoking with the development of lung cancer and other diseases.

 Diversity in Health

Tobacco Drinking?

To North Americans, the phrase "using tobacco" usually means smoking cigarettes, cigars, or pipes. Occasionally we might envision a person using chewing tobacco or placing a pinch of snuff between the gums and cheek. (This practice is called "dipping" snuff.) But various cultures use tobacco in other ways—including some ways that may be new to you.

Drinking liquid tobacco is one of the oldest methods of tobacco use. The members of certain tribal populations in South America, particularly those living in Guiana, the upper Amazon, and the mountainous regions of Ecuador and Peru, drink tobacco juice. The drinking of tobacco has also been reported in other South American regions, including northwestern coastal Venezuela, northwestern Colombia, and a few scattered places in Bolivia and Brazil.

The various groups of people who drink tobacco juice prepare it in different ways. The leaves may be first pounded, chewed, or shredded. Sometimes they are left untreated. Then the tobacco leaves are placed in water; sometimes other ingredients are added such as salt, pepper, or plant materials such as tree bark. The mixture is boiled and then strained to obtain the liquid. Usually it is then set aside to allow much of the water to evaporate. The remaining material has the consistency of a paste, syrup, or jelly. The syrups and jellies are usually liquid enough to drink by mouth or pour in the nose. People from some areas squirt the juice from one person's mouth to another.

Various tribes of the northernmost extension of the Andes in Colombia and Venezuela and in parts of the northwest Amazon make a thick extract of tobacco called ambil that they rub across their teeth, gums, or tongue. This thick, black gelatin is made by boiling tobacco leaves for hours or days and then thickening the extract with starch. Recipes vary; some tribes add pepper, avocado seeds, sugar, or tapioca. Ambil is sometimes ingested with other tobacco products or hallucinogenic drugs.

Using chewing tobacco is practiced by about 2% to 3% of the population in the United States. It is more widely practiced in South America and the West Indies. A person who uses tobacco in this way usually sucks or sometimes chews tobacco quids, which are simply pieces of tobacco made for this purpose. However, the South American and West Indian practices of preparing quids may seem unusual to North Americans. South American and West Indian recipes may include soil, ashes, salt, or honey with the finely crushed tobacco leaves. (North American quids are also flavored in various ways.) South American Indians generally swallow the juices from the tobacco, rather than spit them out.

Another practice among South American Indians that may seem unusual to North Americans is the use of tobacco as an enema or suppository. Generally, these native people use tobacco in this manner to treat constipation or worm infestations. Various tribes of Indians who reside in the mountains of Peru also use tobacco in this way during certain rituals.

People in different cultures often adopt different health-related behaviors. What seems unusual to persons in one culture may not seem unusual at all to individuals from another. In fact, tobacco drinking may be entering the American culture in trendy restaurants. An increasing number are including tobacco items on the menu or in the bar because the law does not allow their customers to light up their favorite cigarettes or cigars. Therefore, restauranteurs have developed alternatives to smoking. In some eateries, tobacco leaves are used as overnight wraps for fish before the fish are smoked. Tobacco juice is being used as an ingredient in sauces and desserts. And an alcoholic beverage has been developed called a Nicotini, which includes "tea" brewed from tobacco leaves.

Tobacco drinking? It may be happening at the table next to yours, and its health effects are still to be determined.

Source: Kuntzman, G. (2003, May 19). Tobacco in your tiramisu? *Newsweek*. Available at http://gershkuntzman.homestead.com/files/tobacco_in_Your_Tiramisu.htm; U.S. Department of Health and Human Services. (1992). *Smoking and health in the Americas: A 1992 report of the Surgeon General, in collaboration with the Pan American Health Organization* (DHHS Publication No. CDC 92-8419). Atlanta, GA: U.S. Department of Health and Human Services, pp. 19–31.

Table 8-8 Typical Symptoms of Nicotine Withdrawal

Restlessness

Eating more than usual

Anxiety/tension

Impatience

Irritability/anger

Difficulty concentrating

Excessive hunger

Depression

Disorientation

Loss of energy/fatigue

Dizziness

Stomach or bowel problems

Headaches

Sweating

Insomnia

Heart palpitations

Tremors

Craving cigarettes

Source: Adapted from Shiffman, S., West, R., & Gilbert, D. (2004). Recommendation for the assessment of tobacco craving and withdrawal in smoking cessation trials. *Nicotine and Tobacco Research, 6*:599–614; Gritz, E. R., Carr, C. R., & Marcus, A. C. (1991). The tobacco withdrawal syndrome in unaided quitters. *British Journal of Addiction, 86*(1):57–69.

Since that famous report, scientists have learned a great deal about the health consequences of smoking and smokeless tobacco use, and the Surgeon General's Office has issued more than 20 reports on smoking and health. In these reports, cigarette smoking is recognized as the leading source of preventable illness and death in the United States. Every year, more than 400,000 people die in the United States as a result of using tobacco products (USDHHS, 2000). Figure 8-8 shows how smoking affects risk for various diseases.

Immediate Effects of Nicotine and Carbon Monoxide After entering the body, nicotine produces a variety of effects. It increases the heart rate and the amount of blood that the heart pumps in a single beat. However, nicotine also constricts, or narrows, the blood vessels. As a result, the blood pressure rises. Nicotine also increases the metabolic rate—the speed at which all the chemical reactions of the body take place. These effects increase the body's demand for oxygen. However, the carbon monoxide in cigarette smoke binds to hemoglobin in the red blood cells, reducing its ability to carry oxygen.

Nicotine and carbon monoxide are not the only components of cigarette smoke that affect the body. There are more than 4,000 chemical compounds in the gases and particles that make up cigarette smoke. Some are poisonous, such as hydrogen cyanide; some are irritating to the lungs and mucous membranes, such as particulate matter; and some cause cancer, such as the tars—sticky substances similar to road tar. The rest of this section describes specific health effects of smoking tobacco and using smokeless tobacco products.

Respiratory Illnesses The windpipe and its major subdivisions are lined with microscopic hairlike structures called *cilia*, which are embedded in a layer of sticky mucus. This mucus traps inhaled particles and microbes. As the cilia beat, the mucus moves upward, sweeping this debris up and out of the air passageways.

Inhaled cigarette smoke paralyzes the cilia. With continued smoking, the cilia are damaged. Cigarette smoke also irritates the airways and tar builds up on the cilia, causing excess mucus to be produced. The chronic cough of smokers, usually called *smoker's cough*, is a result of the body's attempt to remove this excess, stationary mucus.

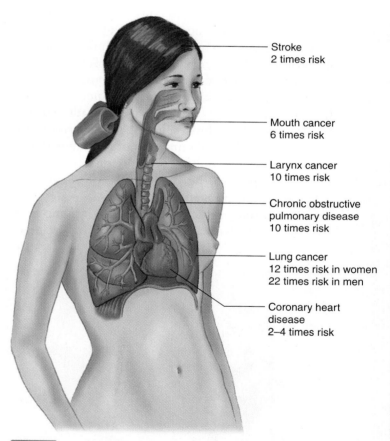

Stroke
2 times risk

Mouth cancer
6 times risk

Larynx cancer
10 times risk

Chronic obstructive pulmonary disease
10 times risk

Lung cancer
12 times risk in women
22 times risk in men

Coronary heart disease
2–4 times risk

Figure 8-8 **The Risk of Smoking Cigarettes.** This illustration compares the increased risk of a smoker to develop certain diseases to the risk of a non-smoker. Sources: Centers for Disease Control and Prevention. (2004, February). *Health effects of cigarette smoking fact sheet.* Available at http://www.cdc.gov/tobacco/factsheets/HealthEffectsofCigaretteSmoking_factsheet.htm; U.S. Department of Health and Human Services. (1989). *Reducing the health consequences of smoking: 25 years of progress. A report of the surgeon general.* Rockville, MD: Office of Smoking and Health.

Acute bronchitis is an inflammation of the mucous membranes of the bronchi, which is usually caused by a viral infection. However, smokers are more susceptible than nonsmokers to acute bronchitis because of their impaired and irritated bronchi. The signs and symptoms of this disease are soreness or tightness in the chest, slight fever, cough, chills, and a vague feeling of weakness or discomfort. Bronchitis with accompanying high fever, breathlessness, and yellow, gray, green, or bloody sputum is serious and the person should seek medical attention immediately.

Chronic bronchitis is usually caused by cigarette smoking, but cigar and pipe smoking may also be causes. Chronic bronchitis is a persistent inflammation and thickening of the lining of the bronchi caused by the constant irritation of smoke. As the lining of these airways thickens, breathing becomes more difficult and coughing increases. The cells lining the bronchi produce additional mucus, causing congestion in the lungs and further hampering breathing. The signs and symptoms of chronic bronchitis are shortness of breath and a chronic cough that produces considerable amounts of mucus. Chronic bronchitis is a serious disease that can result in death. In addition to bronchitis, smoking is also a risk factor for *pneumonia*, an inflammation of the lungs that is caused by a variety of bacteria and viruses.

Smoking is also the main cause of **emphysema** (Figure 8-9), a condition in which the air sacs of the lungs lose their normal elasticity. Some air sacs become overstretched and eventually rupture, resulting in larger air sacs with less surface area over which gas exchange can take place. Under these conditions, the lungs can no longer accommodate normal amounts of air. Also, without the normal elasticity of the lungs, a person can no longer inhale and exhale normally. Breathing becomes a continual effort.

The lung damage of emphysema can never be repaired. As the disease progresses, the heart becomes increasingly overworked. Because the blood it is pumping is oxygen poor, the body sends signals to the heart to pump more blood more quickly. Eventually the person with extensive lung damage dies, usually from heart failure. However, if emphysema is detected early (especially before symptoms develop), its destructive effects can be halted by stopping smoking.

People with chronic bronchitis and emphysema are said to have **chronic obstructive pulmonary disease (COPD).** Cigarette smoking is the major cause of COPD (Croxton et al., 2002); it would probably be a minor health problem if people did not smoke. Smoking is thought to be responsible for approximately 61,000 deaths from COPD per year, or about 82% of all COPD deaths.

Cardiovascular Disease Forty-three percent of people who die from smoking-related causes die from **cardiovascular disease (CVD)**, or dysfunction of the heart and blood vessels. Cardiovascular disease is the number one cause of death in the United States. There are a variety of cardiovascular diseases, including *coronary artery disease (CAD)*, *hypertension* (chronic high blood pressure), and stroke (blood vessel disease of the brain). *Atherosclerosis*, the buildup of fatty deposits in the arteries, is an important cardiovascular disease process that is an underlying cause in CAD and stroke. These diseases are discussed in detail in Chapter 12.

acute bronchitis
a temporary inflammation of the mucous membranes of the bronchi.

chronic bronchitis
a persistent inflammation and thickening of the lining of the bronchi.

emphysema
(EM-fih-SEE-mah) a chronic condition in which the air sacs of the lungs lose their normal elasticity, impairing respiration.

(a)

(b)

Figure 8-9 **A Healthy Lung and Lung from a Person with Emphysema.** (a) The healthy lung is smooth, a deep pink, and relatively uniform in color. (b) Due to emphysema, some of the alveoli have ruptured, creating tiny craters within the lung, which are difficult to see in this picture. Note the blackened tissue as a result of years of smoking.

Cigarette smokers are more than twice as likely as nonsmokers to have a heart attack or stroke, and up to four times as likely to die from a heart attack because of smoking's effects on the cardiovascular system. As many as 20% of CVD deaths in the United States each year are attributable to cigarette smoking (American Heart Association [AHA], 2002). Using smokeless tobacco is a significant CVD risk factor also, but cigar and pipe smoking are less significant.

Women who take oral contraceptives (birth control pills) and who smoke cigarettes increase their risk of heart attack several times. Oral contraceptives increase the risk of developing blood clots, which can block already narrowed arteries in persons with atherosclerosis, a disease that smokers have an increased risk of developing. For these reasons, smoking while taking oral contraceptives also increases the risk of peripheral vascular disease and stroke.

Smokers often think that smoking low-yield ("light") cigarettes poses fewer health risks than smoking regular-strength cigarettes. Light cigarettes, which began to be marketed in the 1960s in response to health concerns, are lower in tar and nicotine. However, research data show that smokers generally puff on these cigarettes longer and inhale more deeply than when smoking regular cigarettes. Also, they often smoke more light cigarettes than they would regular cigarettes, so they may actually take in more tar, nicotine, and other noxious and cancer-causing compounds than if they smoked regular cigarettes. Scientists have found no evidence that smoking low-tar and low-nicotine cigarettes reduces the risk of coronary heart disease.

When a smoker quits, his or her risk of heart disease begins dropping immediately. The time it takes for a former smoker's risk of death from heart attack to reach that of a nonsmoker's varies from three to nine years. The recovery time depends on the number of years a person smoked and how many cigarettes he or she smoked per day. However, if a smoker has already developed heart disease before quitting, the risk of heart attack will not return to that of a nonsmoker, although it will be lower than if he or she had continued smoking.

Cancer Cancer is a group of diseases in which certain cells exhibit abnormal growth. Cancers can arise in various locations in the body and then spread to others. The most prevalent forms of cancer in the United States are discussed in Chapter 13, which also describes lifestyle changes you can make in addition to quitting smoking that will reduce your chances of developing these cancers.

Guidelines for early detection are listed in Chapter 13 (see p. 348).

Cancer is the second biggest killer of Americans, and tobacco use is responsible for about 30% of cancer deaths and 87% of lung cancer deaths annually in the United States (American Cancer Society [ACS], 2004). Tobacco use causes or is related to cancers of the lungs, larynx, oral cavity, esophagus, kidneys, bladder, pancreas, stomach, and cervix. Lung cancer is the most prevalent form of cancer caused by tobacco use.

Periodontal Disease Smoking tobacco and using smokeless tobacco can have serious effects on the oral "cavity." These effects can range from embarrassing problems such as bad breath and stained teeth to life-threatening conditions such as oral cancer (Figure 8-10). People who use tobacco products regularly often develop **periodontal disease**, commonly known as gum disease. Periodontal disease is actually more than just disease of the gums. It is a disease of all the supporting tissues around the teeth, which include the gums, the bone in which the teeth are embedded, and the ligaments that hold the teeth to the bone.

People can develop periodontal disease for a variety of reasons, such as poor dental hygiene, overzealous brushing that damages the gums, and clenching and grinding of the teeth. Using tobacco products is

chronic obstructive pulmonary disease (COPD) a syndrome that includes chronic bronchitis, asthma, and emphysema and that is characterized by extreme difficulty in breathing.

cardiovascular disease (CVD) disorders of the heart and blood vessels.

periodontal disease (PER-ee-oh-DON-tal) a disorder of the tissues that support the teeth.

Figure 8-10   Sean Marsee, before and after Using Smokeless Tobacco. Sean, an Oklahoman and award-winning high school athlete, died of oral cancer caused by his habit of chewing tobacco. His disease developed and killed him in about one year.

especially destructive to the gums and often is a cause of severe periodontal disease. Nicotine narrows the blood vessels in the gums, reducing the amount of oxygen that reaches these tissues. As a result, the gum tissue becomes less resistant to infection. Additionally, good oral hygiene and proper periodontal treatment are often ineffective when a person with periodontal disease continues to use tobacco.

Young people who use smokeless tobacco products often develop periodontal disease. Gum recession most often occurs at places where smokeless tobacco is held in the mouth. Additionally, *leukoplakia*, a disease characterized by precancerous white patches that develop on the mucous membranes of the mouth (Figure 8-11), is common in adolescents who use these products. Approximately 5% of these lesions become cancerous within 5 years. However, if a smokeless tobacco user discontinues use, the leukoplakia regresses and may disappear.

Osteoporosis Osteoporosis, or a loss of bone density, occurs most frequently in postmenopausal white women. This disease is serious because it places women at risk for bone fractures, back pain, and other accompanying problems. Hip fractures are particularly serious; the death rate for women who sustain hip fractures is 15% to 20% higher than for women who do not sustain this injury. (Osteoporosis is discussed in more detail in Chapter 9.)

environmental tobacco smoke (ETS) the smoke emitted from a lit cigarette, cigar, or pipe and the smoke exhaled by smokers.

Figure 8-11   **Leukoplakia.** This precancerous condition often develops on the mucous membranes of the mouths of those who use smokeless tobacco products.

Smoking cigarettes causes a loss of bone density in women and reduces the age at which menopause occurs by about 2 years. Therefore, women who smoke a pack of cigarettes a day throughout their adult lives reach early menopause with bones that are up to 10% less dense than those of nonsmokers.

Environmental Tobacco Smoke

In the past three decades, nonsmokers have become increasingly aware that smoke in their indoor environments could pose a health risk. This smoke, termed **environmental tobacco smoke (ETS)** or *secondhand smoke*, is made up of the sidestream smoke emitted from a lit cigarette, cigar, or pipe and the smoke exhaled by smokers.

In 1986 the National Research Council (NRC) and the United States Surgeon General's Office compiled research data to assess the health effects of exposure to ETS (CDC, 1986; NRC, 1986). Both landmark reports conclude that ETS can cause lung cancer in adult nonsmokers. Researchers estimate that approximately 3,000 lung cancer deaths per year in the United States are attributable to the chronic inhalation of secondhand smoke. The reports also acknowledge that ETS contains the same carcinogenic compounds that have been identified in the mainstream smoke inhaled by smokers.

These conclusions have prompted the designation of governmental and other public buildings, many workplaces, and restaurants in many states as smoke-free environments to reduce the effects of ETS on the public. By 1993 nearly 82% of indoor workers were restricted from smoking in their workplaces (Farrelly et al., 1999), and efforts to increase smoking bans in all public settings was ongoing in 2000 and beyond (McMillen et al., 2003). Workplace smoking bans have also been shown to increase the number of workers who quit smoking (Utsunomiya, 2003; Moskowitz & Hudes, 2000).

Analyses of research data (National Safety Council, 2000) show that chronic exposure to ETS may affect the cardiovascular system and may be linked to the onset of chest pain. Breathing environmental tobacco smoke has other negative effects on nonsmoking adults, such as coughing, mucus production, chest discomfort, and reduced lung function. A person with reduced lung function might become short of breath while performing physical activities.

Children, particularly infants and young children, suffer significant consequences from breathing secondhand smoke. Children of parents who smoke have an increased frequency of respiratory symptoms such as coughing and wheezing, and of lower respiratory tract infections such as bronchitis, influenza, and pneumonia (National Safety Council, 2000). Parents should also note that not all areas designated as smoke free are really safe. Research results show that nonsmoking areas adjacent to smoking areas contain unacceptable levels of airborne pollutants unless the areas have separate ventilation systems (Akbar-Khanzadeh, 2003).

Environmental tobacco smoke is also a risk factor for the development of asthma in children. Exposure to ETS can cause asthmatic attacks and an increased severity of asthma in children who already have the disease. (Chapter 14 discusses asthma in more detail.)

Avoiding secondhand smoke will help you stay healthier. The Managing Your Health box includes tips on how to say no to secondhand smoke.

Quitting

Most smokers want to quit. In a recent Gallup poll, 76% of smokers told Gallup interviewers that they would like to give up cigarettes. Sixty-five percent said that they had made a serious effort to stop smoking in the past. And 95% of smokers reported that they think smoking is harmful to their health. Eighty-three percent of smokers reported that they wish they had never started smoking (Gillespie, 1999).

 Managing Your Health

How to Say No to Secondhand Smoke

If you live with a smoker:

- Ask him or her not to smoke in your home. Discuss how his or her habit puts you and others living there at risk.
- If he or she is unwilling to go outside, suggest ways to limit the exposure to smoke for you and others. Maybe a room could be set aside for smoking—one that is seldom used by other members of the household. Some smokers protect others at home by smoking near an open window or when no one is around.
- Keep rooms well ventilated. Open windows.
- Support smokers who decide to quit.

When visitors come:

- Ask all smokers who visit not to smoke in your house or apartment, but to please smoke outside.
- Do not keep ashtrays around.

In others' homes or in vehicles:

- Tell friends and relatives politely that you would appreciate their not smoking while you are there.
- Let people know when their smoke is causing immediate problems. If it is making your allergies worse, making you cough or wheeze, or making your eyes sting, say so. Some smokers put their cigarettes away when they see the discomfort it causes.

If you have children:

- Insist that babysitters, grandparents, and other caregivers not smoke around your children.
- Help children avoid secondhand smoke if smokers do use tobacco around them. Have them leave the room or play outside while an adult is smoking. Air rooms out after smoking occurs.
- Keep smokers away from places in which children sleep.

When smoking is allowed at the workplace:

- Talk to your employer about the company's smoking policy. Give your employer copies of the Environmental Protection Agency (EPA) report on the harmful effects of environmental tobacco smoke. Call 1-800-438-4318 to obtain this report.
- Ask to work near other nonsmokers and as far away from smokers as possible.
- Ask smokers if they would not smoke around you.
- Use a fan and open windows (if possible) to keep air moving.
- Hang a Thank You for Not Smoking sign in your work area.
- Volunteer to help develop a fair company policy that protects nonsmokers.
- Contact the local Lung Association, the American Cancer Society, or the National Cancer Institute (1-800-4-CANCER) for information concerning smoking cessation programs that can be conducted at your workplace.

When you are in public places:

- Always take the nonsmoking options that are available in rental cars, hotels, and restaurants.
- If a restaurant puts you at a table near smokers (even if you are in a nonsmoking section), ask to move.
- Keep children out of smoking areas.

Source: Adapted from National Cancer Institute. (1993). *I mind very much if you smoke* (NIH Publication No. 93-3544). Washington, DC: National Institutes of Health.

Benefits of Quitting At any age, there are many reasons to stop smoking cigarettes. Five primary reasons to quit are cited in the 1990 report of the Surgeon General (U.S. Department of Health and Human Services) *The Health Benefits of Smoking Cessation:*

1. Smoking cessation has major and immediate health benefits.
2. Former smokers live longer than continuing smokers.
3. Smoking cessation decreases the risk of lung cancer, other cancers, heart attack, stroke, and chronic lung disease.
4. Women who stop smoking before pregnancy or during the first 3 to 4 months of pregnancy reduce their risk of having a low-birth-weight baby to that of women who never smoke.
5. The health benefits of smoking cessation far exceed any risks from the average weight gain of 6 to 9 pounds or any adverse psychological effects that may occur after quitting.

One of the health effects of smoking discussed earlier in this chapter is nicotine addiction. On quitting, an addicted smoker experiences some or all of the nicotine withdrawal symptoms listed in Table 8-8. These unpleasant psychological and physiological conditions peak 1 to 2 days following quitting but subside during the following weeks. The two withdrawal symptoms that last the longest are the urge to smoke and an increased appetite. However, using a nicotine patch, nicotine gum, nicotine inhaler, or buproprion (an antidepressant used to treat nicotine dependence) during the early cessation period may help reduce these symptoms and make quitting easier (Silagy et al., 2004; Hurt, 1998). As these withdrawal symptoms subside, former smokers report that favorable psychological changes occur over time, such as enhanced self-esteem and an increased sense of self-control.

Because smoking cigarettes has negative effects on the respiratory system, a person who quits notices that it is easier to breathe. Smoking cessation reduces the rate at which symptoms such as cough, mucus production, and wheezing occur. It also reduces the incidence of respiratory infections such as bronchitis and pneumonia. (Pneumonia can be deadly for people who have chronic diseases.) Also, after sustained abstinence from smoking cigarettes, persons with COPD have less chance of dying from this disease than they did before they quit.

Quitting also has positive effects on the cardiovascular system. Data show that the smoker who quits cuts his or her elevated risk of cardiovascular disease in half only 1 to 2 years after quitting. The degree of risk that remains then declines gradually. Some data show that a former smoker reaches the risk level of a nonsmoker from 5 to 9 years after quitting. Other data show that the former smoker must wait from 10 to 15 years to achieve this goal (AHA, 2005). The more cigarettes a person smokes and the earlier a person started to smoke, the longer the recovery time. Since the risk of cardiovascular disease increases as the number of cigarettes smoked increases, smoking fewer cigarettes can be a way to lower CVD risk if an individual has little success quitting. However, smoking low-yield (low tar and nicotine) cigarettes does not appear to reduce risk. Among persons diagnosed with cardiovascular disease, smoking cessation markedly reduces the risk of additional heart attacks and cardiovascular death. The benefits of quitting exist for people of all ages. Older individuals should not think that it is "too late" to quit.

Quitting smoking substantially decreases the risk of lung, laryngeal, esophageal, oral, pancreatic, bladder, and cervical cancers (ACS, 2004). However, data suggest that the decrease in risk for cancer is not as rapid as for cardiovascular disease. There appears to be a lag between the time a person quits smoking and the lowering of risk of cancer (Enstrom, 1999; Enstrom & Heath, 1999). Figure 8-12 is a visual summary of the health benefits of quitting smoking.

The Process of Quitting Cigarette smoking is an addiction, and an addicted smoker who is quitting goes through the same process of behavioral change as does anyone addicted to any drug. For a smoker to contemplate quitting, he or she must understand and accept that cigarette smoking is dangerous or must have other reasons for quitting that are important to him or her. Then the smoker begins to see the potential benefits and negative effects associated with quitting. For example, the smoker may realize that nicotine is a drug and that he or she is addicted to this drug. Quitting will stop the addiction. However, along with this positive behavior (stopping the addiction) comes negative consequences: withdrawal symptoms. To be prepared to quit, the smoker should analyze both the negative and positive aspects of change and prepare to deal with the negative aspects. Often, discussion with a medical practitioner is helpful. Also, if a smoker analyzes the reasons he or she smokes (see "Why Do You Smoke?" in the student workbook), the smoker will be better equipped to handle the consequences of quitting (see "Tips for Quitters" on p. 216).

Once the smoker realizes the need to quit, he or she should decide what course of action to take. Should it be quitting "cold turkey" or cutting down at first? (If a person is addicted to nicotine, stopping "cold turkey" may be best. The assessment activity "Why Do

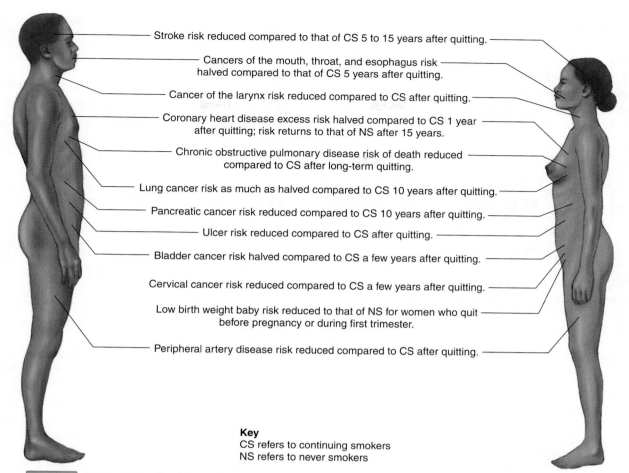

Stroke risk reduced compared to that of CS 5 to 15 years after quitting.

Cancers of the mouth, throat, and esophagus risk halved compared to that of CS 5 years after quitting.

Cancer of the larynx risk reduced compared to CS after quitting.

Coronary heart disease excess risk halved compared to CS 1 year after quitting; risk returns to that of NS after 15 years.

Chronic obstructive pulmonary disease risk of death reduced compared to CS after long-term quitting.

Lung cancer risk as much as halved compared to CS 10 years after quitting.

Pancreatic cancer risk reduced compared to CS 10 years after quitting.

Ulcer risk reduced compared to CS after quitting.

Bladder cancer risk halved compared to CS a few years after quitting.

Cervical cancer risk reduced compared to CS a few years after quitting.

Low birth weight baby risk reduced to that of NS for women who quit before pregnancy or during first trimester.

Peripheral artery disease risk reduced compared to CS after quitting.

Key
CS refers to continuing smokers
NS refers to never smokers

Figure 8-12 **The Health Benefits of Quitting Smoking.** The risks of developing many diseases and conditions drop dramatically, in varied lengths of time, after a person quits smoking. Source: U.S. Department of Health and Human Services. (1990). *The health benefits of smoking cessation: A report of the surgeon general.* Atlanta, GA: Author.

You Smoke?" can help identify addiction.) Will the smoker join a smoking cessation program or stop without group support? Again, the advice of a medical practitioner may be helpful at this stage. A smoker can also call the American Lung Association, the American Heart Association, the American Cancer Society, or the National Cancer Institute for free literature on quitting and information on smoking cessation programs. Many programs are available, and the smoker needs to select the program that suits his or her needs best. Medication may also be helpful at this stage, such as a nicotine patch or nicotine gum to lessen the withdrawal symptoms from nicotine. Also, the smoker may enlist the support of family and friends through the quitting process.

After the first 6 months, which is considered the *quitting period,* the former smoker enters the period of *maintenance,* which lasts 6 months also. Some quitters who join smoking cessation programs continue to attend group meetings for support. Others get con-tinued support from friends, family members, or other former smokers.

As with other addictions, sometimes *relapse* occurs. During a relapse, a former smoker returns to smoking habits. Relapse can be triggered by a variety of factors such as stress, depression, a craving for cigarettes, negative life events, and interpersonal tensions. To quit, the relapsed smoker goes through the stages of behavior change once again.

One barrier to quitting is the smoker's fear of gaining weight. In fact, about 25% of smokers cite this possibility as the reason for not quitting. Likewise, about 25% of people who quit relapse because they begin to gain weight and are afraid of gaining more. This fear is not unfounded—80% of persons who quit smoking gain weight. Data show, however, that the average weight gain is only 6 to 9 pounds and the risk of large weight gain is extremely low. Individuals who smoke heavily gain the most weight after quitting (Heishman, 1998).

People gain weight when they stop smoking for two reasons: They eat more (often to put something other than a cigarette into their mouths) and their metabolism slows slightly. To combat this effect, as part of your smoking cessation plan be sure to include an exercise program to maintain your metabolic rate. Also, keep lots of fat-free, low-calorie snacks handy, such as slices of vegetables with low-fat dip, fruits, pretzels, and sugar-free gelatin.

Prevention

Prevention programs developed in the 1980s reflect an understanding that smoking begins in early adolescence and that young people go through stages in the

Managing Your Health

Tips for Quitters

If you smoke and have not responded to the questions in the assessment activity in the student workbook titled "Why Do You Smoke?" do so now. Then read the suggestions for quitting that specifically address each reason you smoke. If you tailor your plan to quit smoking to match the reasons that you smoke, the cessation process will be easier.

Reason: "Smoking gives me energy."

· Get enough rest to feel refreshed and alert.
· Exercise regularly to raise your overall energy level.
· Take a brisk walk instead of smoking if you start feeling sluggish.
· Eat regular, nutritious meals for energy.
· Drink lots of cold water to refresh you.
· Avoid getting bored, which can make you feel tired.

Reason: "I like to touch and handle cigarettes."

· Pick up a pen or pencil when you want to reach for a cigarette.
· Play with a coin or handle nearby objects.
· Put a plastic cigarette in your hand or mouth.
· Hold a real cigarette if the touch is all you miss.
· Eat regular meals to avoid confusing the desire to eat with the desire to put a cigarette in your mouth.
· Take up a hobby like knitting or carpentry that keeps your hands busy.
· Eat low-fat, low-sugar snacks like carrot sticks or bread sticks.
· Suck on sugar-free hard candy.

Reason: "Smoking gives me pleasure."

· Enjoy the pleasures of being tobacco-free, such as how good foods taste; how much easier it is to walk, run, and climb stairs; and how good it feels to be in control of the urge to smoke.
· Spend the money you save on cigarettes on another kind of pleasure, such as a shopping spree or a night out.
· Remind yourself of the health benefits of quitting. Giving up cigarettes can help you enjoy life's other pleasures for many years to come.

Reason: "Smoking helps me relax when I'm tense or upset."

· Use relaxation techniques to calm down when you are angry or upset. Deep breathing exercises, muscle relax-

ation, and imagining yourself in a peaceful setting can make you feel less stressed.
· Exercise regularly to relieve tension and improve your mood.
· Take action to alleviate situations that cause stress.
· Avoid stressful situations.
· Get enough rest and take time to relax each day.
· Enjoy relaxation. Take a long, hot bath. Have a massage. Lie in a garden hammock. Listen to soothing music.

Reason: "I crave cigarettes and am addicted to nicotine."

· Ask your medical practitioner about using a nicotine patch or nicotine gum to help you avoid withdrawal symptoms.
· Go "cold turkey." Tapering off probably won't work for you, because the moment you put out one cigarette you begin to crave the next.
· Keep away from cigarettes completely. Get rid of ashtrays. Destroy any cigarettes you have. Try to avoid people who smoke and smoke-filled places like bars.
· Tell family and friends you've quit smoking.
· Remember that physical withdrawal symptoms last about 2 weeks. Hang on!

Reason: "Smoking is a habit."

· Cut down gradually. Smoke fewer cigarettes each day or only smoke them halfway down. Inhale less often and less deeply. After several months it should be easier to stop completely.
· Change your smoking routines. Keep your cigarettes in a different place. Smoke with your opposite hand. Do not do anything else while smoking. Limit smoking to certain places, such as outside or in one room at home.
· When you want a cigarette, wait one minute. Do something else instead of smoking.
· Be aware of every cigarette you smoke. Ask yourself, Do I really want this cigarette? You may be surprised at how many you can easily pass up.
· Set a date for giving up smoking altogether and stick to it.

Source: Adapted from National Cancer Institute. (1993). *Learning why you smoke can teach you how to quit.* Washington, DC: U.S. Department of Health and Human Services.

development of smoking behavior (see the section entitled "Psychosocial Reasons for Using Tobacco Products" on pages 206–207). Today's programs also recognize that a child's social environment is the most important determinant of whether he or she will smoke. Therefore, prevention programs now target seventh and eighth graders, reaching children before most start smoking. Their focus is on helping young people develop skills to identify and resist social influences to smoke, such as advertising and peer pressure. Additionally, they educate adolescents about the short-term negative effects of tobacco use. Understanding short-term consequences positively affects adolescent behavior more than knowledge of long-term effects. Data show that several types of prevention programs delay or reduce youth tobacco use for periods of 1 to 5 years and more. Effective prevention programs engage the school, parents, and media (Pentz, 1998).

Other programs have been developed that focus on smokeless tobacco use. The goal of these programs is to counter the perception that smokeless tobacco is a safe alternative to smoking cigarettes.

Reducing the availability of cigarettes to adolescents is another prevention measure. Unfortunately, adolescents can get cigarettes quite easily even though the sale of tobacco products to minors is illegal in all states and the District of Columbia. One of the goals of *Healthy People 2010* is to enforce laws that prohibit sales to minors to reduce the percentage of minors who successfully purchase cigarettes to 5%.

Healthy Living Practices

- If you are a smoker, make a plan for quitting and follow through on your plan. Expect quitting to be difficult at times. Consider using an organized program, medication, or both to help you quit. To combat weight gain when quitting, exercise and keep lots of fat-free, low-calorie snacks handy.

- If you have or plan to have children, consider discussing the health effects of smoking with them when they are very young to discourage them from starting the habit.

- Do not allow your children to be near someone who is smoking. Children are particularly susceptible to the damaging effects of tobacco smoke.

- If you have bronchitis with accompanying high fever, breathlessness, and yellow, gray, green, or bloody sputum, seek medical attention immediately.

- If you have a smoker's cough that produces considerable amounts of mucus and shortness of breath, seek medical attention immediately because you may have chronic bronchitis, a serious disease.

- See your health care provider regularly for an evaluation of your respiratory system.

- If you are a nonsmoker, avoid areas where cigarette smoke is present. Breathing in this smoke increases your risk of developing heart disease, lung cancer, and various respiratory diseases and conditions.

- If you use tobacco products, you can reduce your risk of developing various cancers, cardiovascular disease, and periodontal disease by quitting.

- If you are female and smoke cigarettes, you have a higher risk of developing osteoporosis than nonsmoking women and you may reach menopause early. To reduce this risk, stop smoking.

Across THE LIFESPAN

The Effects of Alcohol and Tobacco Use

Fetuses and infants are significantly affected by the alcohol and tobacco use of their mothers. Approximately 30 years ago, scientists discovered that babies born to alcoholic women exhibited a group of certain abnormal physical and behavioral traits. Together these abnormalities are called **fetal alcohol syndrome (FAS)**.

The predominant feature of FAS is mental retardation. This syndrome is also characterized by retarded growth both before and after birth; central nervous system defects (in addition to mental retardation), such as behavioral problems, and skull or brain malformations; and characteristic facial features that include small eye openings, a broad thin upper lip, and a flattened nose bridge and mid-face (Figure 8-13). Thirty to forty percent of FAS babies are also born with heart defects.

Some babies who were exposed to alcohol before birth are born with only a few FAS abnormalities; these children are said to have **fetal alcohol effects (FAE)** or *alcohol-related birth defects (ARBD)*. The severity and

fetal alcohol syndrome (FAS) a group of abnormal physical and behavioral traits exhibited by babies born to women who consumed alcohol heavily during pregnancy.

fetal alcohol effects (FAE) a condition similar to FAS in which a child exhibits only a few FAS abnormalities.

Child with Fetal Alcohol Syndrome (FAS). This adopted boy exhibits features characteristics of FAS: small eye openings, a broad, thin upper lip, and a flattened nose bridge and mid-face.

extent of the abnormalities appear to be related to the amount a woman drinks during her pregnancy and whether she drinks for the duration of her pregnancy. Scientists have not determined a threshold level beneath which no effects will occur. However, many studies show that pregnant women who drank three alcoholic beverages per day, on average, were more likely to deliver babies with birth defects. Also, binge drinking appears to have high potential for harming an embryo or fetus (Jacobson & Jacobson, 1994; Nevitt, 1996). Moderate drinking may raise the risk of still-birth (Kesmodel, 2002). In 2002 the prevalence of any alcohol consumption in pregnant women was 10.1%, and the prevalence of binge drinking and frequent alcohol use was about 1.9% each (CDC, 2004b).

Maternal smoking during pregnancy can harm not only the fetus, but the pregnant woman as well. *Abruptio placentae* occurs when the placenta separates from the uterus, resulting in hemorrhage (life-threatening bleeding). (The placenta is an organ through which the fetus obtains nutrients and oxygen, and excretes wastes.) Maternal smoking is also associated with *placenta previa,* in which the placenta implants abnormally and covers the opening of the cervical canal. As this opening dilates at the beginning of the birth process, bleeding and severe hemorrhage can occur.

Smoking during pregnancy also reduces the flow of blood in the placenta, limits the nutrients that reach the fetus, and causes an average reduction in birth weight (Larsen et al., 2002). Additionally, the fetuses or infants of women who smoke during pregnancy are 25% to 30% more likely to die between 28 weeks of gestation and 4 weeks after birth than those of women who do not smoke. Babies born of mothers who smoke also have a higher than average incidence of death from sudden infant death syndrome (SIDS) and from respiratory diseases. The sudden, unexpected death of an apparently healthy infant, SIDS occurs while the baby is sleeping. It is the most common cause of death of children between the ages of 2 weeks and 1 year.

The percentage of women who smoke during pregnancy has declined in the past decade, from 18.4% in 1990 to 11.4% in 2002. However, pregnant teenagers 18 and 19 years old had the highest rate of smoking—18.2% (CDC, 2004e).

Another age group of persons strongly affected by alcohol and tobacco use is the elderly. Because the elderly are more physically vulnerable to the effects of alcohol, they may develop alcohol problems even though their formerly unproblematic patterns of drinking have not changed. Alcohol also reacts adversely with many medications. Elderly persons taking medications for various conditions may appear to be reacting adversely to their medications rather than experiencing an alcohol problem. Additionally, if alcohol worsens their health, their health care providers may prescribe additional or different medications. A vicious cycle of drug interactions and health complications may continue until the health care practitioner recognizes that the patient has an alcohol problem.

The elderly face special harm from smoking because most people older than 65 years of age who smoke have been doing so for 30, 40, or 50 years. As a result, a disproportionate number of elderly develop life-threatening diseases such as cancer and emphysema, because these diseases usually take decades to develop.

Among those older than 65, the death rate of current smokers is twice that of people who never smoked. Smoking is associated with a variety of other ailments that are often seen in the elderly, such as cataracts (a loss of transparency of the lens of the eye), delayed healing of broken bones, periodontal problems, ulcers, high blood pressure, brain hemorrhages, and skin wrinkles. From prenatal development to the elderly years, no one who uses alcohol or tobacco products, or breathes in smoke from others' use, can escape their health effects.

Healthy Living Practices

- Do not consume alcoholic beverages when pregnant because alcohol can harm the unborn fetus and is a risk factor for developing life-threatening hemorrhage.

CHAPTER REVIEW

Summary

Drinking alcohol and smoking cigarettes are behaviors that often begin in adolescence. Alcohol use is quite prevalent in the United States; 50.1% of Americans use alcohol. Some people use alcohol responsibly, not allowing their drinking to threaten their health or interfere with their relationships. In contrast, the harmful user drinks alcoholic beverages while knowingly damaging his or her health. The alcohol-dependent person, or alcoholic, additionally develops tolerance to the drug, exhibits withdrawal symptoms when not drinking, compulsively uses alcohol, and may exhibit other behaviors that are a part of the alcohol dependence syndrome.

A cause of alcoholism is unknown. However, studies suggest that alcoholism has a genetic (hereditary) component. People abuse alcoholic beverages and become alcohol dependent for psychological, social, and developmental reasons as well.

When a person drinks alcoholic beverages, various behavioral changes that are commonly called intoxication result from impairment of the central nervous system. The harmful use and abuse of alcohol results in multiple effects on the body that are significant threats to health. Excessive alcohol consumption exerts its most dangerous effects on the liver, cardiovascular system, immune system, reproductive system, and brain. Alcohol use and abuse are also related to serious and even fatal injuries.

Approximately 1.1 million Americans were treated for alcohol abuse and dependence in 2003. Alcohol abuse and dependence are often detected by the use of screening tests. Health care professionals who determine that their patients are alcohol dependent refer them to substance abuse specialists for evaluation and possibly treatment. Patients who show nondependent problem drinking are often encouraged to participate in brief intervention programs. Self-help groups support the alcoholic on a long-term basis to help prevent relapse into abusive or dependent behaviors.

Cigarettes are the most prevalent type of tobacco product used in the United States today. Approximately 25% of Americans smoke cigarettes regularly. Most people who smoke cigarettes and use smokeless tobacco began this habit when they were adolescents. Adolescents initially try tobacco products for a variety of reasons: to do what parents or peers do, to experiment, to feel older and more independent, or to join certain social groups. Adolescents most likely to use tobacco have particular characteristics such as low self-esteem, high susceptibility to peer pressure, and a sensation-seeking nature.

Most teenagers and adults continue to smoke and use smokeless tobacco because they are addicted to the psychoactive drug nicotine. Nicotine, like all psychoactive drugs, acts on certain communication points among nerve cells in the brain.

Cigarette smoking is the leading source of preventable illness and death in the United States because many of the 4,000 chemical compounds in cigarette smoke affect the body adversely. Every year, approximately 400,000 people die in the United States as a result of using tobacco products.

Inhaled cigarette smoke affects the airways by damaging the cilia that sweep debris from this region, by causing the airways to secrete excess mucus, and by irritating and inflaming the airways. As a result, smokers suffer chronic cough and are at high risk for a variety of respiratory infections, such as acute and chronic bronchitis and pneumonia. Smoking is also the main cause of emphysema, a condition in which the air sacs of the lungs have lost their usual elasticity so that a person cannot inhale and exhale normally.

Forty-three percent of people who die from smoking-related causes die from cardiovascular disease. Scientists have found no evidence that smoking low-tar and low-nicotine cigarettes reduces the risk of coronary heart disease.

Cancer is the second-biggest killer of Americans, and tobacco use is responsible for about 30% of cancer deaths annually in the United States. Lung cancer is the most prevalent form of cancer caused by tobacco use. Smokeless tobacco use does not cause lung cancer, but it does cause cancers of the larynx, oral cavity, and esophagus. These cancers are also caused by smoking cigarettes, cigars, and pipes.

People who use tobacco products regularly often develop periodontal disease, which is a disease of the supporting structures of the teeth. Eventually, if periodontal disease is not treated and controlled, the teeth become loose and fall out.

Smoking cigarettes causes a loss of bone density in women. This condition is serious because it places women at risk for bone fractures, back pain, and other accompanying problems. Smoking also reduces the age at which menopause occurs by about two years.

Environmental tobacco smoke (ETS), the sidestream smoke emitted from a lit cigarette, cigar, or pipe and the smoke exhaled by smokers, can cause lung cancer in adult nonsmokers. Chronic ETS exposure is also a risk factor for cardiovascular disease and heart attack. Additionally, children of parents who smoke have an increased frequency of respiratory symptoms such as coughing and wheezing, and lower respiratory tract infections such as bronchitis and pneumonia.

Sixty-five percent of smokers have, at one time, tried to quit smoking. Quitting has major and immediate health benefits for people of all ages.

Cigarette smoking is an addiction, and an addicted smoker who is trying to quit goes through the same process of behavioral change as does anyone addicted to any drug. Quitting is easier if the smoker analyzes why he or she smokes, and develops or chooses a method of quitting that addresses these reasons.

Successful smoking-prevention programs reflect an understanding that smoking begins in early adolescence and that a child's social environment is the most important determinant of whether he or she will smoke. Prevention programs help young people develop the skills to identify and resist social influences to smoke.

Fetuses and infants are significantly affected by the alcohol and tobacco use of their mothers. The syndrome of effects from heavy alcohol consumption during pregnancy is called fetal alcohol syndrome. The predominant feature of FAS is mental retardation. Maternal smoking during pregnancy can harm the pregnant woman as well, placing her at risk for developing several life-threatening conditions.

Another age group of persons strongly affected by alcohol and tobacco use is the elderly. The elderly are more physically vulnerable to the effects of alcohol and are more likely to be taking a variety of medications that may interact negatively with alcohol.

Smoking is associated with a variety of ailments in the elderly. Among those older than 65, the death rate of current smokers is twice that of people who have never smoked.

Applying What You Have Learned

1. Using the information in this chapter, write a paragraph that would describe what you might say to a friend to discourage him or her from abusing alcohol. `Application`

2. Analyze your reasons for smoking or those of a smoking friend or relative by using the assessment "Why Do You Smoke?" located in the student workbook. Then list the essential elements of a smoking cessation program for yourself or for that individual. `Synthesis`

3. For the past two decades or so, researchers have viewed alcoholism from a "biomedical" point of view. Many researchers thought that it was only a matter of time before a gene for alcoholism would be found. Recently, many researchers have agreed that biology plays a role in addiction, but have suggested that biology is only one factor in the development of alcoholism. What other factors are involved? Does Alcoholics Anonymous appear to address this variety of factors in its twelve steps to recovery? State the reasons for your answers. `Evaluation`

4. List all the places where you are regularly exposed to environmental tobacco smoke. Decide whether you should change any of your activities to reduce your exposure to ETS. State the reasons for your answer. `Evaluation`

Key

`Application`	using information in a new situation.
`Synthesis`	putting together information from different sources.
`Evaluation`	making informed decisions.

Reflecting on Your Health

1. Describe your attitudes toward alcoholics before reading this chapter. Have your attitudes changed after reading this chapter? Why or why not?

2. If you drink alcohol, what motivates your use of this drug? Are you comfortable with your patterns of drinking and reasons for doing so? Why or why not? If you are uncomfortable with your drinking patterns, what can you do to change them?

3. If you were out with friends who were drinking, would you attempt to stop someone from driving who was clearly unfit to get behind the wheel? If not, why not? If so, what strategy might be successful? Why do you think this strategy would work?

4. If you are a smoker, what do you do to avoid having others breathe your secondhand smoke? If nothing, what might you do in the future? If you are a nonsmoker, what do you do to avoid breathing others' secondhand smoke? If nothing, what might you do in the future?

5. Do you smoke bidis or clove cigarettes? If so, why did you start smoking these products? After reading the Consumer Health feature in this chapter, do you think you will continue this practice? Why or why not?

References

Akbar-Khanzadeh, F. (2003). Exposure to environmental tobacco smoke in restaurants without separate ventilation systems for smoking and nonsmoking dining areas. *Archives of Environmental Health, 58*(2):97–103.

American Cancer Society. (2004). *Cancer facts and figures 2004.* Atlanta: American Cancer Society.

American Heart Association. (2002). *Heart and stroke statistical update.* Dallas, TX: American Heart Association. Retrieved from http://216.185.112.5/downloadable/heart/101483280946610131909901 23HS_State_02.pdf.

American Heart Association. (2005). *Heart disease and stroke statistics—2005 update.* Dallas, TX: American Heart Association.

Bunout, D. (1999). Nutritional and metabolic effects of alcoholism: Their relationship with alcoholic liver disease. *Nutrition, 15*:583–589.

Castellsague, X., Munox, N., DeStefani, E., Victora, C. G., Castelletoto, R., Rolon, P. A., & Quintana, M. J. (1999). Independent and joint effects of tobacco smoking and alcohol drinking on the risk of esophageal cancer in men and women. *International Journal of Cancer, 82*:657–664.

Centers for Disease Control and Prevention. (1986). *The health consequences of involuntary smoking—a report of the Surgeon General* (DHHS Publication No. [CDC] 87–8398). Rockville, MD: U.S. Department of Health and Human Services, Public Health Service.

Centers for Disease Control and Prevention. (2001). Alcohol involvement in fatal motor-vehicle crashes—United States, 1999–2000. *Morbidity and Mortality Weekly Report, 50*:1064–1065.

Centers for Disease Control and Prevention. (2004a). Alcohol-attributable deaths and years of potential life lost—United States, 2001. *Morbidity and Mortality Weekly Report, 53*(37):866–870.

Centers for Disease Control and Prevention. (2004b). Alcohol consumption among women who are pregnant or who might become pregnant—United States, 2002. *Morbidity and Mortality Weekly Report, 53*(50):1178–1181.

Centers for Disease Control and Prevention. (2004c). Cigarette smoking among adults—United States, 2001. *Morbidity and Mortality Weekly Report, 53*(20):427–431.

Centers for Disease Control and Prevention. (2004d). Cigarette use among high school students—United States, 1991–2003. *Morbidity and Mortality Weekly Report, 53*(23):499–502.

Centers for Disease Control and Prevention. (2004e). Smoking during pregnancy—United States, 1990–2002. *Morbidity and Mortality Weekly Report, 53*(39):911–915.

Croxton, T. L., Weinmann, G. G., Senior, R. M., & Hoidal, J. R. (2002). Future research directions in chronic obstructive pulmonary disease: NHLBI workshop summary. *American Journal of Respiratory and Critical Care Medicine, 165*:838–844.

Cox, D. E., Sadler, D. W., & Pounder, D. J. (1997). Alcohol estimation at necropsy: Epidemiology, economics, and the elderly. *Journal of Clinical Pathology, 50*:197–201.

Dowdall, G. W., & Wechsler, H. (2002). Studying college alcohol use: Widening the lens, sharpening the focus. *Journal of Studies on Alcohol, Supplement,* No. 14:14–22.

Driscoll, T. R., Harrison, J. A., & Steenkamp, M. (2004). Review of the role of alcohol in drowning associated with recreational aquatic activity. *Injury Prevention, 10*(2):107–113.

Ebnet, M. (1998, November 20). Tobacco deal wins unanimous OK by states. *The Seattle Times,* p. A1.

Enstrom, J. E. (1999). Smoking cessation and mortality trends among two United States populations. *Journal of Clinical Epidemiology, 52*:727–729.

Enstrom, J. E., & Heath, C. W. Jr. (1999). Smoking cessation and mortality trends among 118,000 Californians, 1960–1997. *Epidemiology, 10*:500–512.

Farrelly, M. C., Evans, W. N., & Sfekas, A. E. (1999). Impact of workplace smoking bans: Results from a national survey. *Tobacco Control, 8*:272–277.

Gillespie, M. (1999, November 18). *Majority of smokers want to quit, consider themselves addicted.* Princeton, NJ: Gallup News Service. Retrieved from http://www.gallup.com/poll/releases/pr991118.asp.

Ginsberg, E. S. (1999). Estrogen, alcohol, and breast cancer risk. *Journal of Steroid Biochemistry & Molecular Biology, 69*:299–306.

Glindemann, K. E., Geller, E. S., & Fortney, J. N. (1999). Self-esteem and alcohol consumption: A study of college drinking behavior in a naturalistic setting. *Journal of Alcohol and Drug Education, 45*:60–71.

Hanson, G., Venturelli, P. J., & Fleckenstein, A. E. (2004). *Drugs and society.* Sudbury, MA: Jones and Bartlett.

Health Canada. (2001, December). *Canadian tobacco use monitoring survey (CTUMS): Results for first half of 2001.* Retrieved from http://www.hc-sc.gc.ca/hecs-sesc/tobacco/research/ctums_first_2001.html.

Health Canada. (2004, August). *Canadian Tobacco Use Monitoring Survey (CTUMS): Summary of results for 2003.* Retrieved from http://www.hc-sc.gc.ca/hecs-sesc/tobacco/research/ctums/2003/summary_annual_2003.html.

Heishman, S. J. (1998). *Behavioral-cognitive effects of smoking.* A paper presented at National Institutes of Health conference Addicted to Nicotine: A National Research Forum at the Natcher Conference Center in Bethesda, MD, July 27–28.

Hillbom, M., Juvela, S., & Numminen, H. (1999). Alcohol intake and the risk of stroke. *Journal of Cardiovascular Risk, 6*:223–228.

Holder, H. D., Gruenewald, P. J., Ponicki, W. R., Treno, A. J., Grube, J. W., Saltz, R. F., Voas, R. B., Reynolds, R., Davis, K., Sanchez, L., Gaumont, G., & Roeper, P. (2000). Effect of community-based interventions on high-risk drinking and alcohol-related injuries. *Journal of the American Medical Association, 284*:2341–2347.

Hurt, R. D. (1998). *New medications for nicotine dependence treatment.* A paper presented at the National Institutes of Health conference Addicted to Nicotine: A National Research Forum at the Natcher Conference Center in Bethesda, MD, July 27–28.

Jacobson, J. L., & Jacobson, S. W. (1994). Prenatal alcohol exposure and neurobehavioral development: Where is the threshold? *Alcohol Health & Research World, 18*(1):30–35.

Johnson, T. J., & Sheets, V. L. (2004). Measuring college students' motives for playing drinking games. *Psychology of Addictive Behaviors, 18*(2):91–99.

Johnston, L. D., O'Malley, P. M., & Bachman, J. G. (2004a). *Monitoring the Future national results on adolescent drug use: Overview of key findings 2003* (NIH Pub. No. 04–5506). Bethesda, MD: National Institute on Drug Abuse.

Johnston, L. D., O'Malley, P. M., Bachman, J. G., & Schulenberg, J. E. (2004b). *Monitoring the Future national survey results on drug use, 1975–2003: Volume 1, secondary school students* (NIH Publication No. 04-5507). Bethesda, MD: National Institute on Drug Abuse.

Kesmodel, U., Wisborg, K., Olsen, S. F., Henriksen, T. B., & Secher, N. J. (2002). Moderate alcohol intake during pregnancy and the risk of stillbirth and death in the first year of life. *American Journal of Epidemiology, 155*:305–312.

Klein, H. (1992). Self-reported reasons for why college students drink. *Journal of Alcohol and Drug Education, 37*(2):14–27.

Krochanek, K. D., & Smith, B. L. (2004). Deaths: Preliminary data for 2002. *National Vital Statistics Reports, 52*(13). Retrieved from http://www.cdc.gov/nchs/data/nvsr/nvsr52/nvsr52_13.pdf.

Larsen, L. G., Clausen, H. V., & Jonsson, L. (2002). Stereologic examination of placentas from mothers who smoke during pregnancy. *American Journal of Obstetrics and Gynecology, 186*:531–537.

McMillen, R. C., Winickoff, J. P., Klein, J. D., & Weitzman, M. (2003). U.S. adult attitudes and practices regarding smoking restrictions and child exposure to environmental tobacco smoke: Changes in the social climate from 2000–2001. *Pediatrics, 112*(1 Pt 1):e55–60.

Moskowitz, J. M., & Hudes, L. Z. (2000). The impact of workplace smoking ordinances in California on smoking cessation. *American Journal of Public Health, 90*:757–761.

National Institute on Alcohol Abuse and Alcoholism. (2000). *Tenth special report to the U.S. Congress on alcohol and health. Chapter 7. Prevention research.* Washington, DC: National Institutes of Health.

National Research Council. (1986). *Environmental tobacco smoke: Measuring exposure and assessing health effects.* Washington, DC: National Academy Press.

National Safety Council. (2000, June 23). *Fact sheet: Environmental tobacco smoke.* Retrieved from http://www.nsc.org/library/facts/ets.htm.

Nevitt, A. (1996). *Fetal alcohol syndrome.* New York: Rosen Publishing Group.

Pentz, M. A. (1998). *Effective prevention programs for tobacco use.* A paper presented at the National Institutes of Health conference Addicted to Nicotine: A National Research Forum at the Natcher Conference Center in Bethesda, MD, July 27–28.

Pierce, J. P. (1998, July). *Advertising and promotion.* Paper presented at the conference Addicted to Nicotine: A National Research Forum, Bethesda, MD. Retrieved from http://www.nida.nih.gov/MeetSum/Nicotine/Pierce.html.

Pullen, L. M. (1994). The relationships among alcohol abuse in college students and selected psychological/demographic variables. *Journal of Alcohol and Drug Education, 40*(1):36–50.

Silagy, C., Lancaster, T., Stead, L., Mant, D., & Fowler, G. (2004). Nicotine replacement therapy for smoking cessation. *Cochrane Database of Systematic Reviews,* issue 3. Article No. CD0000146. Chichester, UK: John Wiley & Sons.

Smith, G. S., Brana, C. C., & Miller, T. R. (1999). Fatal nontraffic injuries involving alcohol: A metaanalysis. *Annals of Emergency Medicine, 33*:659–668.

Substance Abuse and Mental Health Services Administration. (2004a). *Overview of findings from the 2003 National Survey on Drug Use and Health* (DHHS Publication No. SMA 04-3963). Rockville, MD: SAMHSA Office of Applied Studies.

Substance Abuse and Mental Health Services Administration. (2004b). *Results from the 2003 National Survey on Drug Use and Health: National findings* (DHHS Publication No. SMA 04-3964). Rockville, MD: SAMHSA Office of Applied Studies.

U.S. Department of Health and Human Services. (1990). *The health benefits of smoking cessation: A report of the surgeon general* (DHHS Publication No. [CDC] 90–8416). Atlanta, GA: U.S. Department of Health and Human Services.

U.S. Department of Health and Human Services. (2000). *Reducing tobacco use: A report of the surgeon general.* Atlanta, GA: Centers for Disease Control and Prevention.

U.S. Department of Transportation. (2004). *Traffic safety facts* (DOT HS 809 775). Retrieved from http://www-nrd.nhtsa.dot.gov/pdf/nrd-30/NCSA/TSFAnn/2003/TSF2003-Early.htm.

Utsunomiya, O. (2003). An epidemiological study on the effectiveness of workplace smoking control programs. *Keio Journal of Medicine, 52*(1):30–37.

Wagenaar, A. C., & Toomey, T. L. (2002). Effects of minimum drinking age laws: Review and analyses of the literature from 1960 to 2000. *Journal of Studies on Alcohol, Supplement No. 14*:206–225.

Wechsler, H., Kuo, M., Lee, H., & Dowdall, G. W. (2000). Environmental correlates of underage alcohol use and related problems of college students. *American Journal of Preventive Medicine, 19*:24–29.

Wechsler, H., Lee, J. E., Kuo, M., Seibring, M., Nelson, T. F., & Lee, H. (2002). Trends in college binge drinking during a period of increased prevention efforts: Findings from 4 Harvard School of Public Health college alcohol study surveys: 1993–2001. *Journal of American College Health, 50*:203–217.

Yesavage, J. A., & Leirer, V. O. (1986). Hangover effects on aircraft pilots 14 hours after alcohol ingestion: A preliminary report. *American Journal of Psychiatry, 143*:1546–1550.

What You'll Learn

http://healthyliving.jbpub.com

The Web site for this book offers many useful tools and is a great source for supplementary health information for both students and instructors. Visit the site at http://healthyliving.jbpub.com for information on these topics:

Basic Nutrition Principles
Energy-Supplying Nutrients
Non-Energy-Supplying Nutrients
Planning a Nutritious Diet

Chapter Overview

The basic principles of nutrition
How your body digests and uses the food you eat
The functions and sources of nutrients
How to plan a nutritious diet
How malnutrition affects health

 Diversity in Health
Asian American Food

 Consumer Health
Dietary Supplements

 Managing Your Health
Trimming the Fat from Your Diet

Across
THE LIFESPAN

Nutrition

Student Workbook

Self-Assessment: Assessing the Nutritional Quality of Your Diet/Diabetes Risk Test
Changing Health Habits: Deciding to Change Your Diet

Do You Know?

· *Which foods might help prevent cancer?*
· *How to judge the nutritional adequacy of your diet?*
· *If any vitamins are poisonous?*

Nutrition

Hamburger, cola, french fries, pizza, potato chips, tofu, yogurt, olive oil, nonfat milk, mango, and wheat germ—which of these foods do you eat regularly? Have you eaten chutney, trifle, black beans, calimari, sushi, or hummus? How often do you buy snacks from vending machines? During the past week, how many times did you eat at fast-food restaurants? Why do you eat certain foods and not others? Before deciding what to eat, do you consider the nutritional value of food? When asked if they care about what they eat, three students who were enrolled in a college health class responded:

> Do I care about what I eat? Well, it depends on how hungry I am. If I am hungry enough, I'll eat anything, except some processed meats. I don't care about the amount of fat, calories, or nutritional value in foods. All I care about is how much the food costs and how much it takes to fill me up. I'm young and healthy and have hardly any body fat—I've been eating greasy, cheap, fast foods for years.

> I care about what I eat, but my diet doesn't show it. When I wake up, I don't have time to eat. After class I eat burritos or pizza rolls before going to work. After work, I usually stop at a fast food place. . . I eat lots of french fries. I do want to eat better, but it's hard when you're always on the go.

> I'm not concerned about what I eat. People call me the "fast-food queen" because that's all I eat. I know fast food is not always healthy, but I'm going to school full-time and working. It's hard finding time to buy food and cook it.

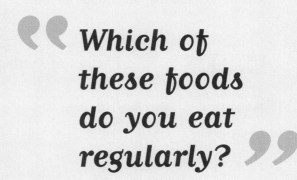

Which of these foods do you eat regularly?

If you are like these students, taste, cost, and convenience are the most important factors that influence your food choices. You may not be aware, however, that many other factors, including food advertising and moods, can also influence your diet. Although people usually associate the term *diet* with losing weight, **diet** actually refers to one's usual pattern of food choices. A healthful diet provides substances that are necessary for life, but most people do not eat simply to satisfy their nutritional needs.

Your diet reflects not only your food likes and dislikes, but also your lifestyle, financial status, and educational, cultural, religious, and ethnic backgrounds. Additionally, certain foods have social significance. When you watch a major sports event at a friend's apartment with a group of people, do you help share the cost of pizzas that are delivered? Other foods have emotional meaning. Eating homemade waffles or blueberry pancakes with real maple syrup may remind you of a grandparent who would take the time to make breakfast for you. Moreover, you may crave sweets to lift your mood when you are feeling sad or distressed. People often use certain foods to fill gaps in their lives. For example, you may head for the kitchen or vending machine not because you are hungry, but because you are bored or lonely. At other times, you may reward yourself for achieving a desired goal by eating a favorite food. Eating food to feel better, substitute for social activity, or to reward yourself can result in a nutritionally inadequate diet and unwanted weight gain.

Poor diet is a major risk factor for serious chronic diseases that are the major killers of Americans: heart disease, stroke, diabetes, obesity, and certain cancers. Sensible lifelong eating habits play important roles in maintaining good health and preventing these chronic diseases. By making specific dietary changes, people can improve their chances of enjoying good health now and later in life.

This chapter highlights the nutrients, their major food sources and roles in the body, and the benefits of choosing a nutritious diet. The information in this chapter will help you evaluate the nutritional adequacy of your diet and plan nutritious menus.

■ Basic Nutrition Principles

What Are Nutrients?

Nutrition is the study of the way the body processes and uses **nutrients**, substances in food that are needed for growth, repair, and maintenance of cells. In addition to these functions, some nutrients regulate cellular activity or supply energy. Table 9-1 lists the six classes of nutrients, describes some of their roles in the body, and identifies their major food sources. In general, carbohydrates and fats supply energy; vitamins and minerals participate in chemical reactions that regulate body processes; and proteins provide the material for tissue growth, repair, and maintenance. Water transports materials in the body and also participates in numerous chemical reactions.

The human body can *synthesize* (produce) certain nutrients. For example, by exposing your skin to sunlight for about 20 minutes, your body can make a day's supply of vitamin D. Other nutrients are essential; that is, the diet must supply nutrients that the body does not make or does not make in the amounts needed for good health. Nutritional deficiency diseases can develop when diets contain inadequate amounts of certain nutrients. These diseases are uncommon in the United States because we have a wide variety of foods available from which to eat. Additionally, many foods are *enriched* or *fortified* with certain vitamins and min-

Table 9-1	The Six Classes of Nutrients	
Nutrient Class	**Major Roles in the Body**	**Rich Food Sources**
Carbohydrates	Energy	Grain products, beans, vegetables, fruits, honey, sugar-sweetened soft drinks, and candy
Lipids	Triglycerides: energy Cholesterol: certain steroid hormones, bile production, skin maintenance, vitamin D synthesis, and nerve function	Vegetable oils, nuts, margarines, fatty meats, cheeses, cream, butter, and fried foods
Proteins	Growth, repair, and maintenance of all cells; production of enzymes, antibodies, and certain hormones	Dried beans, peas, nuts, soy products, meats, shellfish, fish, poultry, eggs, and dairy products (except cream and butter)
Vitamins	Metabolism, reproduction, development, and growth	Widespread in foods: nuts, beans, peas, fruits and vegetables, whole grains, meats, enriched breads and cereals, fortified milk
Minerals	Metabolism, development, and growth	Widespread in foods: nuts and whole grains; meats, fish, and poultry; dairy products; vegetables and fruits; enriched breads and cereals
Water	Essential for life: many chemical reactions require water; it helps maintain normal body temperature, and dissolves and transports nutrients	Water, nonalcoholic and caffeine-free beverages, fruits, vegetables, and milk (nearly every food contributes water to the diet)

erals. As a result of food enrichment and fortification, vitamin and mineral deficiency diseases that were common 100 years ago are rare today.

What Are Non-Nutrients?

Some foods contain substances that you can live without. Many of these *non-nutrients* are naturally found in plants and have beneficial effects on the body. Other non-nutrient substances, such as pesticide residues or lead, enter food unintentionally and can be hazardous to health.

Plants produce a large number of **phytochemicals**, a group of non-nutrients that may have beneficial effects on the body. Many phytochemicals, including beta-carotene, lutein, lycopene, and anthocyanin, are antioxidants. **Antioxidants** prevent or reduce the formation of *free radicals,* unstable and highly reactive atoms or compounds that can cause cellular damage. Such damage may contribute to heart disease and certain cancers. There is no scientific evidence, however, that people benefit from taking pills that contain phytochemicals. Therefore, nutrition experts recommend that people eat a variety of fruits, vegetables, and whole grains daily to obtain a natural array of these substances. Dark green, yellow, orange, red, and purple fruits and vegetables tend to have the most antioxidant phytochemicals, so let color be your key to selecting the richest food sources of antioxidants. Table 9-2 lists some phytochemicals as well as their food sources and possible effects on the body.

Natural, Health, Organic, and Functional Foods

Food manufacturers can label their products as *natural* if they are minimally processed and contain no artificial additives such as synthetic colors or flavors. So-called natural foods are not necessarily more nutritious than foods that do not carry this description. Many consumers think natural foods such as honey, yogurt, herbal teas, and cider vinegar are *health foods* because they have medicinal benefits. Although these foods provide nutrients, there is little or no scientific evidence to support claims that they prevent or treat various health conditions. Regardless of whether it's natural or manufactured, a healthy food contributes to your nutrient needs and is safe to eat. Plants and herbs, for example, may contain beneficial phytochemicals, but many are natural sources of toxic substances and should be avoided.

Food producers can label their fruits, vegetables, and meat and poultry products as *organic* if they meet certain standards. Fruits and vegetables, for example, must be grown without the use of synthetic pesticides and fertilizers. Advertisers sometimes refer to their products as organic to imply that these items are superior. Although organically

diet one's usual pattern of food choices.

nutrients substances in food that are necessary for growth, repair, and maintenance of tissues.

phytochemicals a group of non-nutrients that are produced by plants and may have beneficial effects on the body.

antioxidants compounds that protect cells from free radicals.

Table 9-2	Phytochemicals	
Phytochemicals	**Major Plant Sources**	**Possible Disease-Fighting Properties**
Allium	Garlic, onions, leeks	Enhances immune function, may reduce risk of certain cancers
Indoles, isothiocyanates (includes sulforaphane)	Broccoli, cabbage, watercress, kale, cauliflower, bok choy, collard and mustard greens, brussels sprouts	Inhibit cancer tumor growth
Ellargic acid	Nuts (especially walnuts), grapes, apples, berries	Has antioxidant activity; inhibits tumor growth
Flavonoids (includes anthocyanin)	Soy products, apples, artichokes, red grapes and wines, tea, onions, berries, red cabbage	Have antioxidant activity, may reduce risk of heart disease and certain cancers
Polyphenols	Black and green tea, red wine	Inhibit tumor growth, may reduce risk of heart disease
Monoterpenes	Citrus peel oils, citrus fruits, cherries	Anticancer agents
Carotenoids (includes beta carotene, lutein, and lycopene)	Dark orange, yellow, and green fruits and vegetables; tomatoes	May prevent prostate and other cancers
Phytic acid	Whole wheat (bran and germ)	May reduce risk of certain cancers and heart disease

Source: Dietary flavonoids and risk of coronary heart disease. (1994). *Nutrition Reviews, 52*(2):59–68; Marwick, C. (1995). Learning how phytochemicals help fight disease. *Journal of the American Medical Association, 2 74:*1328–1330; A garden of phytochemicals. (1995). *University of California of Berkeley Wellness Letter, 12*(1):6–7.

grown foods may contain less pesticide residue, they are not nutritionally superior than foods that have been grown using conventional farming methods. Chemists classify compounds as organic if they contain carbon. Carbohydrates, fats, proteins, and vitamins contain carbon; therefore, they are organic compounds. Since foods consist of these nutrients, all foods are organic.

Functional foods, sometimes called *nutraceuticals,* are manufactured foods that have scientifically established medicinal benefits that are not provided by nutrients. A person must eat a certain amount of these foods to obtain the desired effects. For example, a chemical from a plant that can lower blood cholesterol levels has been added to certain margarines and salad dressings. In the future, consumers may be able to buy specially formulated foods that reduce body fat or the risk of cancer.

What Happens to the Food You Eat?

Humans eat a wide variety of plants, animals, and animal products to obtain nutrients and other beneficial substances. In their natural state, many nutrients are in complex forms that the body cannot use. During the process of **digestion**, the digestive system breaks down complex food substances into nutrients (Figure 9-1).

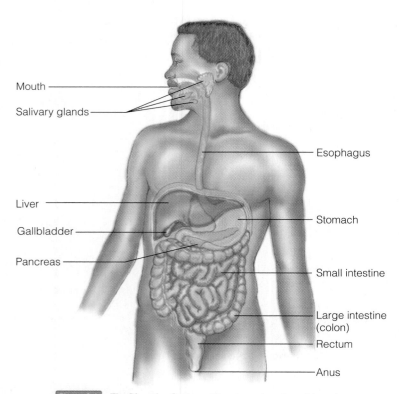

Mouth

Salivary glands

Liver

Gallbladder

Pancreas

Esophagus

Stomach

Small intestine

Large intestine (colon)

Rectum

Anus

Figure 9-1 **The Digestive System.** The stomach and small intestine break down large compounds in foods into smaller molecules that can be absorbed through the intestinal walls.

Various *enzymes,* compounds that speed up chemical changes, participate in the process of digestion.

Absorption is the passage of nutrients through the walls of the intestines and eventually into the blood. After nutrients enter the bloodstream, many circulate to the liver, where they are processed or stored.

By the time any remaining food material enters the large intestine, most of its nutrients have been absorbed. This residue, the *feces* or *stool,* remains in the rectum until the individual has a bowel movement to eliminate the waste. The entire process of digesting the food, absorbing its nutrients, and eliminating fecal residue generally takes about 1 to 3 days.

The kidneys play an important role in maintaining normal nutrient levels by filtering excess water-soluble nutrients from the blood so they can be eliminated in the urine. A *water-soluble* nutrient dissolves in water. Many nutrients such as proteins, B vitamins, and vitamin C are water-soluble. *Fat-soluble* nutrients such as cholesterol and vitamin A do not dissolve in water, and the kidneys cannot eliminate them easily. Since blood has a high water content, the body attaches proteins to fat-soluble nutrients, which enables them to travel in the bloodstream. The kidneys usually do not filter proteins out of the blood, so the fat-soluble nutrients circulate until the liver or fat cells remove them for storage. Health problems occur when the body cannot use or store excess nutrients, especially those that are fat-soluble.

Energy from Foods **Metabolism** refers to all of the chemical reactions that take place in the body. These reactions are necessary to power muscular movements, synthesize and repair tissues, release and use energy, and produce enzymes and hormones. To carry out metabolic activities, cells need the energy stored in certain nutrients. Oxygen, which enters the body from the lungs, is needed to *metabolize* (break down) these substances, releasing the stored energy. This energy powers cell activities and helps maintain body temperature.

The amount of energy in foods is expressed as a number of *kilocalories,* commonly referred to as "calories." A **calorie** is a unit of energy. Foods containing carbohydrates, fats, proteins, and the non-nutrient alcohol provide calories. Proteins and most carbohydrates supply 4 calories per gram, alcohol provides 7 calories per gram, and fat provides 9 calories per gram. Fiber only supplies energy to colon cells; each gram provides about 2 calories (Guenther & Jensen, 2000). The body cannot extract energy from water, vitamins, and minerals; therefore, these nutrients do not provide calories. Food composition tables such as those available online list the caloric value and nutrient content of commonly eaten foods.

Energy-Supplying Nutrients

Carbohydrates

Plant foods supply most of the **carbohydrates** in the diet. The simplest carbohydrates are *sugars* called monosaccharides. *Glucose,* commonly referred to as "blood sugar," is the most important monosaccharide in the human body. All cells, especially nerves, metabolize glucose for energy. Fruits are natural sources of *fructose,* a monosaccharide that the body converts to glucose. *Starches* are complex carbohydrates, long chains of glucose molecules. During digestion, large starch molecules are broken down to release glucose molecules for absorption.

Fruits, vegetables, and corn syrup are rich sources of monosaccharides. Grains, beans, and certain vegetables such as potatoes are rich sources of starch. Except for honey and milk, most animal foods do not contain carbohydrates.

In the United States, carbohydrates constitute about 44% to 47% of the typical person's caloric intake. Many nutrition experts think Americans should increase their total carbohydrate intake to 55% to 60% of calories, primarily from starchy high-fiber foods. Recommendations for simple carbohydrate intake range from 10% to 25% of calories. Foods that contain high amounts of the simple carbohydrates table sugar (*sucrose*) and *high-fructose corn syrup* (*HFCS*) are often poor sources of vitamins and minerals. Thus, eating a lot of sugary foods can displace more nutritious foods from a person's diet.

Most nutrition experts recommend that Americans reduce their intake of sucrose and HFCS by consuming fewer soft drinks, candies, and bakery items. Artificial sweeteners such as aspartame (Nutrasweet), sucralose, and saccharin are often added to sweeten sugar-free gums, candies, and diet soft drinks. When consumed in normal amounts by healthy people, these sweeteners are safe and contribute few or no calories to diets (Henkel, 1999).

Carbohydrates and Health According to the USDA, the average American consumed 90 pounds of carbohydrate sweeteners in 1996 (Kanton, 1999). HFCS and sucrose are the primary sweeteners in soft drinks, candies, desserts, and many processed foods. These simple carbohydrates are blamed for numerous health problems, including diabetes, hyperactivity, mental illness, and criminal behavior. Does scientific evidence support these claims?

Despite popular beliefs, there is no scientific evidence that sugar causes or contributes to hyperactivity, mental illness, or criminal behavior. The only disorder clearly associated with carbohydrate consumption is tooth decay. Carbohydrates can stick to teeth, providing food for bacteria in the mouth. As the bacteria metabolize carbohydrates, they produce acids that destroy the enamel of teeth, and decay results. Good oral hygiene practices, including brushing and flossing after meals and snacks, can reduce the risk of dental decay.

Some people avoid eating white sugar, which is made from sugar beets or sugar cane, but will use honey as a sweetener because they think it is more "natural" and nutritious than sugar. Although honey contains very small amounts of phytochemicals, it has essentially the same nutritional value as table sugar.

Honey should not be added to baby foods because it may contain spores of *Clostridium botulinum,* a bacterium that produces a dangerous toxin. This toxin affects nerves, causing loss of muscle functioning, which can be life threatening when it impairs breathing. Infants who eat contaminated honey are at risk of developing infantile botulism because their stomachs do not produce enough acid to kill the bacterial spores. Children older than 1 year and adults produce sufficient amounts of stomach acid, so they can eat honey safely.

Diabetes Mellitus Diabetes mellitus, often simply called diabetes, is a group of chronic diseases characterized by an inability to metabolize carbohydrates properly. This abnormality also affects metabolism of proteins and fats. A person with diabetes produces no insulin, or insufficient amounts of insulin, or has cells that do not respond normally to insulin. *Insulin,* a hormone that is produced in the pancreas (see Figure 9-1), helps glucose enter cells. Without the normal action of insulin, the cells cannot carry out their metabolic activities properly, and glucose builds up in the blood. High blood glucose levels can lead to serious chronic health disorders, including hypertension, loss of vision, and nerve damage. In the United States, poorly controlled diabetes is a major cause of kidney failure, blindness, and lower limb amputations. Furthermore, having diabetes greatly increases one's risk of heart disease (Lotufo et al., 2001). In 2001, an estimated 16.7 million Americans had diabetes; about one-third of these people were unaware that they had the disease (Mokdad, 2003). Each year, thousands of people die as a result of diabetes; the disease is the sixth leading cause of death in the United States (Mokdad et al., 2003).

digestion the process of breaking down large food molecules into smaller molecules that the intestinal tract can absorb.

absorption the passage of nutrients through the walls of the small and large intestines and eventually into the general circulation of the body.

metabolism all the chemical reactions that take place in the body.

calorie a unit of energy.

carbohydrates a class of nutrients that includes sugars and starches.

The two most prevalent forms of diabetes are *type 1 diabetes*, formerly called type I or insulin-dependent diabetes mellitus, and *type 2 diabetes*, formerly referred to as type II or non-insulin-dependent diabetes mellitus. Table 9-3 lists the common signs and symptoms of each type.

People with type 1 diabetes require daily injections of insulin because the pancreas does not produce the hormone. Medical experts think an inappropriate immune system response to an infection causes this type of diabetes. Although type 1 diabetes is often called juvenile diabetes, the label is misleading because type 1 can strike at any age. The majority of cases, however, are diagnosed in childhood.

Most people with diabetes have type 2. They are usually older than 40 years, overweight, and have a family history of diabetes. Since 1990, the prevalence of type 2 diabetes has increased dramatically in the United States, particularly among black Americans (Mokdad et al., 2003). Moreover, this form of the disease is becoming more common among children and adolescents. Obesity, physical inactivity, and poor diet contribute to the development of type 2 diabetes in both adults and children.

Recently, nutrition scientists determined that the small intestine absorbs monosaccharides from carbohydrate-rich foods at different rates. As a result, carbohydrate-containing foods are assigned values according to their *glycemic index (GI)*. The GI reflects the extent to which a standard amount of the food increases a person's blood glucose level when compared with a standard amount of glucose or white bread.

Foods with high GIs (over 70), such as white, short-grained rice, increase blood glucose levels more than foods with low GIs (under 55), such as kidney beans. When blood glucose levels rise, the pancreas releases insulin in response. People who consume diets that contain more high-GI than low-GI foods may experience an excess of insulin in their blood, which, in turn, may increase the risk of heart disease, obesity, and type 2 diabetes. Among nutrition scientists, however, the overall significance of the glycemic index to health is controversial.

Americans' high intake of HFCS may contribute to the rising prevalence of type 2 diabetes in the United States (Bray et al., 2004). In a study conducted from 1991 to 1999, scientists at Harvard University recorded information about the health and lifestyle practices of over 90,000 women. The researchers found that women who increased their daily consumption of sugar-sweetened soft drinks during the study period gained more weight and had a higher risk of developing type 2 diabetes than women who drank fewer servings of these beverages (Schulze et al., 2004). Soft drinks sweetened with high-fructose corn syrup such as colas and fruit drinks are the primary source of sugar in the typical American's diet (Bray et al., 2004). In the United States, soft drink consumption has increased dramatically since 1970. During this same period, the percentage of Americans who are overweight and have diabetes increased as well. It is difficult to prove that sugar-sweetened soft drinks *cause* excess weight gain and diabetes; more research is needed to support these findings. Nevertheless, you may want to analyze your sugar-sweetened soft drink consumption. These beverages provide few nutrients other than water and carbohydrate. Instead of satisfying your thirst and hunger with sugary soft drinks, consider drinking more nutritious beverages such as nonfat milk and 100% fruit juices.

Type 2 diabetes can often be controlled by dietary modifications and regular exercise, but many affected persons need to take medications that increase the production of insulin by the pancreas. Some people with type 2 diabetes need daily insulin injections. By carefully controlling their blood sugar levels through diet, exercise, and if necessary, medication, diabetics can often lessen the long-term damaging effects of the disease.

It is important to have routine health checkups that include diabetes testing because many people with type 2 diabetes are not aware that they have the disorder. You may want to take the diabetes quiz in your workbook to assess your risk of developing this disease.

Table 9-3	Common Symptoms of Diabetes Mellitus

Type 1 Diabetes
(Generally develops in childhood and young adulthood)

- Lack of energy
- Listlessness
- Frequent urination
- Excessive thirst
- "Fruity" odor in breath
- Increased appetite with weight loss
- Vision problems

Type 2 Diabetes
Usually few symptoms, but when they exist:

- Excessive thirst
- Frequent urination
- Vision problems
- In women, recurrent vaginal infections
- Skin sores that do not heal

Metabolic Syndrome As many as one in four adult Americans have *metabolic syndrome*, a condition that increases a person's risk of cardiovascular disease and type 2 diabetes (Ford et al., 2004). People with metabolic syndrome have excess abdominal fat, slightly elevated fasting blood glucose levels, abnormal blood lipid levels, and hypertension (chronically high blood pressure). Additionally, *C-reactive protein*, a compound in blood that is an indicator of inflammation, tends to be high in people with this syndrome (Grundy et al., 2004). Medical researchers suspect an inflammatory response that occurs within the body can increase the risk of cardiovascular disease. Poor dietary habits such as eating a diet that lacks fruits, vegetables, and other fiber-rich foods contribute to metabolic syndrome. By exercising regularly, maintaining a healthy body weight, and eating plenty of fiber-rich foods, people may be able to avoid this common condition.

Lactose Intolerance Sucrose and *lactose* (milk sugar) are composed of two monosaccharides. During digestion, sucrose and lactose are broken down, releasing their component simple sugars. Many older children and adults, however, cannot digest lactose. Such lactose-intolerant people may experience intestinal bloating, cramps, and diarrhea if they consume milk or other products that contain lactose. Lactose intolerance affects about 25% of the adults in the United States (Inman-Felton, 1999). Members of certain minority groups, especially people with Asian or African ancestry, are more likely to be affected than Caucasians.

Because milk is an excellent source of the mineral nutrient calcium, it is important that lactose-intolerant people consume alternative calcium-rich foods, such as cheese, yogurt, broccoli, turnip and mustard greens, and some types of tofu. People with this condition can add a special enzyme to milk and other foods that contain lactose before consuming them. The enzyme breaks down lactose, reducing the risk of unpleasant side effects. Affected individuals, however, can often consume small amounts of lactose-containing foods without experiencing discomfort.

Fiber and Health Plants make certain carbohydrates and other substances that the human small intestine cannot digest. This material is called **dietary fiber**, or simply fiber. Soluble forms of fiber swell or dissolve in water; insoluble forms remain relatively unchanged in water. Apples, bananas, citrus fruits, carrots, kidney beans, psyllium seeds, and oats are rich sources of soluble fiber. Brown rice, wheat bran, and whole-grain wheat products are rich sources of insoluble fiber. Plants usually contain mixtures of these forms of fiber. Table 9-4

Table 9-4	Fiber-Rich Foods
Whole-grain products	Whole-wheat flour, high-fiber wheat bran cereals, psyllium,* oat bran,* oatmeal,* brown rice, whole-grain crackers, buckwheat groats, barley,* wheat germ
Dried beans and peas	Lentils, pinto beans, lima beans, kidney beans,* navy beans, split peas
Fruits	Bananas,* berries, oranges,* figs, grapefruits,* fruits with edible peels (e.g., apples,* peaches, pears)
Vegetables	Vegetables with edible peels (e.g., potatoes), brussels sprouts, broccoli, okra, cabbage, peas, turnips, spinach, sweet potatoes, carrots*

*Rich source of soluble fiber.

lists fiber-rich foods; note that none are from animal sources.

Fiber provides some important health benefits. By eating more high-fiber cereals, people may reduce their risk of developing metabolic syndrome, a condition that often precedes type 2 diabetes (McKeown et al., 2004). Soluble fiber slows the absorption of glucose from the digestive tract, which is beneficial for people who already have diabetes. Furthermore, eating a high-fiber diet, particularly one with plenty of soluble fiber, can reduce the risk of heart disease (Bazzano et al., 2003; Pereira et al., 2004). Soluble fiber lowers blood cholesterol levels by reducing cholesterol absorption in the small intestine. Elevated blood cholesterol levels are associated with increased risk of heart disease.

Can eating a high-fiber diet reduce your chances of developing certain cancers of the intestinal tract? Over the past few years, several population studies have provided conflicting findings concerning fiber intake and the risk of colon and rectal cancer. Some medical researchers have found no association between high-fiber diets and risk of these cancers, but others have determined that eating such diets lowers the risk. The results of studies involving over 550,000 Europeans and North Americans indicated that high-fiber diets protect against colon and rectal cancer (Peters et al., 2003; Bingham et al., 2003; Slattery et al., 2004). Nevertheless, more research is needed to clarify the role of dietary fiber in gastrointestinal health. Chapter 13 discusses colon and rectal cancer, including risk factors.

Eating fiber-rich foods can prevent *constipation*, infrequent or difficult bowel movements. Insoluble fiber

dietary fiber
indigestible substances produced by plants.

contributes to the formation of softer, larger stools that stimulate the muscles of the colon, producing the urge to have bowel movements more frequently. Many Americans are concerned with their bowel habits; instead of eating more fiber-rich foods, they spend millions of dollars a year on laxatives that promise "regularity." Constipation results when stools are too small and hard to stimulate the colon regularly. A constipated individual often has to strain while having bowel movements, increasing the pressure on veins in the rectum. This pressure can result in **hemorrhoids**, which are painfully swollen veins in the rectal and anal areas. Straining during bowel movements causes **diverticulosis**, a chronic condition in which the lining of the colon forms small pouches called *diverticula* (Figure 9-2). Fecal material that becomes lodged in some of these little pouches can cause serious bleeding and inflammation (*diverticulitis*). Diverticulitis can be life threatening if an inflamed pouch ruptures and spills fecal material into the abdominal cavity. Diverticulosis commonly occurs in Americans over 50 years of age, but the condition often produces no serious symptoms. In addition to eating more fiber-rich foods, you may prevent constipation by consuming adequate amounts of water. Regular exercise is often recommended to improve bowel functioning, but it is not helpful for treating chronic constipation (Meshkinpour et al., 1998). If constipation persists, or if you have intestinal pain, blood in your stools, or rec-

hemorrhoids painfully swollen veins that can form in the rectal and anal areas.

diverticulosis an intestinal disorder that occurs when the colon lining forms small pouches that protrude through the outer wall of the colon.

lipids a class of nutrients, which includes triglycerides and cholesterol, that do not dissolve in water.

triglycerides the most prevalent form of lipids in foods; often called fats or oils.

cholesterol a type of lipid found only in animals.

tal bleeding, check with a physician to rule out serious health problems.

The typical American consumes less than 20 grams of fiber a day. Medical experts think individuals should consume at least 25 grams of fiber by eating more fruits, vegetables, beans, and whole-grain cereal products each day. During processing, grains often lose their vitamin, mineral, and fiber-rich parts. White flour, for example, is a refined grain product made from wheat kernels. Compared to whole-wheat flour, white flour contains very little fiber. Replacing refined flour products, such as white bread, with whole-grain foods is an easy way to increase the fiber content of your diet. Some brown breads contain little fiber; use the nutrient label to compare the fiber content of breads.

Lipids

Dietary **lipids** include cholesterol and triglycerides. About 95% of the lipid content in foods are **triglycerides**, commonly called *fats* and *oils*. Since each cell contains triglycerides, it is not surprising that a small amount of fat is necessary for health. Compared to carbohydrates, fat is a more concentrated source of calories. The body stores energy in its fat deposits, which insulate the body from cold temperatures, give the body shape, and protect internal organs from jarring movements.

Each triglyceride has three fatty acids. Scientists classify fatty acids into three types—*saturated, monounsaturated,* and *polyunsaturated*—according to their chemical structures. Although the triglycerides found in foods contain mixtures of these three types of fatty acids, one type usually predominates. Table 9-5 indicates the amounts of lipid as well as the percentages of saturated, monounsaturated, and polyunsaturated fatty acids in a tablespoon of various fats and oils.

Animal foods generally contain more saturated fat than plant foods. Olive, peanut, and canola oils are rich sources of monounsaturated fat; corn, safflower, cottonseed, and walnut oils are high in polyunsaturated fat. Oils from palm kernels or coconuts, commonly called tropical oils, are unusual in that they are from plants but contain large amounts of saturated fat.

Animal foods also contain **cholesterol**, a compound that is structurally different from a triglyceride. In spite of its reputation for being a troublemaker, cholesterol has several very important functions in the body. Cell membranes contain cholesterol, and the body uses this lipid to produce steroid hormones, vitamin D, and *bile*, a substance needed for proper fat digestion. Even if you could avoid eating foods that contain cholesterol, your liver and small intestine would make this essential compound.

Figure 9-2 **Diverticula.** Diverticula are small pockets of the large intestine's inner lining that protrude through the outer wall of the large intestine. Diverticula can become infected and rupture.

Diverticula

Table 9-5 Fatty Acid Content of Common Fats and Oils*

Source or Type of Fat/Oil	Total Lipid/ Tablespoon (g)	% Saturated	% Monounsaturated	% Polyunsaturated
Safflower oil	14	9	12	74
Sunflower oil	14	11	19	66
Corn oil	14	13	24	59
Soybean oil	14	14	23	59
Soybean/cottonseed oil	14	18	29	48
Olive oil	14	13	73	8
Canola oil	14	7	59	29
Peanut oil	14	17	46	31
Chicken fat	13	30	45	21
Lard (pork fat)	13	39	45	12
Beef fat	13	50	42	4
Coconut oil	14	90	5	1
Hydrogenated vegetable shortening	13	25	45	26
Margarine (hard)	11	20	45	33
Butter	11	65	30	4

*Fatty acid totals are not 100% because other lipids are present in the fat or oil.

Only animals produce cholesterol; therefore, the compound is found in animal and not plant foods. Meats, whole-milk products, and egg yolks supply most of the cholesterol in the typical American diet. Table 9-6 lists cholesterol-rich foods and the amount of cholesterol in each serving.

Lipids and Health If you used to drink whole or reduced-fat (2%) milk, how did you react when you first tasted nonfat milk? Did you think the milk was watery or "thin"? The fat contained in or added to foods makes them taste rich and flavorful. Fat in food also increases the absorption of vitamins A, D, E, and K and many phytochemicals.

Although most people do not eat pure fat, they often have difficulty resisting foods that combine fat with sugar or salt, as in candy bars, cake frostings, or tortilla chips. For the average American, eating a high-fat diet often results in unwanted weight gain. Diets that supply too much saturated fat are associated with an increased risk of heart disease. High intakes of saturated fat can increase blood cholesterol levels. Although eating foods that contain cholesterol may also raise blood levels of this lipid, saturated fat tends to increase blood cholesterol levels to a greater extent.

Diets that contain high amounts of certain unsaturated fatty acids, the *omega-3 fatty acids,* may reduce the risk of heart disease and improve joint mobility of

Table 9-6 Cholesterol in Foods

Food	Serving Size	Cholesterol (mg)
Beef liver	4 oz	545
Egg	1 large	212
Yolk		212
White		0
Shrimp	3 oz	167
Turkey, ground cooked	4 oz	116
Beefsteak	4 oz	94
Ice cream (rich = 16% fat)	1 cup	90
Sherbet (2% fat)	1 cup	10
Yogurt, plain low-fat	1 cup	14
Whole milk	1 cup	33
Reduced-fat (2%) milk	1 cup	18
Nonfat milk	1 cup	4
Butter	1 tablespoon	31
Swiss cheese	1 oz	26
Cream cheese	1 oz	10
Bacon	3 slices	16

people with rheumatoid arthritis (Covington, 2004). Rich food sources of omega-3 fatty acids include canola and soybean oils, walnuts, flax seeds, and fatty fish from cold water, such as wild salmon, herring, tuna, and mackerel. Fish oil supplements, however, are not recommended because high intakes of omega-3 fatty acids can interfere too much with blood clotting, making excessive bleeding likely. Instead of taking fish oil supplements, try to include cold-water fish in your meals a couple of times each week.

Unlike the typical American (*Western*) diet, traditional food choices of Mediterranean populations supply smaller amounts of meat, fried foods, and sweets and larger amounts of plant foods, fish, and olive oil (see the inside back cover). The risk of heart disease is lower for individuals who consume the traditional Mediterranean diet ("Eating Mediterranean," 1999). The Diversity in Health essay discusses the traditional Asian diet, which also contains less animal protein and saturated fat than Western diets.

Not all foods made with vegetable oil have healthful properties. *Hydrogenation* is a food-processing technique that partially hardens the oil so it can be made into shortening and sticks of margarine. This process alters the natural chemical structure of some unsaturated fatty acids in vegetable oils, forming *trans fatty acids*. In the body, trans fatty acids behave like saturated fats, raising blood cholesterol levels (Ascherio et al., 1999). Late in 1999 the Food and Drug Administration (FDA) proposed new labeling regulations that would require food manufacturers to add information about a product's trans fat content on the label. By January 1, 2006, food manufacturers must display this information on the label. To reduce your intake of trans fatty acids, use soft or liquid margarines, eat less commercial cake frostings, and avoid baked goods and fried foods, which are often made with hydrogenated fats. Other factors besides dietary lipids contribute to heart disease; Chapter 12 discusses in depth this number one killer of Americans.

Fat Substitutes Engineered compounds such as Olestra, Oatrim, and Simplesse are used to replace some or all of the fat in certain processed foods. Olestra, for example, supplies no calories because it cannot be digested and absorbed. A one-ounce serving of regular tortilla chips supplies 130 calories and contains 6 grams of fat; the same amount of chips fried in Olestra contains 76 calories and no fat. For consumers demanding a

Diversity in Health

Asian American Food

For centuries, the Chinese culture has had a major influence on other Asian populations. These populations consume large quantities of rice, wheat noodles, and vegetables combined with eggs or a small amount of meat (usually poultry, fish, or pork). The traditional Asian diet is high in starch and fiber and usually low in fat, especially saturated fat. Stir-frying vegetables and meats in a lightly oiled wok and steaming foods are popular Oriental cooking methods that add fewer calories than deep-fat frying and preserve more vitamins and minerals than boiling. To season their foods, most Asian cooks use low-fat items such as garlic, ginger, and sauces made from mustard and soybeans.

Not all features of the traditional Asian diet are healthful. Asian meals contain little or no dairy products; therefore, the amount of calcium in these diets is usually low. Compared to Caucasians and Africans, people of Asian ancestry have a higher risk of osteoporosis. Among the residents of northern Japan, the consumption of soy sauce as well as fermented and pickled foods may contribute to the relatively high incidence of certain cancers and hyper-

tension. After immigrating to the United States, many Asians adopt Western food preferences and preparation practices. For example, American-style Chinese meals often include larger portions of meat and breaded, deep-fat fried foods.

Some people experience an adverse reaction when they eat Asian or other foods to which the flavor enhancer *monosodium glutamate (MSG)* has been added. After eating food that contains MSG, persons who are sensitive to the compound may report a "tight" sensation in the face and chest, headache, and pain and reddening of skin, especially on the face. Clinical studies, however, fail to indicate that MSG consistently causes adverse reactions in the general population (Geha et al., 2000).

You can still enjoy eating meals in Chinese, Japanese, Thai, and other Asian American restaurants by selecting menu items carefully. Choose plenty of steamed vegetables and rice or noodles to accompany the entrée. Avoid dishes containing foods that have been dipped in batter and fried, avoid or limit your intake of fried wontons and egg rolls, and do not add soy sauce to your food. If you react adversely to MSG, many cooks, upon request, will prepare your food without it.

variety of fat-free snack foods that taste good, Olestra seems to be a good fat substitute. However, eating foods made with Olestra may produce some unpleasant side effects. Additionally, the substance interferes with the absorption of certain vitamins. Food scientists are currently developing fat replacers that taste good, do not cause side effects, and are chemically stable when heated.

Setting Limits The typical American diet contains too much fat, especially saturated and trans fats from dairy products, meats, baked goods, and processed snack foods. College students and other busy people often consume more fat than is necessary by eating greasy snacks and fast foods regularly. Popular fast foods, such as cheeseburgers, pizza, fried chicken and fish, french fries, and milk shakes, contain large amounts of fat. Many fast-food restaurants, however, offer less fatty items such as roast chicken, low-fat yogurt, bean burritos, and meatless salads. Nutrition experts recommend that healthy adults reduce their total fat consumption to 20% to 35% of calories, limit their saturated fat consumption to less than 10% of calories, and limit their cholesterol intake to no more than 300 milligrams per day (USDA/USDHHS, 2005).

Currently, about one-third of the calories in the average adult American's diet are from fat. The Managing Your Health feature "Trimming the Fat from Your Diet" provides some practical ways to reduce your intake of fat.

Most food labels provide nutrition information concerning the amounts of total fat, saturated fat, and cholesterol in food products. A later section of this chapter will show you how to use this information to control the amount and type of fat in your diet.

Proteins

Your body needs **proteins** to build, maintain, and repair cells; to form structural components such as hair and nails; and to make enzymes, antibodies, and numerous hormones. Although carbohydrates and fats are its primary fuels, the body derives a small amount of energy from protein. Most foods, even plant foods, contain some protein.

Proteins consist of **amino acids**. During digestion, proteins in plant or animal foods are broken down, releasing amino acids for absorption. Human cells use about

proteins a class of nutrients that build, maintain, and repair cells.

amino acids the molecules that compose proteins.

Managing Your Health

Trimming the Fat from Your Diet

Americans are reducing the amount of fat in their diets by changing the ways they select and prepare their food. The following tips can help you trim much unnecessary and unwanted fat from your diet.

- Stir fry or steam vegetables, or eat them raw.
- Avoid breaded and fried vegetables, chicken, fish, and meats.
- Avoid sausage, bacon, and fatty luncheon meats.
- Eat boiled or baked instead of fried potatoes.
- Trim all visible fat from meats before cooking them.
- Bake, roast, boil, or broil meats instead of frying them.
- Remove and discard the skin before cooking poultry (about one-half of the fat is in the skin).
- Chill cooked chili, stews, soups, sauces, and gravies. Then, skim off the fat before reheating and serving these foods.
- Substitute nonfat milk for whole or reduced-fat (2%) milk.

- Substitute reconstituted, nonfat dry milk in recipes that use milk or cream.
- Eat low-fat or fat-free frozen yogurt, ice milk, and cheese made from nonfat milk.
- When making omelets, use only one egg yolk.
- Substitute fat-reduced cream cheese for regular cream cheese.
- Use a light coating of an oil spray when baking, instead of large amounts of fats or oils.
- Eat more chicken and fish and less beef.
- Use low-fat or fat-free salad dressings.
- Substitute plain low-fat or fat-free yogurt for sour cream in recipes.
- Skim frostings from cakes; commercial frostings are often made with hydrogenated shortening, which is 100% fat and contains trans fats.
- When eating two-crust pies, eat the filling and only one crust; discard the remaining crust.
- Reduce by one-fourth the amount of fat (margarine, butter, oils, or shortening) in recipes.

20 different amino acids to synthesize the thousands of proteins in the body. The cells can make 11 of these amino acids; the other 9 amino acids are essential and must be supplied by the diet. If the diet lacks the essential amino acids, the body is unable to grow properly or carry out vital functions.

Most animal foods contain adequate amounts of each essential amino acid; these foods are *complete* or high-quality protein sources. Plants are sources of *incomplete* or low-quality protein because they either contain insufficient amounts or lack one or more of the essential amino acids. The best plant sources of essential amino acids are soybeans, whole grains, seeds, nuts, peas, and lentils. Fruits do not contain appreciable amounts of essential amino acids.

Proteins and Health Most adult Americans consume about 14% to 18% of their calories from protein, which is about twice the amount required by the body. Animal products, especially meat, fish, poultry, and dairy foods, contribute about 70% of the protein in the American diet (Smit et al., 1999). Although eating large amounts of protein does not harm most healthy individuals, generous portions of animal foods contribute excessive amounts of saturated fat to the diet. Diets that contain high amounts of saturated fat are associated with increased risk of heart disease, the number one killer of Americans.

Many athletes and bodybuilders think it is necessary to consume large quantities of animal foods and protein supplements to increase their muscle mass. This practice does not build bigger muscles; instead, the body must metabolize the extra amino acids for energy or convert them into body fat. Additionally, the kidneys need more water to eliminate the excess amino acid by-products. The most effective way to enhance muscle mass is to combine a nutritionally adequate diet with a program of muscle-strengthening exercises.

Animal foods are among the most expensive items on the typical American's grocery list. You can reduce your food costs and decrease your saturated fat intake by substituting certain plant foods for meat and other animal protein sources. The following section discusses vegetarianism, a way to reduce your animal protein intake without sacrificing the nutritional adequacy of your diet.

Vegetarianism A growing number of Americans are consuming plant-based, or *vegetarian*, diets that contain little or no animal foods. Many people associate meat with protein, but processed soybean foods, such as tofu, soymilk, and soy nut butter; various beans, peas, and lentils; nuts; seeds; and foods made from cereal grains (for example, wheat, and oats) are among the best sources of protein from plants.

There are several types of vegetarian diets. The *vegan*, or total vegetarian, diet consists of plant foods only. Other vegetarian diets include some animal foods. For example, the *lacto-vegetarian* diet contains dairy products, and the *lacto-ovo-vegetarian* diet includes eggs as well as dairy products. Some people who eat fish or poultry still call themselves vegetarians because they do not eat *red* meats. There are so many different plant-based diets, it is difficult to estimate the number of Americans practicing some form of vegetarianism.

Are vegetarian diets nutritious? Plant-based diets may promote good health because they contain more fiber, antioxidants, and phytochemicals and less saturated fat and cholesterol than the traditional meat-rich Western diet. Generally, the nutritional adequacy of a vegetarian diet varies according to the degree of its dietary restrictions. Animal foods are rich sources of essential amino acids as well as certain minerals and vitamins. Plant foods, on the other hand, generally lack one or more essential amino acids. In the past, nutrition experts advised vegans to consume mixtures of plant foods that supplied all the essential amino acids in one meal, because it was believed the body did not save essential amino acids and was unable to make proteins unless all of them were available at one time. Now it is known that the body can conserve essential amino acids after a meal or snack and use them for protein production later in the day. Although it is not necessary to combine plant foods to obtain the proper mix of amino acids, combinations such as peanut butter on toast or red beans and rice make vegetarian meals nutritious, inexpensive, and easy to prepare. Most vegetarians can obtain adequate amounts of essential amino acids and other nutrients by eating a variety of plant foods, consuming dairy products, and taking a multiple vitamin/mineral supplement.

Thus, with careful planning, most plant-based diets can be nutritionally adequate (American Dietetic Association, 1997). If you are interested in learning specific details about vegetarian cookery and menu planning, you can obtain this information from hospital dietitians or University Outreach Extension nutritionists in your area.

Food Allergies A 3-year-old child develops *hives*—small, itchy, swollen, reddened areas on her skin—soon after she eats eggs. Her older brother must avoid peanuts and foods that may contain peanuts because he can experience *shock*, a drop in blood pressure and loss of consciousness that can be deadly if not treated immediately. These reactions are the result of food allergies, the immune system's inappropriate response to harmless proteins (allergens) in certain foods. In the United States, an estimated 8% of children and 2% of adults are allergic to one or more foods (American Academy of Allergy, Asthma, and Immunology, 2003). Proteins in cows' milk, eggs, peanuts, tree nuts (such as cashews and walnuts), wheat, soybeans, fish, and shellfish are most likely to cause allergic reactions in susceptible people.

Hives are the most common sign of food allergy; other signs include *eczema*, a scaly skin rash; asthma symptoms, such as wheezing and difficulty breathing; and vomiting and diarrhea. Shock (anaphylaxis) occurs when the entire body reacts to the allergen. As mentioned earlier, shock can be fatal.

If you think you or someone you know has a food allergy, consult an allergist/immunologist, a physician who specializes in the diagnosis and treatment of allergies. Alternative medical procedures to diagnose allergies, such as hair analysis, cytotoxic or electrodermal testing, and kinesiology, are not useful (Niggemann & Gruber, 2004). In the case of a true food allergy, the best treatment is to avoid the offending food. Additionally, the allergic person should be prepared to treat shock by taking antihistamines or administering injectable epinephrine, a naturally produced substance that raises blood pressure. Parents of children with food allergies must read labels carefully to check ingredients for allergens. They should inform their children's adult caretakers, teachers, and the parents of their children's friends about the allergy and the importance of not offering foods that may contain allergens to their children. Although most children outgrow milk, egg, and wheat allergies, they are likely to remain allergic to peanuts, tree nuts, fish, and shellfish throughout their lives. Contact with substances other than foods can also produce allergies. Chapter 14 discusses the immune system, including the allergic response.

Healthy Living Practices

- To reduce your risk of obesity, heart disease, type 2 diabetes, and certain digestive tract disorders, consume at least 25 grams of fiber each day by eating more fruits, vegetables, beans, and whole-grain cereal products.
- To lower your risk of diabetes and heart disease, reduce your fat intake to less than 20% to 35% of your daily calories, limit your intake of saturated fat to less than 10% of daily calories, and reduce your cholesterol intake to 300 or fewer milligrams per day.

- You can reduce the amount of cholesterol and saturated and trans fat in your diet by consuming low-fat yogurt and nonfat milk and by eating less cheese, fatty meat, fried food, and fat-laden bakery goods and snack foods.
- Many fast foods are high in fat. If you eat at fast-food restaurants regularly, reduce your intake of fried foods by selecting salads or grilled chicken or fish items.
- If you eat large amounts of red meat and other animal foods, consider eating less of it and consuming more beans, nuts, and whole-grain cereals instead.

■ Non-Energy-Supplying Nutrients

Vitamins

The human body needs **vitamins** to regulate growth; release energy from carbohydrates, fats, and proteins; and maintain tissues. Although many vitamins participate in the chemical reactions that release energy, they do not provide calories.

Scientists classify vitamins according to their ability to dissolve in water or fat. Vitamin C and the eight B vitamins are water-soluble; vitamins A, D, E, and K are fat-soluble. The body does not store most water-soluble vitamins to any appreciable extent, whereas fat-soluble vitamins are stored in the liver and body fat and can accumulate. Table 9-7 lists most of the vitamins as well as their major roles in the body and rich food sources.

vitamins a class of nutrients that participates in a variety of chemical reactions, such as energy production, growth regulation, and tissue maintenance.

Compared to the energy-supplying nutrients and water, the body requires very small amounts of vitamins. Diets that include a wide variety of foods can meet the vitamin needs of healthy individuals. Some persons, however, take nutrient supplements that provide several times the recommended levels of vitamins to treat or prevent illness. More of a nutrient is not necessarily better. Cells use limited amounts of each vitamin daily. In many instances, excessive amounts of these nutrients accumulate in the body and cause harmful side effects. Vitamins A, D, B_6, and niacin are very toxic when taken in large doses. Table 9-7 provides information concerning the signs and symptoms of vitamin toxicity disorders.

Table 9-7 | Major Vitamins

Vitamin	Major Functions	Rich Food Sources	Deficiency Signs/Symptoms	Toxicity Signs/Symptoms
A and provitamin A (beta-carotene)	Vision in dim light, growth, reproduction, maintains immune system and skin, antioxidant	Liver, milk, dark green and leafy vegetables; carrot, sweet potato, mango, oatmeal, broccoli, apricot, peach, and romaine lettuce	Poor vision in dim light, dry skin, blindness, poor growth, respiratory infections	Intestinal upset, liver damage, hair loss, headache, birth defects, death (beta-carotene is less toxic than A)
D	Bone and tooth development and growth; immune system functioning	Few good food sources other than eggs, fortified milk, and orange juice	Weak, deformed bones (rickets)	Growth failure, loss of appetite, weight loss, death
E	Antioxidant: protects cell membranes	Vegetable oils, whole grains, wheat germ, sunflower seeds, almonds	Anemia (rarely occurs)	Intestinal upsets, bleeding problems
C	Scar formation and maintenance, immune system functioning, antioxidant	Citrus fruits, berries, potatoes, broccoli, peppers, cabbage, tomatoes, fortified fruit drinks	Frequent infections, bleeding gums, bruises, poor wound healing, depression (scurvy)	Diarrhea, nosebleeds, headache, weakness, kidney stones, excess iron absorption and storage
Thiamin	Energy metabolism	Pork, liver, nuts, dried beans and peas, whole-grain and enriched breads and cereals	Heart failure, mental confusion, depression, paralysis (beriberi)	No toxicity has been reported
Riboflavin	Energy metabolism	Milk and yogurt, eggs and poultry, meat, liver, whole-grain and enriched breads and cereals	Enlarged, purple tongue; fatigue; oily skin; cracks in the corners of the mouth	No toxicity has been reported
Niacin	Energy metabolism	Protein-rich foods, peanut butter, whole-grain and enriched breads and cereals	Skin rash, diarrhea, weakness, dementia, death (pellagra)	Painful skin flushing, intestinal upsets, liver damage
Vitamin B_6	Protein and fat metabolism	Liver, oatmeal, bananas, meat, fish, poultry, whole grains, fortified cereals	Anemia, skin rash, irritability, elevated homocysteine levels	Weakness, depression, permanent nerve damage
Folate (folic acid)	DNA production	Leafy vegetables, oranges, nuts, liver, enriched breads and cereals	Anemia, depression, spina bifida in developing embryo, elevated homocysteine levels	Hides signs of B_{12} deficiency; may cause allergic response
B_{12}	DNA production	Animal products	Pernicious anemia, fatigue, paralysis, elevated homocysteine levels	No toxicity has been reported

Antioxidants The chemical structures of certain compounds, particularly polyunsaturated fatty acids, make them vulnerable to damage by free radicals. Free radical formation produces chemical changes in cells that may contribute to the development of cardiovascular disease (diseases of the heart and blood vessels), certain cancers, degenerative changes in the eye, and other chronic health conditions.

Many foods contain antioxidants that can protect cells by preventing or reducing the formation of free radicals. These antioxidants include vitamins E and C, and a variety of phytochemicals such as beta-carotene, a yellow pigment in plants that the body converts to vitamin A. Table 9-2 lists some phytochemicals and their major food sources; Table 9-8 lists fruits and vegetables with high antioxidant activity.

Table 9-8

Table 9-8 Rich Fruit and Vegetable Sources of Antioxidants*

Fruits	Vegetables
Prunes	Kale
Raisins	Spinach
Blueberries	Brussels sprouts
Blackberries	Alfalfa sprouts
Strawberries	Broccoli florets
Raspberries	Beets
Plums	Red bell peppers
Oranges	Onions
Red grapes	Corn
Cherries	Eggplant

*The fruits and vegetables in the table are ranked according to their score on the ORAC (Oxygen Radical Absorbance Capacity) assay.

Source: Antioxidant foods: Foods that score high in antioxidant assay ORAC (Oxygen Radical Absorbance Capacity). (1999). *Food and Nutrition Research Briefs.* U.S. Department of Agricultural Research Service. www.ars.usda.gov/is/np/fnrb/.

Since the 1980s, scientists have been investigating the possible risks and benefits of eating diets rich in antioxidants or taking antioxidant supplements. Although there is no strong scientific data to support the popular belief that vitamin C prevents colds, vitamins C and E may reduce the risk of developing heart disease, certain cancers (Hercberg et al., 1999), and Alzheimer's disease (Engelhart et al., 2004).

Should you take large doses of vitamins, especially antioxidant vitamins, to prevent disease? Nutrition experts are divided over the issue of antioxidant vitamin supplementation. The cells in your body make antioxidants. Some scientists think modern humans are exposed to much higher levels of environmental hazards, such as air pollution and pesticide residues, than their ancestors. These conditions may increase the body's need for antioxidants beyond the amounts that are made or can be obtained from food, making supplementation necessary. Other scientists think plant foods are the best source of antioxidants. Unlike nutrient supplements, plant foods contain mixtures of vitamins and phytochemicals that collectively may provide healthful benefits (Polidori, 2003). Taking large doses of antioxidant vitamins may have harmful side effects, including promoting the growth of cancer cells (Hercberg et al., 1999).

Many adult Americans take high-dose vitamin supplements; vitamin C, vitamin E, and the B vitamins are the most popular (Murphy et al., 2002; Radimer et al., 2004). Unless medically necessary, taking these supplements is an economically wasteful and risky practice. By eating a variety of whole-grain products and fruits and vegetables daily, you are less likely to encounter toxicity problems because these foods naturally supply vitamins in smaller quantities.

Minerals

Minerals are a group of elements such as calcium, iron, and sodium that can function as free atoms or as parts of *chemical* compounds. Minerals have a wide variety of roles in the body. Many mineral elements such as magnesium regulate chemical reactions; others are structural components contained in certain organic molecules, like the calcium in bones. The body needs very small amounts of minerals, compared to the energy-supplying nutrients and water. Excesses of any mineral can create imbalances with other minerals or can be toxic.

Table 9-9 lists some essential minerals, describes their major roles, and identifies foods that contain high amounts of these substances. The following section provides information about calcium and iron, two minerals that have considerable health importance.

Calcium Calcium is the most plentiful mineral in the body. You may be aware that calcium is necessary for the development of strong bones and teeth, but this mineral has other important roles as well, such as regulating blood pressure and participating in muscular movements. The body carefully maintains the level of calcium in the blood within a specific range. When the level is too high, the bones can remove and store the excess. If the amount of calcium in the blood begins to drop below normal levels, the bones release some of the mineral from storage, returning the level to normal.

As it adjusts to the demands of bearing the body's weight, bone tissue undergoes a continual process of being built, torn down, and rebuilt. After about 40 years of age, the bones of most people begin to break down at a faster rate than they rebuild. As bones gradually lose mineral density, they become weak and brittle. Fragile bones break easily, and sometimes shatter due to being unable to support the body. Although any bone can be affected, bones in the hip, spine, and wrist are most likely to break. This condition, **osteoporosis**, threatens the health of millions of aging Americans, especially menopausal women. One of every two women and one in eight men over 50 years of age will have a fracture that is the result of osteoporosis (National Institutes of Health [NIH], 2002). Men usually have

minerals a class of inorganic nutrients that includes several elements, such as iron, calcium, and zinc, that have a wide variety of functions in the body.

osteoporosis an age-related condition in which bones lose density, becoming weak and breaking easily.

Table 9-9 Some Essential Minerals

Mineral	Roles	Rich Food Sources	Deficiency Signs/Symptoms	Toxicity Signs/Symptoms
Calcium	Builds and maintains bones and teeth, regulates muscle and nerve function, regulates blood pressure and blood clotting	Milk products; fortified orange juice, tofu, and soy milk; fish with edible small bones such as sardines and salmon; broccoli; hard water	Poor bone growth, weak bones, muscle spasms, convulsions	Kidney stones, calcium deposits in organs, mineral imbalances
Potassium	Maintains fluid balance, necessary for nerve function	Whole grains, fruits, and vegetables, yogurt, milk	Muscular weakness, confusion, death	Heart failure
Sodium	Maintains fluid balance, necessary for nerve function	Salt, soy sauce, luncheon meats, processed cheeses, pickled foods, snack foods, canned and dried soups	Muscle cramping, headache, confusion, coma	Hypertension
Magnesium	Regulation of enzyme activity, necessary for nerve function	Green leafy vegetables, nuts, whole grains, peanut butter	Loss of appetite, muscular weakness, convulsions, confusion, death	Rare
Zinc	Component of many enzymes and the hormone insulin, maintains immune function, necessary for sexual maturation and reproduction	Meats, fish, poultry, whole grains, vegetables	Poor growth, failure to mature sexually, improper healing of wounds	Mineral imbalances, gastrointestinal upsets, anemia, heart disease
Selenium	Component of a group of antioxidant enzymes, immune system function	Seafood, liver, and vegetables and grains grown in selenium-rich soil	May increase risk of heart disease and certain cancers	Hair and nail loss
Iron	Oxygen transport involved in the release of energy	Clams, oysters, liver, red meats, and enriched breads and cereals	Fatigue, weakness, iron-deficiency anemia	Iron poisoning, nausea, vomiting, diarrhea, death

denser bones than women, which may explain why most aging men are not affected by osteoporosis to the same extent as aging women.

Fractures are associated with an increased risk of permanent disability or death, particularly if the fracture immobilizes the person; immobility increases the likelihood that fatal blood clots or pneumonia will develop. A painful and disabling condition known as "dowager's hump" can occur when bones in the upper spine are so weak that they experience small compression fractures over time while trying to support the weight of the skull. As these bones heal into wedge shapes, the upper spine assumes an abnormal curvature (Figure 9-3). As a result, people with spinal osteoporosis often "shrink"—they lose some of their height.

As one ages, a calcium-rich diet and weight-bearing physical activity help build and maintain strong bones. After menopause, however, such practices may not be enough to prevent osteoporosis or slow its progress. Within the first 5 to 10 years after menopause, even healthy women are susceptible to losing a large percentage of their bone mass. Why?

The hormone *estrogen* stimulates bones to maintain their mass and retain calcium. A sign of normal estrogen production is regular menstrual cycles. A woman has reached *menopause* when her estrogen levels drop dramatically and her menstrual cycles have ceased. As women approach this time of life, those who have a history of regular menstrual cycles are more likely to maintain their bone mass than those who had irregular or absent menstrual cycles.

Besides being a postmenopausal woman, other characteristics increase one's risk of osteoporosis. The condition may be inherited, and members of certain racial groups are more susceptible to osteoporosis than others. African Americans tend to have larger bone masses that afford some protection against osteoporosis. On the other hand, slender, small-boned people of European

Figure 9-3 **Dowager's Hump.** In people with osteoporosis, the bones in the upper spine develop small compression fractures. These bones heal into wedge shapes, and the upper spine assumes a deformed, curved shape known as "dowager's hump."

and Asian ancestry are more likely than people with large bones to develop osteoporosis.

Certain lifestyle choices can increase a person's risk of osteoporosis. Young people with low-calcium diets are likely to have less dense bones that are susceptible to osteoporosis as they grow older. Cigarette smoking and alcohol consumption can accelerate bone loss. Furthermore, young women who exercise excessively may disrupt their body's normal estrogen production and menstrual cycles. This reduction in estrogen levels can lead to premature bone loss.

Special x rays are used to diagnose bone loss clinically. To treat menopausal women who are at risk of osteoporosis, physicians often prescribe hormone replacement therapy, that is, synthetic hormones that contain estrogen or a combination of estrogen and progesterone. Nonhormonal treatments are available also. Women who are approaching menopause should consult their physicians about their risks of developing osteoporosis and their treatment options.

Most medical experts recommend that young men and women adopt behaviors that maximize their bone mass. If you are concerned about your risk of developing osteoporosis, consume foods that supply calcium such as those shown in Figure 9-4 . If you do not consume dairy products or foods fortified with calcium, ask your physician about alternative ways to obtain this mineral, such as calcium-containing supplements or antacids. In addition to calcium, vitamin D and the mineral magnesium are important for bone health. Adopting healthful lifestyles, such as refraining from smoking, reducing alcohol consumption, and engaging in physical activities that place stress on your bones, such as walking, weight lifting, or jogging, can help maintain your skeleton's structural integrity.

Osteoporosis can occur at any age. If you think your risk of developing this condition is high, ask your doctor to perform a bone density test. By treating osteoporosis in its early stages, substantial bone loss can be prevented.

Iron Most of the body's iron is found in the *hemoglobin* molecules within the red blood cells. Hemoglobin combines with oxygen in the lungs and transports it to cells throughout the body. Oxygen is necessary to release the energy stored in glucose.

Anemia results when the body produces abnormal red blood cells. In cases of iron-deficiency anemia, the bone marrow forms red blood cells that are smaller and contain less hemoglobin than normal cells. Without sufficient hemoglobin, the red blood cells carry less oxygen than usual as they circulate. Anemic individuals often report feeling tired because their cells are unable to obtain adequate amounts of energy.

Iron deficiency is one of the most prevalent nutritional disorders in the United States. Many individuals, especially premenopausal women, are at risk of becoming iron deficient because they do not consume enough iron-rich food to replace the iron lost each month in menstrual blood. Individuals undergoing

Figure 9-4 **Calcium-Rich Foods.** Some of the richest food sources of calcium are low-fat milk and yogurt, and greens. Although most cheeses are high in fat, they are good sources of calcium.

rapid growth, such as infants, children, teenagers, and pregnant women, have high needs for iron and are at risk of iron deficiency. If untreated, severe iron deficiency can cause iron-deficiency anemia. This type of anemia often occurs in people who lose a lot of blood.

To ensure adequate iron intake, you can eat the iron-rich foods listed in Table 9-9. Normally, the small intestine does not absorb much of the iron in foods, especially the iron in plants. You can enhance the absorption of plant sources of iron by eating them with meat or vitamin C–rich foods. In addition to eating more foods that contain iron, people with iron-deficiency anemia may need to take iron supplements.

Annually, thousands of young children unintentionally poison themselves, a few of them fatally, after ingesting toxic amounts of iron-containing supplements. Many of these cases involve unsupervised young children who take overdoses of flavored vitamin/mineral supplements, thinking they are candy. To prevent such tragedies, store nutrient and other dietary supplements like other medications, making them inaccessible to children.

As many as 1 in 250 Americans has a genetic condition that increases the intestinal absorption of dietary iron (Brandhagen et al., 2002). The iron accumulates in their organs and reaches toxic levels by the time they are middle-aged. These people are often unaware that they have the potentially fatal condition called *hemochromatosis*, or iron overload, until it causes serious conditions such as diabetes, liver damage, and heart disease. A simple blood test can detect this treatable disorder. People with hemochromatosis should not take supplements that contain iron and should limit their intake of iron-rich foods.

Water

Water is essential for life on earth. You can survive weeks, months, and even years without one of the other nutrients, but you cannot survive for more than a few days without water. Water has many functions in the body: dissolving and transporting materials, eliminating wastes, lubricating joints, and participating in numerous chemical reactions.

About 60% of an adult's body is water. To function properly, the body maintains its fluid levels within specific limits, generally by increasing or decreasing urine production. Although it carefully conserves water, the body loses water when one perspires, urinates, exhales, and defecates. Drinking plain water and fluids such as milk, juices, and soft drinks replenishes the body's water. Most foods, especially fruits and vegetables, also supply water.

Advertisements often promote beer as a thirst quencher; however, drinking alcoholic beverages does not replace body water. Alcohol acts as a *diuretic*, a compound that increases urinary losses of water. Caffeine is also a diuretic.

According to a report issued by an expert panel of the National Institute of Medicine, the daily recommended amounts of water from food and beverages are about 16 cups for men and 11 cups for women (Food and Nutrition Board [FNB], 2004). In general, Americans' water intake is adequate. *Dehydration* occurs when the normal level of body water declines, and the affected individual does not consume replenishing fluids. The symptoms of dehydration include weakness, confusion, and irritability. During prolonged fevers or bouts of diarrhea or vomiting, the body can lose substantial amounts of water, causing dehydration. These conditions cause the loss of minerals such as sodium and potassium as well. If untreated, severe dehydration is usually fatal. Chapter 11 provides more information about dehydration and heat-related illnesses.

Healthy people can become dehydrated while working or exercising in hot conditions. Is it helpful to consume sports drinks under these situations? In addition to water and glucose, sports drinks contain small amounts of the minerals sodium and potassium; therefore, these beverages may be beneficial for individuals engaging in prolonged, strenuous physical activities in which considerable sweating occurs. Most people, however, can maintain their fluid and mineral balance by eating a variety of foods and by drinking water before and during the activity.

Healthy Living Practices

- To obtain all of the vitamins and minerals you need, eat a wide variety of foods each day; include whole grains, dairy products, fruits, and vegetables.
- Store dietary supplements like other medications, making them inaccessible to children.
- If you are hot or exercising heavily, to prevent dehydration, drink plenty of water and other beverages that do not contain caffeine or alcohol.
- To increase the likelihood that you will maintain your bone mass as you age, consume adequate amounts of calcium-rich foods, drink less alcohol, do not smoke, and engage in weight-bearing exercise regularly.

Planning a Nutritious Diet

The Keys to a Nutritious Diet

When you eat a milk-chocolate candy bar or some french-fried potatoes, you probably know that these foods contain carbohydrate and fat, but you may be surprised to learn that they also supply some protein, water, and even vitamins and minerals. Most foods are mixtures of nutrients that contain relatively large quantities of water, carbohydrate, fat, or protein, with much smaller quantities of vitamins and minerals. Candy bars and french fries are commonly called "junk" foods because they contain considerable calories from fat and sugar. Dietitians, however, generally refer to such foods as "empty-calorie" rather than junk foods.

A nutritious diet has two key features: nutrient adequacy and nutrient balance. The foods in a nutritionally adequate and balanced diet contain all essential nutrients in the proper proportions. By selecting a wide variety of foods, you can usually obtain the essential nutrients. Many people upset the nutritional balance of their diets by consuming more food than they need, by making poor food choices, or by taking massive doses of nutrient supplements. Eating too much food can make one overweight; eating too much saturated fat may clog one's arteries, ingesting too many supplements can cause nutrient toxicity disorders. "Everything in moderation" is the best approach to planning nutritionally adequate and well-balanced diets.

How much of each nutrient do you need for optimal health? How can you be certain that your diet is nutritionally adequate? The following information provides answers to these questions.

Nutrient Requirements and Recommendations

A **nutrient requirement** can be defined as the minimum amount that prevents an average person from developing the nutrient's deficiency disease. A required level of a nutrient, however, is not necessarily an optimal amount. By obtaining only the required levels of most vitamins, for example, the body does not have amounts to store in various tissues. The body relies on its nutrient reserves if nutritious food becomes unavailable. Thus, nutrition experts recommend that people consume more than just the required amounts of many nutrients.

To determine whether a diet supplies amounts of certain nutrients that can prevent deficiency diseases, nutritionists now use a complex set of standards called the **Dietary Reference Intakes (DRIs)**. The DRIs are com-posed of four different recommendations for nutrient intake levels, including the *Recommended Dietary Allowances (RDAs)*, which at one time were the only standards for planning nutritious diets and analyzing the nutritional adequacy of diets. At this point, many nutrients do not have a complete set of DRIs, so their RDAs are still used. Appendix C provides a table of RDAs or other DRI values for several vitamins and minerals.

To establish the RDA for a nutrient, scientists take the required level and add a certain amount to provide a margin of safety. For example, the current RDA for vitamin C is 90 milligrams for men and 75 milligrams for women (nonsmokers). The average person, however, requires only about 8 to 10 milligrams of vitamin C each day to prevent scurvy, the vitamin's deficiency disease. Therefore, most people will not develop scurvy even if their intake does not meet 100% of the RDA.

You can evaluate the nutritional adequacy of your diet by using the RDAs or other DRI values. Complete the activity "Assessing the Nutritional Quality of Your Diet" in the student workbook. If your usual intake of a nutrient is between 75% and 100% of the RDA, you probably are not at risk of developing that nutrient's deficiency disease. If you need to boost your intake of one or more nutrients, you can identify foods that are rich sources of the nutrient by using food composition tables, such as those at the "healthyliving" Web site for this section of the chapter, and eat more of these foods.

nutrient requirement the minimum amount of a nutrient that prevents that nutrient's deficiency disease.

Dietary Reference Intakes (DRIs) a new set of standards for evaluating the nutritional quality of diets.

The Healthy Eating Pyramid

In addition to eating a nutritionally adequate diet, exercising regularly is crucial for optimal health. The recommendations of the Healthy Eating Pyramid, shown in Figure 9-5 , incorporate recent scientific evidence concerning the role of diet and exercise in disease. Note that this food guide recommends a small amount of alcohol because of its effects on heart health. However many people, such as pregnant women, should not drink alcohol.

The Dietary Guidelines

Every 5 years the U.S. Department of Agriculture (USDA) and the Department of Health and Human Services issue the *Dietary Guidelines for Americans*, a list of general recommendations that focus attention on the association between diet and chronic diseases, such as type 2 diabetes and cardiovascular disease. These guidelines provide basic advice concerning

Figure 9-5 The Healthy Eating Pyramid.
The Healthy Eating Pyramid incorporates recent medical evidence concerning the role of diet in disease. Plant oils and foods rich in fiber and complex carbohydrates form the foundation of the pyramid; foods high in animal fat and low in fiber form its small top.
Source: Willett, W. C. (2001). *Eat, drink, and Be Healthy*. New York: Simon and Schuster.

lifestyle behaviors that relate to nutritional health, such as choosing nutrient-dense foods, being more physically active, and following food safety practices (see Table 9-10). The next section discusses the MyPyramid Plan that incorporates recommendations from the latest edition of the *Dietary Guidelines* into a diet planning tool.

Table 9-10 Key Recommendations from *Dietary Guidelines for Americans 2005*

1. Manage your weight at a healthy level.
2. Be physically active daily.
3. Consume a nutritionally adequate diet.
4. Consume fruits, vegetables, whole grains, and fat-free or low-fat dairy foods.
5. Keep foods safe to eat.
6. Consume 20% to 35% of calories from fat and limit your cholesterol intake to 300 mg daily.
7. Consume fiber-rich foods and limit your intake of sugary foods.
8. Restrict salt intake to less than 1 teaspoon daily.
9. If you drink alcohol, do so in moderation. Avoid alcohol if you are pregnant, breastfeeding, under 21 years of age, driving, or operating other machinery.

Source: Retrieved January 12, 2005, from http://www.healthierus.gov/dietaryguidelines/.

The MyPyramid Plan

In spring 2005, the USDA replaced the Food Guide Pyramid with the MyPyramid Plan, a more specific guide for planning healthful diets. The MyPyramid Plan has 6 food groups, each of which is depicted by a different colored band. Orange, green, red, yellow, blue, and purple represent the grain, vegetables, fruits, oils and discretionary calories, milk, and meat and beans groups, respectively (Figure 9-6). The left side of the pyramid has a stylized human figure climbing steps to show the need for daily physical activity.

The MyPyramid Plan suggests amounts of foods to include in meals and snacks from the food groups to meet recommended nutrient intakes at 12 different calorie levels, ranging from 1,000 to 3,200 calories/day. Thus, a person can use this guide to plan menus that meet his or her energy and nutrient needs. For example, a very physically active 22-year-old male may need 3,000 calories/day, whereas his physically inactive 20-year-old female friend might only need 1,600 calories/day. Appendix D provides the 12 food intake patterns as well as sample menus for a 2,000-calorie/day food pattern.

To obtain more information about the MyPyramid Plan, access the USDA's interactive Web site (www.MyPyramid.gov). By clicking on each of the color-coded stripes, you will learn more about the foods in each group. If you click on the figure that is climbing the steps, you will see that the Plan recommends engaging in at least 30 minutes of physical activity, in addition to one's regular activities, most days of the week. If you fill in the box that requests your age, gender, and daily physical activity level, the program will suggest specific amounts of foods that you should eat daily to have a nutritious diet.

Discretionary Calories Each of the MyPyramid Plan's 12 dietary patterns includes allowances for oils and *discretionary calories*, extra calories that remain after a person eats the recommended amounts of foods in each food group. Most physically inactive people have only a small number of discretionary calories to use for eating extra foods, generally between 100 and 300 calories daily. People can "spend" these calories by eating additional nutrient-dense low-fat foods from the other food groups, but they often consume fatty meats, high-fat cheeses, and empty-calorie foods such as sweets and alcoholic drinks instead. Diets that contain too much high-fat and empty-calorie foods may contribute to excess body fat, heart disease, cancer, and alcoholism. Additionally, these items can displace more nutrient-dense foods from your diet (Kant, 2000). Consuming a reasonable amount of empty-calorie foods may be acceptable, if your diet is nutritionally adequate and you are physically active and need the extra calories to fuel physical activity. The workbook includes an activity that enables you to use the MyPyramid Plan to evaluate the nutritional adequacy of your daily food choices.

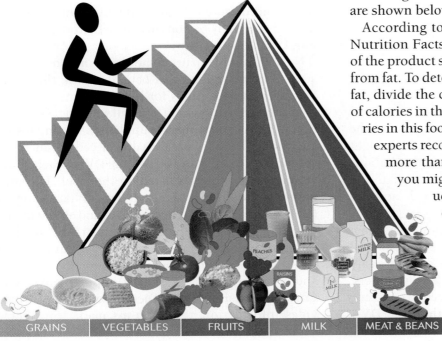

Figure 9-6 **The MyPyramid Plan.** The USDA's MyPyramid Plan is a more specific tool for planning healthful diets than the original Food Guide Pyramid. (The yellow band depicts Oils.)

GRAINS   VEGETABLES   FRUITS   MILK   MEAT & BEANS

Using Nutritional Labeling

The FDA requires nearly every packaged food to have nutritional labeling. Consumers can use food labeling to determine and compare the nutritional value of most packaged foods. **Figure 9-7** illustrates the Nutrition Facts portion of a food label.

Many consumers want to know how many grams of fat and calories are in a serving of food. This information appears at the top of the Nutrition Facts label. People can also monitor the amounts of cholesterol, sodium, and fiber in packaged foods. The Nutrition Facts label indicates these amounts by weight and as percentages of established nutrient labeling standards called the Daily Values (DVs).

Health officials at the FDA used various sources of nutritional information to determine the DVs for many nutrients and for fiber. As you can see in Figure 9-7, the lower part of the Nutrition Facts label shows two sets of DVs. One set of DVs is for people who consume 2,000 calories each day; the other set is for those who consume 2,500 calories daily. The DVs for total fat, saturated fat, cholesterol, and sodium are maximum amounts. Most Americans should keep their daily intake of these nutrients *below* these amounts.

Specific information concerning the nutritional content per serving of the food product appears on the upper half of the label. In addition to showing amounts of fat, saturated fat, cholesterol, sodium, total carbohydrate, fiber, sugar, and protein by weight, the Nutrition Facts label displays most of this information as percentages of the DVs for a 2,000-calorie diet. Percentages of the DVs for key vitamins and minerals are shown below the second bold line.

According to the information near the top of the Nutrition Facts label shown in Figure 9-7, a serving of the product supplies 360 calories, 120 of which are from fat. To determine the percentage of calories from fat, divide the calories from fat (120) by the number of calories in the serving (360). One-third of the calories in this food (33%) are from fat. Since most health experts recommend that healthy Americans eat no more than 35% of their total calories from fat, you might decide to purchase other food products that contain similar percentages of calories from fat.

Nutrition Facts

Serving size 10 1/2 oz (298 g)
Servings per Container 2

Amount per serving

Calories 360	Calories from Fat 120

	% Daily Value*
Total Fat 13 g	20%
Saturated Fat 8 g	40%
Trans Fat 0 g	
Cholesterol 60 mg	20%
Sodium 800 mg	33%
Total Carbohydrate 37 g	12%
Dietary Fiber 0 g	
Sugars 10 g	
Protein 24 g	

Vitamin A 10%	•	Vitamin C 15%	• Iron 6%

*Percent Daily Values are based on a 2,000-calorie diet. Your daily values may be higher or lower depending on your calorie needs.

	Calories	2,000	2,500
Total Fat	Less than	65 g	80 g
Sat Fat	Less than	20 g	25 g
Cholesterol	Less than	300 mg	300 mg
Sodium	Less than	2,400 mg	2,400 mg
Total Carbohydrate		300 g	375 g
Dietary Fiber		25 g	30 g

Calories per gram: Fat 9 • Carbohydrate 4 • Protein 4

Figure 9-7 **Nutrition Facts.** Most packaged foods have nutrient facts on their labels. People can use this information to evaluate the nutritional quality of their food.

Another approach to controlling your fat intake is to eat foods with a variety of fat contents, but your intake should not exceed 65 grams of fat per day, the DV for a 2,000-calorie diet. For example, you might eat a 1-oz. serving of corn chips that contains 6 grams of fat and supplies 40% of its calories from fat. The other foods eaten on this day should provide no more than 59 grams of fat.

Not everyone thinks that the Nutrition Facts label is easy to use or helpful. Since the percentage of total calories from fat is not listed, people cannot easily compare the fat content of packaged food products. Additionally, many adult Americans need to consume lower amounts of calories and fat than the DVs. Furthermore, most people eat a variety of foods, some of which is fresh, or prepared in restaurants. As a result, these people will probably underestimate the amounts of calories and nutrients in their diet if they rely only on the information provided by food labels.

Do You Need Vitamin or Mineral Supplements?

Do you buy dietary supplements such as the ones listed in Table 9-11 ? If your answer is yes, why do you take them? Millions of Americans purchase dietary supplements, especially individual vitamin pills and multiple vitamin-mineral pills that contain mixtures of vitamins and minerals. According to the 2000 National Health Interview Survey, approximately one-third of adult Americans take a vitamin or mineral supplement or both (Millen et al., 2004). In 2002, sales of dietary supplements, which include vitamin and mineral pills, herbal products, and certain hormones, were estimated to be almost $19 billion in the United States (Beales, 2004).

Many people take vitamin and mineral supplements to reduce the risk of heart disease, osteoporosis, and other serious chronic diseases. By carefully selecting a variety of foods and eating recommended amounts from the major food groups, healthy adults should be able to obtain enough nutrients without supplementation. Some people, however, need to supplement their diets with certain nutrients. Pregnant and breastfeeding women need more iron, calcium, and folic acid than what is available in foods. Some vegetarians need more calcium, iron, zinc, and vitamins B_{12} and D. Elderly persons may benefit from extra vitamin D and B_{12}.

Nutrient supplements do not contain all of the substances found in food that benefit health; therefore, they are not substitutes for nutrient-dense foods. If your diet is nutritious and you still want to take a multiple vitamin and mineral supplement as an "insurance policy," choose a reasonably priced product that contains no more than 100% of the DV for each of the vitamins and minerals listed on the label. The supplement should meet United States Pharmacopeia (USP) standards for strength, purity, and ability to dissolve. Vague advertising statements or labeling declarations, such as "meets laboratory standards for quality," do not guarantee product quality. Vitamin and mineral pills are dietary supplements. The Consumer Health feature "Dietary Supplements" provides information about claims made for dietary supplements.

Table 9-11 | Nutritional Dietary Supplements

Supplement	Major Claims	Health Risks/Benefits
Apple cider vinegar	Cures arthritis, promotes weight loss, reduces blood cholesterol level	No scientific evidence to support claims.
Beta-carotene	Reduces risk of cancer and heart disease; antioxidant	Acts as antioxidant, but supplements may stimulate cancer cell growth.
Choline	Improves memory	No scientific evidence to support claims.
Chondroitin sulfate	Treats arthritis (often combined with glucosamine)	No scientific evidence to support claims.
Coenzyme Q-10	Reverses signs of aging and disease; antioxidant	Helps cells generate energy and may have medicinal benefits, but more research is needed.
DHEA	Slows aging process, increases muscular strength, and cures numerous ailments	Does not slow rate of aging or cure ailments; long-term effects of taking this naturally occurring hormone are unknown.
Fish oil	Prevents heart disease and stroke, cures rheumatoid arthritis, reduces risk of Alzheimer's disease	Reduces inflammation by suppressing the body's immune response and lowers elevated triglyceride levels. May interfere with blood clotting, increasing the risk of hemorrhagic stroke. Cod liver oil contains vitamins A and D, which are toxic when taken in large doses.
Garlic	Lowers blood cholesterol levels	Does not lower cholesterol consistently, and can cause allergic reaction and unpleasant body odor and interfere with prescription blood thinners.
Glucosamine sulfate	Treats arthritis	May slow the destruction of cartilage in knee joint.
Lysine	Prevents herpes simplex viral outbreaks from recurring	No scientific evidence to support claim.
Melatonin	Treats insomnia and jet lag	Scientific evidence suggests this hormone can treat certain sleep disorders, but information about its long-term safety is lacking.
SAM-e	Relieves pain and depression	More research is needed to support claims and determine health risks; may increase risk of heart disease.
Yogurt (containing live bacterial cultures)	Slows aging process, prevents and cures vaginal yeast infections	No scientific evidence to support these claims, but it may improve intestinal health.

Healthy Living Practices

- To plan well-balanced, nutritious daily menus, you can follow the recommendation, of the latest dietary guidelines and the new MyPyramid Plan.
- Use the Nutrition Facts on food labels to compare the nutritional content of packaged foods and plan nutritious meals and snacks.
- If you want to take a multiple vitamin and mineral supplement, choose a product that meets USP standards and supplies no more than 100% of each nutrient's DV.

Malnutrition: Undernutrition and Overnutrition

Malnutrition results when a person's usual food intake supplies inadequate or excessive amounts of nutrients. *Under*nutrition occurs when a diet does not contain enough nutrients; *over*nutrition results from consuming excessive amounts of nutrients. Undernutrition can be especially devastating for children. Undernourished youngsters often develop nutritional deficiency diseases; as a result, they may not grow properly or perform physical and mental tasks optimally. Undernutrition exists in the United States. At some time during 2002, 11%

malnutrition
overnutrition or undernutrition that results when diets supply improper amounts of nutrients.

Dietary Supplements

Provisions of the 1994 Supplement and Health Education Act allow manufacturers to classify vitamin and mineral pills, protein or amino acid preparations, and certain hormones as "dietary supplements." As mentioned in Chapter 1, the FDA does not regulate dietary supplements as extensively as it regulates medicinal drugs. For example, a pharmaceutical company that's developing a new drug to treat diabetes must submit the medication to thorough testing and provide scientific evidence of its safety and effectiveness as a treatment before the drug can be introduced into the marketplace. Thus, the process of approving a new medication generally takes several years. When the medication finally becomes available, purchasing it is likely to require a physician's prescription.

Dietary supplement manufacturers, however, do not need to provide the FDA with scientific evidence that a supplement is safe for humans or provides measurable health benefits before they can market the product. As a result, many supplements contain ingredients that have not been scientifically tested for safety or effectiveness. Even if an ingredient in a dietary supplement is known to cause serious side effects, the product can still be sold through Internet outlets or in health food stores, pharmacies, and supermarkets without a prescription. If the FDA collects enough convincing evidence that a dietary supplement is dangerous, then the agency can ask manufacturers to remove the product from the marketplace voluntarily or require them to stop distributing it. Table 9-11 lists popular nutritional dietary supplements and their claimed health benefits and notes their potential risks.

The FDA requires manufacturers to provide certain information on dietary supplement labels. The label must show the product's name, state that it is a supplement, provide a list of ingredients, and indicate the net weight of the product's contents. The label also needs to display the name and address of the product's packer, distributor, or manufacturer. Additionally, supplements must have a Supplement Facts label that lists the product's ingredients and includes other information, such as the suggested daily dose.

The FDA allows manufacturers to make certain claims about a dietary supplement's nutrient content, health benefits, and structure/function usefulness. If manufacturers indicate that a dietary supplement treats a specific nutritional deficiency, supports health in some manner, or reduces the risk of a health condition, such claims must be followed by the disclaimer "This statement has not been evaluated by the Food and Drug Administration. This product is not intended to diagnose, treat, cure, or prevent any disease." To learn which health claims have been approved by the FDA, see www.cfsan.fda.gov/~dms/flg-6c.html.

According to the FDA, many consumers of dietary supplements want to know if health claims for these products on labels or in advertisements and printed material are truthful. Such claims do not require FDA approval before they can be used, but manufacturers are supposed to provide evidence to support the claims if the agency asks them to do so. The FDA, however, lacks sufficient funding and personnel to investigate questionable or misleading claims.

Consumers need to be aware that herbal dietary supplements may be contaminated with pesticides or toxic metals. Additionally, herbal products may not contain ingredients from the plants listed on the label. In many instances, supplement pills are not standardized, which means amounts of active ingredients in each dose may be more or less than the label indicates. In 2003, the FDA proposed guidelines that would require dietary supplement manufacturers to label their products accurately. Nevertheless, consumers should be wary of health claims used to promote a dietary supplement and thoroughly investigate the risks of using the product before purchasing it.

---

of U.S. households were uncertain about having or unable to obtain enough food for all members because of the lack of resources (Nord et al., 2003). Even some people with adequate incomes are marginally nourished because they choose diets that supply barely enough calcium, zinc, iron, vitamin E, and the B vitamin folate. Such individuals may experience more frequent infections and take longer to recover from illnesses than those who are well nourished.

People living in countries with high standards of living are more likely to suffer from the ill effects of overnutrition rather than undernutrition. Individuals who eat too much fat, for example, may develop obesity, diabetes, and heart disease. The following chapter discusses obesity and weight management.

Across
THE LIFESPAN

Nutrition

From conception until birth, the developing embryo/fetus depends on its mother to supply the nutrients it needs for development and growth. Women often

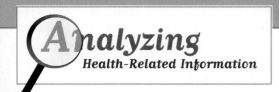

Analyzing
Health-Related Information

 The following advertisement promotes a dietary supplement, garlic oil tablets, to relieve fatigue. Read the ad and evaluate it using the model for analyzing health-related information. The main points of the model are noted below; the model is fully explained on pages 13–15.

1. Which statements are verifiable facts, and which are unverified statements or value claims?

2. What are the credentials of the person who wrote the ad? Does the author appear to have appropriate background and education in the topic area? If it is difficult to tell if the author has specific health expertise, what can you do to check his or her credentials?

3. What might be the motives and biases of the author?

4. What is the main point of the ad? Which information is relevant to the issue or main point, and which information is irrelevant?

5. Is the source reliable, or does it have a reputation for publishing misinformation? Does the ad present both the pros and cons of the product?

6. Does the ad attack the credibility of conventional scientists or medical authorities?

Based on your analysis, do you think that this ad is a reliable source of health-related information? Summarize your reasons for coming to this conclusion.

RUSSIAN SCIENTISTS DISCOVER NEW TREATMENT FOR FATIGUE!

Kiev, Russia—Russian researchers working under the direction of famed doctor Igor X. Ivanamiraculsky of Minsk have discovered that Russian garlic oil is a safe and effective treatment for chronic fatigue. In hundreds of double-blind studies performed at the Minsk Institute of Food Research, college students, athletes, and even elderly persons who took the garlic oil capsules reported having 25% more energy than those persons taking placebos. These results are nothing short of amazing!

Now, you can benefit from Dr. Ivanamiraculsky's discovery. For the first time, the doctor's energy-boosting garlic oil pills are available in the United States. No prescription is needed for this 100% completely natural energizer. Just ask for odor-free GARGOIL at your local pharmacy or health-food store. Satisfaction guaranteed! If you are not completely satisfied after taking GARGOIL, return the unused portion to the place of purchase for a refund. Remember to be careful and follow the label's instructions; some people report feeling too energized after taking GARGOIL! Accept no garlic oil substitutes—ask for GARGOIL.

become more health-conscious during pregnancy, and as a result, they may select more nutritious diets. A woman's nutritional status prior to conception, however, has a significant impact on the health of her baby. By consuming a nutritious diet before becoming pregnant, a woman can build optimal nutrient reserves that prepare her body for the nutritional demands of pregnancy. During pregnancy, undernourished women have a higher risk than well-nourished mothers-to-be of miscarrying, having premature or underweight infants, and delivering babies with birth defects.

Consuming diets that supply adequate folate is critical, especially during the first four weeks of pregnancy when the *neural tube,* the embryonic region that forms the brain and spinal cord, develops. Occasionally, the neural tube fails to develop properly, resulting in *spina bifida* and related defects. Spina bifida occurs when a section of the spinal bones does not fuse to form the channel that encases and protects the spinal cord. In severe cases, the spinal cord protrudes from the infant's back, seriously impairing the child's ability to control the lower part of its body.

Many pregnant women are not even aware of their pregnancy when the neural tube is forming. To maximize the amount of folate in their tissues, women should eat plenty of folate-rich foods, especially enriched breads and cereals, lentils, fruits, and green leafy vegetables (see Table 9-7), before pregnancy.

During pregnancy, women should eat nutritious diets, obtain medical care, and take their *prescribed* doses of prenatal vitamin and mineral supplements. Before taking other supplemental nutrients, pregnant women should always check with their physicians. Consuming excessive amounts of nutrient supplements during pregnancy increases the risk of certain birth defects.

Current infant feeding recommendations include the following: provide breastmilk and a supplement that contains vitamin D and iron for at least the first 12 months of life; do not feed solid foods before 4 months of age; and do not feed fresh whole or reduced-fat cows' milk before the first birthday. Iron-fortified infant formulas are acceptable alternatives, but every healthy pregnant woman should consider the benefits of breastfeeding her baby. Breastmilk is the most suitable food for infants.

Breastmilk offers many advantages to infants and their mothers (National Women's Health Information Center, 2002). It is formulated properly and requires no bottles. Breastfed infants have fewer intestinal and respiratory tract infections. The proteins in human milk will not cause allergies like those in formulas. Breastfeeding is economical and convenient; mothers can breastfeed anywhere they feel comfortable doing

so. Moreover, breastfeeding may reduce a woman's risk of breast cancer. Individuals who are interested in breastfeeding can obtain educational materials and advice from members of the La Leche League, an organization with groups in many U.S. communities.

Many women do not breastfeed because they want to return to a job, they lack the support of family and friends, or they are uncomfortable with this practice. These women should follow their pediatrician's advice concerning the use of commercially prepared infant formulas.

Parents often describe their preschool-aged children as picky eaters because they do not seem to be as hungry or interested in eating as when they were infants. However, most children eat enough calories to maintain their normal growth pattern. During this period, children often establish their food preferences and eating habits; well-informed, responsible adults can serve as role models, teaching youngsters how to choose nutrient-dense foods.

Eating a nutritious breakfast is an important habit to develop early in life. The child who routinely skips breakfast and eats too many sugary snacks can develop borderline or overt nutritional deficiencies. This child often lacks energy, has difficulty concentrating on school work, and experiences behavioral problems. In severe cases, a malnourished child fails to grow properly.

Adolescents experience rapid growth during puberty, and their appetites increase accordingly. Teenagers often become overly concerned with their body size and shape. As a result, boys may experiment with dietary supplements to increase muscle mass. To lose weight, girls may skip meals or choose diets that limit nutritious foods, such as calcium-rich dairy products. Growing adolescents require plenty of calcium to maximize bone mass. An obsession with body size can foster poor eating practices and eating disorders that last into adulthood.

Aged persons who consumed a nutritious diet and have exercised regularly since their youth are more likely to enjoy good health than those who ate poor diets and were inactive. However, physical, psychological, social, and economic factors often influence the quality and quantity of the elderly person's food intake. As one ages, production of acid and other stomach secretions decreases, reducing the ability of the small intestine to absorb calcium, iron, and vitamins D and B_{12}. Therefore, older adults should ask their physicians about the need to take certain nutrient supplements.

Many elderly persons are unable to shop for groceries or prepare foods because of arthritis and strokes. Older individuals who are psychologically depressed, socially

Figure 9-8 Many elderly Americans participate in congregate meal programs within their community.

mobile aged individuals can participate in congregate meal programs in which they visit community centers where hot meals are served five days a week (Figure 9-8). Besides providing a nourishing meal, these sites enable elderly participants to interact socially. Frequent contact with other people can reduce an elderly person's risk of depression, a health problem that often affects isolated aged people.

isolated, or financially impoverished often lack the interest or the resources to prepare nutritious meals. These people are at risk of becoming malnourished. Many communities offer federally subsidized nutrition programs such as Meals-on-Wheels and congregate meals for those who are at least 60 years old. The Meals-on-Wheels program relies on community volunteers to deliver a hot meal, milk, and fresh fruit to homebound people as often as five days a week. More

Healthy Living Practices

- To increase your chances of having a healthy baby, improve the quality of your diet before you become pregnant.
- Excesses of certain nutrients can produce birth defects, so ask your physician for advice before you take nutrient supplements during pregnancy.
- If you are a woman who plans to have children, consider the benefits of breastfeeding, especially during their first 12 months of life.

CHAPTER REVIEW

Summary

Nutrients are substances in foods that supply energy; regulate body processes; and provide material for growth, maintenance, and repair of tissues. The six classes of nutrients are carbohydrates, lipids, proteins, vitamins, minerals, and water. Many foods also contain non-nutrients, substances that are not essential but may have healthful benefits. Phytochemicals may prevent various chronic diseases, including certain cancers.

During digestion, food is broken down into nutrients that can be absorbed. Cells metabolize carbohydrates, fats, and proteins for energy. The amount of energy stored in food is measured in calories. Cells cannot release energy from water, vitamins, and minerals.

Carbohydrates, the sugars and starches, are a major source of energy for the body. The only disorder that is clearly associated with excessive carbohydrate consumption is tooth decay. Plant foods supply dietary fiber and phytochemicals. Diets rich in fiber may reduce the risks of diverticulosis, hemorrhoids, constipation, colon and rectal cancer, and heart disease.

Many medical experts think Americans eat too much fat, saturated fat, trans fat, and cholesterol. Eating excessive amounts of these lipids is associated with an increased risk of obesity, heart disease, and certain cancers.

Protein is essential for tissue growth, repair, and maintenance; and for producing enzymes, antibodies, and certain hormones. The average American consumes more than twice the amount of protein needed, particularly from animal foods. One way to reduce the amount of animal foods in the diet is to eat more protein from plants. Vegetarian diets are associated with lower risks of chronic conditions such as heart disease.

Vitamins and minerals regulate body processes; some minerals are structural components of tissues. Overdoses of many vitamins and most minerals can cause nutritional imbalances and be toxic; therefore, unless medically indicated, people should avoid taking high doses of nutrient supplements.

A lifetime of inadequate calcium intake coupled with low estrogen levels after menopause increases a woman's risk of osteoporosis. Iron deficiency is a common nutritional problem, especially among women of childbearing ages. Dehydration is a serious condition that results when water intake is inadequate or water losses are excessive.

The key features of a nutritious diet are nutrient adequacy and nutrient balance. By selecting a variety of foods and by avoiding the indiscriminate use of nutrient supplements, one's diet can be nutritionally adequate and balanced.

A requirement for a nutrient is the smallest amount that prevents a deficiency disease. Dietary Reference Intakes (DRIs) are standards for planning nutritious diets and determining the nutritional adequacy of diets. The Healthy Eating Pyramid, MyPyramid Plan, and the dietary guidelines are practical daily menu-planning guides. Nutrient labeling can help consumers select nutritious foods. Malnutrition occurs when diets supply too little or too many nutrients.

The quality of a woman's diet before and during pregnancy has an impact on the health of her developing child. During the first year of life, human milk is the best food for infants; solid foods should not be fed to babies until they are 4 months old. Without proper supervision, children and teenagers may skip meals or select inadequate diets. Physical, psychological, economic, and social factors contribute to the risk of malnutrition in the elderly.

Applying What You Have Learned

1. Explain how you would use nutrient labeling information to choose food products that are low in fat. `Application`
2. Keep a food record for one day. Analyze this day's food choices by using the MyPyramid Plan. `Analysis`
3. Plan a menu for a day (meals, snacks, and beverages) that meets the MyPyramid Plan's recommended amounts of foods for a person of your age, sex, and physical activity level. You'll need to visit www.mypyramid.gov to do this activity. `Synthesis`
4. Use a computer dietary analysis program to evaluate the nutritional quality of your diet. Which foods can you eat to improve your diet? `Evaluation`

Key

`Application`	using information in a new situation.
`Analysis`	breaking down information into component parts.
`Synthesis`	putting together information from different sources.
`Evaluation`	making informed decisions.

Reflecting on Your Health

1. After reading this chapter, what changes can you make to improve your diet? How is your present diet different from what you ate as a child or while in high school? Why do you think your present diet is better or worse than your past diet?
2. What factors influence your food choices? How willing are you to try new foods? What new foods have you eaten in the past year?
3. Do you use nutrition labels? If you do, which information do you think is most important? How does nutritional labeling help you be a better consumer? If you don't use nutrition labels, why not?
4. Do you take dietary supplements? If you do, which supplements do you take? Why do you take them?
5. Females: Would you or did you breastfeed your children? Explain why you would or did breastfeed your children. Males: Would you want or did the mother of your children breastfeed them? Why or why not?

References

American Academy of Allergy, Asthma, and Immunology. (2003). Tips to remember. Retrieved August 20, 2004, from http://www.aaaai.org.

American Dietetic Association. (1997). Position of the American Dietetic Association: vegetarian diets. *Journal of the American Dietetic Association, 97*(11):1317–1321.

Ascherio, A., Katan, M. B., Zock, P. L., Stampfer, M. J., & Willett, W. C. (1999). Trans fatty acids and coronary heart disease. *New England Journal of Medicine, 340*(25):1994–1998.

Bazzano, L. A., Ogden, L. G., Loria, C. M., Whelton, P. K., et al. (2003). Dietary fiber intake and reduced risk of coronary heart disease in U.S. men and women: The National Health and Nutrition Examination Survey I Epidemiological Follow-Up Study. *Archives of Internal Medicine, 163*(16):1897–1904.

Beales, J. H. (2004). *Prepared statement of the Federal Trade Commission before the Committee on Energy and Commerce, Subcommittee on Oversight and Investigations, United States House of Representatives.* Washington, DC. Retrieved September 12, 2004, from http://www.ftc.gov/os/2004/06/040616dietarysupptestimony.pdf.

Bingham, S. A., Day, N. E., Luben, R., Ferrari, P., et al. (2003). Dietary fibre in food and protection against colorectal cancer in the European Prospective Investigation into Cancer and Nutrition (EPIC): An observational study. *Lancet, 361*(9368):1496–1501.

Brandhagen, D. J., Fairbanks, V. F., & Baldus, W. (2002). Recognition and management of hereditary hemochromatosis. *American Family Physician, 65*(5):853–860, 865–866.

Bray, G. A., Nielsen, S. J., & Popkin, B. M. (2004). Consumption of high-fructose corn syrup in beverages may play a role in the epidemic of obesity. *American Journal of Clinical Nutrition, 79*(4):537–543.

Covington, M. B. (2004). Omega-3 fatty acids. *American Family Physician, 70*(1):133–140.

Eating Mediterranean. (1999). *Mayo Clinic Health Letter, 17*(6):4.

Engelhart, M. J., Geerlings, M. I., Ruitenberg, A., van Swieten, J. C., Hofman, A., Witteman, J. C., & Breteler, M. M. (2002). Dietary intake of antioxidants and risk of Alzheimer's disease. *Journal of the American Medical Association, 287*(24):3223–3229.

Food and Nutrition Board, National Institute of Medicine. (2004). *Dietary reference intakes for water, potassium, sodium, chloride, and sulfate.* Washington, DC: National Academy Press. Retrieved September 10, 2004, from http://www.nap.edu/openbook/0309091691/html.

Ford, E. S., Giles, W. H., & Mokdad, A. H. (2004). Increasing prevalence of the metabolic syndrome among U.S. adults. *Diabetes Care, 27*(10):2444–2449.

Frazao, E. (1999). *American's eating habits: Changes and consequences* (Agricultural Information Bulletin No. 750). Washington, DC: U.S. Department of Agriculture.

Geha, R. S., Beiser, A., Ren, C., Patterson, R., Greenberger, P. A., Grammer, L. C., Ditto, A. M., Harris, K. E., Shaughnessy, M. A., Yarnold, P. R., Corren, J., & Saxon, A. (2000). Review of alleged reaction to monosodium glutamate and outcome of a multicenter double-blind placebo-controlled study. *Journal of Nutrition, 130*:1058S–1062S.

Grundy, S. M., Brewer, H. B., Cleeman, J. I., Smith, S. C., & Lenfant, C. (2004). Definition of metabolic syndrome: Report of the National Heart, Lung, and Blood Institute/American Heart Association conference on scientific issues related to definition. *Circulation, 109*(3):433–438.

Guenther, P. M., & Jensen, H. H. (2000). Estimating energy contributed by fiber using a general factor of 2 vs 4 kcal/g. *Journal of the American Dietetic Association, 100*(8):944–946.

Henkel, J. (1999). Sugar substitutes: Americans opt for sweetness and lite. *FDA Consumer, 33*(6):12–16.

Hercberg, S., Galan, P., & Preziosi, P. (1999). Antioxidant vitamins and cardiovascular disease: Dr. Jekyll or Mr. Hyde? *American Journal of Public Health, 89*(3):289–291.

Inman-Felton, A. E. (1999). Overview of lactose maldigestion (lactase non-persistence). *Journal of the American Dietetic Association, 99*(4):481–489.

Kant, A. K. (2000). Consumption of energy-dense, nutrient-poor foods by adult Americans: Nutritional and health implications. The third National Health and Nutrition Examination Survey, 1988–1994. *American Journal of Clinical Nutrition, 72*:929–936.

Kanton, L. S. (1999). A comparison of the U.S. food supply with the Food Guide Pyramid recommendations. In E. Frazão (Ed.), *America's eating habits: Changes and consequences* (Agricultural Bulletin No. 750). Washington, DC: U.S. Department of Agriculture.

Lotufo, P. A., Gaziano, J. M., Chae, C. U., Ajani, U. A., Moreno-John, G., Buring, J. E., & Manson, J. E. (2001). Diabetes and all-cause and coronary heart disease mortality among U.S. male physicians. *Archives of Internal Medicine, 161*(2):242–247.

McKeown, N. M., Meigs, J. B., Liu, S., Saltzman, E., Wilson, P. W. F., & Jacques, P. F. (2004). Carbohydrate nutrition, insulin resistance, and the prevalence of the metabolic syndrome in the Framingham cohort. *Diabetes Care, 27*(2):538–546.

Meshkinpour, H., Selod, S., Movahedi, H., Nami, N., James, N., & Wilson, A. (1998). Effects of regular exercise in management of chronic idiopathic constipation. *Digestive Diseases and Science, 43*(11): 2379–2383.

Millen, A. E., Dodd, K. W., & Subar, A. F. (2004). Use of vitamin, mineral, nonvitamin, and nonmineral supplements in the United States: The 1987, 1992, and 2000 National Health Interview Survey results. *Journal of the American Dietetic Association, 104*(6):942–950.

Mokdad, A. H., Ford, E. S., Bowman, B. A., Dietz, W. H., et al. (2003). Prevalence of obesity, diabetes, and obesity-related health risk factors, 2001. *Journal of the American Medical Association, 289*(1):76–79.

Murphy, S. P., Wilkens, L. R., Hankin, J. H., Foote, J. A., Monroe, K. R., Henderson, B. E., & Kolonel, L. N. (2002). Comparison of two instruments for quantifying intake of vitamin and mineral supplements: A brief questionnaire versus three 24-hour recalls. *American Journal of Epidemiology, 156*(7):669–675.

National Women's Health Information Center. (2002). *Benefits of breastfeeding.* Office on Women's Health, U.S. Department of Health and Human Services. Retrieved May 31, 2002, from http://www.4woman.gov/breastfeeding/index.htm.

National Institutes of Health, Osteoporosis and Related Bone Diseases National Resource Center. (2002). *Osteoporosis overview.* Washington, DC: NIHORBDNNRC. Retrieved June 3, 2002, from www.osteo.org/.

Niggemann, B., & Gruber, C. (2004). Unproven diagnostic procedures in IgE-mediated allergic diseases. *Allergy, 59*(8):806–808.

Nord, M., Andrews, M., & Carlson, S. (2003). *Household food security in the United States, 2002* (Food Assistance and Research Report No. 35). Washington, DC: Food and Rural Economics Division, Economic Research Service, U.S. Department of Agriculture. Retrieved September 26, 2004, from http://www.ers.usda.gov/publications/fanrr35/fanrr35fm.pdf.

Pereira, M. A., O'Reilly, E., Augustsson, K., Fraser, G. E., et al. (2004). Dietary fiber and risk of coronary heart disease: A pooled analysis of cohort studies. *Archives of Internal Medicine, 164*(4):370–376.

Peters, U., Sinha, R., Chatterjee, N., Subar, A. F., et al. (2003). Dietary fibre and colorectal adenoma in a colorectal cancer early detection program. *Lancet, 36*(9369):1491–1495.

Polidori, M. C. (2003). Antioxidant nutrients in the prevention of age-related diseases. *Journal of Postgraduate Medicine, 49*(3):229–235.

Radimer, K., Bindewald, B., Hughes, J., Ervin, B., Swanson, C., & Picciano, M. F. (2004). Dietary supplement use by U.S. adults: Data from the National Health and Nutrition Examination Survey, 1999–2000. *American Journal of Epidemiology, 160*(4):339–349.

Schulze, M. B., Manson, J. E., Ludwig, D. S., Colditz, G. A., Stampfer, M. J., Willett, W. C., & Hu, F. B. (2004). Sugar-sweetened beverages, weight gain, and incidence of type 2 diabetes in young and middle-aged women. *Journal of the American Medical Association, 292*(8):927–934.

Slattery, M. L., Curtin, K. P., Edwards, S. L., & Schaffer, D. M. (2004). Plant foods, fiber, and rectal cancer. *American Journal of Clinical Nutrition, 79*(2):274–281.

Smit, E., Nieto, F. J., Cresp, C. J., & Mitchell, P. (1999). Estimates of animal and plant protein intake in U.S. adults: Results from the third National Health and Examination Survey, 1988–1991. *Journal of the American Dietetic Association, 99*:813–820.

U.S. Department of Agriculture and U.S. Department of Health and Human Services. (2005). *Dietary guidelines for Americans 2005.* Retrieved January 12, 2005, from http://www.healthierus.gov/dietaryguidelines/.

What You'll Learn

http://healthyliving.jbpub.com

The Web site for this book offers many useful tools and is a great source for supplementary health information for both students and instructors. Visit the site at http://healthyliving.jbpub.com for information on these topics:

Overweight and Obesity
The Caloric Cost of Living
Weight Management

Chapter Overview

The definitions of overweight and obesity
How your body uses the energy from foods
How to determine your percentage of body fat
The causes of obesity
How to manage your weight

Diversity in Health
The Plight of the Pima

Consumer Health
Dietary Supplements: Weight Loss Aids

Managing Your Health
General Features of Reliable Weight Reduction Plans

Across
THE LIFESPAN

Weight Management

Student Workbook

Self-Assessment: How Much Energy Do You Use Daily?
Changing Health Habits: Altering Caloric Intake and Physical Activity

Do You Know?

· *How to shed fat and gain muscle?*
· *What causes "middle-age spread"?*
· *How to lose weight and keep it off?*

Body Weight and Its Management

"I've always been fat," says 20-year-old college student Justin Godin. "I weighed over 10 pounds at birth. In elementary school, kids made fun of me for being so fat. When I was in high school PE classes, I couldn't do a single push up. It was so embarrassing. I didn't date . . . girls wouldn't look at me and I didn't have the confidence to ask one out. Now when I look back, I realize my diet was terrible. I snacked on white rice and ate fast food and drank regular soft drinks regularly. If my mom brought home chips, cookies, or ice cream from the store, I would eat it all. I didn't eat breakfast, but I'd eat two big meals late in the day and then gorge on pizza before going to bed."

By the time Justin was 18, he weighed 225 pounds, far too much for his 5′9″ body frame. Today, Justin weighs 180 pounds, and only about 10% of his body is fat. As you can see in the photo, Justin not only lost a lot of fat, he beefed up his muscle mass too. What made him decide to shed the excess weight and how did he do it?

After graduating from high school, Justin enrolled in courses at a community college and worked part-time at a clothing store. "I had lost 10 pounds and was feeling pretty good about my progress. Then during a meeting of store employees, one of the girls who worked with me commented that my suit jacket was too tight. Everyone heard her . . . I was really embarrassed." This experience triggered Justin's motivation to lose weight. "I started working out on a treadmill . . . and I noticed my weight began going down."

" *. . . changing my eating habits made losing weight easier.* **"**

"At that point, I decided to eat healthier foods . . . then I noticed how changing my eating habits made losing weight easier." Justin stopped eating fast food and started eating breakfast and low-fat foods; grilled chicken, peas, and green beans became some of his favorite choices. After 8 months, his weight dropped to 145 pounds. Family members who hadn't seen him in a year were amazed by his trim appearance. "They thought I looked great," he says, beaming with pride. "To build up my muscles, I experimented with different training methods and got into power lifting. My training routine now includes stretching, jogging on the treadmill, and weight lifting." Recently, Justin was accepted to a 4-year school where he'll major in sports medicine so he can become an athletic trainer. More confident around people now, Justin has shown that it's possible for people to change health-related habits and improve the quality of their lives. He has the following advice for people who want to lose weight: "Keep going—results will come if you're determined and have a set goal in mind."

Overweight and **obesity** are conditions characterized by excessive and unhealthy amounts of body fat. People who do not have "weight problems" often think overweight individuals lack the willpower to control their eating and weight. It is true that a person gains body fat by eating more food energy (calories) than needed and that losing the excess weight involves a considerable amount of motivation and commitment. Overweight and obesity, however, result from a complex combination of biological, psychological, environmental, cultural, and socioeconomic influences. Thus, shedding excess fat to achieve a healthy body weight is not an easy task for people who are overweight. Most medical experts now view obesity as a chronic metabolic disease that is extremely difficult to treat.

The majority of adult Americans have too much body fat—overweight is the most common nutritional disorder in the United States (Yanovski & Yanovski, 2002). Overweight and obesity often result from a combination of two behavioral risk factors—poor diet and physical inactivity. In this country, an increasing number of people are dying of causes related to these risk factors (Mokdad et al., 2005). In 2003, the total medical costs of treating health conditions associated with obesity were estimated to be $75 *billion* (Finkelstein et al., 2004).

This chapter examines factors that contribute to the development of excess body fat, identifies health problems associated with this condition, and discusses various weight loss methods. Some individuals are underweight and want to increase their muscle mass; therefore, this chapter also provides information concerning healthy ways to gain weight.

obesity a condition in which the body has an excessive and unhealthy amount of fat. Obese people have BMIs of 30 or more.

body mass index (BMI) a standard that correlates body weight with the risk of developing chronic health conditions associated with obesity.

overweight a condition in which the body has too much fat. Overweight people have BMIs of between 25 and 30.

■ Overweight and Obesity

A healthy body is not fat free; a small amount of fat is essential for the normal functioning of all cells. Additionally, the body has specialized cells *adipose cells* that store the extra energy from food as triglyceride (fat). If a person eats more food energy than is needed, his or her fat cells continue storing fat and increasing in size. Under certain conditions, additional fat cells can develop, further enlarging the fat mass, and this person soon notices that his belts are too small or her slacks are too tight as a result.

How much extra fat must a person have to be considered overweight? At what point does an overweight person become obese? Definitions for these terms used to rely on height/weight tables. In the late 1950s, the Metropolitan Life Insurance Company introduced a set of height/weight tables that were widely used in the United States for more than two decades. The tables indicated an "ideal" weight range for a particular height. Although the tables were popular, they had limited usefulness. The insurance company developed them by using measurements from healthy nonsmokers who were 25 to 59 years old and had purchased certain life insurance policies. Therefore, the tables' height and weight ranges could not be applied to the general population. Most health experts now use the **body mass index (BMI)** instead of height/weight tables to determine if an individual weighs too much.

The BMI correlates body weight with the risk of developing chronic health conditions associated with excess body fat. To estimate your BMI, multiply your weight in pounds by 705. Then divide that number by your height in inches squared. For example, if you weigh 150 lb and are 67″ tall, multiplying your weight times 705 equals 105,750 and squaring your height equals 4,489. Dividing 105,750 by 4,489 produces approximately 23.56. Thus, your BMI is 23.56.

Adults with BMIs below 18.5 are classified as *underweight*. Adults with BMIs between 25.0 and 29.9 are **overweight**; those with BMIs of between 30.0 and 39.9 are obese. People who have BMIs of 40 or more are often referred to as *morbidly extreme* or *super obese*.

Using BMIs as a guide, you can determine if your weight is healthy for your height (Table 10-1). The median BMI for adult Americans is 25.5, which is in the overweight range (Kuczmarski et al., 1997).

You can use the graph shown in Figure 10-1 to determine if your weight is within the healthy BMI range. Find your height, without shoes, on the left-hand side of the graph and place your left index finger on that point. Then find your weight, without clothing, on the bottom line of the graph, and place your right index finger on that point. Move your left finger to the right and your right finger up until they meet. Note which range that point is in. Is your weight in the healthy BMI range?

Table 10-1 Classifying Body Weight Based on BMIs

Height (in.)	Overweight (BMI 25.0 to 29.9) Lower Limit (lb)	Obese (BMI 30 or more) Lower Limit (lb)
58	119	143
59	124	148
60	128	153
61	132	158
62	136	164
63	141	169
64	145	174
65	150	180
66	155	186
67	159	191
68	164	197
69	169	203
70	174	207
71	179	215
72	184	221
73	189	227

Source: *Clinical guidelines on the identification, evaluation, and treatment of overweight and obesity in adults.* (1998). Bethesda, MD: National Institutes of Health, National Heart, Lung, and Blood Institute.

Defining *overweight* and *obese* as certain BMIs can produce inaccurate conclusions. For example, athletic individuals may have a BMI of 26 and be overweight according to Figure 10-1. Since muscle is denser than fat, an athletic muscular person can be heavier but healthier than a physically inactive (*sedentary*) individual who is the same height.

The Prevalence of Overweight and Obesity

The prevalence of excess body fat has reached epidemic proportions in the United States. In 1980 almost 50% of American adults were overweight or obese. By 2002, 65% of Americans 20 years of age or older were too fat (Hedley et al., 2004). In the past couple of decades, the percentage of American adults who were obese increased from 15% to 30%. Thus, nearly 1 in 3 adults are obese. American children are growing fatter too. According to the Centers for Disease Control and Prevention (CDC), the percentage of American children who are overweight has doubled since 1980. In 2002, 16% of children between the ages of 6 and 19 years were too fat, and 31% were at risk of becoming overweight (Hedley et al., 2004).

An objective of *Healthy People 2010* is to reduce the prevalence of overweight to 15% of the adult American population (U.S. Department of Health and Human Services [USDHHS], 2000). It is unlikely that Americans will meet this objective by 2010. A later section of

Figure 10-1 **BMI Graph.** Find your BMI by following the instructions provided in the text. Source: *Nutrition and your health: Dietary guidelines for Americans,* 5th ed. (2000). Washington, DC: U.S. Departments of Health and Human Services and Agriculture. Retrieved August 16, 2002, from http://www.health.gov/dietaryguidelines/.

this chapter discusses factors that contribute to the rising prevalence of overweight in America.

The United States is not the only country experiencing a rapid increase in the prevalence of overweight people. The World Health Organization (WHO) recognizes obesity as a global health problem (WHO, 2002). The worldwide prevalence of obesity (*globesity*) is rising rapidly, especially in nations with developed market economies such as those in Western Europe. According to WHO estimates, about 20% of the adult population in developed countries were obese in 2000. In the least developed nations, only about 2% of the population were obese. Globally, about 300 million people were obese; remarkably, there were far more obese adults in the world than there were severely underweight adults in 2000.

How Does Excess Body Fat Affect Health?

Excess body fat contributes to many serious and disabling health problems. Compared to people who have healthy body weights, obese individuals are more likely to die prematurely (Flegal et al., 2005). Overweight people have greater risks than lean people of developing gout, a condition that affect joints; carpal tunnel syndrome, a painful nerve disorder involving the wrist and hand; and sleep apnea, a condition in which one stops breathing periodically while sleeping. Overweight people are also more likely to suffer from metabolic syndrome, gallbladder disease, hypertension, diabetes, and heart disease. Obesity significantly increases the risk of cancers of the large intestine (colon), breast (postmenopausal women), uterus, kidney, and esophagus (Calle & Thun, 2004). In the United States, excess body fat contributes to more than 90,000 cancer deaths each year (Calle et al., 2003).

Surgery is riskier for obese people because physicians have more difficulty estimating the amount of anesthesia needed. Obese men and women are more likely to experience fertility problems than people whose weights are in the healthy range. Overweight women who are pregnant with their first child have greater risks of developing diabetes (*gestational diabetes*) and a form of severe hypertension during pregnancy, as well as giving birth prematurely (Baeten et al., 2001). Furthermore, being too fat can interfere with one's ability to perform daily activities that require walking, carrying, kneeling, and stooping.

Few obese individuals are free of physical health problems. Excess body weight can stress joints, especially weight-bearing joints in the knees and hips, so they wear out sooner. Obese people often have breathing problems because the excess fat interferes with lung expansion when they inhale. Additionally, obesity may upset the body's normal hormonal balance, which can interfere with fertility.

At one time, scientists thought adipose cells were simply storage sites for fat. Today, researchers are learning more about the roles these cells play in health and disease. When fat cells become too large, they lose their ability to respond to the hormone insulin, and the overweight person develops diabetes as a result. Fat tissue also contains cells called *macrophages*. Although these cells play a role in immune system processes that protect an individual from disease, they may multiply excessively and malfunction in people who have too much body fat. Scientists think macrophages found in fat tissue produce chemicals that cause inflammation, resulting in damage to the heart and blood vessels (Weisberg et al., 2003).

An overweight person does not have to become slim to reap some benefits of losing weight. Losing 10% of body weight and maintaining that loss often reduce risks of heart disease and stroke. Additionally, an overweight or obese person who loses modest amounts of fat can save thousands of dollars that would have been spent on treating medical conditions related to excess body fat (Oster et al., 1999).

Besides affecting physical health, excess body fat can have a negative impact on psychological health. Obese people, particularly obese women who seek weight loss treatment, often suffer from depression and low self-esteem (Friedman et al., 2002). An obese individual may develop these psychological problems after being discriminated against or having humiliating and embarrassing experiences while obtaining an education or seeking a job. Additionally, lean people often perceive obese individuals as physically unattractive, lacking willpower, and lazy. Not surprisingly, many overweight or obese individuals are dissatisfied and preoccupied with their body image (Friedman et al., 2002).

What are the factors that contribute to the development of excess body fat? Why are so many Americans too fat? Is it possible to control one's weight?

■ The Caloric Cost of Living

Energy for Basal (Vital) Metabolism

Metabolism refers to all chemical changes that take place in cells. Human cells use energy (calories) from food to perform vital activities such as building and repairing tissues, circulating and filtering blood, and producing and transporting substances. Nevertheless, cells release much of the calories from food as heat, which is necessary for maintaining one's body temperature. Every day the body expends the largest portion of calories (50% to 70%) to carry out these vital activities. The **metabolic rate** is the amount of energy required to fuel cellular activities within a specified time.

Metabolic rates vary; genetic factors probably play a major role in setting these rates. Hormones, especially thyroid hormone produced in the thyroid gland, regulate metabolism (Figure 10-2). In some people, the thyroid gland does not function properly, and as a result the organ produces too much or too little thyroid hormone. An individual who produces too much thyroid hormone has a higher than normal metabolic rate. This person feels warm, is nervous and shaky, has chronic diarrhea, and loses weight despite eating large amounts of food. People with overactive thyroid glands can take medication or have surgery to reduce the amount of hormone produced by the organ. A person who suffers from lack of thyroid hormone has a lower than normal metabolic rate. This individual feels cold, has little energy, is constipated, and gains weight easily. People suffering from underactive thyroid glands can increase their metabolic rates by taking thyroid hormone pills. The vast majority of overweight people, however, have normal thyroid hormone levels and normal metabolic rates.

The proportion of muscle and fat tissue also influences the metabolic rate. Muscle cells use more energy than fat cells; therefore, people with greater amounts of muscle mass have higher metabolic rates than those with more fat tissue. Testosterone is a hormone that stimulates muscle mass development. Since men normally produce more testosterone than women, they usually have more muscle and less fat. On average, men have higher metabolic rates than women.

Age also influences the metabolic rate. Because they are growing rapidly, infants and children have higher metabolic rates than adults. After 20 years of age, metabolic rates decline about 1% to 2% each decade. As a result of this gradual slowdown, aging people need less energy. If older people continue to eat the same amount of food as they did when younger, they gain weight. Between the ages of 20 and 50, the average American gains 20 to 30 pounds! Although the declining metabolic rate is a contributing factor, many health experts think physical inactivity is more responsible for "middle-age spread" than is overeating. As one grows older, exercising regularly can help retain muscle mass and slow the decline in the metabolic rate.

metabolism all chemical reactions that take place in the body.

metabolic rate the amount of energy the body requires to fuel cellular activities during a specified time.

Energy for Physical Activity

In addition to the caloric cost of vital metabolic activities, the body expends energy to contract skeletal muscles. The amount of energy needed for physical activity depends on the type of activity, the time spent performing the activity (its duration), and the intensity at which it is performed. Although it is not related directly to physical activity, a person's body size influences the amount of physical effort needed to move. A person who weighs 120 pounds and another who weighs 175 pounds might spend the same amount of time playing a game of tennis. If both of them play tennis with the same intensity, the muscles of the heavier person require more energy to move than those of the lighter person.

Health experts recommend that adults perform at least 30 minutes of moderate-intensity physical activity nearly every day. According to a recent survey, most adult Americans do not engage in enough moderate-intensity physical activity to meet this recommendation (Ham et al., 2004). About one in four adults are physically inactive even during their leisure time. Chapter 11 identifies physical activities that are moderately intense.

People can increase the amount of energy expended during physical activity by increasing its duration or intensity. Furthermore, the metabolic rate often remains elevated for several hours after one discontinues vigorous physical activity. This elevation may result

Thyroid gland

Windpipe

Figure 10-2 **The Thyroid Gland.** The thyroid gland produces hormones that control the metabolic rate.

from an increase in the metabolic activity of muscle cells that occurs after physical exertion. Therefore, individuals who engage in regular vigorous activity may be able to raise their resting metabolic rates (Speakman & Selman, 2003).

Some health experts classify physical activities as sports types of exercise, movement for daily living, or spontaneous muscular movements. *Sports types of exercise* are physical activities that are planned and carried out for the purpose of improving health and well-being. Swimming, brisk walking, and lifting weights are sports types of exercises. *Movement for daily living* includes various unstructured physical activities such as housework, gardening, walking, and leisure-time physical activities that are not associated with sports, eating, or sleeping (Levine, 2004). Each day, the typical American expends more energy for physical activities associated with daily living than for sports types of exercise. *Spontaneous muscular movement* includes fidgeting and maintaining balance and body posture. Movements for daily living and spontaneous muscular movements are referred to as *non-exercise activity thermogenesis (NEAT)*. As a result of NEAT, people can reduce the risk of gaining body fat by being restless and busy, because they will metabolize far more energy each day than people who spend much of their day engaging in sedentary activities such as lying down or sitting still. Nevertheless, more research is needed to determine the role of NEAT in weight maintenance.

thermic effect of food (TEF) the small amount of energy that the body uses to digest, absorb, and process the nutrients from foods.

Table 10-2 lists some common physical activities and the number of calories people expend per minute of performing each activity. Note that the number of calories used for an activity varies according to body weight. For most people, the total number of calories expended daily for physical activity is *less* than the number expended for basal metabolism.

Energy for the Thermic Effect of Food

Together, metabolic and physical activity energy needs constitute more than 90% of a person's energy expenditure. After eating a meal, the body requires a small amount of energy to digest, absorb, and process the nutrients from food. This use of energy, the **thermic effect of food (TEF)**, accounts for a very small portion, less than 10%, of one's total energy expenditures.

How many calories does your body need daily? To estimate your daily caloric expenditures, you can add the number of calories needed for basal metabolism, physical activity, and TEF. The assessment activity in the student workbook can help you estimate the number of calories you expend in a day.

| Table 10-2 | Approximate Energy Costs of Various Physical Activities |

Physical Activity	Calories per Pound of Body Weight per Minute	
	Range for Women	Range for Men
Sedentary Sitting quietly, playing a musical instrument	up to .017	up to .017
Light Playing pool, bowling, golf, volleyball, walking (3 mph)	.017 to .033	.017 to .035
Moderate Badminton, canoeing, gymnastics, hockey, cycling, swimming, dancing, tennis, skiing	.033 to .050	.035 to .052
Vigorous/Heavy Basketball, climbing, cross-country running, rowing	.050+	.052+

To estimate the number of calories you expend while performing a particular physical activity, multiply the calories per pound per minute by your weight. Use the figures in the left-hand column if you are a woman, and in the right-hand column if you are a man. Then multiply that number by the number of minutes spent performing the activity. For example, if you are a woman who weighs 120 lb, and you spent 40 min cycling: .033 × 120 = 3.96 calories per minute; 3.96 × 40 minutes = about 158 calories spent. (The rates of caloric expenditure per minute are given as ranges. For example, if you cycled intensely, use a rate at the high end of the range.)

Source: Adapted from Durnin, J. V. G. A., & Passmore, R. (1967). *Energy, work, and leisure*. London: Heinemann.

The Basics of Energy Balance

In general, people maintain, gain, or lose body weight according to the basic principles of energy balance, as illustrated in Figure 10-3. When the caloric intake from food equals the number of calories expended for energy needs, no change in body weight occurs. When caloric intake is less than caloric expenditures, the body loses weight as cells burn stored fat. If caloric intake is more than caloric expenditures, the body conserves much of the excess calories as fat, and weight gain occurs. Each pound of body fat represents about 3,500 calories of potential energy; therefore, consuming as little as 100 extra calories per day for a year can result in a 10-pound weight gain.

Figure 10-3 **Energy Balance.** (a) When energy expenditure equals energy intake, the body maintains its weight; (b) when energy expenditure is greater than energy intake, the body loses weight; (c) when energy expenditure is less than energy intake, the body gains weight.

■ Body Composition

How Much Fat Is Normal?

When you step on a scale, you can determine your body weight as a number of pounds or kilograms. That weight, however, does not specify how much water, muscle, or fat is in your body. Fat-free body weight consists of water, proteins, and minerals found in the bones, muscles, and organs (*lean tissues*). About 60% of a healthy adult's weight is water; 6% to 22% is protein, and 3% is minerals. Most of the remaining weight is fat.

About one-half of an average person's body fat is located in a layer under the skin (*subcutaneous* fat). Small amounts of fat are stored in muscles, which rely on the fat for energy. Besides subcutaneous and muscle fat, regions of the abdomen, thighs, hips, and buttocks store considerable amounts of fat.

Every year Americans spend money on useless treatments to eliminate "cellulite." Many people think cellulite is an abnormal type of fat that appears as lumpy dimpled skin on the buttocks and thighs. Cellulite fat, however, does not exist. There is no difference between the fat cells in so-called cellulite and those in other parts of the body (Rosenbaum et al., 1998). Strands of connective tissue hold subcutaneous fat in place. If these strands hold the fat in an irregular pattern, the fat tissue can extend into layers of skin, giving the skin a lumpy appearance. Women are more likely than men to have irregular connective tissue under their skin. The best way to improve the appearance of thighs and buttocks is to exercise and lose excess weight.

Obesity can begin at any age. However, the number and size of fat cells increase dramatically when this condition occurs during childhood and other periods of rapid growth (Robertson et al., 1999). People who become overweight in adulthood usually have normal numbers of fat cells, but their fat cells are larger than normal. The number of fat cells, however, can increase when extreme obesity occurs during the adult years.

Once fat cells form, there is little evidence that they can disappear with short-term weight reduction efforts. Under these conditions, most fat cells shrink as they release stored fat to meet the energy needs of other tissues. After shrinking, fat cells may send chemical signals to the nervous system that stimulate the urge to eat, making it difficult for people to maintain their reduced body weights.

Estimating Body Fat

Many health experts use the percentage of body fat to determine if a person is obese. The average healthy young woman has more body fat than the average healthy young man, because the fat is needed for hormonal and reproductive purposes. Although people tend to gain fat as they age, the increase does not necessarily cause health problems.

A variety of methods are used to determine one's percentage of body fat, including hydrostatic weighing, bioelectrical impedance, near-infrared interactance, dual-energy x-ray absorptometry, skinfold thicknesses, and ultrasound. The following sections discuss these techniques.

Hydrostatic weighing (underwater weighing) is one of the most reliable methods to estimate an individual's percentage of body fat. Body fat is less dense than lean tissues or water; therefore, extra fat makes the body more buoyant. Underwater weighing, however, is not a practical or convenient way to determine one's percentage of body fat.

Bioelectrical impedance uses electrical currents to estimate the percentage of body fat. Water and certain mineral elements conduct electrical currents, whereas fat is a poor conductor of electricity. The equipment shown in Figure 10-4 safely measures the body's electrical conductivity to determine the percentage of body fat. When subjects have normal amounts of body water, bioelectrical impedance provides reliable estimates of their percentage of body fat.

Near-infrared interactance testing estimates the percentage of body fat by using a small device to pass infrared light quickly through the biceps muscle of the upper arm. Near-infrared testing, however, often underestimates percentage of body fat, especially as body fatness increases. This error limits its usefulness as a reliable measurement (Wagner & Heyward, 1999).

Dual-energy x-ray absorptiometry (DEXA or DXA) is often used in clinical studies to measure body fat as well as bone density, which is useful for diagnosing osteoporosis. Although the technique is very accurate for measuring body composition, the equipment is very expensive and requires trained x-ray technicians to use it.

Skinfold Thicknesses Several years ago, advertisements for a breakfast cereal asked people to "pinch an inch" as a method of determining their amount of body fat. If people could pinch a fold of abdominal skin that was more than an inch wide, they were too fat. This crude technique of measuring skinfold thicknesses relied on the principle that one-half of an average person's fat is located beneath the skin.

Using skinfold thicknesses to assess body composition is not as accurate as the underwater weighing and bioelectrical impedance techniques, but it is more practical and less costly. Instead of using fingers to pinch a section of skin and its underlying layer of fat, a trained person uses special calipers to measure skinfold thickness more precisely. Skinfold measurements should be taken at three or more body sites; averaging these measurements accounts for individual differences in body fat distribution.

The reliability of using skinfolds to estimate the percentage of body fat depends on the accuracy of the calipers, the number of skinfolds measured, and the skill of the person performing the measurements. Although measuring skinfolds is a popular technique, some health experts challenge the value of skinfold thicknesses to determine the degree of body fat in obese individuals. Unlike average persons, obese individuals have less than half of their body fat under their skin, and they store considerable amounts of fat in their abdomens. Therefore, researchers are testing the accuracy of other assessment methods such as ultrasound.

Waist-to-Hip Circumference The distribution rather than the percentage of body fat may be a more important risk factor for the health conditions that are associated with excess body fat. Men and women who have large body fat depots centrally located in their waists and backs tend to have higher blood cholesterol levels and a greater risk of developing diabetes, hypertension, and heart disease than individuals with the same amount of fat located below the waist (Pi-Sunyer, 2004). Why? The abdominal fat cells of some obese people may be more likely to release their stores of fatty acids into the blood than fat cells found in the hips and thighs. Excessive amounts of fatty acids in the blood may promote cardiovascular disease, increase blood pressure, and interfere with normal blood glucose metabolism, resulting in diabetes. More research is needed, however, to determine the link between abdominal fat and these chronic diseases (Klein, 2004).

Figure 10-4 **Bioelectrical Impedance.** This woman is having her percentage of body fat determined by the bioelectrical impedance method.

Figure 10-5 **Typical Fat Distribution in Overweight Persons.** Men and women who have large body fat depots centrally located in their waists and backs tend to have a higher risk of chronic health problems than individuals with the same amount of fat located below the waist. (a) Overweight males typically have central fat deposits ("apple-shaped bodies"); (b) Overweight females often have excess body fat below the waist ("pear-shaped bodies").

(a)   **(b)**

As both men and women grow older, they usually add body fat in their abdominal regions, which often increases their **waist-to-hip circumference ratio (WHR)** to unhealthy levels. Figure 10-5 shows a man with central obesity ("apple-shaped") and a woman whose excess body fat is located primarily below the waistline ("pear-shaped").

The only equipment you need to determine your WHR is a flexible but nonstretchable tape measure. Figure 10-6 illustrates where to place the tape measure. To measure your waistline, place the tape around your body just below the ribcage and at the top of the hip-

bone. The proper way to measure your hip circumference is to place the tape around your buttocks at the widest point. Divide your waist measurement by the hip measurement to calculate the ratio of your waist circumference to your hip circumference. What is your WHR? Men who have WHRs greater than .90 and women with WHRs greater than .80 have increased risks of developing the health problems associated with being overweight. According to a report published by the National Institutes of Health (National Heart, Lung, and Blood Institute, 1998), high-risk waistlines measure greater than 40 inches for males and 35 inches for females.

waist-to-hip circumference ratio (WHR) the relationship between waist and hip circumferences that is used to predict the health risks associated with excess body fat.

— Waist measurement (top of hipbone)

Navel —

— Hip measurement (widest portion of buttocks)

Figure 10-6 **Measuring Waist and Hip Circumferences.** To determine one's waist and hip circumferences, measure the waist directly above the hipbone; measure the hips at the widest point of the buttocks.

■ What Causes Obesity?

In most cases, there is no single cause for obesity. According to the principles of energy balance, the body gains fat when it has an excess of energy; the body loses weight when energy intake does not meet its needs. Overweight people often claim that they gain weight by eating small amounts of food. Underreporting caloric intake, however, is common, especially by overweight individuals (Livingstone & Black, 2003). The following section examines factors that contribute to weight gain.

Biological Influences

Genes control the development of many physical characteristics, including height, fat distribution, and body frame size. Genes may also code for weight gain by determining the production of hormones that regulate one's metabolic rate and appetite. As a result, cases of obesity are more likely to occur in certain families. When one or both parents are obese, they are more likely to have offspring who gain excessive amounts of body fat than two parents of normal weights. Could a person benefit from inheriting genes that code for gaining weight easily?

Thousands of years ago, "fat" genes were vital to human survival. Our early ancestors probably endured long periods of fasting, interrupted by shorter periods of feasting. When food was plentiful, our ancestors thrived on the bounty. Some members of the population may have inherited metabolisms that "burned off" the excess food energy as body heat. Others had "thrifty" metabolisms that enabled them to store much of the excess energy as body fat. When food was scarce, individuals with thrifty metabolisms were more likely to survive than those with metabolisms that did not store as much excess energy as fat. Today, most Americans have access to a steady supply of tasty fattening food. Therefore, persons who have thrifty metabolisms find it difficult to control their weight in such environments. The Diversity in Health essay "The Plight of the Pima" discusses the harmful effects that genetic and environmental factors have had on the Pima Indian population of southern Arizona.

set point a theoretical level of body fat that resists weight loss efforts.

hunger the physiological drive to seek and eat food.

appetite the psychological desire to eat foods that are appealing.

satiety the feeling that enough food has been eaten to relieve hunger and turn off appetite.

The Set Point Theory Although body weight usually fluctuates slightly from day to day, most people report that their weight remains fairly stable for months, even years. This observation led some medical experts to propose that the level of body fat is genetically preset. Once the level of body fat reaches this **set point**, the metabolic rate and other internal mechanisms maintain the degree of fatness, like a thermostat can be set to maintain the temperature of a room. Lean persons may have lower set points than overweight individuals. For example, when lean people deliberately overeat to gain weight, they usually lose the extra weight after resuming their normal eating habits. Although having a high set point may result in an unhealthy percentage of body fat, that amount of fat may be normal for the person. As a result, the person's fat cells may resist efforts to lose storage fat. Furthermore, an obese person who loses weight is likely to regain some or all of it within a few years. Why? Some scientists think "slimmed down" fat cells send messages to the brain that are interpreted as hunger. As a result, the person overeats and his or her fat cells expand again.

Appetite Regulation Nearly everyone knows what it feels like to be hungry. **Hunger** is the physiological drive to seek and eat food. **Appetite** is the psychological desire to eat specific foods, which is not the same as being hungry. **Satiety** is the feeling that enough food has been eaten to relieve hunger and turn off appetite.

The digestive system, brain, and fat cells play important roles in controlling hunger and satiety. While a person is eating, the intestinal tract releases several chemicals that signal the brain to eat less food. Additionally, the sensation of stomach fullness results in termination of eating. Leptin, a hormone produced by fat cells, and insulin, the pancreatic hormone that lowers blood sugar levels, affect the *hypothalamus*, a region of the brain that regulates eating behavior (Figure 10-7). Leptin and insulin play important roles in regulating eating behavior, but in obese people, these hormones seem to lose their effectiveness (French & Castiglione, 2002).

Scientists recently discovered *ghrelin*, a compound produced primarily by the stomach that stimulates feeding behavior in certain laboratory animals (Eisenstein & Greenberg, 2003). More research is needed to determine how ghrelin affects human appetites and metabolisms.

Composition of the Diet An excess of calories from carbohydrate, protein, fat, and alcohol can result in weight gain. However, high-fat diets are associated with overeating and gaining body fat (Tremblay, 2004). An ounce of fat supplies more than twice the number of calories as an ounce of carbohydrate or protein. Furthermore, the body stores more fat when the excess

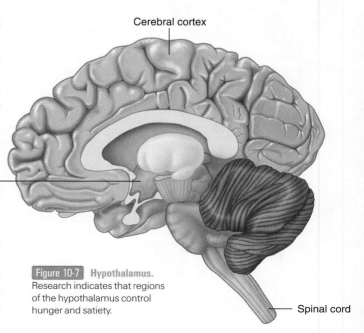

Cerebral cortex

Hypothalamus

Spinal cord

Figure 10-7 **Hypothalamus.** Research indicates that regions of the hypothalamus control hunger and satiety.

of calories is supplied by dietary fat rather than carbohydrate or protein (Hill & Peters, 1998).

No specific calorie-restricted diet enhances weight loss and maintenance. However, overweight people often lose weight when following a low-fat, high-carbohydrate diet because the food plan includes generous servings of fruits, vegetables, beans, and whole-grain cereals. These nutrient-dense, high-fiber foods are quite filling, and dieters may fail to eat enough to meet their total permissible number of calories. Why do overweight people blame carbohydrates for their weight problem?

Carbohydrate-rich foods often taste better when they are fried or when fats such as butter, sour cream, or gravy are added to them. Most desserts and snack foods contain refined carbohydrates and fat; mixtures of sugar and fat are almost irresistible. Thus, the typical American diet promotes overeating because it provides an interesting, tasty, and enjoyable variety of fatty foods.

Many people are unaware of the number of calories that are in their snacks and meals. Calorie and fat-counting guides are helpful if you are trying to control your weight. Keeping a record of everything you eat and drink each day can also be useful for identifying problem foods and poor eating habits. By eating more fruits and vegetables and fewer sugary and fatty foods, you can control your caloric intake.

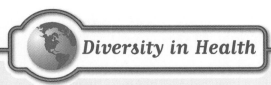

Diversity in Health

The Plight of the Pima

After the July rains, the Sonora Desert of southwestern Arizona becomes transformed for a brief time into a natural fast-food restaurant. For hundreds of years, the Pima Indians residing in this harsh environment harvested the seasonal bounty of mesquite pods, acorns, wolfberries, prickly pears, tepary beans, and cholla blossoms to supplement their regular diet of hunted animals and cultivated maize (corn) and lima beans. The Pima were slim, but they flourished while enduring this cycle of feast and famine.

By the 1930s, the Arizona Pima had discontinued eating most of their ancient fare and adopted Western foods that provided generous amounts of lard (pork fat), refined starches, and sweets. Within a couple of decades, an alarming number of Pima had become obese and developed type 2 diabetes. Today, nearly 70% of Arizona Pima are obese (Valencia et al., 1999). Obesity is a risk factor for type 2 diabetes; more than 40% of Arizona Pima suffer from this condition. This is the highest known incidence of the disease in the world. Why are the Pima so severely affected by obesity and type 2 diabetes?

Medical experts suspect certain biological and environmental factors influence the development of obesity and diabetes in this population. Experts think the Pima have thrifty metabolisms that allow them to survive their harsh desert environment with its natural cycles of feast and famine. Although their current dietary habits have made the need for such metabolisms obsolete, the Pima are still genetically programmed to conserve a major share of their food intake as fat. Additionally, most Arizona Pima lead more sedentary lives than their ancestors or relatives living in Mexico. The typical Mexican Pima Indian has fewer labor-saving devices and performs more physical work than the typical Arizona Pima.

The Arizona Pima's abandonment of ancient dietary practices may contribute to their current health problems. Besides being lower in fat, traditional Pima foods provide more complex carbohydrates than typical modern menus. Furthermore, the ancestral diet supplied substances that may have protected the Pima from diabetes. Many desert plants contain significant amounts of amylose, a digestible carbohydrate, as well as gums and mucilages, two forms of soluble fiber. Eating foods rich in these substances slows digestion and delays the absorption of glucose from the small intestine. This delay prevents sharp increases in blood levels of insulin, the hormone that signals cells to remove glucose (blood sugar) from the blood. Under normal circumstances, the body can prevent sharp increases or decreases of blood glucose. However, individuals who suffer from type 2 diabetes are unable to avoid dramatic fluctuations in blood glucose or insulin levels, which can damage the body.

Today medical experts are studying the Pima to determine what steps can be taken to reduce their prevalence of obesity and diabetes. Some scientists think tribal members should return to their former dietary practices; many of these ancestral foods are still available. By eating desert plant foods rich in amylose and soluble fibers, the Pima may reduce their risk of developing type 2 diabetes. If the Pima are to survive as a population, they may need to recover their traditional "roots."

Sources: Boyce, V. L., & Swinburn, B. A. (1993). The traditional Pima Indian diet: Composition and adaptation for use in a dietary intervention study. *Diabetes Care, 16*(51):369–371.

Cowen, R. (1990). Seeds of protection: Ancestral menus may hold a message for diabetes-prone descendants. *Science News, 137*:350–351.

Valencia, M. E., Bennett, P. H., Ravussin, E., Esparza, J., Fox, C., & Schultz, L. O. (1999). The Pima Indians of Sonora, Mexico. *Nutrition Reviews, 57*(5):S55–S58.

Environmental, Social, and Psychological Influences

A variety of environmental, social, and psychological factors promote overeating in the United States. Since the early 1900s, typical portions of many popular foods have increased (Young & Nestle, 2003). When the Hershey chocolate bar was introduced in 1906, it weighed a little over half an ounce; today the smallest Hershey bar weighs 1.6 ounces. Compared with original bakery bagels, an average bakery bagel now weighs three times as much and provides three times the amount of energy. Fast-food hamburgers and standard servings of french fries and soft drinks are often considerably larger than those served when these popular restaurants first opened in the 1950s and 1960s. Many fast-food and family-style restaurants promote their "super-size" portions as being bargains. Such food production practices encourage overeating. The average American man consumes 7% more calories, and the average American woman 22% more calories, than 30 years ago (Wright et al., 2004).

Advertisers know the value of making foods look appealing. To stimulate sales, for example, fast-food restaurants show hamburgers topped with crisp lettuce and bacon extending beyond the bun. Actors in food ads appear to be happy and satisfied with their food choices. Many fast-food restaurants as well as supermarkets are open 24 hours. You do not even have to leave home to buy food; pizza, Chinese, and other food can be delivered to your front door.

Many people respond to certain social situations by overeating. For example, you may be "stuffed" after eating a Thanksgiving dinner, but when you see pumpkin pie topped with whipped cream, you can find "room" in your stomach for dessert. Additionally, events that mark important milestones of life usually include big meals and special foods. Imagine a birthday party or wedding celebration that does not include a frosted layer cake!

Work and home environments often do not provide opportunities for Americans to be physically active. Modern technology enables machines, instead of our muscles, to do much of our work. At home, many people spend their leisure time engaged in sedentary activities such as watching television or using a computer. Physically inactive people are likely to gain weight unless they restrict their food intake.

Psychological state can influence eating behavior. Some people eat long after satisfying their hunger, because they are excited, anxious, or bored. Many depressed individuals seek comfort from eating, especially foods that are fatty and sugary. The following personal reflection written by an overweight young woman illustrates how emotions can affect eating behavior:

> I gained 20 pounds between the ages of 16 and 18. At the time I was in an abusive relationship with my boyfriend. I felt like dirt and the only thing that made me feel good was food. I was totally devastated when he was killed in a car accident when I was 18. I ate even more. I went to a nutritionist for a diet. I tried to stay on it but failed. Looking back, every time I gained weight it was due to stress. When I am stressed, I need to get out of the house, take my mind off things.

In developed nations, bulimia nervosa and binge eating disorder affect considerable numbers of people, especially girls and women. These conditions are associated with serious psychological disturbances; therefore, they are discussed in Chapter 2.

■ Weight Management

According to a survey conducted in 1998, 24% of American men and 38% of American women were trying to lose weight (Kruger et al., 2004). Dissatisfaction with body size is common, particularly among women. Almost 25% of the women who were making an effort to lose weight had normal weights. Only one-third of the people who wanted to lose weight had tried reducing their caloric intakes and increasing their exercise levels. In a survey of American college students, nearly 60% of females and 30% of males reported that they were attempting to lose weight at the time of the survey ("Youth Risk," 1997).

Even though they may have gained the weight gradually, overweight individuals who want to lose weight often seek methods that promise quick and dramatic results. These people are likely to believe advertisements for weight loss methods or products that guarantee pounds will "melt fast without sweating or dieting." As a result, most people lose more than just body fat by using various weight loss products and services. Each year, Americans spend over $33 billion on various weight control efforts (Kruger et al., 2004). These efforts include joining weight loss programs or spas and buying special foods, books, pills, and gadgets. Do these products and services enable people to lose weight? How can you judge the value of a weight loss method? The following sections answer these questions.

Weight Reduction Diets

As mentioned earlier, the body loses weight when its caloric intake is less than its energy needs. In this situation, the body relies primarily on stored fat for energy. To lose weight, overweight individuals should eat fewer calories than they need or expend more calories. Most reliable weight reduction regimens incorporate both of these features by combining a low-calorie diet with a plan that increases physical activity.

Some of the more popular weight loss diets of the last three decades have included a variety of recommendations such as fasting, counting calories, not counting calories, avoiding certain food combinations, eating plenty of protein and little carbohydrate, or eating only a few foods (Table 10-3). Such diets are often referred to as **fad diets** because they remain popular for a period of time and then quickly lose their widespread appeal. The low-carbohydrate "Atkins diet," for example, gained many followers when it was first introduced in 1973, but dieters soon lost interest in its restrictive food choices. When the Atkins diet was reintroduced about 25 years later, its renewed popularity resulted in the marketing of a wide array of "low-carb" foods. By the fall of 2004, however, most American dieters had lost their enthusiasm for the low-carbohydrate diet fad. Fad diets usually have a few common features—gimmicks and caloric restriction. A *gimmick* is a promotional feature that makes a fad weight loss diet appear to be new, unique, and more effective than other diet plans. Some fad diets, including the Atkins diet, use carbohydrate restric-

tion as a gimmick. Other fad diets use gimmicks such as prescribed food combinations based on your blood type, dietary supplements that "melt fat while you sleep," and "secret" food ingredients that allow you to eat all your favorite foods or retain fat in desirable places (the breasts of women, for example) while shedding it from the hips, abdomen, and thighs. Although such claims are untrue and not based on scientific evidence, they attract people who are seeking quick and easy ways to lose their excess fat. Overweight people can lose weight while following fad diets because the diet plans that accompany the gimmicks usually provide fewer calories than the level of energy supplied by typical American diets. Regardless of the type of diet they used to lose excess fat, the majority of formerly overweight people find it difficult to maintain their new body weights.

Very low-calorie diets may provide fewer than 800 calories per day and be nutritionally inadequate because they limit food choices. Diets that provide 400 or fewer calories daily are often called *fasts*. Fasts are essentially starvation regimens. Some fasts permit only fruit juices and nutrient supplements. Fasting accelerates the loss

fad diets
eating plans that are popular for a time, then quickly lose their widespread appeal.

Table 10-3	Some Fad Diets	
Diet	**Approach**	**Possible Problems**
Dr. Atkins Diet Revolution Enter the Zone The Doctor's Quick Weight Loss Diet Protein Power Calories Don't Count The Complete Scarsdale Medical Diet Sugar Busters	Restrict carbohydrate intake while increasing protein and fat intake	High animal fat intake may contribute to heart disease. Although initial weight loss can be impressive, long-term results are similar to other calorie-reduced plans.
Pritikin Diet Macrobiotic Diet (certain types) The Rice Diet Eat More, Weigh Less T-Factor Diet Stop the Insanity The Pasta Diet The McDougall Plan The Maximum Metabolism Diet	Limit food choices; very low fat	Boredom with limited food choices; feeling of deprivation since favorite foods are limited or prohibited. High fiber intake results in increased intestinal gas and may interfere with mineral absorption; dieter often feels deprived and hungry.
Cabbage Soup Diet The New Beverly Hills Diet Dr. Berger's Immune Power Diet Bloomingdale's Diet Eat to Win Two-Day Diet Spirulina Diet Vinegar Diet Grapefruit Diet	Promote certain nutrients, substances, foods, or food combinations as having special "fat-burning" or weight loss abilities	Boredom with limited food choices; may result in nutritional deficiencies if followed for long periods.

Source: Adapted from Wardlaw, G. M. (1999). *Perspectives in nutrition.* Boston: McGraw-Hill.

of fat and lean body tissue, creating unhealthy metabolic by-products. Healthy individuals should not fast for more than a day without medical supervision.

Initially, obese people typically lose substantial amounts of weight while following a low-calorie diet or fast. When caloric intake is very low, the body burns fat as well as lean tissue for energy. Since fat and lean tissue store water, using these tissues for energy creates a surplus of water in the body. The kidneys eliminate the excess water, causing a dramatic loss of weight that often encourages dieters during the early phase of their weight reduction efforts. Within a few weeks, however, the body regains its normal water balance, and the rate of weight loss slows.

Very low-calorie diets or fasts trigger energy-conserving mechanisms in the body that are designed to help people survive starvation. The metabolic rate decreases with caloric restriction, especially when individuals consume fewer than 800 calories a day. Thus, dieters must cut their caloric intakes even further to continue losing weight, which often makes adhering to their diets even more difficult.

In spite of their efforts, most individuals experience a decline in their rate of weight loss after several weeks of following a calorie-reduced diet. Some of this slowdown occurs because the body expends fewer calories to maintain the new weight. As the body adjusts to the reduced caloric intake, it metabolizes less fat and lean tissue for energy, slowing the rate of weight loss. Additionally, dieters who follow restrictive diet plans for more than a few weeks often become bored with the regimens and gradually return to their old eating habits. Most people who have lost weight regain some or all of it—and often, even more weight—after a period of caloric restriction. Frustrated dieters often blame themselves for lack of self-control. Episodes of losing and regaining weight are referred to as *yo-yo dieting* or *weight cycling*. Some medical experts think weight cycling is more harmful to one's health than maintaining an excessive but stable amount of body fat. Current research, however, indicates that yo-yo dieting does not increase the risk of hypertension or other risk factors for heart disease (Graci et al., 2004). Obesity clearly poses more health risks than weight cycling. Rather than endure periodic fad dieting, overweight people should consider other, more successful methods of losing weight—changing eating and exercise patterns for life.

Physical Activity

Many American adults are less active physically than when they were younger, partly because they have occupations that require little physical effort. Men who had trim, athletic builds during adolescence often develop bulging waistlines by the time they are 40. As they reach middle age, women often blame "gravity" or pregnancy for the expanding dimensions of their waists, hips, and thighs. Can adopting more physically active lifestyles reverse these changes?

> I gained 20 pounds before my wedding. My husband bought me a stepper for a wedding present (that's what I wanted), and I use it with an exercise video. Now, I exercise more than ever, but I haven't lost much weight.

This student has discovered that exercising to lose body fat often does not produce the desired change in body weight. Physical activity alone is not as effective as low-calorie diets for treating obesity, because most overweight individuals cannot perform enough exercise to create a significant deficit of calories. This does not mean that overweight people should abandon physical activity as a means of losing excess body fat. Exercise retains lean tissue and builds muscle mass, which may stabilize or even increase one's body weight. Thus, what appears to be a lack of progress while restricting food intake and exercising may be the result of a healthy increase in muscle mass.

Rather than tracking changes in body weight, physically active overweight individuals can keep weekly records of waist and chest circumferences (men) or waist and hip circumferences (men and women). People who become more physically active while dieting often report that their clothing fits better, or they can wear smaller sizes, even though they have not lost much weight. Besides improving physical appearance, exercise reduces elevated blood pressures and lipid levels. Furthermore, individuals who exercise for 200 to 300 minutes per week are more likely to maintain their weight loss than those who are less active (Jakicic et al., 2001).

Most overweight individuals can safely increase their physical activity by walking, bicycling, or swimming for at least 30 minutes, preferably on a daily basis. Regardless of the activity, it should be enjoyable and practical to perform on a year-round basis. Before beginning a vigorous physical activity program, inactive people over 40 years of age should obtain the approval of their health care practitioners.

Surgical Procedures

Most severely obese individuals experience little success following low-calorie diet plans and exercising to lose weight. *Gastric bypass* surgeries are sometimes used to treat extremely obese individuals. Figure 10-8 illustrates the appearance of the stomach and small intestine after one type of gastric bypass surgery. A sur-

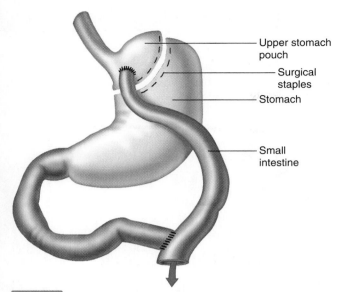

Figure 10-8 **Gastric Bypass Surgery.** Gastric bypass is a surgical procedure used to treat severe obesity. After surgery, the obese person experiences discomfort after overeating and is less likely to overeat.

geon drastically reduces the capacity of the stomach by creating a small pouch in the upper part of the stomach for food to enter. After having this procedure, the overweight person can no longer eat large portions of food without vomiting or uncomfortable feelings of fullness. Most people who have had gastric bypasses are able to lose 50% or more of their presurgery weight, achieving long-term weight maintenance and improving their overall health (Herron, 2004).

Liposuction, vacuuming subcutaneous fat out of the body, is the most common type of cosmetic surgery in the United States. Before removing the fat, the area is injected with an anesthetic-containing fluid or treated with ultrasound *(ultrasound-assisted lipoplasty).* This technique has cosmetic value when used to remove small areas of fat that create unsightly bulges such as "saddlebag thighs" or double chins (Figure 10-9). Liposuction can be hazardous; infections, blood clots, disfigurement, and even death can result. For most overweight individuals, liposuction is not an acceptable weight loss method.

Medications

Overweight people who are trying to follow low-calorie diets often lose control over their appetites and as a result overeat. For decades, medical researchers have been testing various compounds to determine if they can help people adhere to their diet plans more easily or lose weight faster. The FDA has approved only two drugs to treat obesity; these medications generally reduce food intake by suppressing appetite or hinder fat absorption from the small intestine. Medications that increase the metabolic rate are not approved for weight reduction in the United States (Yanovski & Yanovski, 2002).

Prescription weight loss drugs are not useful unless added to a plan that includes a calorie-reduced diet and an exercise regimen. Furthermore, people who have lost weight with the help of "diet drugs" usually regain it when they discontinue taking the medications.

Additionally, weight loss medications can cause serious side effects. In 1997 fenfluramine and dexfenfluramine were withdrawn from the market after some individuals using either drug or Fen/Phen, a non-FDA-approved combination of fenfluramine and phentermine, developed a rare heart valve defect or a deadly form of high blood pressure. Sibutramine (Meridia) is the only appetite suppressant that has FDA approval for long-term (two years) use with a calorie-reduced diet (FDA, 2001). Sibutramine, however, can increase blood pressure in some patients. In 2002 Italian health officials removed the drug from the market after two deaths and several reports of serious side effects were linked with its use (Wooltorton, 2002). Thus, physi-

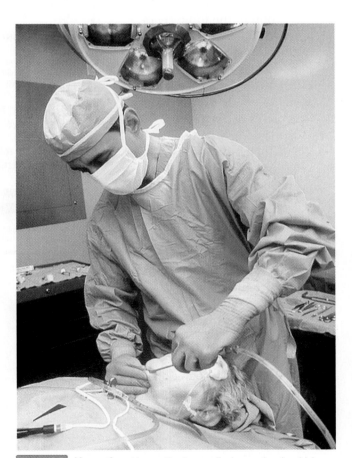

Figure 10-9 **Liposuction.** Liposuction is a medical procedure in which a special instrument is inserted into body fat through an incision made in the skin, and the fat is vacuumed from the body.

This advertisement promotes a weight loss product. Read the ad and evaluate it using the model for analyzing health-related information. The main points of the model are noted below; the model is explained fully on pages 13–15.

1. Which statements are verifiable facts, and which are unverified statements or value claims?

2. What are the credentials of the person who wrote the ad? Does the author appear to have appropriate background and education in the topic area? If it is difficult to tell if the author has specific health expertise, what can you do to check his or her credentials?

3. What might be the motives and biases of the author?

4. What is the main point of the ad? Which information is relevant to the issue or main point, and which information is irrelevant?

5. Is the source reliable, or does it have a reputation for publishing misinformation? Does the ad present both the pros and cons of the product?

6. Does the ad attack the credibility of conventional scientists or medical authorities?

Based on your analysis, do you think that this ad is a reliable source of health-related information? Summarize your reasons for coming to this conclusion.

FINALLY!

a weight-loss product that lives up to your expectations!

Pond scum, grapefruit pills, cabbage soup, stimulants, prepackaged foods, cellulite creams—you name the diet or diet product—you probably have tried it and have been disappointed. The fat didn't budge, and what's worse, you may have gained even more weight as a result of your efforts. You are not alone. There are millions of victims of diet failure—people, like you, who wasted their money and hope on diets and diet products that promised so much and delivered so little.

New and improved FLAB-BE-GONE speeds up your cells' natural fat-burning potential by 68%.

Now you can stop dieting and get the slim, trim figure that you've always wanted.

HOW? Take FLAB-BE-GONE, the revolutionary new method of weight loss that uses your cells' own fat-burning ability to shed unwanted pounds of ugly fat from your body. FLAB-BE-GONE enables you to lose weight effortlessly, while you sleep or watch TV. There's no need for exercise that makes you sweat and damages your joints. You don't have to count calories, grams of carbs or fat, or starve yourself. Just take two FLAB-BE-GONE tablets with meals or snacks. Want an ice cream sundae? Go ahead, eat it. Just take FLAB-BE-GONE with it! Within hours, watch as those pounds of fat and cellulite melt off your body!

Can you believe it? Yes, it's true.
The unique formulation of FLAB-BE-GONE makes it possible to lose up to 10 pounds overnight. Guaranteed!
If you don't lose weight after 1 week of using FLAB-BE-GONE as directed, we will refund your money. You can't lose!

For a month's supply, send $59.95 to:

LOSE UP TO: 10 inches off your waistline
6 inches off your hips
8 inches off your thighs.

Warning: We must ask you to consult your physician before taking this product. If your weight drops too quickly while taking FLAB-BE-GONE, simply reduce the dose.

cians in countries where sibutramine is still available, such as the United States and Canada, need to inform patients of its risks as well as its benefits.

Orlistat (Xenical) is a prescription drug that does not suppress appetite but interferes with fat digestion. As a result, some of the fat in foods is not digested and is eliminated in feces. Fat-soluble vitamins are generally found in fats and oils, so a person taking orlistat will not absorb as many of these nutrients from foods, and therefore should take a vitamin supplement.

Dietary supplements such as those containing chitosan, chromium picolinate, and conjugated linoleic acid are available without prescriptions. Medical experts, however, do not recommend these products for weight loss because reports of their safety and effectiveness are not based on well-designed clinical studies (Yanovsky & Yanovsky, 2002). The Consumer Health feature "Dietary Supplements: Weight Loss Aids" provide's information about some popular over-the-counter weight loss products. The Analyzing Health-Related

Consumer Health

Dietary Supplements: Weight Loss Aids

Anyone who has tried to lose weight knows it can be a frustrating effort. Hunger seems to be a constant companion. For years, overweight people have taken various pills and dietary supplements sold over the counter to promote weight loss and prevent hunger. Stimulant drugs, including *phenylpropanolamine (PPA)* and ephedra, are mild stimulants that suppress hunger over a short period. Recently, the FDA requested manufacturers of weight loss aids to remove PPA from their products, and the agency banned the sale of dietary supplements and weight loss aids that contained ephedra. The FDA took

these actions after evaluating medical reports that associated PPA and ephedra with dangerous and sometimes deadly side effects. (See Chapter 1 for more information about ephedra.)

Certain dietary supplements promoted for weight loss purposes are still available. Table 10-A includes several of the more popular supplements that people take to lose weight and provides information concerning the scientific support for health-related claims associated with the product.

Individuals should not use any weight loss drug or dietary supplement without the advice and monitoring of their physician. If you experience any side effects while taking a weight loss medication or product, report the problem to the FDA's MedWatch hotline by calling 1-800-332-1088.

Table 10-A Dietary Supplements: Weight Loss

Dietary Supplement	Claims	Scientific Findings
Garcinia	Reduces body fat	The evidence to support the claim is weak.
Bitter orange	Enhances weight loss	Bitter orange can increase heart rate and blood pressure; therefore, its use is risky.
Blue-green algae (spirulina)	Promotes weight loss, boosts immune system functioning, and treats asthma, depression, and several other common disorders	No evidence to support claims. Algae may be contaminated with toxins that are in their environment.
Chitosan (chitin)	Enhances weight loss, reduces blood lipid levels	No evidence to support weight loss claim. Chitosan may reduce cholesterol levels, but the effect is minimal.
Chromium picolinate	Increases metabolic rate, facilitates weight loss	May result in slight reduction in body weight, but the loss is not impressive.
Glucomannan	Enhances weight loss	Some evidence to support claim, but more research is needed.
Yerba maté	Enhances weight loss	Results of one study suggest that a combination of yerba maté, guarana, and damiana may assist weight loss, but more research is needed.

Sources: Swartzberg, J. E., Margen, S., et al. (2001). *The complete home wellness handbook*. New York: Health Letter Associates; Pittler, M. H., & Ernst, E. (2004). Dietary supplements for body-weight reduction: A systematic review. *American Journal of Clinical Nutrition, 79*(4):529–536.

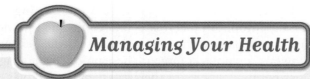

Managing Your Health

General Features of Reliable Weight Reduction Plans

Use the following features to judge the quality of weight loss programs.

The diet plan is medically sound if it

- provides recommendations that are safe and supported by scientific evidence.
- suggests receiving a physician's approval prior to initiating the plan.
- encourages gradual weight loss.

The diet is nutritionally sound if it

- meets nutritional needs.
- includes foods from each food group.
- encourages eating smaller portions of nutritious foods.
- encourages self-control over problem foods such as sweets.
- considers individual food preferences.
- includes reasonable amounts of fiber and complex carbohydrates.
- reduces caloric intake to no lower than 1,000 calories per day.
- recommends losing $\frac{1}{2}$ lb to 2 lb per week.
- avoids requiring special or costly supplements and foods.
- avoids claims about the superiority of the plan.
- avoids guarantees concerning weight loss.

The diet plan considers physical fitness needs if it

- recommends an exercise plan that is tailored to the individual's needs, time constraints, interests, and capabilities.
- includes practical suggestions for altering sedentary behaviors.
- encourages daily aerobic activities that last at least half an hour.
- avoids promoting costly exercise equipment, joining exercise clubs, or buying special gadgets to shed pounds.
- recommends physical activities that are safe and enjoyable.
- considers special health concerns of the individual.

The diet plan meets psychological and social needs if it

- provides practical suggestions for modifying food-related attitudes and behaviors.
- educates about the need to set realistic weight loss goals.
- includes techniques to monitor progress (such as weekly recording of waist-to-hip ratios).
- builds self-esteem.
- includes tips to control eating in social situations.
- includes foods that family and friends eat.
- provides strategies for coping with setbacks, difficult situations, and nonsupportive people.
- offers opportunities for group support.

Source: Adapted from Dwyer, J. T. (1992). Treatment of obesity: Conventional programs and fad diets. In P. Björntorp & B. N. Brodoff (Eds.), *Obesity* (pp. 662–676). Philadelphia: Lippincott.

Information feature in this chapter includes an advertisement for a dietary supplement that is marketed for weight loss.

Strategies for Successful Weight Loss

Overweight individuals can lose body fat and maintain their new weight by following sensible and safe weight loss plans, which have four major characteristics:

1. They are medically and nutritionally sound.
2. They include practical ways to engage in regular physical activity.
3. They are adaptable to one's psychological and social needs.
4. They can be followed for a lifetime.

Nutritionally sound weight reduction diets emphasize nutrient-dense foods, and they are nutritionally well balanced and adequate. Without being overly restrictive, such diets supply fewer calories than overweight people need. No special foods are necessary; the recommendations of the dietary guidelines and MyPyramid Plan form the basis of nutritious calorie-reduced daily menus.

Reasonable and reliable diet plans recommend ways to increase physical activity such as by adding 30 to 90 minutes of walking, swimming, or bicycling to one's routine on most days of the week. Additionally, weight loss plans should meet the psychological and social needs of overweight persons. A reliable plan, for example, helps a person set an achievable weight loss goal, recognize faulty eating habits, build self-esteem, and obtain family or group support. You can use the criteria listed in the Managing Your Health tips entitled "General Features of Reliable Weight Reduction Plans" to judge the effectiveness of most weight-reduction methods.

Effective weight loss plans usually emphasize *behavior modification*. Behavior modification involves learning to identify behaviors that contribute to one's inability to lose weight, such as eating too much fatty food and not engaging in enough physical activity. Additionally, the overweight person learns to modify inappropriate behaviors so that weight loss and its maintenance are possible. Table 10-4 lists key behaviors, such as not watching television while eating, that can

help overweight people achieve their weight loss goals. By identifying and modifying behaviors that resulted in weight gain, an overweight person can develop a weight loss and maintenance plan that works best for him or her.

To avoid regaining weight, successful dieters must make lifestyle changes they can follow throughout their lifetimes, such as exercising regularly and controlling caloric intake. Small incremental changes that are implemented gradually are easier to adopt than extreme exercise regimens and overly restrictive diets. Most fad diets do not focus on behavior modification. However, even reliable weight loss programs that promote behavior modification do not offer guarantees for long-term suc-

Table 10-4	Examples of Behavior Modification for Weight Management
Behavior	**Actions to Modify Behavior**
Identify faulty eating behaviors and eliminate or ignore improper eating cues.	· Keep daily food records to identify problem foods. · Use a shopping list and do not buy problem foods. · Eat fruit or a meal before shopping for food. · Discard problem foods. · While at home, restrict eating to the kitchen or dining room. · Do not eat while watching TV, reading, or talking on the phone. · Avoid places with vending machines. · Avoid fast-food restaurants that do not sell low-fat foods.
Reduce caloric intake.	· Serve meals on smaller plates. · Prepare smaller amounts of foods to reduce the likelihood of "seconds." · Avoid buffet-style or all-you-can-eat restaurants. · Eat a low-fat high-fiber snack such as a piece of fruit or vegetable before a meal. · Keep fruit and vegetables on hand to snack on when hungry. · Ask for salad dressing "on the side" at restaurants. · Prepare low-calorie lunches and snacks to take to work or school. · Substitute fresh fruit or yogurt for rich desserts. · Read nutrition labels to identify high-calorie foods. · Learn to leave some food on your plate.
Stay focused on weight-loss goal.	· Set reasonable incremental goals, such as losing 5 pounds in 5 weeks. · Place a picture of yourself on the refrigerator, pantry door, or bedroom mirror. · Measure your waistline once a week. · Place exercise equipment and walking shoes where you can see them. · Buy new pants that are one size smaller and hang them where you can see them. · Ask your friends and family to support your efforts. Give them examples of how they can help.
Practice appropriate behaviors.	· Find ways to move around while at work, school, or home. For example, take the stairs instead of the elevator. · If you relapse, tell yourself that this is normal. Do not label yourself a failure. Ask yourself what you can learn from the experience so it is less likely to affect your eating again. Minor occasional indulgences will not affect your weight. Continue to focus on your weight loss goal. · Set aside at least 30 minutes each day to engage in an enjoyable physical activity. Gradually increase the duration of the activity to 45 to 60 minutes daily.
Use nonfood rewards for behaviors.	· Praise yourself frequently for exercising or taking smaller servings of high-calorie appropriate foods. · Buy a desired item such as a new CD, DVD, or an item of clothing. · Take a walk or ride a bike through a park.

cess. The process of changing behaviors takes education, practice, time, and perseverance.

The majority of people who have lost weight through nonsurgical methods experience relapse, regaining some or all of the weight within 1 to 5 years ("Position of the ADA," 1997). Relapses occur when overweight persons fail to modify eating behaviors and physical activity patterns permanently and have unrealistic weight loss expectations. Individuals who lose weight while following fad diets are prone to relapse when they return to their usual food habits.

Presently, there is no safe or effective treatment that "cures" being overweight. Therefore, one should strive to prevent excessive weight gain by making permanent lifestyle changes that include reducing the size of food portions, especially fatty foods, and increasing physical activity.

Weight Gain

Although it may seem nearly everyone is on a diet to lose weight, some people are underweight and trying to gain weight. Many health experts think underweight individuals should avoid gaining body fat unless their condition is the result of chronic illness. Nevertheless, thin individuals are often just as dissatisfied with their body sizes as overweight people.

To gain lean tissue, underweight persons need to consume at least 700 to 1,000 more calories per day than they usually eat and perform muscle-building exercises. To obtain the extra calories, underweight people can eat more than three meals a day and snack on nutrient-dense foods such as dried fruit, whole-wheat muffins, granola bars, yogurt and fruit smoothies, peanut butter, and nuts. You can find other nutritious foods that are high in food energy by consulting food composition tables. Since fatty foods are a source of considerable calories, physically active underweight individuals can eat as much as 35% of their caloric intake from these items. Because of the association with cardiovascular disease, people trying to gain weight should avoid eating excessive amounts of saturated fats. Avocados, olives, and nuts are high in unsaturated fat, which is healthier than saturated fat. For people trying to gain weight, the effort must be maintained over the long term, just as it is for people trying to lose weight.

If you are thinking about losing or gaining weight, complete the Changing Health Habits activity for this chapter in the student workbook. This activity can help you decide if you are ready to make the lifestyle changes needed to modify your weight and maintain a new, healthier weight for the rest of your life.

Healthy Living Practices

- If you want to lose weight, modify your lifestyle. For example, eat less fat by replacing high-fat snacks with more nutrient-dense foods.
- To lose or control your body weight, engage in vigorous physical activity such as jogging, brisk walking, cycling, or swimming for at least 30 minutes, preferably every day.
- To judge whether a weight loss plan or program is sensible and safe, determine if it is medically and nutritionally sound, includes a plan to increase regular physical activity, is adaptable to your psychological and social needs, and can be followed for a lifetime.
- If you want to gain weight, add at least 700 to 1,000 calories to your usual daily intake and exercise to build muscle mass. To boost the caloric content of meals and snacks, eat more nutrient-dense foods such as dried fruit, whole-wheat muffins, granola bars, peanut butter, and nuts.

Across THE LIFESPAN

Weight Management

The amount of weight a woman gains during pregnancy affects the health of her baby. The average woman should gain about 25 to 35 pounds by the end of pregnancy (Wardlaw, 2004). This weight gain includes not only the fetus's weight, but also the weight of the pregnant woman's additional body fluids, fat stores, and breast and uterine tissues. Women who are underweight when they become pregnant can expect to gain more weight; those who are overweight may gain a few pounds less than average.

Some pregnant women restrict their food intake to limit their weight gain because they do not want to struggle with losing the extra pounds after the baby arrives. However, caloric restriction during pregnancy may be hazardous to the developing fetus. The time to lose weight is before or after pregnancy and not during this period. Nevertheless, within two years after giving birth, many women remain several pounds heavier than those who have not been pregnant.

Infancy is a period characterized by rapid gains in both weight and height. Many babies who are overweight at their first birthday slim down by the time they enter school. Because dietary fat is essential for normal growth and development, low-fat or calorie-restricted diets are not recommended for children under 2 years of age.

As mentioned in the beginning of this chapter, the percentage of overweight school-age children is increasing in the United States (Figure 10-10). Children and adolescents need adequate amounts of energy for physical development and activity, but they often eat more calories and fat than recommended by dietitians. Besides dietary factors, preoccupation with sedentary activities such as watching television contributes to the increase of childhood obesity (Crespo et al., 2001).

No one can predict whether an overweight child will become an overweight adult. However, fat children and adolescents are more likely to remain obese into adulthood (Guo et al., 2002). Thus, preventing childhood obesity has become a national health priority.

Childhood and adolescent obesity often becomes a problem that affects the entire family. Overweight children may develop eating disorders and low self-esteem when parents, other adults, or peers treat them negatively. An effective program that helps overweight children lose weight should not interfere with their normal physical development and should not encourage the development of eating disorders. Successful treatment involves teaching children and their parents how to make appropriate dietary modifications, increase physical activity, and resolve conflicts that may involve eating habits.

By 65 years of age, most people have experienced a decline in their lean mass and an increase in their fat mass. This change occurs to a lesser extent in individuals who maintain a high degree of physical activity as they grow old. Some elderly persons may benefit from having moderate amounts of body fat, particularly if they lose their appetites during illness. In most instances, however, the same health problems that plague younger overweight individuals can affect the overweight elderly.

Overweight elderly persons can follow the same recommendations for losing weight as do younger overweight individuals: Select nutrient-dense foods, reduce intakes of fatty and sugary foods, and become more physically active. Even modest increases in physical activity, such as walking, swimming, or light exercise, can benefit most elderly people.

Figure 10-10 **Childhood Obesity.** The percentage of overweight children is increasing in the United States.

Healthy Living Practices

- Weight gain is necessary during pregnancy, so if you are pregnant, do not try to lose weight at this time.
- Restrictive diets can interfere with a child's normal development. Check with a health care practitioner before placing your child on a fat- or calorie-restricted diet.
- To avoid becoming overweight as you grow older, select nutrient-dense, low-fat foods and maintain moderate to high degrees of physical activity.

Summary

Recent health surveys indicate that more Americans are overweight than in previous decades. More than 60% of the adult U.S. population is too fat. Excess body fat is associated with low self-esteem and increased risks of chronic health conditions such as osteoarthritis, sleep apnea, gallbladder disease, gout, hypertension, diabetes, certain cancers, and heart disease.

The body uses the energy in foods to power vital metabolic activity, to move skeletal muscles, and to process nutrients after meals. According to the principles of energy balance, the body requires a certain number of calories to maintain its weight. When one consumes more calories than needed, weight gain occurs; when one ingests fewer calories than needed, weight loss occurs. Since each pound of body fat represents about 3,500 calories, consuming 500 fewer calories a day than needed should result in a weight loss of about one pound per week.

Methods of determining the percentage of body fat include measuring subcutaneous fat (skinfold thicknesses), hydrostatic weighing, bioelectrical impedance, and near-infrared interactance. To determine if they are overweight, many people rely on skinfold measurements, waist-to-hip ratios (WHR), and body mass indices (BMI). Risks of chronic health problems and death increase as the WHR and BMI increase.

Obesity is not simply the result of a lack of willpower. The development of obesity is a complex process involving interactions among biological, psychological, social, and environmental factors. These factors include genetics, responses to social situations, food availability and composition, and levels of physical activity.

Obesity is a chronic condition. Most people who have lost weight will regain much or all of it within 5 years. To lose weight and maintain the loss, overweight individuals need to decrease their caloric intake by eating less food and increase their caloric expenditures by increasing their levels of physical activity. A reliable weight loss regimen should include a well-balanced, nutritionally adequate but calorie-reduced diet and an exercise regimen that can be followed for life.

To increase her chances of having healthy babies, a healthy pregnant woman needs to gain about 25 to 35 pounds. While pregnant, women should not consume low-calorie diets because caloric restriction may harm the fetus. After birth, infants need some fat in their diets; therefore, physicians do not recommend that parents restrict the fat intake of children under 2 years of age.

Children and adolescents need adequate amounts of energy for physical development and activity. In the United States, the percentage of children and teenagers who are overweight is growing. Experts think that this increase is primarily the result of sedentary lifestyles and poor eating habits. It is difficult to predict whether an overweight child will become an overweight adult. Overweight adolescents, however, are at risk of remaining overweight when they reach adulthood. Overweight elderly individuals tend to experience the same health problems as younger overweight adults.

Applying What You Have Learned

1. Develop a day's menu, including meals and snacks, for a nutritionally adequate weight loss plan. Your plan should include foods from all major food groups. **Application**
2. You see an advertisement for a special drink that is supposed to eliminate excess body fat while you sleep. According to the ad, this product helps you lose weight "fast" by increasing your metabolic rate; there is no need to eat less food or exercise more often. Explain why you think this ad is a source of reliable or unreliable health-related information. **Synthesis**
3. A man has been maintaining his weight by consuming 2,500 calories a day. If he does not alter his physical activity level, how many calories should he consume daily to lose 4 pounds in a month? **Application**

4. Compare your present weight to your weight of 2 years ago. If you have gained or lost weight over the past couple of years, explain how you reached your present weight by evaluating your lifestyle. What factors might account for the weight change? If you have not gained or lost weight during this period, explain why this situation has occurred. **Evaluation**

Key

Application	using information in a new situation.
Synthesis	putting together information from different sources.
Evaluation	making informed decisions.

Reflecting on Your Health

1. "Fat people could lose weight if they would just push themselves away from the dinner table." After reading this chapter, what have you learned about obesity and weight control that might cause you to react differently to this statement than you might have prior to reading this chapter?
2. As mentioned in this chapter, normal-weight people often have negative feelings toward obese individuals. What were your feelings about obese people before you read this chapter? After reading this chapter, have your feelings about obese persons changed? If so, describe how your feelings changed.
3. How would you respond if a close friend or relative told you that you needed to lose weight? If

someone you know is trying to lose weight, what would you do to help them in their weight loss efforts?
4. Recently the U.S. National Transportation Safety Board (NTSB) proposed reducing the weight limit of each airline passenger and his or her luggage because of concern that the excess load could result in plane crashes. Explain your reaction to this proposal.
5. How does the media influence your satisfaction with your body size and shape? Do you think the media should encourage people to be more satisfied with their body sizes and shapes? If you think the media should take such steps, how could this affect people's health?

References

Baeten, J. M., Bukusi, E. A., & Lambe, M. (2001). Pregnancy complications and outcomes among overweight and obese nulliparous women. *American Journal of Public Health, 91*(3):436–440.

Calle, E. E., & Thun, M. J. (2004). Obesity and cancer. *Oncogene, 23*(38):6365–6378.

Calle, E. E., Rodriguez, C., Walker-Thurmond, K., & Thun, M. J. (2003). Overweight, obesity, and mortality from cancer in a prospective studied cohort of U.S. adults. *New England Journal of Medicine, 348*(17):1625–1638.

Crespo, C. J., Smit, E., Troiano, R. P., Bartlett, S. J., Macera, C. A., & Andersen, R. E. (2001). Television watching, energy intake, and obesity in U.S. children. *Archives of Pediatric and Adolescent Medicine, 155*:360–365.

Eisenstein, J., & Greenberg, A. (2003). Ghrelin: Update 2003. *Nutrition Reviews, 61*(3):101–104.

Finkelstein, E. A., Fiebelkorn, I. C., & Wang, G. (2004). State-level estimates of annual medical expenditures attributable to obesity. *Obesity Research, 12*(1):18–24.

Flegal, K. M., Graubard, B. I., Williamson, D. F., & Gail, M. H. (2005). Excess deaths associated with underweight, overweight, and obesity. *Journal of the American Medical Association, 293*(15):1861–1867.

Food and Drug Administration. (2001). *Meridia*. Retrieved June 11, 2002, from http://www.fda.gov/cder/foi/label/2001/20632s8s11LBL.pdf.

French, S., & Castiglione, K. (2002). Recent advances in the physiology of eating. *Proceedings of the Nutrition Society, 61*(4):489–496.

Friedman, K. E., Reichmann, S. K., Costanzo, P. R., & Musante, G. J. (2002). Body image partially mediates the relationship between obesity and psychological distress. *Obesity Research, 10*(1):33–41.

Graci, S., Izzo, G., Savino, S., Cattani, L., et al. (2004). Weight cycling and cardiovascular risk factors in obesity. *International Journal of Obesity and Related Metabolic Disorders, 28*(1):65–71.

Guo, S. S., Wu, W., Chumlea, W. C., & Roche, A. F. (2002). Predicting overweight and obesity in adulthood from body mass index values in childhood and adolescence. *American Journal of Clinical Nutrition, 76*(3):653–658.

Ham, S. A., Yore, M. M., Fulton, J. E., & Kohl, H. W., III. (2004). Prevalence of no leisure-time physical activity—35 states and the District of Columbia, 1988–2002. *Morbidity and Mortality Weekly Report, 53*(4):82–86.

Hedley, A. A., Ogden, C. L., Johnson, C. L., Carroll, M. D., Curtin, L. R., & Flegal, K. M. (2004). Prevalence of overweight and obesity among U.S. children, adolescents, and adults, 1999–2002. *Journal of the American Medical Association, 291*(23):2847–2850.

Herron, D. M. (2004). The surgical management of severe obesity. *Mount Sinai Journal of Medicine, 71*(1):63–71.

Hill, J. O., & Peters, J. C. (1998). Environmental contributions to the obesity epidemic. *Science, 280*:1371–1374.

Jakicic, J. M., Clark, K., Coleman, E., Donnelly, J. E., Foreyt, J., et al. (2001). American College of Sports Medicine position stand: Appropriate intervention strategies for weight loss and prevention of weight regain for adults. *Medicine & Science in Sports and Exercise, 33*(12):2145–2156.

Klein, S. (2004). The case of visceral fat: Argument for the defense. *Journal of Clinical Investigation, 113*(11):1530–1532.

Kruger, J., Galuska, D. A., Serdula, M. K., & Jones, D. A. (2004). Attempting to lose weight: Specific practices among U.S. adults. *American Journal of Preventive Medicine, 26*(5):402–406.

Kuczmarski, R. J., Carroll, M. D., Flegal, K. M., & Troiano, R. P. (1997). Varying body mass index cutoff points to describe overweight prevalence among U.S. adults: NHANES III (1988 to 1994). *Obesity Research, 5*:532–548.

Levine, J. A. (2004). Non-exercise activity thermogenesis. *Nutrition Reviews*, 62(7):S82–S98.

Livingstone, M. B. E., & Black, A. E. (2003). Markers of the validity of reported energy intake. *Journal of Nutrition*, 133(Suppl 3):L895S–920S.

Mokdad, A. H., Marks, J. S., Stroup, D. F., & Gerberding, J. L. (2005). Correction: Actual causes of death in the United States, 2000. *Journal of the American Medical Association*, 293(3):293–294.

National Heart, Lung, and Blood Institute. (1998). *Clinical guidelines on the identification, evaluation, and treatment of overweight and obesity in adults*. Bethesda, MD: National Institutes of Health.

Oster, G., Thompson, D., Edelsberg, J., Bird, A. P., & Colditz, G. A. (1999). Lifetime health and economic benefits of weight loss among obese persons. *American Journal of Public Health*, 89(10):1536–1542.

Pi-Sunyer, F. X. (2004). The epidemiology of central fat distribution in relation to disease. *Nutrition Reviews*, 62(7):S120–S126.

Position of the American Dietetic Association: Weight management. (1997). *Journal of the American Dietetic Association*, 97(1):71–74.

Robertson, S. M., Cullen, K. W., Baranowski, J., Baranowski, T., Hu, S., & de Moor, C. (1999). Factors related to adiposity among children aged 3 to 7 years. *Journal of the American Dietetic Association*, 99(8):938–943.

Rosenbaum, M., Prieto, Y., Hellmer, J., Boschmann, M., Krueger, J., Leibel, R. L., & Ship, A. G. (1998). An exploratory investigation of the morphology and biochemistry of cellulite. *Plastic and Reconstructive Surgery*, 101(7):1934–1939.

Speakman, J. R., & Selman, C. (2003). Physical activity and resting metabolic rate. *Proceedings of the Nutrition Society*, 62(3):621–634.

Tremblay, A. (2004). Dietary fat and body weight set point. *Nutrition Reviews*, 62(7):S75–S77.

U.S. Department of Agriculture and U.S. Department of Health and Human Services. (2005). *Dietary guidelines for Americans 2005*. Retrieved January 12, 2005, from http://www.healthierus.gov/dietaryguidelines/.

U.S. Department of Health and Human Services, National Center for Health Statistics, Public Health Service. (2000). *Healthy People 2010*. Washington, DC: Government Printing Office.

Wagner, D. R., & Heyward, V. H. (1999). Techniques of body composition assessment: A review of laboratory and field methods. *Research Quarterly for Exercise and Sport*, 70(2):135–149.

Wardlaw, G. M. (2004). *Nutrition perspectives*. New York: McGraw-Hill.

Weisberg, S. P., McCann, D., Desai, M., Rosenbaum, M., et al. (2003). Obesity is associated with macrophage accumulation in adipose tissue. *Journal of Clinical Investigation*, 112(12):1796–1808.

Wooltorton, E. (2002). Obesity drug sibutramine (Meridia): Hypertension and cardiac arrhythmias. *Canadian Medical Association Journal*, 166(10):1307–1308.

World Health Organization. (2002). *Nutrition data banks: Global database on obesity and body mass index (BMI) in adults*. Geneva, Switzerland. Retrieved June 10, 2002, from http://www.who.int/nut/db_bmi.htm.

Wright, J. D., Kennedy-Stephenson, J., McDowell, M. A., & Johnson, C. L. (2004). Trends in intake of energy and macronutrients—United States, 1971–2000. *Mortality and Morbidity Weekly Report*, 53(4):80–82.

Yanovski, S. Z., & Yanovski, J. A. (2002). Obesity. *New England Journal of Medicine*, 346(8):591–601.

Young, L. R., & Nestle, M. (2003). Expanding portion sizes in the U.S. marketplace: Implications for nutrition counseling. *Journal of the American Dietetic Association*, 103(2):231–234.

Youth Risk Behavior Surveillance: National College Health Risk Behavior Survey—United States, 1995. (1997). *Weekly Morbidity and Mortality Report*, 46(SS-6):1–54.

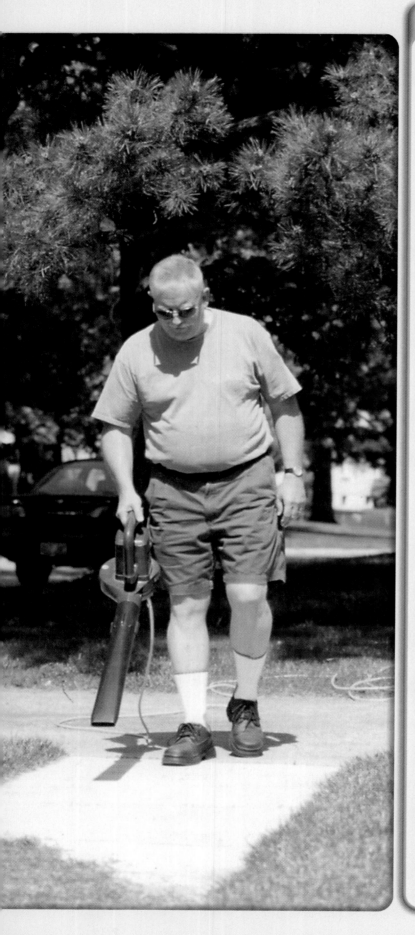

Chapter Overview

The principles of physical fitness
The health-related components of fitness
Exercising for optimal health
Preventing and managing exercise injuries
Developing your own exercise program

Diversity in Health
New Interest in an Ancient Approach to Fitness

Consumer Health
Choosing a Fitness Center

Managing Your Health
Assessing the Intensity of Your Workout: Target Heart Rates

Across
THE LIFESPAN

Physical Fitness

Student Workbook

Self-Assessment: Cardiorespiratory Fitness: Check Your Physical Activity & Heart Disease IQ/The Rockport Fitness Walking Test

Changing Health Habits: Do You Want to Be More Physically Active?

Do You Know?

· *How to calculate your target heart rate?*
· *How to bulk up safely?*
· *If muscles can turn into fat?*

Physical Fitness

*I*f you look around your home, you will see many devices and products that make your life easier: electric can openers, microwave ovens, permanent-press clothes, dishwashers, garage-door openers, and remote controls. Outside of your home, there are more labor-saving machines. You can use a leaf blower instead of a rake, drive a car rather than walk to places, use elevators and escalators rather than climb stairs, and take moving walkways rather than walk through some of the larger airports. You can even make your leisure time less physically demanding by using a motorized cart to get around a golf course or a motorboat to get around a lake. Besides using labor-saving products, you can have other people perform your physical work. For example, you can pay a team of people to mow your grass, wash your car, or clean your house.

A hundred years ago Americans often performed hard physical work at home and on the job. By the end of the twentieth century, a variety of machines, products, and services had become available that made our daily lives less physically demanding. Today, we generally have more leisure time than our great-grandparents, but many of us spend it performing activities that do not contribute to our physical health.

Regardless of age and physical condition, nearly everyone can achieve health benefits by exercising regularly and becoming more physically active. Many people are aware of the beneficial effects of exercise on the functioning of the heart and skeletal muscles. In 2002, however, 25% of U.S. adults did not exercise during their leisure time (Ham et al., 2004). Each year, lack of regular physical activity (a *sedentary* lifestyle) contributes to thousands of American deaths, primarily from heart disease, stroke, and diabetes. An objective of *Healthy People 2000* was that at least 30% of Americans who are 6 years old and older would be engaging in light to moderate exercise for a minimum of 30 minutes, preferably every day, by the year 2000. In 1985, 22% of Americans who were at least 6 years of age engaged in light to moderate exercise regularly. According to the *Healthy People 2000* final review (U.S. Department of Health and Human Services [USDHHS], 2001), 30% of this population were performing light to moderate exercise regularly in 2000. Thus, Americans met this important health objective. New physical activity objectives established for *Healthy People 2010* state that the

> *. . . many devices . . . make your life easier . . .*

percentage of adults who do not engage in leisure time physical activity should decrease to 20% by 2010 (USDHHS, 2000). Additionally, the percentage of adults who perform moderate-intensity physical activity for at least 30 minutes, preferably daily, should increase from 15% to 30% by 2010. According to a recent survey, over 50% of American adults do not engage in enough physical activity to meet this recommendation (Macera et al., 2003).

A physically fit person has the physical strength, endurance, flexibility, and balance as well as energy to perform various daily living activities, including typical occupational responsibilities and recreational interests that require physical movement. This chapter discusses the basic principles of fitness, including the health benefits of exercise and a physically active lifestyle, and how to design a basic fitness program that you can follow for the rest of your life.

■ Principles of Physical Fitness

The Body in Motion

Physical movement involves the interrelated functioning of the muscular and skeletal systems. The functioning of the muscular system is so closely associated with the skeletal system that the two are often referred to as the *musculoskeletal system*.

The *skeletal muscles* provide shape, support, and movement for your body. Figure 11-1 identifies the major skeletal muscle groups of the human body. A skeletal muscle consists of hundreds of muscle cells called *muscle fibers*. Movement occurs when the muscle fibers contract, shortening the length of the muscle. **Tendons**, tough bands of fibrous tissue, connect skeletal muscles to bones and play an important role in muscular movement. **Joints** are places where two or more bones

Figure 11-1 Major Skeletal Muscles of the Human Body. (a) Front view. (b) Back view.

(a) FEMALE

- Facial muscles
- Sternocleidomastoid
- Trapezius
- Deltoid
- Pectoralis major
- Biceps
- External oblique
- Finger and wrist flexors
- Sartorius
- Quadriceps
- Anterior tibial
- Foot and ankle flexors
- Pectoralis minor
- Intercostals
- External oblique
- Rectus abdominus
- Internal oblique
- Gluteus maximus
- Adductors of thighs
- Vastus muscle (part of quadriceps)

(b) MALE

- Trapezius
- Deltoid
- Triceps
- External oblique
- Hip adductor muscles
- Hamstrings
- Sartorius
- Gastrocnemius

come together. Most joints are movable; therefore, such joints permit the movement between bones. **Ligaments** are tough bands of connective tissue that hold bones together at the joints.

The Circulatory and Respiratory Systems

Optimal functioning of the circulatory and respiratory systems (sometimes referred to as the *cardiorespiratory system*) is necessary to achieve a high degree of physical fitness. The circulatory system includes the heart, blood, and blood vessels. The lungs are the major structures of the respiratory system. As Figure 11-2 illustrates, the functioning of the heart and lungs is interrelated.

The heart is a muscular pump that usually beats about 70 to 80 times each minute. Its job is to circulate blood throughout the body's vast network of blood vessels: the arteries, veins, and capillaries. Blood transports oxygen and nutrients to cells and carries waste products such as carbon dioxide away from them.

Cells need oxygen to release the energy stored in glucose and fats. As the heart pumps blood through microscopic blood vessels in the lungs, carbon dioxide leaves the blood and is exhaled. While in the lungs, hemoglobin in the red blood cells picks up oxygen from the inhaled air. The oxygen-rich blood returns to the heart, which pumps it to the rest of the body. As the blood moves through tiny capillaries in tissues, oxygen and nutrients move out of the bloodstream and into muscle fibers and other cells. Waste products move out of cells and into the blood. The blood then circulates through veins back to the heart. This cycle repeats itself with every heartbeat and breath.

Defining Physical Activity and Exercise

Physical activity is movement that occurs when skeletal muscles contract; everyone engages in some physical activity as part of their daily living routines. These activities include shopping, housekeeping, and walking pets. **Exercise** is physical activity that is usually planned and performed to improve or maintain one's physical condition. For example, doing biceps curls is an exercise that develops upper arm strength.

How does physical activity affect health? Before reading the following section, check your knowledge by taking the physical activity and heart disease quiz in the workbook.

tendons tough bands of tissue that connect many skeletal muscles to bones.

joints the places where two or more bones come together.

ligaments tough bands of connective tissue that hold bones together at joints.

physical activity movement that occurs when skeletal muscles contract.

exercise physical activity that is usually planned and performed to improve or maintain one's physical condition.

■ Physical Activity and Health

Being physically active can substantially reduce your risks of serious chronic diseases including heart (*coronary artery*) disease, certain forms of cancer, type 2 diabetes, obesity, hypertension, and osteoporosis (USDHHS, 2002). Regular physical activity helps maintain muscle strength and joint function. Furthermore, elderly people can improve their balance and reduce their risk of falls by performing certain exercises regularly. Men and women who are physically fit have a lower risk of dying prematurely from cardiovascular disease than people who are not physically fit (Laukkanen et al., 2001). Making small lifestyle adjustments that increase your level of physical activity can lower your risk of premature death significantly (Lee & Skerrett, 2001).

In addition to improving physical health, regular exercise and physical activity can enhance psychological health and sense of well-being. According to *Physical Activity and Health: A Report of the Surgeon General* (USDHHS, 1996), physical activity "reduces symptoms of anxiety and depression and fosters improvements in mood and feelings of well-being." This does not mean that physical inactivity *causes* mental health problems or that exercising will cure these conditions. Additionally, regular physical activity can

O_2
Air
CO_2

Carbon dioxide leaves the blood.

CO_2 O_2

The blood carries the carbon dioxide back to the lungs.

Blood picks up oxygen in the lungs.

The circulatory system carries the oxygenated blood to cells.

Oxygen moves out of the blood and into cells. Waste products move out of cells and into blood.

Figure 11-2 **Cardiorespiratory System.** The functioning of the heart and lungs is interrelated. The heart pumps blood to the lungs, where it picks up oxygen. The oxygenated blood returns to the heart, which pumps it throughout the body.

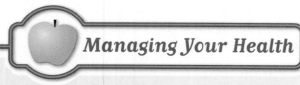
Assessing the Intensity of Your Workout: Target Heart Rates

To maximize the cardiorespiratory benefits of aerobic activity, you should work out at the level of intensity that raises your heart rate to within your target heart rate zone. To estimate your target heart rate zone, you need to take your pulse. Figure 11-A illustrates where you can feel your pulse using the carotid artery in your neck or radial artery in your wrist. Although locating the carotid artery pulse can be easier than the radial pulse, applying pressure to the carotid artery can reduce the heart rate, which interferes with obtaining a reliable measurement. For some people with cardiovascular disease, applying pressure to the carotid artery can be dangerous. Many medical experts advise using gentle pressure on your carotid artery to measure your pulse. Practice finding your radial pulse, so you can take it quickly while exercising.

To obtain the most accurate heart rate, measure your pulse while you are still engaging in the physical activity or within 10 seconds after discontinuing the muscular movement. This timing is necessary because your pulse declines rapidly when you stop exercising. Count your pulse for 10 seconds, then multiply that number by 6 to obtain your heart rate per minute.

To estimate your target heart rate zone, obtain your *age-predicted maximum heart rate* by subtracting your age from 220. For example, if you are 21 years old and healthy, your age-predicted maximum heart rate is 199 beats per minute. Exercising at your age-predicted maximum heart

Figure 11-A **Taking Your Pulse.**
(a) Carotid site. (b) Radial site.

(a) (b)

improve the quality of sleep (Holbrook et al., 2000), which benefits psychological health.

Many people experience short-term psychological benefits during or immediately after exercising. Strenuous physical activity produces chemical changes in the body that can improve psychological health. For example, the central nervous system releases *beta-endorphins* during exercise. Beta-endorphins are pain-killing substances that may provide natural relaxing and mood-elevating effects. Also, exercise can divert a person's attention away from distressing thoughts and negative emotions, which relieves anxiety. Long-term psy-

chological benefits of exercise may include boosting self-esteem (Maltby & Day, 2001). Additionally, people who exercise with others can experience psychological benefits from the social interaction.

The Health-Related Components of Physical Fitness

Cardiorespiratory fitness, muscular strength, muscular endurance, flexibility, and body composition are the health-related components of physical fitness. These rate is undesirable and uncomfortable; this extreme level of intensity is unnecessary for achieving cardiorespiratory fitness. Healthy people should exercise with enough intensity to raise their heart rates to within 65% and 90% of their age-predicted maximum heart rates. This interval is the *target heart rate zone*. People in excellent physical condition may calculate their target heart rates at the 85% to 90% intensity level. Most experts do not recommend that individuals raise their heart rates more than 90% of their age-predicted maximum levels.

If you are healthy and exercise regularly, multiply your age-predicted maximum heart rate by 0.65 and 0.90 to obtain a heart rate interval that is 65% to 90% of your maximum. For example, a healthy 21-year-old person would multiply 199 by 0.65 to determine the lowest heart rate (65% level) and by 0.90 (90% level) to find the highest rate. If you are out of shape, multiply your age-predicted maximum heart rate by 0.55 (55% of the maximum). Figure 11-B illustrates target heart rate zones for fit and unfit people. If you are sedentary and just starting an exercise program, strive for a maximum heart rate at the low end of your target zone. As your physical condition improves, you will need to recalculate your target heart rate so that it is in "the zone."

While exercising, if you can raise your heart rate to a value in your target zone, and maintain this rate for 30 to 60 minutes, you are giving your heart and lungs a beneficial aerobic workout. During aerobic activity, you should measure your pulse about every 10 minutes without stopping the activity. If your heart rate is higher than the maximum value of your target heart rate zone, it is possible that you underestimated your zone, or you may be overexerting yourself at your present level of fitness. You may need to reduce your muscular work load. On the other hand, if your heart rate during aerobic exercise is less than the target range, you may not be working hard enough to achieve cardiorespiratory benefits.

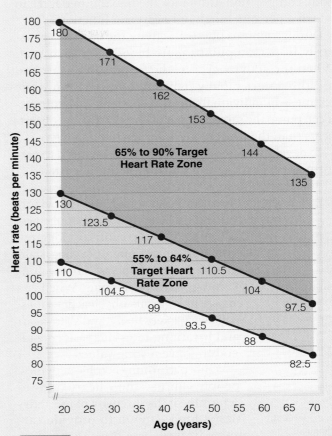

Figure 11-B **Target Heart Rate Zones.** The shaded areas include pulse rates within the 55% to 64% and 65% to 90% intensity ranges.

physical characteristics provide support for the body, sustain its effective and efficient movement, and influence overall health and well-being.

Cardiorespiratory Fitness

During intense physical activity, skeletal muscles need large quantities of oxygen to release enough energy to sustain movement. To supply more oxygen for working muscles, the heart and breathing rates increase as the intensity of physical activity increases. However, the lungs and heart have a maximum capacity to distribute an adequate supply of oxygen throughout the body within a certain time. Once the lungs and heart reach this maximum capacity, the skeletal muscles cannot obtain the additional oxygen needed to sustain their intense level of activity, and they become fatigued.

Individuals with high degrees of **cardiorespiratory fitness** (or *endurance*) can perform muscular work more intensely and longer without becoming fatigued than persons with low levels of cardiorespiratory fitness. Young physically fit individuals can raise their heart rates to about 200 beats per

cardiorespiratory fitness the ability to perform muscular movements intensely and for long periods without becoming fatigued.

minute while engaging in intense aerobic activities. As people grow older, their maximum heart rates decline. In addition to physical condition and age, other personal characteristics, including heredity, gender, and body composition, influence the maximum degree to which a person's lungs and heart can function.

During vigorous physical activity, the heart of a physically fit person pumps more blood with each beat. When the activity ceases, the fit person's heart and breathing rates rapidly return to normal. Even while resting, a fit individual's heart is efficient; each minute, it can pump the same amount of blood with fewer heartbeats than the heart of an unfit person.

To develop cardiorespiratory fitness, you need to perform **aerobic** (oxygen-requiring) activities. An aerobic activity lasts longer than 2 minutes, increases heart and breathing rates, and involves vigorous movements of large muscles. Popular aerobic activities include running, jogging, race-walking, lap swimming, cycling, stair-stepping, aerobic dancing, cross-country skiing, and rope skipping. When you engage in vigorous physical activities, you sweat excessively, and your heart and breathing rates increase considerably above resting values.

While performing aerobic activities, people can use their heart rates to determine if the intensity of the activities is high enough to provide cardiorespiratory benefits. To be very effective, a physical activity should be vigorous enough to raise your heart rate to within a certain range, the *target heart rate zone*. After raising your heart rate to the target zone, you should continue performing the aerobic activity, maintaining the level of intensity for at least 20 minutes. According to the American College of Sports Medicine (ACSM), healthy adults should perform moderate-intensity aerobic activities 3 to 5 days a week, from 55% to 90% of their maximum heart rates, continuously for 20 to 60 minutes (Pollock et al., 1998). The Managing Your Health box "Assessing the Intensity of Your Workout: Target Heart Rates" on pages 286-287 describes how to measure your heart rate and calculate your target heart rate zone.

You do not have to jog 6 miles daily to reap the health benefits of a physically active lifestyle; most people can improve their health by performing a minimum of 30 minutes of moderately intense physical activity, preferably every day (Stofan et al., 1998). People can even benefit from intermittent episodes of aerobic activity that last 8 to 10 minutes and accumulate to at least

30 minutes in one day (Schmidt et al., 2001). Most sedentary and overweight people can integrate more physical activity into their daily routines, for example, by climbing stairs instead of taking elevators and walking to nearby places instead of driving. By exercising more vigorously, however, people can achieve even greater health benefits. Table 11-1 lists some physical activities classified as light, moderate, and intense.

If you have heart disease or other serious chronic conditions, are out of shape, or are 40 years old or older, obtain the approval of a physician before beginning an exercise program, especially if the program includes aerobic activities.

Assessing Cardiorespiratory Fitness You can judge your level of cardiorespiratory fitness by answering the following questions. While engaging in strenuous exercise, can you carry on a conversation with others, or are you panting for air and unable to talk? How long does it take you to catch your breath or for your heart to stop racing after you stop the activity? If you are unable to talk while exercising and it takes you a long time to recover your normal breathing and heart rates when you finish the physical activity, you probably have a relatively low degree of cardiorespiratory fitness. The assessment activity for this chapter involves a simple test that you can perform to determine your level of cardiorespiratory fitness (see the student workbook).

Many formerly out-of-shape people discover that their resting heart rates have declined after a few months of regular aerobic exercise. Observing such a decline in resting heart rate not long after beginning a regular aerobic exercise program is usually an indication that cardiorespiratory fitness has improved.

To track your aerobic fitness progress, record your resting heart rates before and after initiating an exercise regimen. Determine your resting heart rate by measuring your pulse when you first wake up, before getting out of bed, on 3 consecutive days. Calculate your average resting heart rate over this 3-day period, and record it and the date. After a few months of engaging in a vigorous exercise program, repeat the procedure to determine your resting heart rate and compare the before and after measurements.

Muscular Strength

Muscular strength is an important aspect of muscular fitness. **Muscular strength** is the ability of muscles to apply maximum force against an object that is resisting this force. Many individuals perform specific resistance exercises to increase muscular strength because they want to lift heavy objects with ease or improve their appearance. (Figure 11-3). Other people are interested in devel-

aerobic oxygen-requiring.

muscular strength the ability to apply maximum force against an object that is resisting this force.

hypertrophy a condition in which muscles become larger and stronger.

atrophy a condition in which muscles lose size and strength.

detraining a condition characterized by atrophied and weak muscles, which occurs when skeletal muscles are not used regularly.

Table 11-1   Physical Activities: Intensity Levels

Light Activity (less than 3 calories/kg/hr)	Moderate Activity (3 to 6 calories/kg/hr)	Intense/Vigorous Activity (more than 6 calories/kg/hr)
Walking slowly (1 to 2 mph)	Walking briskly (3 to 4 mph)	Walking briskly uphill with a load
Cycling, stationary bike	Cycling for pleasure or transportation	Cycling, fast or racing
Swimming, slow treading	Swimming, moderate effort	Swimming, fast treading, or crawl
Conditioning exercises: light stretching	Conditioning exercises: general calisthenics	Conditioning exercises: ski or stair-climbing machine
—	Racket sports: table tennis	Racket sports: racketball, singles tennis
Golf, using power cart	Golf, pulling cart or carrying clubs	—
Bowling	—	—
Fishing, sitting	Fishing, standing and casting	—
Boating (power boat)	Canoeing leisurely (2 to 3.9 mph)	Canoeing rapidly (≥4 mph)
Carpet sweeping	General housecleaning	Moving furniture
Carpentry	Housepainting	—

Source: Adapted from Pate, R. R., et al. (1995). Physical activity and public health. *Journal of the American Medical Association, 273*:402–407.

oping larger, stronger muscles because they want to compete in sporting events that require strength. How do the strength and size of a muscle increase?

To develop a high degree of strength, muscles need to be overloaded by moving heavy objects repeatedly, particularly objects that become progressively heavier over time. For example, using a weight-lifting machine regularly can increase the size and strength of the biceps muscle in the upper arm. This response is called the *training effect*. Under these conditions, the individual fibers of the biceps muscle can enlarge, or **hypertrophy**, making the entire muscle stronger and larger. Once muscle cells enlarge, they require a regular program of resistance exercise to maintain their size and strength.

The saying "Use it or lose it" generally applies to skeletal muscles. Muscular **atrophy**, a condition of a muscle that has lost size and strength, results from a few weeks of **detraining**. If you have ever had a broken arm or leg, you may recall that after the cast was removed, the muscles of the recovered limb were atrophied and weak. When you first used the limb, the weakened muscles ached for a brief time, but within days they became stronger. Eventually, using these muscles enabled them to regain their full strength and original size.

Exercising for Muscular Strength A safe and effective way to increase muscle strength and size is to perform repetitive exercises that overload a particular muscle group, such as lifting weights. A *repetition* is the completion of a particular exercise, for example,

lifting a handheld weight one time and returning to the resting position. A *set* involves performing the same resistance exercise movement usually 8 to 12 times. During a workout session, healthy people can train their major muscle group by performing a single set of

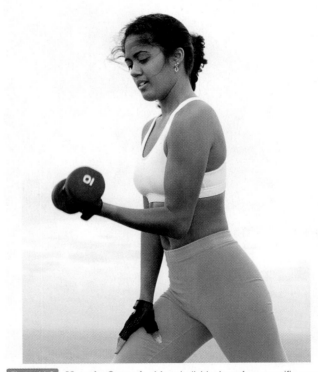

Figure 11-3   **Muscular Strength.** Many individuals perform specific exercises to improve their appearance or to develop larger, more well-defined muscle groups.

exercises for each group of muscles (Feigenbaum & Pollock, 1999). For best results, a person should do the resistance workout three times a week. Two forms of exercise that increase muscular strength are isometric and isotonic exercises. In an **isometric** exercise an individual exerts muscular force against a fixed, immovable object of resistance. For example, applying a constant amount of force while pushing against an immovable door frame is an isometric exercise. During isometric contraction, the muscle does not shorten, so it does not bulge. Although isometric exercises can increase muscular strength, they do not increase muscular endurance or flexibility effectively. Furthermore, muscles can apply excessive pressure on certain arteries during isometric contractions, raising blood pressure. Therefore, many medical practitioners do not recommend isometric exercises for people older than 35 or those suffering from cardiovascular disease.

Figure 11-4 **Isotonic Contraction.** While performing isotonic exercise, the muscle contracts, shortening in length.

When performing **isotonic** exercises, a person exerts muscular force against a movable but constant source of resistance. During isotonic exercise, the muscle shortens and bulges. Isotonic exercises include lifting barbells, performing push-ups, or using weight machines (Figure 11-4). Instead of describing the exercises as isotonic, some fitness experts prefer to use the term *dynamic constant external resistance* because it reflects the nature of these movements more accurately. An exercise is dynamic if the skeleton moves during the activity.

Muscular Endurance

Muscular endurance is another important aspect of muscular fitness. **Muscular endurance** is the ability of a muscle to contract repeatedly without becoming fatigued easily. For example, many people perform "crunches" to strengthen their abdominal muscles. A sedentary person may experience muscular fatigue after the third crunch and not be able to do another one. If this person, however, continues to perform crunches regularly and increases the number performed during each exercise session, he or she will develop muscular endurance in the abdominal muscles. As a result, this person can do numerous crunches with ease.

To achieve muscular endurance, you need to train skeletal muscles by contracting them repeatedly. Furthermore, the ability to sustain muscular contractions over a relatively long period requires a constant source of energy. Glucose is skeletal muscles' preferred fuel for high-intensity endurance exercise. Muscles metabolize glucose derived from the bloodstream or from glycogen that is stored in muscle tissue. Additionally, muscle fibers can use fatty acids and amino acids for energy.

Flexibility

A third aspect of muscular fitness is flexibility. Movement is limited if joints are damaged or muscles cannot extend themselves fully. **Flexibility** refers to the ability to extend muscles, enabling a person to position a movable joint anywhere in its normal range of motion. Flexibility allows people to perform a variety of skeletal movements with ease, including bending, gliding, rotating, and twisting. Many daily tasks require the ability to extend muscles and move joints easily: reaching for an item stored on a high shelf, stretching to pull up a back zipper, or bending to pick up a tennis ball. Having fully extendible muscles and flexible joints enables you to care for yourself and to participate in enjoyable activities.

Figure 11-5 **Stretching to Improve Flexibility.** Flexible muscles enable one to make a variety of skeletal movements occur with ease. People can develop flexibility by performing stretching exercises such as the (a) low back stretch, (b) calf stretch, (c) modified hurdle, (d) lunge stretch, (e) supine hamstring stretch, and (f) groin stretch.

People can develop flexibility by performing yoga, Pilates, or stretching exercises such as those shown in Figure 11-5. The proper stretching technique, *static stretching*, involves slowly and fully extending the muscle and nearby joints throughout their natural ranges of motion. When performing a static stretch, gently extend the muscle until you feel tension; if you feel discomfort, relax the muscle slightly. While stretching, breathe normally, do not hold your breath. You should be comfortable holding this position for 15 seconds. Roberts and Wilson (1999) determined that maintaining the stretched position for 15 seconds during three separate stretching intervals achieves greater improvements in flexibility of the leg muscles than holding the stretch for only 5 seconds during nine separate intervals.

Most fitness experts do not recommend *ballistic stretching* activities that involve bouncing. Additionally, you should not use unnatural stretching motions that injure muscles and tendons or extend joints beyond their normal ranges of motion. If pain occurs while stretching, discontinue the activity immediately. The Analyzing Health-Related Information activity on pages 292–293 describes safe alternatives to outdated stretching exercises.

Healthy joints control the ability of muscles to move bones. Joints are susceptible to *dislocation,* that is, becoming displaced by force. Dislocation can result when joints and their supportive tissues are torn or worn after engaging in certain strenuous physical activities. When a joint becomes damaged, the injury reduces its normal range of motion, and movement often becomes painful. Although involvement in certain sports, like American football, increases the risk that the participants will damage their joints, any physically active person can experience joint injuries. Furthermore, most people experience painful arthritic changes in their joints as they age. A later section of this chapter describes injuries that can occur to the muscles, joints, and related structures.

Low Back Pain The majority of Americans encounter low back pain during their lives (Speed, 2004). As its name implies, low back pain occurs in the lumbar region of the spine (the lower back, above the hips), and it can be disabling (Figure 11-6). People with this condition are unable to perform activities essential to daily living comfortably, if at all. Furthermore, low back pain is responsible for a significant percentage

The accompanying article describes safe alternatives to outdated exercises. Read the article and evaluate it using the model for analyzing health-related information. The main points of the model are noted below; the model is explained fully on pages 13–15.

Safe Alternatives for Outdated Exercises

Bryant Stamford, Ph.D.

Stretching and strengthening exercises are, of course, good for you. As a part of a complete fitness program, they help you stay flexible and avoid injury.

Not all exercises, though, are good for all people. Healthy young people can do almost any exercise with little risk. And older people who have exercised all their lives can exercise safely under most circumstances. But middle-aged and older people who have been inactive need to know that some of the old standbys—such as sit-ups and toe touches—can result in injury.

So how do you get the important benefits of stretching and strengthening but avoid the injuries? You need to choose exercises carefully, especially if you are getting up in years and haven't exercised regularly. To help you, potentially troublesome exercises are cited below, with recommended alternatives.

If you aren't very flexible or have had back problems, it's best to consult a doctor before starting an exercise program. You may be more susceptible to injury because of a number of factors, including past injuries, fitness, body type, flexibility, technique, and age.

Regardless of the exercises you select, apply the following principles for maximum safety:

- Use strict technique. Stop using an exercise when physical limitation prevents you from performing it well. Also stop when you are tired.
- Use a slow, deliberate approach. Never bounce: The momentum can make a safe exercise dangerous.
- Hold stretches at least 6 seconds initially, building gradually to 30 seconds, then to 2 minutes. Holding a stretched position is more effective than doing many repetitions.
- Reject the "no pain, no gain" philosophy. Pain means something is wrong, so stop immediately.

Many popular exercises stress the lower back. High on the list is the standing toe touch, which stretches the ham-string muscles at the back of your thighs. This is a bad exercise even if done slowly, but it's even worse if you bounce. A safer option is the one-legged stretch (Figure 1).

Figure 1: One-legged stretch.

Sit-ups are popular, supposedly for stomach toning. But full sit-ups stress the lower back, and they work the hip muscles more than the abdominal muscles. The "crunch" is better (Figure 2).

Figure 2: The crunch.

The double-leg lift while lying on your back places tremendous stress on the lower back. Movements of this type cause your back to arch, placing your lower spine and back muscles in a vulnerable position. Scissoring the legs while in this position also places the lower back in a dangerous position. Again, the crunch is a safe alternative.

The donkey kick can also be dangerous, especially to your neck and lower back. It involves being on all fours and lifting one leg as high as possible in a kicking fashion. An alternative to the donkey kick is the rear-thigh lift (Figure 3).

Exercises that involve twisting can be especially dangerous. Windmills, in which you bend over and try to touch one hand to the opposite foot, are very stressful on the lower back. But in some sports—like golf—twisting plays a major part. Therefore, when recovering from a low-back injury, perform mild, pain-free twisting movements under professional supervision.

Figure 3: Rear-thigh lift.

Some exercises can harm the neck. Head rolls, in which you roll your head in a complete circle, are very stressful to the upper spine. Do neck stretches instead (Figure 4).

Figure 4: Neck stretch.

People do the yoga plow to stretch upper and lower back muscles by lying on their back and bringing their feet up and over until they touch the floor beyond their head. Unfortunately, this forces the disks in the neck to bulge, risking injury. For the same reason, avoid the "bicycle," in which you lie on your back, raise your hips, and "pedal" your feet. An excellent alternative is the fold-up stretch (Figure 5).

Figure 5: Fold-up stretch.

Full squats or deep knee bends can damage your knees, especially when you bounce out of the squat. Partial squats done slowly and under control are safer.

Jumping jacks involve considerable forces on your legs, particularly the knees. If you land on your toes, the Achilles tendons at the back of your heels bear a major load and could rupture if your legs aren't in the best of shape. Gently running in place provides a lower-impact way to warm up.

Less Risky Business

No matter what your age or physical condition, choosing safer exercise options will lower your risk of injury. And remember that whatever the exercise, good technique is essential.

Remember: This information is not intended as a substitute for medical treatment. Before starting an exercise program, consult a physician.

Dr. Stamford is director of the Health Promotion and Wellness Center and Professor of Allied Health in the School of Medicine at the University of Louisville, Kentucky.

Source: Stamford, B. (1995). Safer alternatives to outdated exercises. *The Physician and Sportsmedicine*, 23(6):87–88. Reproduced with permission from The McGraw-Hill Companies. All rights reserved.

1. Which statements are verifiable facts, and which are unverified statements or value claims?
2. What are the credentials of the person who wrote the article? If this information is available, does the author's background and education qualify him as an expert in the topic area?
3. What might be the motives and biases of the person who wrote the article? State reasons for your answer.
4. Which information in the article is relevant to the topic? Which information is irrelevant?
5. Is the source reliable? Does it have a reputation for publishing misinformation?
6. Does the article attack the credibility of conventional scientists or medical authorities?

Based on your analysis, do you think this article is a reliable source of health-related information? Explain why you would or would not use the information. Summarize your reasons for coming to this conclusion.

Figure 11-6 **Spinal Disks.** (a) Normal disk position. (b) Bulging disk pressing on spinal cord.

Lumbar region

Spinal cord

(a) Normal disk

Vertebra

(b) Bulging disk

shock absorbers, protecting the bones from striking each other. As people age, their spinal disks become worn and sometimes bulge out of their normal position. Pounding, twisting, and lifting place physical stress on the spine and are likely responsible for displacing or damaging some disks. Such movements include jogging on a sidewalk, swinging a golf club, carrying a heavy backpack, and picking up a heavy box or a child. Additionally, people who have poor posture, sit for hours in awkward positions, wear high-heeled shoes, or have too much body fat are susceptible to low back pain, especially if they have weak abdominal muscles.

Although medical experts agree that exercising to strengthen the abdominal, hip, upper leg, and back muscles can prevent or treat many cases of low back pain, they do not agree on which exercises to recommend. Some health care practitioners recommend aerobic exercises; others promote various stretching activities. Figure 11-7 shows various exercises designed to strengthen the weak muscles that contribute to low back pain and improve the flexibility of the spinal joints.

You can reduce your risk of developing low back pain by changing some behaviors; for example, lose excess

of worker absenteeism and workers' medical compensation claims.

Weak abdominal, back, and leg muscles as well as worn *spinal disks* often contribute to the development of low back pain. The spinal disks are flexible pads that separate the bones of the spine and act as

Figure 11-7 Exercises to Prevent Low Back Pain.

Figure 11-8 Practices to Protect Your Low Back. (a) To bend safely, bend your knees, not your back. (b) When lifting a child or heavy object, hold it close to your body, at chest level, and do not make twisting motions. (c) To protect your lower back while sitting, rest your lower back against the chair's back and avoid bending forward. Use an adjustable seat and prop up your feet so that you sit with your hips slightly lower than your knees.

body fat, exercise regularly, and wear shoes with low or no heels. Additionally, you can often prevent low back pain by following the lifting and sitting practices recommended in Figure 11-8.

Over-the-counter pain medicines and heat treatments can often relieve low back pain. After the discomfort subsides, people should perform exercises that strengthen the lower back, hip, and abdominal muscles. If the pain is intense or persists, however, the person should obtain a complete medical evaluation to determine the source of the pain. In some cases, surgery may be necessary.

Body Composition

As mentioned in Chapter 10, a healthy body contains large quantities of water and smaller amounts of fat and lean tissues (bones, muscles, and organs). Body composition, the percentages of body weight contributed by lean tissue and fat mass, is a major factor in health. Although a small amount of body fat (about 4% in men and 10% in women) is essential, too much fat contributes to a variety of chronic diseases, including cardiovascular disease, hypertension, and diabetes. Regular exercise builds and maintains muscle mass and helps keep the amount of body fat at healthy levels.

The cells that comprise lean tissues, particularly muscle cells, are more metabolically active than fat cells. Therefore, muscle cells burn more calories than fat cells. By exercising and increasing muscle mass, you can increase your metabolic rate (Binzen et al., 2001).

Aging muscle cells eventually wear out and die. Unfortunately, the body does not replace these cells. As a result, people usually lose muscle mass and gain fat as they age. Many people think that unused or dying muscle cells can "turn into" fat cells. Muscle cells, however, do not transform themselves into fat cells. A muscle cell is very different from a fat cell; each type of cell has specific structures and functions. Nevertheless, you can preserve more of your muscle mass as you get older if you continue to follow a regular exercise program.

Although regular physical activity can help a person maintain muscle mass while losing weight, "spot" exercising, such as performing 100 crunches daily to shrink the abdominal area, does not reduce the amount of fat stored there. During physical activity, fat deposits throughout the body release fatty acids into the bloodstream to supply energy for the vigorously moving muscles. Exercising a specific muscle group, however, can improve physical fitness and appearance by increasing the strength of the exercised muscles and improving their ability to hold in the underlying fat mass.

Engaging in moderate- to vigorous-intensity aerobic activities for about 60 minutes nearly every day, while not exceeding your calorie needs, is an effective method of "burning" body fat for energy (USDA/USDHHS, 2005). Even performing 30 minutes of moderate-intensity physical activity each day can help you control your weight. For example, walking 2 miles at a brisk pace expends about 200 calories, which is about the number of calories in four chocolate chip cookies ($2\frac{1}{4}$-inch diameter) or 1 plain cake doughnut ($3\frac{1}{4}$-inch diameter). This may seem to be a small amount of energy, but a person who consumes 200 more calories a day than necessary can gain more than 20 lb in a year. As mentioned in the previous chapter, increasing physical activity and eating a sensible calorie-restricted diet is the most effective way to control weight.

- Engaging in intense aerobic activity regularly can improve your cardiorespiratory fitness and burn excess body fat.
- Engaging in regular resistance exercises, such as lifting weights, can increase the size and strength of your muscles.
- Stretching muscles can improve their flexibility.

Athletic Performance

The Sports-Related Components of Fitness

Although genetic factors contribute to cardiorespiratory fitness, training is essential for athletes to develop their inborn physical capabilities and compete successfully in sports. The sports-related components of fitness include *speed, power, coordination, agility, balance,* and *reaction time.* Speed is the rate of movement; power is the ability to concentrate a considerable amount of force, usually from a particular group of muscles, when performing work. Coordination is the ability to perform a series of complicated muscular movements in a continuous manner. Agility enables a person to make quick precise movements, such as changing direction, with ease. Balance enables one to maintain a poised upright body position. Reaction time is the time it takes a person to adjust his or her body position to a changing environment. Although athletes often focus on improving the sports-related components of fitness that are associated with their specific sports, they also need to develop the health-related components of fitness.

ergogenic aid a product or device that enhances physical development or performance.

Diet and Performance

Most athletes are on the lookout for something—a diet, supplement, or drug—that may give them the competitive edge. The best advice for all athletes is to drink adequate amounts of water and choose a well-balanced diet composed of a variety of foods. By eating more servings of fruits and vegetables, athletes can obtain safe quantities of vitamins and minerals without taking supplements. There is no scientific evidence that protein-rich diets build bigger muscles, so eating large servings of meat or taking protein supplements is unnecessary. High protein intakes may cause dehydration and accelerate the loss of calcium from bones. Furthermore, protein-rich foods often contain a lot of fat, especially saturated fat.

Carbohydrate is the preferred fuel of the body, and a diet that supplies plenty of complex carbohydrates from starchy foods is recommended. Starchy foods usually contain more vitamins and minerals than sugary foods. Some athletes practice "carbohydrate loading" to maximize the amount of carbohydrate stored in their muscles. A few days before an event, for example, the athlete gradually increases the amount of carbohydrate eaten to about 70% of calories and gradually decreases the amount of time working out. Two to four hours before the competitive event, the athlete eats a light meal composed of starchy foods such as bagels, pasta, or breads and cereals. Not all athletes find that carbohydrate loading helps their performance. Thus, one should test the effects of the diet when not preparing for competition.

Ergogenic Aids

Ergogenic (work-producing) **aids** include a variety of products such as dietary supplements, stimulant drugs, and mechanical devices that supposedly enhance physical development or performance. Some of these aids are beneficial and harmless, but others are dangerous and illegal. Chromium picolinate, for example, is a popular dietary supplement that some people use to build lean body mass. The results of numerous scientific studies, however, fail to provide evidence that it improves physical performance. Furthermore, results of animal studies indicate that high doses of chromium picolinate may damage DNA, which increases the risk of cancer (Stearns et al., 2002). Creatine, an amino acid, is another popular ergogenic aid. Although people can gain small amounts of body weight while taking creatine supplements, scientific studies do not support claims that the amino acid improves endurance or performance; indeed, such supplements may have negative health effects (Terjung et al., 2000). Table 11-2 lists some dietary supplements, claims about their ergogenic effects, and information concerning whether scientific studies support these claims. For information about other dietary supplements, see Tables 1-4, 9-11, and 10-A.

Anabolic Steroids Both men and women may lift weights during their workout sessions to build stronger, more well-defined muscles. Men, however, are capable of developing larger muscles and having greater

Table 11-2 Dietary Supplements as Ergogenic Aids

Aid	Claim	Current Scientific Findings
Caffeine	Improves strength; Enhances fat metabolism	Increases alertness, but at high doses causes nervousness; raises free fatty acid levels during exercise; might provide modest improvement of performance.
Creatine	Enhances release of energy during exercise	May enhance performance during resistance exercise; more research is needed.
Carnitine	Enhances fat metabolism	No significant improvement in performance, but more research is needed.
Wheat-germ oil	Increases oxygen uptake by cells, improving stamina	Results of well-designed studies do not support ergogenic claims.
Lecithin and choline	Increase production of a neurotransmitter, resulting in more muscular strength	Results of well-designed studies do not support ergogenic claims.
Omega-3 fatty acids	Makes blood flow better, stimulates muscle growth	Results of well-designed studies do not support ergogenic claims; large doses may increase the risk of stroke.
Amino acids, brewer's yeast, enzymes, and DNA supplements	General performance-enhancing effects	Results of well-designed studies do not support ergogenic claims; large doses of amino acids can inhibit amino acid absorption and increase water requirement.
CoQ$_{10}$ (coenzyme Q or ubiquinone)	Improves heart function	Results of well-designed studies do not show consistent improvement in performance; more research is needed. Long-term safety is unknown.
Bee pollen	Shortens recovery time	Results of well-designed studies do not support ergogenic claims; may cause allergic responses in some individuals.
CLA (conjugated linoleic acid)	Increases lean body mass	Results of well-designed studies do not support ergogenic claims. Long-term safety is unknown.

overall strength because their testosterone levels are higher than those of women. Testosterone is an *anabolic* (tissue-building) hormone.

Anabolic steroids are a group of synthetic and natural substances that are chemically related to testosterone and may have muscle-building properties. Although certain anabolic steroids are classified as controlled substances, they can be prescribed by physicians for legitimate medical uses. These drugs, however, are often illegally obtained and abused by athletes and others who want to enhance their physical performance or muscle development or both. In the United States, it is difficult to estimate the prevalence of anabolic steroid abuse because people are often unwilling to admit to taking the substances. Nevertheless, as many as 3 million Americans, many of them young adults and adolescent males involved in organized sports, are estimated to have abused anabolic steroids at some point in their lives (Kutscher et al., 2002).

Why is there so much concern over the abuse of anabolic steroids? Athletes who abuse these drugs to improve their physical strength can have an unfair competitive advantage over athletes who choose not to use them. Additionally, anabolic steroids can have serious irreversible effects on the body (Figure 11-9). Male anabolic steroid abusers often experience shrunken testicles and infertility. Women who abuse these drugs may become bald, grow facial hair, and experience menstrual irregularities. Anabolic steroid abuse increases the risks of developing heart and kidney diseases, certain cancers, and liver tumors. In some cases, damage to the liver or kidneys is so severe that death occurs. Additionally, anabolic steroids can affect personality. People who abuse anabolic steroids may act more aggressive, hostile, and irritable than usual. Regular resistance exercise is the only safe way to increase the size and strength of a muscle.

anabolic steroids a group of drugs that can have muscle-building effects on the body.

Anabolic steroids may cause:

Male

Premature balding
Severe acne, greasy skin
Sleep disturbances
Aggressive, hostile, and irritable behavior

Increased blood pressure
Reduced HDL levels, increasing the risk of heart disease
Liver tumors and liver failure

Reduced testosterone secretion and sperm production
Testicle shrinkage

Female

Scalp hair loss
Severe acne, greasy skin
Sleep disturbances
Aggressive, hostile, and irritable behavior
Increased body hair, including facial hair

Increased blood pressure
Breast shrinkage
Reduced HDL levels, increasing the risk of heart disease
Liver tumors and liver failure

Ovaries malfunction
Menstrual irregularities

Figure 11-9 **Possible Effects of Anabolic Steroids on the Body.** To increase their muscle mass, some men and women abuse anabolic steroids or other chemicals that are promoted for their muscle-building properties. These drugs can have serious irreversible effects on the body.

Healthy Living Practices

- Do not use anabolic steroids to build your muscles; they can be very harmful.

◼ Exercising for Health

People often engage in a particular *type* of exercise because of its healthful benefits. Aerobic activities increase cardio-respiratory fitness and muscular endurance. Additionally, performing high-impact aerobic activities, including basketball and jogging, can build stronger bones (Jakes et al., 2001). Although isometric and isotonic exercises develop muscular strength, these activities may not increase cardiorespiratory fitness significantly. Many people combine aerobic and muscle-strengthening activities in their daily workouts to improve their overall physical condition; others perform isotonic and aerobic workouts on alternate days. For example, one day's workout session would be devoted to weightlifting; the following day's session would involve race-walking.

The frequency, duration, and intensity of exercise also influence the degree of health benefits a person derives from it. Exercise *frequency* is the number of times an individual exercises, usually reported as the number of days or exercise sessions in a week. People who exercise at least three times a week generally experience more rapid improvements to their overall fitness than people who exercise less often.

The *duration* of exercise refers to the total time the person is physically active during each exercise session. For example, people who jog for 40 minutes, 3 days a week, experience more cardiorespiratory benefits than those who jog for 10 minutes, 3 days a week (Lee & Paffenbarger, 2000). Sedentary people can develop cardiorespiratory fitness if they engage in an aerobic exercise program that gradually increases the duration of the activity, usually over several weeks.

A relatively easy way to assess and increase your physical activity level is to measure the number of steps you take in a day. You will need to purchase a pedometer; inexpensive ones sell for under $30 (Figure 11-10). Before you begin a typical day's activities, place the pedometer on your belt or waistband. Then check the pedometer before going to bed and record the number of steps you took that day. If you have a sedentary lifestyle, you probably will have taken fewer than 3,000 steps. Gradually increase the number of steps you take by making a conscious effort to be more active. A brisk walking routine, for example, can increase the number of steps you take daily and increase your cardiorespiratory fitness level. Your goal should be to record *at least* 8,000 steps each day.

The *intensity* of an exercise reflects the amount of physical exertion a person uses while performing the activity. Fitness experts use several methods to estimate the intensity of exercise, including the rate of oxygen consumption during exercise, heart rate, and personal perceptions of physical exertion. For the average person, playing nine holes of golf while using a power golf cart or bowling for 30 minutes are light activities; playing tennis or walking briskly for a half-hour are moderate activities; and jogging for 6 miles or playing racquetball for 30 minutes are intense activities (see Table 11-1).

The frequency, duration, and intensity of aerobic physical activities influence fitness. For example, you can exercise intensely for 20 minutes or moderately for 30 minutes and achieve similar cardiorespiratory benefits.

The Exercise Session

People should *warm up* before and *cool down (warm down)* after intense exercise. Warming up reduces the physical stress that vigorous exercise can place on the body. While warming up, the person's skeletal muscles become warm and extend easily, joints become more flexible, and heart and breathing rates increase gradually. Warming up may reduce the likelihood of injuries, but more research is needed (Parkkari et al., 2001). Cooling down facilitates the circulation of blood, especially in the leg muscles, enabling the body to recover from intense physical activity.

To warm up the entire body before engaging in a vigorous physical activity, you can walk at an easy pace, then gradually increase your speed until you have walked for 5 to 10 minutes. At this point, your muscles should be warm enough to perform stretching exercises such as those shown in Figure 11-5. Stretching muscles before the warm-up session is usually not recommended because extending "cold" muscles may injure them. According to current research findings, however, stretching does not protect against sports injuries (Thacker et al., 2004).

After stretching, many persons perform *active, task-specific* activities to warm up specific muscles. For example, a jogger would jog slowly for a few minutes, gradually increasing the pace until reaching his or her usual training speed.

Warming up before exercising is essential for people with heart disease. Abnormal functioning of the heart may occur when sedentary, middle-aged people begin to exercise suddenly without warming up. Warm-up activities increase the blood flow to the heart gradually, reducing the risk of heart attack during physical exertion.

After exercising vigorously, people should cool down by gradually reducing the intensity of their activity and by stretching. Many types of strenuous exercise increase the blood supply to the leg muscles; suddenly stopping these intense muscular movements can cause blood to accumulate in the leg veins, which can reduce the blood flow to the brain, causing dizziness, faintness, or loss of consciousness. Cooling down by engaging in 5 to 10 minutes of light exercise gradually decreases the blood flow to the leg muscles. Figure 11-11 illustrates a 50-minute workout session that consists of 10 minutes of warm-up activities, 30 minutes of jogging, and 10 minutes of cool-down exercises.

Figure 11-10 Pedometer. A pedometer is a relatively easy way to assess your physical activity level.

| 0 | 5 | 10 | 15 | 20 | 25 | 30 | 35 | 40 | 45 | 50 |

Slow pace or light activity | Stretching exercises | | | | | | | Slackened pace | Stretching exercises

Warm-up | Aerobic activity Pulse within target heart rate zone | Cool-down

Figure 11-11 **A Suggested Workout Session.** A reasonable 50-minute workout session may consist of 10 minutes of warm-up activities, 30 minutes of jogging, and 10 minutes of cool-down exercises.

Exercise Danger Signs

Exercise improves the functioning of the heart and reduces the risk of heart disease. Sudden and intense physical exertion, however, can strain the heart, especially the heart of an unfit individual or someone with cardiovascular disease.

To reduce the risk of overtaxing your cardiovascular system during vigorous exercise, warm up first, then exercise at a reduced intensity level for about 10 to 15 minutes. Keep records of your activity level and any discomfort that you experience. Discontinue the activity and consult a physician if any of the following signs or symptoms of heart disease occur during or after exercising:

strain generally refers to an injured muscle or tendon.

sprain generally refers to an injured ligament.

- Heart abnormalities, such as irregular rhythms, a feeling that your heart is pounding in your throat, or fluttering in your chest
- Pain or pressure in your chest, throat, or arms
- Shortness of breath, dizziness, sudden loss of coordination, cold sweating, or fainting

■ Preventing and Managing Exercise Injuries

Everyone should be concerned about personal safety while exercising. People should check their exercise equipment for defects and wear the proper clothing, shoes, and protective gear for the activity. Additionally, people should use some common sense about when and where they exercise. Bicyclists and joggers, for example, should obey traffic signals and avoid busy roads that have narrow or rocky shoulders. Engaging in physical activity outdoors at night is especially dangerous; people should wear clothing with reflective strips to become more visible.

Although engaging in regular physical activity is essential for optimal health, some activities are likely to result in musculoskeletal injuries. Suddenly raising the intensity level or duration of a physical activity may damage muscles or supportive tissues or aggravate existing injuries. Physically active people can use some general precautions to minimize their risk of musculoskeletal injury. Sudden, awkward movements are likely to injure muscles, tendons, and joints; therefore, people should avoid physical activities that involve exaggerated twisting.

Strains and Sprains

Almost everyone who is physically active has experienced muscle soreness or musculoskeletal injuries such as strains and sprains. Although there are no clear clinical definitions for strain or sprain, a **strain** generally refers to the damage that a muscle or tendon sustains when overextended rapidly. A **sprain** usually refers to a damaged ligament. Although these two types of injuries often occur together, a sprain tends to be more serious than a strain. The sprained ligament may be partially or completely torn, and the nearby muscle, joint, or bones may be damaged; therefore, severe sprains generally require immediate medical attention.

RICE, the acronym for rest, ice, compression, and elevation, is often effective for treating strains and sprains.

- *Rest* can reduce the pain, but light exercise or activity that uses the injured muscles is usually recommended, as long as the discomfort is tolerable.

- *Ice* treatments should be limited to 20-minute sessions and can be repeated every 2 hours (while the injured person is awake) for 2 to 3 days. Do not place ice directly on the skin.

- *Compression,* an external source of pressure, can prevent swelling. Apply a pressure bandage on the injury to produce compression. Make sure the bandage is not tight enough to interfere with circulation.

- *Elevation* also reduces swelling. When an injured limb is elevated, gravity helps the veins of the limb return blood to the heart, reducing the amount of blood and other fluids that accumulates in the damaged tissue.

With RICE and over-the-counter pain medicines, muscle soreness usually disappears within a day or two. If an injured area does not improve with RICE and the pain persists or worsens, consult a physician.

Temperature-Related Injuries

When exercising in sunny weather, the body gains heat from the environment and from its active muscles. To cool itself, the body perspires heavily, transferring heat to the environment. *Dehydration* (lack of body water) can occur if a person does not replace the fluid lost by perspiration. The muscles of a person suffering from dehydration are less able to work efficiently. It is essential that people replace the water lost in sweat by consuming adequate amounts of fluids, especially plain water. Soups, fruits, vegetables, and nonalcoholic drinks contribute water to the diet also.

Hyperthermia, higher than normal body temperature, can result from dehydration. If a person becomes hot and dehydrated, heat cramps, heat exhaustion, or heat stroke may occur. The signs and symptoms of **heat cramps** include muscular tightening and pain in the limbs or abdomen. The affected individual usually recovers after stopping the activity, resting in a shady area, stretching the cramped muscles, and drinking several ounces of water. After recovering, this person should not exercise for the remainder of the day.

Heat exhaustion and **heatstroke** are more serious conditions than heat cramps. People suffering from heat exhaustion have pale and clammy skin; sweat profusely; and feel nauseated, tired, and weak. They need to move to a cooler area and drink plenty of cool water. If heat exhaustion is not recognized and treated, heatstroke can develop. The signs and symptoms of heatstroke include hot, dry, reddened skin; rapid pulse; fever; and loss of consciousness. Heatstroke is a life-threatening

emergency; victims should be removed from the heat and receive immediate medical attention.

When the weather is hot and humid, avoid exerting yourself outdoors during the hottest time of the day. If you must be outdoors when it is hot, follow a few precautions to reduce the likelihood of heat-related injury. Two hours before exercising, drink about 16 oz. of water; during exercise, drink 4 to 8 oz. of water every 15 to 20 minutes (Convertino et al., 1996). Your goal is to consume enough fluids to replace the amount lost by sweating.

When the weather first becomes hot, individuals should begin working or exercising outdoors at a reduced intensity, then gradually increase the intensity over a 2-week period to become *acclimatized,* that is, physically adjusted to the extreme temperature change. Wearing light-colored, loose clothing in sunny, hot, and humid weather helps people stay comfortable because light colors reflect sunlight and loose clothing allows perspiration to evaporate more easily. When environmental temperature and humidity are very high, most individuals should consider reducing the intensity and duration of their outdoor workouts to reduce the risk of heat-related illness.

People who perspire excessively can lose considerable amounts of sodium chloride in their sweat. Most of these individuals can drink more water and fruit juices and consume foods to replace the lost nutrients. While engaging in strenuous exercise that lasts an hour or more, people can also consume sports drinks for fluid replacement (Coyle, 2004). In addition to water, these drinks contain sodium chloride and energy-supplying carbohydrate. Most physically active people do not need to take salt tablets (Williams, 2005). Individuals should not consume alcoholic beverages to replenish body fluids, because alcohol is a *diuretic.* A diuretic increases urine production; therefore, people lose even more body water when they drink alcohol-containing beverages. Although caffeine is also a diuretic, recent results of scientific studies indicate caffeinated beverage consumption does not produce major urinary losses of body water (Paluska, 2003).

Participating in outdoor activities during the winter months increases the risk of cold injury. Exposed to cold temperatures, the body reduces its blood flow to the skin, conserving body heat. The chilled person shivers and feels tingling, numbness, or burning in

hyperthermia a condition that occurs when body temperature rises above the normal range.

heat cramps in a dehydrated and hot person the signs and symptoms of heat cramps include muscular tightening and pain in the limbs or abdomen.

heat exhaustion extreme fatigue that results from exercise or work in hot temperatures.

heatstroke a life-threatening condition that can occur when people exercise or work in hot temperatures.

exposed skin or body parts. *Frostbite* occurs when ice crystals form in the deeper tissues of the skin, damaging them. Blood flow to the affected area slows, causing clots to form. Unable to obtain oxygen and nutrients, the tissue dies. The damage may be so extensive that the frostbitten areas must be amputated. A person's fingers, toes, nose, ears, and face are most susceptible to frostbite, but any exposed skin can become frostbitten. Frostbite requires immediate and proper medical treatment. Avoid rubbing frostbitten skin because it can further damage cold tissues. To prevent frostbite, people need to wear gloves or mittens, thick socks, hats that can be pulled down over the ears, and scarves when outdoors in cold weather.

Hypothermia occurs when the body's core temperature drops below 95°F (Kanzenbach & Dexter, 1999). (A rectal thermometer is used to measure core body temperature.) As body temperature declines, the person shivers, feels tired, displays poor judgment, acts disoriented, and eventually loses consciousness. Death can occur when the core temperature falls below 82°F, and breathing and circulation are too weak to support life.

As in cases of frostbite, hypothermia requires prompt medical treatment. It is important to shelter people suffering from hypothermia from the cold and remove their wet clothing. Covering them in dry blankets keeps them warm until they can be taken to a hospital. To protect against hypothermia, wear a hat and layers of warm, dry clothing when you are in cold environments.

Healthy Living Practices

- If you have musculoskeletal injuries, use RICE as treatment. If pain and swelling persist, contact your health care practitioner.
- If you develop heat cramps or heat exhaustion while working or exercising, stop the activity immediately, get out of the heat, and drink plenty of water.
- If you plan to exercise or work in hot conditions, wear loose, light clothing and take an ample supply of water, fruit juices, or sports drinks with you.
- When you exercise or work in cold conditions, protect yourself against hypothermia and frostbite by wearing layers of warm, dry clothing, a hat or ski mask, gloves or mittens, and thick socks.
- Avoid drinking beverages that contain alcohol to replace body water that is lost during exercise or exposure to hot temperatures.

Developing a Personal Fitness Program

A basic personal physical fitness program should include activities that enhance cardiorespiratory fitness, muscular strength and endurance, and flexibility. To develop an effective program, determine your needs, interests, and limitations (Holly & Shaffrath, 1998). Answering the following questions can help you accomplish this step:

- How can I schedule my day's activities so I have time to exercise?
- Which physical activities am I most likely to enjoy and practice regularly for the rest of my life?
- Do I want to develop or enhance specific sports-related skills?
- Would I rather work out alone or with others?
- Where will I exercise?
- Do I have physical limitations that require special equipment or rule out certain activities?

The Changing Health Habits activity for this chapter can help you determine if you are ready to improve your level of physical fitness (see student workbook).

After completing the first step, make a list of your general fitness goals. One of them should be to enhance the health-related components of fitness, for example, improving your cardiorespiratory fitness or flexibility. Other goals may be changing your appearance or building agility. Although your list may include several goals, choose one or two to work on at a time.

At this point, you need to choose enjoyable physical activities that will help you meet your fitness goals. As mentioned earlier, aerobic exercise is necessary for achieving cardiorespiratory fitness. Resistance training is important for increasing lean body mass and maintaining muscular strength and endurance. Warm-up and cool-down stretching exercises can improve range of motion. Faculty who conduct personal fitness classes in the physical education department at your college can answer your questions concerning the need for special equipment or how to perform activities safely.

If you are overweight or have been sedentary, give your body time to adapt to the fitness program. For the first 2 weeks, do not try to exercise at a high intensity level or for more than 15 minutes. Some people keep an exercise log or diary to track their progress. Stop when you experience signs of exercise intolerance, such as pain or breathlessness, and note this in your log. A common problem encountered by enthusiastic but out-of-shape people is trying to do too much too soon.

When you do not experience fatigue or discomfort as a result of the activity, you are ready to move on to the improvement stage of the program. By gradually increasing the intensity and duration of your physical activity, you can progressively overload your muscles and achieve your fitness goals. For example, add 5 minutes to the time of your aerobic workout session each week, until you are exercising for 45 to 90 minutes most days of the week. If you are walking at 2 mph, gradually increase the pace until you are able to walk between 3 and 4 mph without effort. To acquire the fitness benefits of aerobic exercise, a person must engage in the activity for at least 10 minutes at a time, at least 2 days a week, and at a minimum of 55% to 64% of his or her maximum heart rate (Pollock et al., 1998). However, engaging in aerobic exercise more often, for longer periods, and at higher intensity levels develops much higher degrees of fitness.

You can enhance muscular size and strength with a weightlifting program that gradually overcomes the resistance of progressively heavier weights. As your muscles adapt to the workload, you should be able to develop strength by adding resistance while performing fewer repetitions. After each bout of heavy training, muscles engaged in resistance exercises need about 48 hours to recover, to repair themselves, and to grow. Thus, experts often recommend alternating the days of the week in which you perform cardiorespiratory and strength training activities. Table 11-3 shows a sample aerobic and weight resistance program that includes stretching exercises. By the end of 6 months, you should be ready to move on to the maintenance stage of the program.

A major feature of the maintenance stage of your fitness program is sustaining your fitness level and interest. Adding new activities prevents boredom with the workout program and develops different muscle groups or skills. Cross-training, incorporating a variety of aerobic activities into a fitness program, is an excellent way to maintain enthusiasm and interest. Working out in different environments can also add interest. Walking in parks or hiking on trails, for example, can be more interesting than walking around indoor tracks. By working out with friends or family members, you can enhance your physical as well as social health.

Once people achieve high degrees of physical fitness, they need to continue exercising to maintain the healthful benefits gained during their training program. Sometimes physically fit individuals discontinue intensive regular exercise regimens for a variety of reasons, such as experiencing injuries or losing motivation. Detraining can occur within a couple of weeks after exercise sessions are discontinued. Even if they have to reduce the frequency of their exercise sessions, people can usually maintain their high level of physical fitness as long as they do not stop working out.

Healthy Living Practices

- When you perform isometric or isotonic exercises to increase muscular strength, also engage in aerobic exercises to enhance your cardiorespiratory fitness.
- You can enhance your muscular strength, muscular endurance, and flexibility by increasing the frequency, duration, and intensity of your exercise sessions.
- If you have heart disease or other serious chronic conditions, are out of shape, or are over 40 years of age, obtain the approval of a physician before beginning an exercise program, especially if the program includes aerobic activities.

Active for a Lifetime

People are more likely to engage in physical activity regularly if they enjoy it, recognize the health benefits, and make it a priority. Some sedentary people dislike vigorous exercise because they do not feel competent performing the activity; others may associate the activity with sweating, strain, and pain. Adults who enjoy being active make exercise and physical movement integral parts of their daily routines.

Many people find it easier to be physically active while in college than when they are out of school and working full time. In a nationwide survey, nearly 40% of college students reported participating in vigorous physical activities during the week prior to the survey ("Youth Risk," 1997). Male students were more likely to engage in vigorous physical activity than female students, and students between 18 and 24 years old were more active than students 25 years of age and older. Additionally, black students were more likely than white students to engage in moderate physical activities and muscle-strengthening exercises.

Most college and university campuses have physical education departments that offer a variety of sports and fitness courses; some of these departments have

hypothermia
a condition that occurs when the body's core temperature drops below 95°F.

cross-training
incorporating a variety of aerobic activities into a fitness program.

Table 11-3 A Sample Four-Week Combined Workout Program

Week 1	Warm-Up* (min.)	Workout	Cool-Down* (min.)	Week 3	Warm-Up* (min.)	Workout	Cool-Down* (min.)
Monday	5 to 10	Brisk walking 15 min.	5 to 10	Monday	5 to 10	Brisk walking 25 min.	5 to 10
Tuesday	5 to 10	Resistance training, beginning load Reps: 5, Sets: 4	5 to 10	Tuesday	5 to 10	Resistance training, beginning load Reps: 5, Sets: 4	5 to 10
Wednesday	5 to 10	Brisk walking 15 min.	5 to 10	Wednesday	5 to 10	Brisk walking 25 min.	5 to 10
Thursday	5 to 10	Resistance training, beginning load Reps: 5, Sets: 4	5 to 10	Thursday	5 to 10	Resistance training, beginning load Reps: 5, Sets: 4	5 to 10
Friday	5 to 10	Brisk walking 15 min.	5 to 10	Friday	5 to 10	Brisk walking 25 min.	5 to 10
Saturday	5 to 10	Resistance training, beginning load Reps: 5, Sets: 4	5 to 10	Saturday	5 to 10	Resistance training, beginning load Reps: 5, Sets: 4	5 to 10
Sunday	5 to 10	Brisk walking 15 min.	5 to 10	Sunday	5 to 10	Brisk walking 25 min.	5 to 10

Week 2	Warm-Up* (min.)	Workout	Cool-Down* (min.)	Week 4	Warm-Up* (min.)	Workout	Cool-Down* (min.)
Monday	5 to 10	Brisk walking 20 min.	5 to 10	Monday	5 to 10	Brisk walking 30 min.	5 to 10
Tuesday	5 to 10	Resistance training, beginning load Reps: 5, Sets: 4	5 to 10	Tuesday	5 to 10	Resistance training, beginning load Reps: 10, Sets: 4	5 to 10
Wednesday	5 to 10	Brisk walking 20 min.	5 to 10	Wednesday	5 to 10	Brisk walking 30 min.	5 to 10
Thursday	5 to 10	Resistance training, beginning load Reps: 5, Sets: 4	5 to 10	Thursday	5 to 10	Resistance training, beginning load Reps: 10, Sets: 4	5 to 10
Friday	5 to 10	Brisk walking 20 min.	5 to 10	Friday	5 to 10	Brisk walking 30 min.	5 to 10
Saturday	5 to 10	Resistance training, beginning load Reps: 5, Sets: 4	5 to 10	Saturday	5 to 10	Resistance training, beginning load Reps: 10, Sets: 4	5 to 10
Sunday	5 to 10	Brisk walking 20 min.	5 to 10	Sunday	5 to 10	Brisk walking 30 min.	5 to 10

*Slow walking and stretching.

Choosing a Fitness Center

Every year millions of Americans join health clubs, gyms, and exercise and fitness centers. Thousands of these people complain about their membership to states' attorneys general, Better Business Bureaus, and other consumer protection groups. The following tips can help you avoid becoming another dissatisfied health and fitness center consumer:

- Determine if you can afford to join the center.
- Inspect the center for cleanliness, type and quality of equipment, and especially staff qualifications. Ask if staff are certified as aerobics instructors, weight trainers, or athletic trainers. Are they trained in cardiopulmonary resuscitation (CPR) and first aid?
- Ask current members if they are satisfied with the center's facilities and why or why not.

- Ask your local Better Business Bureau about the number and nature of complaints against the organization.
- Ask for a trial period to use the facilities before joining.
- Never sign a contract under pressure at the center. Many centers use confusing and misleading advertising, including prizes or special short-term offers to spark your interest. Once you are in the facility, aggressive sales staff engage in high-pressure sales tactics to convince you to sign a contract.
- Before signing, take a few days to read the contract carefully. Make certain that you understand the details concerning payment options, membership restrictions, cancellation terms, and the membership period. If a staff member makes additional promises, have the individual record it in writing, on the contract.

---

well-equipped fitness centers. Additionally, the staff of the physical education department may conduct intramural athletic programs that are open to students, and at certain times, they may open the college's gyms and athletic fields to all students. While in school, students should take advantage of the fitness opportunities available on their college or university campuses.

After leaving college, individuals can continue to build or maintain their fitness level by exercising at home or by joining fitness centers or clubs. Although large resistance exercise machines are highly effective for building muscular strength, their expense and size make them unlikely to be found in most homes. However, you can buy barbells and smaller handheld weights at most department or sporting goods stores for use at home. To improve cardiorespiratory fitness, rowing machines, stationary bikes, and cross-country skiing machines can be purchased for home fitness centers. Before buying any large piece of fitness equipment, you should visit a gym or fitness club to test the machine and discuss its value with qualified fitness experts. For additional information, check popular consumer magazines that occasionally rate exercise equipment.

Building or maintaining physical fitness does not require a long-term commitment with a gym or fitness club, but many people enjoy the social aspects of exercising at these facilities. The quality and cost of gyms and fitness clubs vary, so you may want to consider the

points listed in the Consumer Health feature "Choosing a Fitness Center" before joining one.

Unless you have a job that requires physical exertion or you work at a company that provides a worksite fitness center for its employees, you need to find ways to be more physically active at work. If your office building has stairways, climb the stairs rather than ride the elevators. Instead of eating lunches in restaurants, bring your lunches from home to eat at your desk, and use the remaining time to go outside and walk. You might consider buying two pairs of athletic shoes— one for your office and one for home. You may like walking with others better than walking alone; ask someone to walk with you. Colleagues, spouses, or friends can provide the valuable social support you may need to maintain your motivation to exercise at work or home. In addition to increasing your physical activity at work, you can move around more at home. Child care, housework, and gardening chores often require contracting large muscle groups, which expends energy and strengthens the muscles. How many times a week do you go up and down steps, walk a pet, or go shopping? What lifestyle changes can you make to increase your physical activity?

Like many people, you may want to be more active, but you cannot seem to find the time to exercise. It is important to remember that you do not have to spend hours each day engaging in strenuous exercises to improve your health. Even 10 to 20 minutes of

THE ACTIVITY PYRAMID

CUT DOWN ON

IF YOU'RE INACTIVE
(Rarely active)

Increase daily activities at the base of the pyramid.

◆ Walk whenever you can.
◆ Make leisure time as active as possible.

IF YOU'RE SPORADIC
(Active some of the time, but not regularly)
Become more consistent with activities in the middle of the pyramid.

◆ Plan activity in your day.
◆ Set realistic goals.

IF YOU'RE CONSISTENT
(Active most days of the week)
Choose activities from all levels of the pyramid.

◆ Change your routine if you start to get bored.
◆ Explore new activities.

Sitting
Watching TV
Computer time

3+ TIMES A WEEK

Stretch & Strengthen Your Muscles

Periodic stretch breaks
Yoga
Tai Chi
Weight lifting

Tension bands
Pushups
Curl ups

3-5 TIMES A WEEK

Give Your Heart & Lungs A Workout

Biking
Hiking
Brisk walking
Running / Jogging

Swimming
Water aerobics
Basketball
In-line skating

EVERY DAY

Walk Often & Stay Active

Walking the dog
Doing yard work

Golfing
Bowling

Parking your car farther away
Taking the stairs instead of the elevator

Figure 11-12 **The Activity Pyramid.** This physical activity pyramid includes recommendations for healthy lifestyles. Source: © Park Nicollet Health Innovations, Minneapolis, U.S.A. 1-888-637-2675. Reprinted wih permission.

vigorous aerobic activity can boost your fitness level. Determine how you spend your leisure time. Each day, how much time do you spend engaging in sedentary activities such as watching TV, communicating with others in a chat room, or playing computer games? Can you set aside at least 30 minutes each day to engage in some moderately intense physical activities? The pyramid shown in Figure 11-12 illustrates physical activity recommendations for healthy lifestyles. Canada's *Physical Activity Guide* is shown in Appendix E.

Many aerobic and resistance activities do not require extensive time, complex skills, or special and costly equipment. For example, people can exercise by dancing to music or videos, or by performing tai chi in the privacy of their homes. The main objective is to select physical activities that you enjoy and can perform regularly for the rest of your life.

As mentioned earlier, if you are out of shape or older than 40 years, you should consult a physician before beginning a physical fitness program that includes moderate-intensity activities. This precautionary measure can determine whether you have serious health

problems. If you have a chronic condition, consult your physician for an exercise prescription. Most adults can begin a regular walking program to get into shape; after a few weeks, they can add more intense forms of physical activity to boost their cardiorespiratory fitness.

Healthy Living Practices

• To become physically fit or to maintain a high degree of fitness, design a personal fitness program that includes activities that you enjoy and can perform regularly while you are in college and throughout your lifetime.

• If you have a sedentary lifestyle, find ways to become more physically active at work and home, such as walking some of the way to work, using the stairs instead of elevators, doing housework, and walking during your leisure time.

Physical Fitness

The health habits that a person adopts in childhood, including physical and sports activities, are likely to be practiced and enjoyed for a lifetime. Children who are physically active have better measures of all health-related fitness components than those who are sedentary. Since sedentary lifestyles are associated with heart disease in adults, many health care practitioners are concerned that children may begin to develop this disease, especially if they do not engage in physical activities regularly. To improve the overall health and well-being of children, parents and schools need to find ways to encourage youngsters who are physically unfit to increase their fitness levels.

Another major concern of health and fitness experts is the proportion of American children and adolescents who spend a considerable amount of time engaged in sedentary activities, such as playing computer games or viewing television. In 2003, about 56% of American high school students were enrolled in physical education classes; only about 28% of students attended such classes daily (Lowry et al., 2004). More research is needed to determine the long-term effects of childhood and adolescent activity habits on their future health.

Regular exercise is just as important during pregnancy as in the other times of a woman's life. Healthy, physically fit women can continue engaging in a program of mild to moderate physical activity throughout their pregnancies (American College of Obstetricians and Gynecologists [ACOG], 2002). However, performing strenuous exercise (e.g., jogging) five or more times per week increases the risk of having a low-birth-weight baby (Campbell & Mottola, 2001). The ability to engage comfortably and safely in many physical activities often becomes limited in the latter stage of pregnancy. During this time, a woman's weight usually increases dramatically, especially in the center and front part of her body. As a result, she often feels awkward while engaging in many physical activities, and her risk of injury increases.

A pregnant woman should avoid activities if they pose a risk to her health and that of her developing fetus. Physical activities that might result in falls or injuries to the abdominal area and exhaustive exercises such as contact sports, heavy weightlifting, or training and participating in competitive events are generally not recommended for pregnant women. Additionally, exercising while lying down may inter-

Figure 11-13 **Exercising During Pregnancy.** Nearly all pregnant women can safely walk, swim, or ride a stationary bicycle.

fere with blood flow to the uterus and is not recommended. It is important for pregnant women to be well hydrated before, during, and after exercise and to avoid overheating. Physicians do not recommend that pregnant women exercise in hot, humid conditions or use hot tubs and saunas because these activities can raise the woman's body temperature, endangering the fetus.

It is a good idea for pregnant women to discuss their exercise plans with their physicians. Nearly all pregnant women can safely walk, swim, or ride a stationary bicycle (Figure 11-13). Healthy pregnant women should engage in at least 30 minutes of moderate-intensity exercise daily on most or all days of the week (ACOG, 2002). Those who are obese or severely underweight, are sedentary, or have histories of health problems should consult their physicians before following an exercise program.

As people age, they experience numerous changes that indicate a decline in their physical conditions. For example, the maximum heart rates of elderly people are lower during exercise, and their hearts pump less blood with each beat. Compared to when they were young adults, most aged persons have more body fat. Although exercise training of the elderly does not prevent these physical changes, it can limit the extent of the decline.

Most Americans become less active as they age. In 2001, about 31% of women and 25% of men 65 years of age and older did not engage in leisure-time physical activities or exercise (CDC, 2001). It is important for people to continue exercising as they age (Figure 11-14). Physically fit aged persons usually have healthier hearts and body compositions than unfit persons of the same age. Even by performing light physical activities regularly, elderly people can reduce their blood pressure, resting heart rate, and body mass index (Mensink et al., 1999). Additionally, physical activity helps maintain or improve the flexibility of joints as well as the strength and endurance of muscles. The

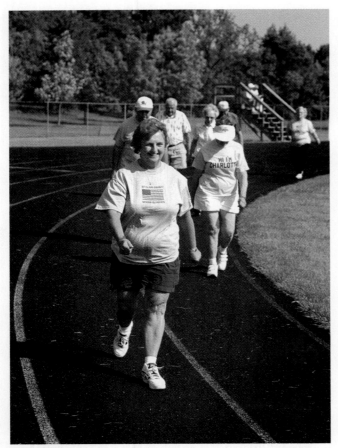

Figure 11-14 **Exercise Is for Everyone.** It is important for people to continue exercising as they age.

A minor fall that would not injure a healthy 23-year-old person can have dire consequences for a frail 85-year-old one. An elderly person who falls is more likely to suffer a disabling bone fracture or die from the injury than a younger person. Aged people who survive falls often experience some degree of immobility and pain that limits their ability to care for themselves and interact socially. By participating in exercise classes that improve balance and muscular strength, elderly people can reduce their risk of falls (Tsang & Hui-Chan, 2004). The Diversity in Health essay on page 309 describes the benefits of *tai chi*, a form of martial arts that helps some elderly people become healthier.

It is never too late to become physically fit. By increasing physical activity, even very old people can gain healthful benefits such as improved muscular strength and endurance, flexibility, and psychological well-being. To achieve these benefits, participation in strenuous formal exercise programs is not necessary; most elderly people can improve their overall health by engaging in light to moderate physical activities regularly such as walking, gardening, or mall-walking every day.

Healthy Living Practices

- If you have children, consider limiting the amount of time they spend watching television or playing computer games. Encourage your children to be physically active.
- If you are pregnant, consult your physician to determine which physical activities are safe to perform during this time.
- As you age, exercise regularly and be physically active.

results of some studies suggest that regular exercise improves the cognitive functioning and mood of elderly people (Kritz-Silverstein et al., 2001; Yaffe et al., 2001). Older adults can enjoy the social aspects of exercising by joining mall-walking, dancing, or fitness classes that are designed for the elderly.

People lose their ability to maintain their balance as they age, which increases their risk of falling.

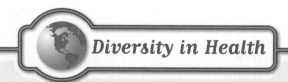

New Interest in an Ancient Approach to Fitness

*In motion
all parts of the body must be
light,
nimble,
and strung together.*
**From T'ai chi ch'uan
by Chang San-feng (1279–1386 A.D.)**

To people outside of China, it may seem difficult to believe that the graceful dancelike movements of t'ai chi chu'uan (tie-jee-chwahn), commonly called "tai chi," is a form of exercise. Unlike Western physical activities that often require rapid, forceful, and extensive motions, tai chi involves gentle gliding muscular movements that do not overextend body parts. According to its promoters, tai chi promotes good health, physical fitness, and longevity.

The exact origins of traditional tai chi are unknown. For more than 2,000 years, the Chinese have practiced qigong (ch'i-kung), a series of simple exercises that focus on breathing, maintaining certain body postures, and relaxing. These features are also emphasized in tai chi. In fact, the word *chi* means "breath energy." Thus, the ancient practice of qigong may have set the stage for the development of tai chi.

In addition to qigong, the Chinese martial arts probably contributed to the development of tai chi ch'uan. Ch'uan means "the joy of fighting with bare fists." Originally tai chi ch'uan may have been used for self-defense or boxing. However, a major principle of tai chi ch'uan is to overcome brute force and harshness with softness, gentleness, and smoothness.

Chang San-feng, the thirteenth century Taoist priest whose writing appears above, is usually credited with creating tai chi. Taoism is an ancient Chinese religion and philosophy that emphasizes living in harmony with nature. To Taoists, the harmonious functioning of the body is important if one is to achieve good health and live a long life. Today, tai chi is growing in popularity with Western exercise enthusiasts who are interested in achieving its potential health benefits (Figure 11-C). Promoters of tai chi claim that the physical exercises improve digestion and circulation, as well as increase alertness. People who practice tai chi often report that the exercises reduce stress (see Chapter 3).

While performing the specific sequential exercises, the upper part of the body remains loose; the knees are slightly bent, but firmly supporting the weight of the body.

Movements flow from one to another. Opposing arms and legs move in harmony; for example, as one arm gracefully arches upward, the other moves down in the same fashion. According to those who teach tai chi, if one body part does not follow another, the body is not in harmony. The series of vertical and horizontal movements continues until the sequence of exercises has been completed.

An important aspect of tai chi is mental concentration. As individuals engage in these exercises, they focus their attention on the sensations associated with the sequential movements; such attention requires silence.

As with other physical activities, practicing tai chi every day improves flexibility, muscular strength, and balance. Since tai chi does not require rapid, forceful muscular movements, it is a beneficial form of physical activity for elderly people or anyone who cannot engage in aerobic exercises.

A specially trained instructor is necessary to teach the proper posture, sequences of coordinated movements, and breathing technique of tai chi. Therefore, if you are interested in learning the exercises, check with the physical education department at your college or university to see if it offers tai chi instruction. Fitness centers in your community, such as the YMCA, might also offer tai chi classes.

Source: Lie, F. T. (1988). *T'ai chi ch'uan: The Chinese way.* New York: Sterling.
The essence of t'ai chi ch'uan. (1979). Translated and edited by Lo, B. P. J., Inn, M., Amacker, R., & Foe, S. Richmond, CA: North Atlantic Books.

Figure 11-C **Tai Chi.** Practicing tai chi improves flexibility, muscular strength, and balance.

CHAPTER REVIEW

Summary

Regardless of age and physical condition, nearly everyone can achieve numerous health benefits by engaging in physical activity and exercise. Performing regular, vigorous exercise and physical activity can build, maintain, and preserve skeletal muscles; improve the circulation and functioning of the heart; and regulate the amount of body fat. Additionally, weight-bearing exercises such as walking, dancing, and jogging strengthen bones, which can prevent or delay the development of osteoporosis.

Besides improving physical health, exercise can have short-term and long-term psychological benefits. Physical activity can reduce symptoms of anxiety and depression and improve mood and well-being.

The health-related components of physical fitness are cardiorespiratory fitness, muscular strength, muscular endurance, flexibility, and body composition. Many fitness experts consider cardiorespiratory fitness the most important health-related element of physical fitness.

Regular aerobic exercise enhances cardiorespiratory fitness, increasing the stroke volume of the heart and reducing the resting heart rate. To develop cardiorespiratory fitness, a person needs to perform aerobic activities for 30 to 60 minutes at least three times a week. Examples of popular aerobic activities include running, jogging, race-walking, lap swimming, cycling, stair-stepping, aerobic dancing, cross-country skiing, and rope skipping.

To develop muscular strength, muscles need to be overloaded by repeatedly moving objects that become progressively heavier. When muscles are overloaded, they hypertrophy; when muscles are not used, they atrophy or detrain. Detraining can occur within a couple of weeks after people discontinue their exercise training regimen. Thus, people must maintain their exercise programs to avoid detraining.

Immediate first aid for most musculoskeletal injuries includes RICE, the combination of rest, ice, compression, and elevation. Hypothermia and hyperthermia are serious temperature-related injuries that can occur when the body is unable to maintain its temperature in the normal range. Exercising in hot weather can produce heat cramps, heat exhaustion, or heatstroke. If untreated, heat cramps or heat exhaustion can lead to heatstroke, which can be fatal. Maintaining adequate hydration and avoiding overexertion in hot and humid conditions can reduce the risk of heat-related illnesses. To avoid frostbite or hypothermia, people should dress warmly while outdoors in cold and windy conditions, keeping their skin well covered.

When planning an effective overall fitness regimen, people need to consider the type, frequency, duration, and intensity of their exercise activities. Additionally, individuals should design personal fitness programs that provide health benefits, satisfy their needs and interests, and can be followed for a lifetime. Before beginning fitness regimens that include aerobic activities, people with heart disease or other serious chronic conditions and people who are out of shape or older than 40 years should obtain the approval of their physicians.

Regular physical activity is just as important for youngsters as for adults. Performing certain activities may be risky during pregnancy; therefore, pregnant women should discuss their physical activity with their physicians. In most cases, it is never too late for people to begin fitness programs. By engaging in light to moderate physical activities regularly, such as walking or gardening every day, elderly individuals can improve their overall health.

Applying What You Have Learned

1. Calculate your target heart rate zone. **Application**
2. For 3 days, record the amount of time you spend engaging in various physical activities, such as walking to class, playing racquetball, or riding a bike. Use Table 11-1 to classify your physical activities as being light, moderate, or intense. **Analysis**
3. Plan an exercise program that you can follow for a lifetime. **Synthesis**
4. Use the step test in the assessment activity to evaluate your current level of cardiorespiratory fitness. **Evaluation**

Key

Application — using information in a new situation.

Analysis — breaking down information into component parts.

Synthesis — putting together information from different sources.

Evaluation — making informed decisions.

Reflecting on Your Health

1. Are you satisfied with your level of physical fitness? Why or why not? If you are dissatisfied, what ideas did you get from reading this chapter that will help you improve your fitness? If you are satisfied, how will you maintain your fitness?
2. What benefits would you derive from adopting a more physically active lifestyle? What factors interfere with and what factors reinforce your efforts to become more physically fit?
3. Before reading this chapter, how did you feel about ergogenic aids such as dietary supplements or anabolic steroids to enhance athletic performance? Based on what you have read in this chapter, has your attitude changed? Why or why not?

4. If you have children or are thinking about having children, how would you encourage them to maintain a balance between the time they spend engaging in sedentary activities such as watching TV and in activities that develop physical fitness?
5. Which labor-saving devices would you be willing to stop using so you could use your muscles to do the work? Why did you choose these devices or machines? Describe practical steps you can take to increase your physical activity level.

References

American College of Obstetricians and Gynecologists. (2002). ACOG committee opinion: Exercise during pregnancy and the postpartum period. *International Journal of Gynaecology and Obstetrics, 77*(1):79–81.

Binzen, C. A., Swan, P. D., & Manore, M. M. (2001). Postexercise oxygen consumption and substrate use after resistance training in women. *Medicine & Science in Sports & Exercise, 33*:932–938.

Campbell, M. K., & Mottola, M. F. (2001). Recreational exercise and occupational activity during pregnancy and birth weight: A case-control study. *American Journal of Obstetrics and Gynecology, 184*(3):403–408.

Centers for Disease Control and Prevention. (2001). U.S. physical activity statistics: 2001 state physical activity comparison by demographic group. Retrieved November 8, 2004, from http://www.cdc.gov/nccdphp/dnpa/physical/stats/us_physical_activity/index.htm.

Convertino, V. A., Armstrong, L. E., Coyle, E. F., Mack, G. W., Sawka, M. N., Senay, L. C., Jr., & Sherman, W. M. (1996). Exercise and fluid replacement. *Medicine & Science in Sports & Exercise, 28*:i–vii.

Coyle, E. F. (2004). Fluid and fuel intake during exercise. *Journal of Sports Sciences, 22*(1):39–55.

Feigenbaum, M. S., & Pollock, M. L. (1999). Prescription of resistance training for health and disease. *Medicine & Science in Sports & Exercise, 31*(1):38–45.

Ham, S. A., Yore, M. M., Fulton, J. E., & Kohl, H. W., III. (2004). Prevalence of no leisure-time physical activity—35 states and the District of Columbia, 1988–2002. *Morbidity and Mortality Weekly Report, 53*(4):82–86.

Holbrook, A. M., Crowther, R., Lotter, A., Cheng, C., & King, D. (2000). The diagnosis and management of insomnia in clinical practice: A practical evidence-based approach. *Canadian Medical Association Journal, 162*(2):216–220.

Holly, R. G., & Shaffrath, J. D. (1998) Cardiorespiratory endurance. In: *ACSM's Resource Manual for Guidelines for Exercise Testing and Prescription,* 3rd ed. American College of Sports Medicine. Baltimore: Williams & Wilkins.

Jakes, R. W., Khaw, K., Day, N. E., Bingham, S., Welsh, A., Oakes, S., Luben, R., Dalzell, N., Reeve, J., & Wareham, N. J. (2001). Patterns of physical activity and ultrasound attenuation by heel bone among Norfolk cohort of European Prospective Investigation of Cancer (EPIC Norfolk): Population based study. *British Medical Journal, 322*(7279):140–143.

Kanzenbach, T. L., & Dexter, W. W. (1999). Cold injuries: Protecting your patients from the dangers of hypothermia and frostbite. *Postgraduate Medicine, 105*(1):72–78.

Kritz-Silverstein, D., Barrett-Connor, E., & Corbeau, C. (2001). Cross-sectional and prospective study of exercise and depression mood in the elderly: The Rancho Bernardo study. *American Journal of Epidemiology, 153*(6):596–603.

Kutscher, E. C., Lund, B. C., & Perry, P. J. (2002). Anabolic steroids: A review for the clinician. *Sports Medicine, 32*(5):285–296.

Laukkanen, J. A., Lakka, T. A., Rauramaa, R., Kuhanen, R., et al. (2001). Cardiovascular fitness as a predictor of mortality in men. *Archives of Internal Medicine, 161*(6):825–831.

Lee, I. M., & Paffenbarger, R. S., Jr. (2000). Associations of light, moderate, and vigorous intensity physical activity with longevity. The Harvard Alumni Health Study. *American Journal of Epidemiology, 151*(3):293–299.

Lee, I. M., & Skerrett, P. J. (2001). Physical activity and all-cause mortality: What is the dose-response relation? *Medicine & Science in Sports & Exercise, 33*(6 Suppl):S459–471.

Lowry, R., Brener, N., Lee, S., Epping, J., Fulton, J., & Eaton, D. (2004). Participation in high school physical education—United States, 1991–2003. *Morbidity and Mortality Weekly Report, 53*(36):844–847.

Macera, C. A., Jones, D. A., Yore, M. M., Ham, S. A., Kohl, H. W., et al. (2003). Prevalence of physical activity, including lifestyle activities among adults—United States, 2000–2001. *Morbidity and Mortality Weekly Report, 52*(32):764–769.

Maltby, J., & Day, L. (2001). The relationship between exercise motives and psychological well-being. *Journal of Psychology, 135*(6):651–660.

Mensink, G. B., Ziese, T., & Kok, F. J. (1999). Benefits of leisure-time physical activity on the cardiovascular risk profile at older age. *International Journal of Epidemiology, 28*(4):659–666.

Paluska, S. A. (2003). Caffeine and exercise. *Current Sports Medicine Reports, 2*(4):213–219.

Parkkari, J., Kujala, U. M., & Kannus, P. (2001). Is it possible to prevent sports injuries? Review of controlled clinical trials and recommendations for future work. *Sports Medicine, 31*(14):985–995.

Pollock, M. L., Gaesser, G. A., Butcher, J. D., Després, J., Dishman, R. K., Franklin, B. A., & Garber, C. E. (1998). American College of Sports Medicine position stand: The recommended quantity and quality of exercise for developing and maintaining cardiorespiratory and muscular fitness, and flexibility in healthy adults. *Medicine & Science in Sports & Exercise, 30*(6):975–991.

Roberts, J. M., & Wilson, K. (1999). Effect of stretching duration on active and passive range of motion in the lower extremity. *British Journal of Sports Medicine, 33*(4):259–263.

Schmidt, W. D., Biwer, C. J., & Kalscheuer, L. K. (2001). Effects of long versus short bout exercise on fitness and weight loss in overweight females. *Journal of the American College of Nutrition, 20*(5):494–501.

Speed, C. (2004). Low back pain. *British Medical Journal, 328*(7448): 1119–1121.

Stearns, D. M., Silveira, S. M., Wolf, K. K., & Luke, A. M. (2002). Chromium III tris (picolinate) is mutagenic at the hypoxanthine (guanine) phosphoribosyltransferase locus in Chinese hamster ovary cells. *Mutation Research, 513*(1–2):135–142.

Stofan, J. R., DiPietro, L., Davis, D., Kohl, H. W., III, & Blair, S. N. (1998). Physical activity patterns associated with cardiorespiratory fitness and reduced mortality: The Aerobics Center longitudinal study. *American Journal of Public Health, 88*(12):1807–1813.

Terjung, R. L., Clarkson, P., Eichner, E. R., Greenhaff, P. L., Hespel, P. J., Israel, R. G., Kraemer, W. J., Meyer, R. A., Spriet, L. L., Tarnopolsky, M. A., Wagenmakers, A. J., & Williams, M. H. (2000). American College of Sports Medicine roundtable: The physiological and health effects of oral creatine supplementation. *Medicine & Science in Sports & Exercise, 32*(3):706–717.

Thacker, S. B., Gilchrist, J., Stroup, D. F., & Kimsey, C. D., Jr. (2004). The impact of stretching on sports injury risk: A systematic review of the literature. *Medicine in Science, Sports & Exercise, 36*(3):371–378.

Tsang, W. W. N., & Hui-Chan, C. W. Y. (2004). Effect of 4- and 8-week intensive tai chi training on balance control in the elderly. *Medicine & Science in Sports & Exercise, 36*(4):648–657.

U.S. Department of Agriculture and U.S. Department of Health and Human Services. (2005). *Dietary guidelines for Americans 2005.* Retrieved January 12, 2005, from http://www.healthierus.gov/dietaryguidelines/.

U.S. Department of Health and Human Services. (1996). *Physical activity and health: A report of the Surgeon General.* Atlanta, GA: Centers for Disease Control and Prevention, National Center for Chronic Disease Prevention and Health Promotion.

U.S. Department of Health and Human Services, Office of Disease Prevention and Health Promotion. (2000). *Healthy People 2010.* Washington, DC: Government Printing Office. http://www.health.gov/healthypeople/.

U.S. Department of Health and Human Services, National Center for Health Statistics, Public Health Service. (2001). *Healthy People 2000: Final review.* Washington, DC: Government Printing Office.

U.S. Department of Health and Human Services. (2002). *Physical activity fundamental to preventing disease.* Retrieved October 27, 2004, from http://aspe.hhs.gov/health/reports/physicalactivity/index.shtml.

Williams, M. H. (2005). *Nutrition for health, fitness, and sport.* (7th ed.), New York: WCB McGraw-Hill.

Yaffe, K., Barnes, D., Nevitt, M., Lui, L. Y., & Covinsky, K. (2001). A prospective study of physical activity and cognitive decline in elderly women who walk. *Archives of Internal Medicine, 161*(14):1703–1708.

Youth Risk Behavior Surveillance: National College Health Risk Behavior Survey: United States, 1995. (1997). *Weekly Morbidity and Mortality Report, 46*(SS-6):1–54.

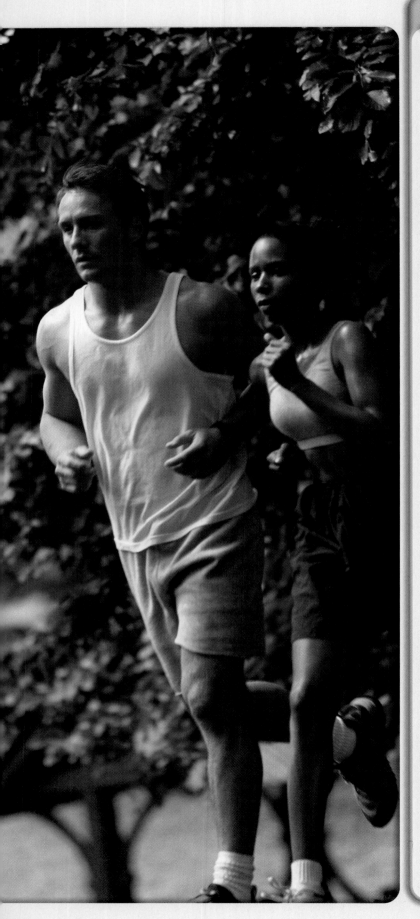

The Web site for this book offers many useful tools and is a great source for supplementary health information for both students and instructors. Visit the site at http://healthyliving.jbpub.com for information on these topics:

The Cardiovascular System and How It Works
Cardiovascular Diseases
Risk Factors for Cardiovascular Disease
Maintaining Cardiovascular Health

Chapter Overview

How the cardiovascular system works

Symptoms of and treatments for cardiovascular disease

Risk factors for cardiovascular disease

How to maintain your cardiovascular health

Diversity in Health
The Italian Gene: A Hope for Reversing Atherosclerosis?

Consumer Health
Vitamin Pills for a Healthier Heart?

Managing Your Health
Heart Attack Symptoms: What to Do in an Emergency

Across
THE LIFESPAN

Cardiovascular Health

Student Workbook

Self-Assessment: Check Your Cholesterol and Heart Disease IQ

Changing Health Habits: Reducing Your Risk of Cardiovascular Disease

Do You Know?

· *What to do to keep your heart and blood vessels healthy?*

· *What to do if you or someone you know is having a heart attack?*

· *If you are likely to have a heart attack or stroke?*

Cardiovascular Health

Do you think that you are immune from cardiovascular disease—dysfunction of the heart and blood vessels—because you are young? If so, think again! Even though cardiovascular disease (CVD) does not normally occur in young adults, unhealthy lifestyle patterns practiced and ingrained during this stage of life predispose a person to cardiovascular disease. Metabolic processes leading to cardiovascular disease *can* begin in childhood and accelerate at adolescence (Kohn & Jacobson, 2004).

In one large multicenter study (McGill & McMahan, 1998), medical researchers examined the relationship of the risk factors for cardiovascular disease (such as smoking, obesity, poor diet, and lack of exercise) to the development of fatty deposits in the arteries, which is one process that occurs in the development of this condition. They studied nearly 3,000 persons aged 15 to 34 years who died from accidents, homicides, and suicides. The results of the study revealed that young persons with risk factors for CVD began developing fatty streaks within their arteries in their teenage years. By age 25, young persons with risk factors also had developed raised lesions in the major blood vessels of the heart. The results of this and other studies (Brox et al., 2002; Yarnell et al., 2000; Berensen et al., 1998; Oalmann et al., 1997) show that reducing the likelihood of developing cardiovascular disease later in life involves controlling risk factors early in life. Behaviors in adolescence and young adulthood *do* matter: They can influence your health for years to come and can affect your lifespan.

Research results also show that adolescents are aware of cardiovascular risk factors, but many do not put this knowledge into practice. In other words, their understandings of heart-healthy behaviors and their lifestyles do not match (Steptoe et al., 2002). For example, in a study of cardiovascular disease risk factor attitudes and habits, three-fourths of those aged 17 to 18 years acknowledged the role of cigarette smoking in cardiovascular disease, yet one-third of this group smoked (Smalley et al., 2004).

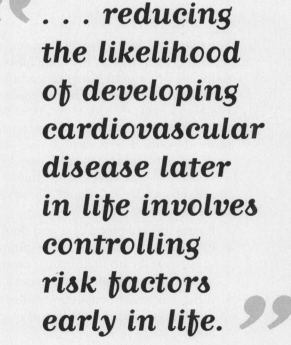

". . . reducing the likelihood of developing cardiovascular disease later in life involves controlling risk factors early in life."

As mentioned in Chapter 1, having knowledge about positive health practices does not always result in healthy lifestyles. The motivation to make positive changes in heath habits must accompany knowledge of what those changes should be. After reading this chapter, read the Changing Health Habits feature "Reducing Your Risk of Cardiovascular Disease" in the workbook that accompanies this textbook to help you develop motivation to implement heart-healthy lifestyle changes.

This chapter describes the causes of cardiovascular diseases and hypertension—noninfectious diseases in which hereditary, environmental, and lifestyle factors interact to create an individual's risk level for developing any one of them. It also describes the interrelatedness of these diseases and how the development of one affects the development of another. Last, it explores the factors critical to maintaining cardiovascular health, to help you preserve the fitness of your heart and blood vessels throughout your lifetime. First, let us explore the cardiovascular system and how it works.

The Cardiovascular System and How It Works

You may have heard the cardiovascular system also referred to as the circulatory system. These terms are often used interchangeably. The term *cardiovascular* refers to the heart (*cardio-*) and blood vessels (*vascular*). The term *circulatory* refers to the circulation of the blood. In practical use, both terms describe a body system that pumps blood enclosed in blood vessels to all parts of the body.

Blood is a somewhat viscous fluid made up of cells suspended in a liquid. Blood performs many functions:

- It contains red blood cells and fluid (plasma) that transport the respiratory gases (oxygen and carbon dioxide), nutrients, hormones, enzymes, and waste products.

- It helps regulate body temperature by distributing the heat generated by chemical reactions in the body.

- It contains blood clotting factors (including pieces of cells called *platelets*) that protect the blood supply from excessive losses and help in tissue repair.

- It contains white blood cells (including the lymphocytes of the immune system) that help protect the body from infection (see Chapter 14).

The blood is pumped by the heart, a muscular, fist-sized organ that lies in the chest cavity about midway between the shoulders and the waist, and slightly to the left of the midline (Figure 12-1). The heart consists of four chambers: two upper chambers called *atria* and two lower chambers called *ventricles*. The upper chambers receive blood and then push it into the lower chambers, which pump blood to the lungs and the rest of the body.

Blood flows within a vast network of blood vessels. **Arteries** carry blood away from the heart. They have muscular, elastic walls that bulge slightly when the left ventricle contracts and pushes blood through them, and they recoil at the end of the beat. Arteries branch into smaller vessels called *arterioles*. When these vessels become so small that they allow the passage of only one blood cell at a time, they are called **capillaries**.

Left common carotid artery

Left subclavian artery

Aorta

Heart

Abdominal aorta

Iliac arteries

Femoral arteries

Figure 12-1 **The Major Arteries of the Body.** The heart is located to the left of the midline in the chest cavity. The arteries take blood away from the heart and are shown in red. Veins return blood to the heart and are shown in blue.

The capillaries permeate tissues. These tiny blood vessels have walls that are only one cell thick. The thinness of capillary walls allows substances such as nutrients and oxygen to move out of the blood, and other substances such as waste products and carbon dioxide to move into the blood. Capillaries join to form larger vessels called *venules,* which in turn join to form still larger vessels, the veins.

Veins return blood to the heart. By the time the blood reaches the veins it has lost most of the force (pressure) of its push from the heart. Therefore, veins have thinner walls than do arteries; they contain less muscle and elastic tissue. In addition, veins have one-way valves along their length, which help prevent the backflow of blood. Blood returning to the heart from the head, neck, and shoulders is helped along by the force of gravity. Blood returning to the heart from the arms, legs, and torso combats the force of gravity but is pushed along as the skeletal muscles squeeze the veins in these areas.

Many adult women and men develop varicose veins. (The prevalence in one Belgian study [Van den Oever et al., 1998] is estimated to be 10% to 15% of men and 20% to 25% of women and in one French study [Carpentier et al., 2004] to be 50.5% of women and 30.1% of men.) *Varicose veins* are distended or stretched veins and are found most frequently in the legs or the trunk (Figure 12-2). They have a variety of causes, including defective valves, continual and prolonged sitting or standing, pregnancy, family history, lack of physical activity, and obesity (Kroeger et al., 2003; Jawien, 2003; Lee et al., 2003). Therapy for varicose veins includes elevating the legs, wearing elastic stockings, and, in severe cases, surgery. Lasers have been used successfully to shrink a type of varicose vein called spider leg veins (McDaniel et al., 1999). Spider veins are groups of stretched, small blood vessels that form a spiderlike pattern on the skin.

Coronary arteries arise from the base of the aorta and bring freshly oxygenated blood to the heart muscle itself. (Although blood flows in and out of the heart's chambers, the heart muscle is not nourished by the blood while it is in the chambers.) There are two main coronary arteries: the left and the right coronary arteries (see Figure 12-8). Both of these arteries branch into multiple vessels that supply the entire heart with blood.

Cardiovascular Diseases

A person with blocked coronary arteries is said to have **coronary artery disease (CAD)**, one type of cardiovascular disease. (Coronary artery disease is also commonly called coronary heart disease [CHD].) Coronary artery disease may result in a heart attack in which a portion of the heart muscle dies, or in **angina pectoris** (chest pain).

Coronary artery disease is only one type of **cardiovascular disease (CVD)**, or dysfunction of the heart and blood vessels. Other major cardiovascular diseases are hypertension (chronic high blood pressure), stroke (blood vessel disease of the brain), and rheumatic heart disease (a complication of strep throat). Atherosclerosis (blood vessel disease) is an important cardiovascular disease process that is an underlying cause of CAD and stroke. Other cardiovascular diseases are described throughout this chapter. About 70 million Americans (1 in 5) are estimated to have one or more forms of CVD (American Heart Association [AHA], 2005b). As Figure 12-3 shows, cardiovascular disease kills more people in the United States than any other disease.

After coronary artery disease, stroke and hypertension (in that order) produce the next highest death rates due to cardiovascular diseases. Stroke is the third leading

arteries blood vessels that carry blood away from the heart.

capillaries (KAP-ih-LAIR-eez) microscopic blood vessels that permeate tissues, connecting small arteries to small veins.

veins blood vessels that return blood to the heart.

coronary arteries blood vessels that arise from the base of the aorta and bring freshly oxygenated blood to the heart muscle.

coronary artery disease (CAD) a condition in which the coronary vessels are blocked partially or completely by fatty deposits, blood clots, or both. Also commonly called coronary heart disease (CHD).

angina pectoris (an-JEYE-nah PECK-tor-iss) chest pain due to insufficient oxygen in a portion of the heart.

cardiovascular disease (CVD) (KAR-dee-oh-VAS-ku-lar) disorders of the heart and blood vessels.

Figure 12-2 Close-up of Varicose Veins on a Woman's Thigh.

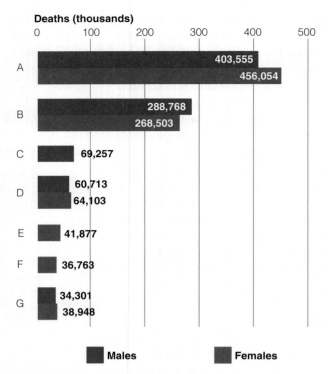

Deaths (thousands)

A	403,555 / 456,054
B	288,768 / 268,503
C	69,257
D	60,713 / 64,103
E	41,877
F	36,763
G	34,301 / 38,948

■ Males ■ Females

A Total cardiovascular (including cerebrovascular) diseases
B Cancer
C Accidents
D Chronic lower respiratory diseases
E Alzheimer's disease
F Pneumonia/influenza
G Diabetes mellitus

Figure 12-3 **Leading Causes of Death, United States, 2002.** This graph shows that cardiovascular disease is the number one cause of death for both men and women (all races, all ages). Source: National Center for Health Statistics. (2004). *Health, United States 2004*. Washington, DC: U.S. Government Printing Office.

cause of death in the United States (National Center for Health Statistics [NCHS], 2004). (Cancer is second; see Chapter 13.) These big killers—coronary artery disease and stroke—result from the development of yet another cardiovascular disease: atherosclerosis.

Atherosclerosis

In 99% of CAD cases, the blood supply to portions of the heart is reduced because the coronary arteries are blocked by fatty deposits. These fatty deposits, or **plaques**, develop as part of a disease of the arteries called **atherosclerosis**. (Arterial plaque is not the same as dental plaque.) An *atheroma* is a deteriorated, thickened area on the inner lining of a large or medium-sized artery. *Sclerosis* refers to loss of elasticity, or hardening of these arteries.

plaques
(plaks) fatty deposits in artery walls.

atherosclerosis
(ATH-er-oh-skle-ROW-sis) disease of large and medium-sized arteries in which the inner lining has areas that are deteriorated, thickened, and inelastic.

Atherosclerosis is one form of *arteriosclerosis* (hardening of the arteries).

Atherosclerosis may begin with an injury to the lining of a blood vessel. Factors such as high blood pressure, for example, can damage this lining, or the immune system may play a role. Lipids, especially cholesterol, accumulate at injury sites and cling to the interior of blood vessel walls. These plaques thicken blood vessel walls, which narrows the interiors of arteries (Figure 12-4) and interferes with arterial cells' ability to obtain nutrients. Eventually, the wall beneath a plaque degenerates. Scar tissue forms and calcium is often deposited there, "hardening" the artery. Blood clots sometimes develop there, too, and may be the ultimate cause of a heart attack or stroke.

Although the incidence of atherosclerosis increases with age, not all elderly people have extensive plaques. Conversely, *some young people do* (see chapter opening story).

Atherosclerosis occurs most often in the aorta, and in the coronary, femoral, iliac, internal carotid, and cerebral arteries. Most of these vessels are labeled on Figure 12-1. As you can see, these arteries supply blood to the heart, torso, legs, and head. The cerebral arteries, not shown in the diagram, branch from the carotid arteries and other vessels to supply large portions of the brain with blood. Atherosclerosis is most serious when it develops in the vessels that supply the heart, which can lead to heart attacks, and in the vessels that supply the brain, which can result in strokes.

Any blockage of vessels other than those to the heart is often referred to as **peripheral vascular disease**. This disease affects the organs and tissues that blocked vessels serve. One result of peripheral vascular disease, for example, can be erectile dysfunction (impotence) in men (see Chapter 6).

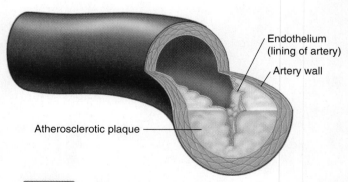

Endothelium (lining of artery)

Artery wall

Atherosclerotic plaque

Figure 12-4 **A Plaque in an Artery.** A plaque is formed by a buildup of fatty material on an artery wall. This illustration shows the interior of an affected artery that has been narrowed by plaque.

Coronary Artery Disease

In CAD, coronary vessels may become partially or completely blocked by one or more of the following: fatty deposits, which narrow blood vessels (see "Atherosclerosis"), a blood clot that develops at the site of fatty deposits, or a floating blood clot that lodges in a vessel. A stationary blood clot, called a **thrombus**, can block a vessel already narrowed by fatty deposits. Blood clots frequently form in vessels in which blood flow is slowed by fatty deposits. The development of a thrombus that blocks a coronary artery is called **coronary thrombosis**.

A thrombus may dislodge from the place in which it forms and become a floating blood clot, or **embolus**. An embolus can block a coronary artery downstream from where it was formed, producing a **coronary embolism**. In the early stages of CAD, coronary arteries may also become narrowed by muscle spasms of these vessels, frequently triggered by exposure to cold, physical exertion, or anxiety. Usually such muscle spasms are short lived and do not damage the heart muscle.

Angina Pectoris Spasms, partial blockage, or complete blockage of one or more of the coronary vessels can cause insufficient blood to reach part of the heart, which is called **ischemia**. When this happens, the heart does not receive sufficient oxygen and a person experiences angina pectoris, or chest pain. Angina is felt beneath the breastbone and extends to the left shoulder and down the left arm. (Pain in the arm may help you distinguish between angina and heartburn or other gastric distress.) Angina pain may also be felt in the jaw and neck and, infrequently, in the back. The pain is described as aching, squeezing, burning, heaviness, or pressure. Some people experience *silent* (painless) *angina*, which consists of strange feelings at angina sites without pain. Silent angina can be diagnosed by exercise testing or by wearing a portable device that monitors the electrical activity of the heart during a 24-hour period.

Angina attacks may come and go, brought on by physical exertion or by mental or emotional stress, but they are signs of serious coronary artery disease. Angina should not be ignored; a person experiencing angina attacks should seek medical attention immediately. Rest and drugs that dilate, or widen, the blood vessels (such as nitroglycerin) relieve attacks of angina. Other drugs used to treat angina include those to reduce blood pressure or those that slow the heart rate. Both types of drugs reduce the workload of the heart and its need for oxygen.

In cases of angina, a physician may suggest assessing the degree and location of vessel blockage to determine whether further treatment is necessary to reduce symptoms and avoid a heart attack. One common technique to visualize the coronary blood vessels is *coronary angiography*.

An *angiogram* is an x-ray image of blood vessels after they have been injected with a fluid called a *contrast medium*. The contrast medium used in angiography is composed primarily of iodine because it absorbs x rays, making visible the interiors of blood vessels. To perform coronary angiography, physicians first thread a thin plastic tube called a *catheter* through an artery in the arm or the groin until it reaches the coronary arteries. After injecting the contrast medium into the catheter, they take high-speed x-ray movies of blood flowing through the arteries. Figure 12-5 shows frames of such a movie and indicates where physicians are able to detect irregularities and narrowing of the coronary arteries.

Other tests such as magnetic resonance imaging (MRI) are also performed at many medical centers to create images of the heart and its vessels for various diagnostic purposes. MRI uses magnetic fields and radio waves to visualize structures.

If a patient has atherosclerosis in many coronary vessels, a physician may recommend coronary artery bypass graft surgery. If only one of a patient's coronary arteries is narrowed significantly, a physician may recommend widening the interior of the artery with a type of **angioplasty**, the reconstruction of damaged blood vessels. In balloon angioplasty, the physician threads a catheter through an artery in the arm or the groin until it reaches the coronary arteries, as done when performing an angiogram. However, instead of injecting dye into the catheter, the physician threads a second, balloon-tipped catheter through the first. When the second catheter reaches the area of blockage, the balloon is inflated, breaking up the plaque while compressing it against the arterial wall (Figure 12-6). This balloon technique also stretches the artery somewhat. Two newer techniques are atherectomy and stenting.

Atherectomy refers to methods that remove plaque from the interior of an artery. The procedure is performed like balloon angioplasty, but the second catheter

---

peripheral vascular disease any blockage of vessels other than those to the heart.

thrombus (THROM-bus) a stationary blood clot.

coronary thrombosis (throm-BOW-sis) the development of a stationary blood clot that blocks blood flow in an artery that brings blood to the heart muscle.

embolus (EM-bow-lus) a floating blood clot.

coronary embolism (EM-bow-lizm) a floating blood clot that lodges in an artery that brings blood to the heart muscle, blocking blood flow.

ischemia (is-KI-me-ah) insufficient blood in part of the heart.

angioplasty (AN-jee-oh-PLAS-tee) the reconstruction of damaged blood vessels.

atherectomy (ATH-er-EK-toe-me) the removal of plaque from the interior of an artery.

Figure 12-5 **Coronary Angiogram.** The arrows on the top angiogram point out some of the irregularities and areas of narrowing of this coronary artery. This same vessel is shown in the bottom image, taken minutes after balloon angioplasty.

Figure 12-6 **Balloon Angioplasty.** In balloon angioplasty, a thin tube containing a balloon is threaded through an artery until it reaches the area of plaque that is narrowing the vessel. The balloon is inflated, compressing the plaque against the artery wall and stretching the artery.

contains a cutting and collecting tip instead of a balloon tip.

Stenting is similar to balloon angioplasty in that a catheter device first compresses plaque against the artery wall. A springlike mesh device, the stent (Figure 12-7) is then implanted within the artery, covering the compressed plaque, supporting the artery, and smoothing the artery wall. After a time, tissue may grow around a stent, however, increasing the risk of the artery reclogging. One type of stent invented recently continues to expand inside the blood vessel in which it is placed. As it expands, it continues to widen the blood vessel, reducing the risk of reclogging. Additionally, drug-coated stents have been developed; they appear to inhibit reclogging in most patients (Rogers, 2004).

One technique that is used frequently to treat coronary artery disease is bypass surgery. In the United States in 2002 an estimated 515,000 of these procedures were performed on 306,000 patients (AHA, 2005b).

The phrase *bypass surgery* usually means **coronary artery bypass graft surgery (CABG)**. The coronary arteries are blood vessels that supply oxygen-rich blood to the heart muscle. When these vessels become blocked, blood flow is slowed and the heart muscle does not get enough oxygen.

People who have chronic angina, blockage in the vessels that supply the left side of the heart (the side that pumps blood to the body), or blockage in multiple

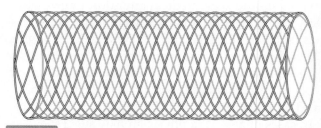

Figure 12-7 **An Arterial Stent.** This springlike mesh device is implanted in an artery after balloon angioplasty to cover the compressed plaque, smooth the artery wall, and support the vessel.

coronary arteries are often candidates for bypass surgery. To perform this operation, surgeons first open the chest cavity. Using a blood vessel taken from another part of the patient's body (usually the leg), they graft one end of the new vessel to the aorta, the major artery that carries blood away from the heart and to the body. Heart surgeons graft the other end of the new vessel to the damaged coronary artery, past the area of blockage (Figure 12-8). The grafted vessel thus bypasses the blocked portion of the diseased vessel.

An emerging therapy aimed at increasing blood flow to the heart muscle is transmyocardial laser revascularization (TMLR). In TMLR, surgeons use a laser to bore narrow channels from the heart chamber into the heart muscle. The idea behind this technique was that blood would flow through the heart muscle via these channels. Medical researchers now think that this procedure may work by stimulating the growth of new vessels (Galli et al., 1999; Korkola et al., 1999). Although TMLR does not help a heart patient live longer, it reduces the frequency of recurrent heart pain and increases the quality of life (Spertus et al., 2001). In addition, TMLR is being used in conjunction with CABG. Together, these procedures appear to provide results superior to CABG alone (Frazier et al., 2004).

Heart Attack Victims of coronary artery disease are often unaware that the arteries supplying their heart with blood have become blocked. They may have no signs or symptoms of CAD or may not notice any. For this reason, one-third to one-half of persons with CAD are stricken suddenly and unexpectedly with a **heart attack**, which health care practitioners call a *myocardial infarction (MI)*. Myocardial simply means heart (*cardium*) muscle (*myo-*). An infarction is an area of heart muscle that dies because it does not receive enough oxygen due to insufficient blood. As heart muscle dies, it may trigger abnormal electrical activity that causes the ventricles to beat irregularly. Abnormal heartbeats are called **arrhythmias**. Heart failure, cardiac arrest, and death may occur during ventricular arrhythmia.

Heart failure is sometimes called *congestive* heart failure because the veins bringing blood to the heart become congested, or overfilled, with blood when the heart cannot pump effectively. Heart failure (ineffective pumping) may be the result of all forms of cardiac disease, including CAD, structural heart defects, and rheumatic heart disease, and may also be a chronic condition, resulting in shortness of breath, retention of fluid, congestion of the lungs, and fatigue. A person experiencing severe cardiac failure may be a candidate for a heart transplant or the implantation of a left ventricular assist device (which has replaced the artificial heart) while waiting for a donor heart. The pump is implanted in the abdomen and is connected to the main pumping chamber of the heart, the left ventricle. The power source for the pump is located outside of the patient's body on a rolling cart, or is a portable battery that hangs by a strap from the shoulder.

Sudden cardiac death (cardiac arrest) may also occur as a result of a heart attack. During cardiac arrest, the heart suddenly stops beating. Getting immediate medical care is crucial in such a situation because the heart must be *defibrillated* (given electric shock) within a few minutes of its stopping to cause it to begin beating again and avoid heart, lung, kidney, and brain damage and to avoid death. Sudden cardiac death is the result of an unresuscitated cardiac arrest.

About 335,000 persons in the United States die each year from sudden cardiac death (AHA, 2005b). The average age for sudden cardiac death in the United States is 60 years. Eighty percent of the time the underlying cause of cardiac arrest is coronary artery disease. The other 20% of cases are due to a variety of other

stenting the implantation of a spring-like mesh device within an artery to cover compressed plaque, support the artery, and smooth the artery wall.

coronary artery bypass graft surgery (CABG) a surgical procedure in which healthy blood vessels are used to redirect blood flow around blocked vessels of the heart.

heart attack myocardial infarction (MI); an area of heart muscle that dies because it does not receive enough oxygen due to insufficient blood.

arrhythmias (uh-RITH-me-uhs) abnormal heartbeats.

heart failure ineffective pumping of the heart, which results in the overfilling of the veins that bring blood to the heart.

sudden cardiac death (cardiac arrest) cessation of the heartbeat.

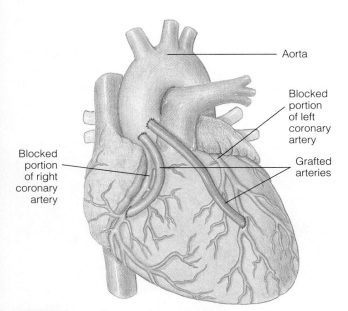

Figure 12-8 **Vessel Position in a Coronary Artery Bypass Graft.** In a coronary artery bypass graft, blood vessels taken from another part of the body are grafted to the aorta, the large artery emerging from the heart. The other ends of these vessels are grafted to the coronary arteries (those that serve the heart) beyond the area of blockage.

Aorta

Blocked portion of left coronary artery

Grafted arteries

Blocked portion of right coronary artery

Figure 12-9   A Heart Attack Prematurely Ended the Life of Former All-Star Third Basemen Ken Caminiti. Caminiti fought drug and alcohol problems for much of his adult life. The drugs he took are thought to have weakened his heart; he died of a heart attack at age 41 in October 2004.

stroke
a brain injury that occurs when arteries that supply the brain become blocked and prevent blood flow, or become damaged and leak blood onto or into the brain.

cerebral thrombosis
a stroke due to a stationary blood clot.

conditions such as an inflammation of the heart caused by infection, rheumatic fever, or medications; heart muscle disorders having unknown causes; congenital heart defects; and drug abuse (Figure 12-9). (Rheumatic fever is a disorder that sometimes occurs as a result of strep throat. It affects the heart.) One of these conditions is often the reason a young, physically fit person such as an athlete dies suddenly on the basketball court, track, or skating rink.

Learn the warning signs of a heart attack and what to do if you or someone you are with experiences them (see the Managing Your Health feature on page 323). You can distinguish a heart attack from angina by the severity of the pain: Heart attack pain is much more severe and lasts longer than that of angina. The pain of a heart attack is usually described as pressure (heaviness), burning, aching, and tightness, which is felt in the same locations as angina pain. The person suffering a heart attack may also experience shortness of breath, profuse sweating, weakness, anxiety, or nausea.

If you experience some or all of these signs and symptoms or are with someone who does, obtain emergency medical care *immediately*. Many heart attack victims die because they do not seek medical attention quickly, denying that they are having a heart attack. Today, 35% of people who suffer an MI die before they reach the emergency room. However, if you call for help quickly, an emergency response team trained to provide prompt medical care can keep a heart attack victim alive and help reduce damage to the heart while transporting him or her to the hospital.

Most heart attacks are results of coronary artery thrombosis. Blood clots often form suddenly when the plaque in an artery breaks apart and blood platelets clump at that site (Figure 12-10). Therefore, in the emergency room, heart attack patients are quickly given clot-dissolving drugs intravenously.

Most patients who survive a heart attack do not experience complications after the attack if they receive appropriate medical treatment. Some may not even have detectable heart abnormalities if their MI involved only a small portion of the heart muscle. Unfortunately, some patients do experience life-threatening complications. If a substantial portion of the heart was involved, the MI victim may develop cardiogenic shock, in which the left ventricle of the heart does not pump sufficient blood to sustain the body. Although physicians can treat this condition with angioplasty or surgery, cardiogenic shock is fatal 50% to 80% of the time (Krost, 2004).

After an MI, the physician evaluates the health of the patient's heart. Using measurements of enzymes released from the heart and techniques to visualize the heart and blood vessels, such as an angiogram or MRI, the physician assesses cell damage and ventricular function (the ability of the heart to pump blood to the body) to select a patient's post-MI therapy. Such therapy may include surgical procedures, medications, and lifestyle changes.

Figure 12-10   An Occluded (Blocked) Vessel. This coronary artery is totally blocked with plaque and a blood clot (dark area).

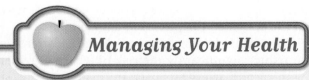

Managing Your Health

Heart Attack Symptoms: What to Do in an Emergency

IF YOU THINK YOU ARE HAVING A HEART ATTACK, CALL YOUR EMERGENCY MEDICAL SYSTEM IMMEDIATELY.

Common or "classic" signs of heart attack
- Uncomfortable pressure, fullness, squeezing, or pain in the center of the chest that lasts more than a few minutes, or goes away and comes back
- Pain that spreads to the shoulders, neck, or arms
- Chest discomfort with light-headedness, fainting, sweating, nausea, or shortness of breath

Less common warning signs of heart attack
- Atypical chest pain, stomach, or abdominal pain
- Nausea or dizziness (without chest pain)
- Shortness of breath and difficulty breathing (without chest pain)
- Unexplained anxiety, weakness, or fatigue
- Palpitations, cold sweat, or paleness

Not all of these signs occur in every heart attack. Sometimes they go away and return. If some occur, get help fast. IF YOU NOTICE ONE OR MORE OF THESE SIGNS IN ANOTHER PERSON (OR YOU HAVE THEM YOURSELF),

DON'T WAIT. CALL 911 OR YOUR EMERGENCY MEDICAL SERVICES AND GET TO A HOSPITAL RIGHT AWAY!

Be prepared
- Keep a list of emergency rescue service numbers next to the telephone and in your pocket, wallet, or purse.
- Find out which area hospitals have 24-hour emergency cardiovascular care.
- Know (in advance) which hospital or medical facility is nearest your home or office.

Take action
- If you have heart attack symptoms that last more than a few minutes, don't delay! Immediately call 911 or the EMS number so an ambulance (ideally with advanced life support) can quickly be sent for you.
- If ambulance service isn't available in your area, immediately have someone drive you to the nearest hospital emergency room (or another facility offering 24-hour life support).
- If you're with someone who may be having heart attack symptoms, immediately call 911 or the EMS. Expect the person to protest—denial is common. Don't take "no" for an answer. Insist on taking prompt action.
- Give CPR (mouth-to-mouth breathing and chest compression) if it's needed and you're properly trained.

Stroke

A **stroke** occurs when arteries that supply the brain with blood become blocked, preventing blood flow. The primary cause of stroke is the same as that for heart attacks or angina pectoris: atherosclerosis—the buildup of plaque or a blood clot that blocks arteries bringing blood to the organ. Blood clots are a common cause of a stroke. If the stroke is due to a stationary clot, the condition is called a **cerebral thrombosis**. If the blood clot was formed elsewhere and becomes lodged in a cerebral artery, blocking flow, it is called a **cerebral embolism**.

A stroke may also occur if an artery supplying the brain bursts. This situation is called a **cerebral hemorrhage** and may occur when atherosclerosis and high blood pressure are present. Cerebral hemorrhage may also occur from a head injury or from a burst **aneurysm** (a swollen, weakened blood vessel).

During a stroke, the brain cells normally supplied by the blocked or burst vessel do not receive oxygen.

Brain cells, like heart cells, die when they do not receive the oxygen they need. A cerebral hemorrhage affects the brain in an additional way: Pressure builds in the brain due to blood that has leaked out of the burst vessel. When this blood clots, it can damage brain tissue, causing physical disability.

The signs and symptoms of a stroke vary (Table 12-1), depending on the location of the damage. In most cases, one side of the body becomes weak, numb, or paralyzed.

One group at highest risk for a stroke is people with **atrial fibrillation**. Atrial fibrillation is a type of arrhythmia. During atrial fibrillation, the upper chambers of the heart contract with no set pattern, which upsets the normal rhythm of the heartbeat. This arrhythmia can result in the formation of floating

cerebral embolism a stroke due to a floating blood clot that becomes lodged in a cerebral artery, blocking blood flow.

cerebral hemorrhage (HEM-ah-rij) a stroke due to a burst artery that supplies the brain.

aneurysm (AN-you-rizm) a swollen, weakened blood vessel.

atrial fibrillation (fih-brih-LAY-shun) a type of arrhythmia in which the upper chambers of the heart contract with no set pattern.

Table 12-1	Signs of Stroke

Some or all of these signs accompany a stroke

Weakness, numbness, or paralysis on one side of the body

Loss or dimming of vision, particularly in one eye

Loss of speech, or difficulty speaking or understanding speech

Sudden, severe headache

Sudden dizziness, unsteadiness, or episodes of falling

blood clots (emboli) that can travel to the brain, block a blood vessel, and result in a stroke.

More than 1 million Americans have atrial fibrillation. Its incidence increases with age because its primary underlying causes, hypertension and coronary artery disease, also increase with age.

Another group at high risk for strokes is persons with *stenosis* (narrowing) of one or both of the carotid arteries. The right and left carotid arteries branch off major vessels leaving the heart and bring blood up the neck to the brain (see Figure 12-1). Physicians diagnose carotid artery stenosis by using ultrasound (a tech-

nique that uses sound waves to visualize soft tissues of the body; see Chapter 5) or angiography.

Physicians often recommend *carotid endarterectomy* to reduce significantly the risk of stroke in patients with carotid artery stenosis. In this procedure, surgeons remove the inner lining of the partially blocked carotid artery along with the plaque. Also, physicians may prescribe long-term aspirin therapy or anticoagulant drugs for treatment of either carotid artery stenosis or atrial fibrillation.

In the hospital, physicians usually perform computed tomography (CT) scans (detailed x rays of cross-sectional slices of body structures) or MRI scans of the brain of the stroke victim to confirm the diagnosis and determine the location and extent of injury (Figure 12-11). Until recently, no good treatment for stroke existed. The first drug that has shown promising results is a clot-dissolving drug called tissue plasminogen activator (tPA). If given within 3 hours of a stroke's onset, it raises the chances that no permanent brain damage will occur (Felberg et al., 2002). Poststroke therapy focuses on helping patients redevelop motor skills that may have been lost due to damage to part of the brain.

Just as heart attacks may be preceded by smaller angina attacks, major strokes may be preceded by minor strokes called **transient ischemic attacks (TIAs)**. Ischemic attacks are similar to strokes, usually cause no permanent damage, and have signs that last only a short time. A TIA is a serious warning that a stroke may occur within weeks or months. Persons experiencing a TIA should see their physicians immediately. Often, blood-thinning drugs such as aspirin are prescribed to lessen the possibility of a stroke.

Figure 12-11 **CT Scan of a Stroke Victim.** The darkened area on the left side of the brain scan reveals dead tissue due to a lack of oxygen during a stroke.

Healthy Living Practices

- Any person who experiences chest pain, especially pain beneath the breastbone that extends to the neck, shoulders, and/or arms, should seek medical attention immediately.
- Any person experiencing weakness, numbness, or paralysis on one side of the body; loss or dimming of vision; loss of speech, or difficulty speaking or understanding speech; a sudden, severe headache; or sudden dizziness or unsteadiness should seek medical attention immediately.

Risk Factors for Cardiovascular Disease

Medical researchers have identified several risk factors for cardiovascular disease, traits that have been shown to be associated with the incidence of CVD. In general, people with more than one of these traits, which are listed in Table 12-2, have a greater probability of developing atherosclerosis and suffering a heart attack or stroke than people with one or none of these risk factors. Many of these risk factors are modifiable. In other words, people can often reduce their risk of cardiovascular disease by changing one or more health-related behaviors.

The major risk factors for the development of CVD are male gender (the average man with CAD has his first heart attack in his mid-50s; the average woman with CAD in her mid-60s), increasing age (the incidence of coronary artery disease rises in both men and women with each decade from age 40 to age 79), family history of cardiovascular disease, cigarette smoking, obesity, hypertension, elevated blood cholesterol levels, and lack of physical activity. All these risk factors are important in the development of CAD. However, hypertension is the most important risk factor for stroke; high blood cholesterol levels play only a small role in the development of this disease.

Family History

A family history of atherosclerosis, stroke, or coronary artery disease indicates a genetic predisposition to these conditions or reflects similar diets, stresses, and lifestyles among family members. A person with a family history of premature CAD is twice as likely to suffer a heart attack as a person with no family history. A history of premature atherosclerosis (MI or sudden death before 55 years of age in the father or other male first-degree relative, or before 65 years of age in the mother or other female first-degree relative) is more meaningful than having relatives who developed atherosclerosis in the elderly years. The genetic effect decreases at older ages. Unfortunately, you cannot change your family history, but you can monitor other factors to reduce your risk in other ways.

Elevated Blood Cholesterol

Another major risk factor in the development of atherosclerosis, coronary artery disease, and stroke is elevated blood cholesterol levels (also called serum cholesterol). The American Heart Association states that the desirable range of total blood cholesterol is

Table 12-2	Risk Factors for Cardiovascular Disease

Cigarette smoking

Diabetes mellitus

Blood cholesterol above 200 mg/dl

A ratio of total cholesterol to high-density lipoprotein (HDL) cholesterol above 5:1 (optimum ratio is 3.5:1)

High levels of low-density lipoprotein (LDL) cholesterol

Physical inactivity

Family history of cardiovascular disease

Obesity

Uncontrolled, persistent high blood pressure

Heavy alcohol use

Gender (women are at lower risk of heart attack until menopause)

Age (risk increases with age)

Anxiety disorders (increased risk of fatal heart attack in men)

Elevated C-reactive protein*

*Elevated C-reactive protein is an indicator of inflammation and is not specific to CAD.

less than 200 milligrams per deciliter (200 mg/dl). Only 49.3% of American adults have total blood cholesterol levels within this range. The borderline high range is 200 to 239 mg/dl, a category encompassing 32.4% of American adults. The high range is 240 mg/dl and higher, a category that includes 18.3% of adult Americans (Table 12-3); (AHA, 2005b).

What is cholesterol? This substance is a *steroid*, a type of lipid. The most abundant steroid in the human body, cholesterol is used to make the sex hormones and composes part of the membranes of the body's cells. We take in cholesterol in most animal foods, such as egg yolks, fatty meats, and butter, but our bodies also make this chemical.

The blood levels of lipid-carrying molecules called lipoproteins are also critical to cardiovascular health. The major lipoproteins are **high-density lipoproteins (HDL)** and **low-density lipoproteins (LDL)**. HDL carries cholesterol from the cells and to the liver for removal from the body. LDL carries cholesterol to the cells, including the cells that line the blood vessel walls. You may have heard these molecules referred to as "good" cholesterol and "bad" cholesterol, respectively.

transient ischemic attacks (TIAs) (is-KI-mik) minor strokes that usually cause no permanent damage and have signs that last for only a short time.

high-density lipoproteins (HDL) (LIP-oh-PRO-tea-in) "good" cholesterol that carries cholesterol from the cells and to the liver for removal from the body.

low-density lipoproteins (LDL) "bad" cholesterol that carries cholesterol to the cells, including the cells that line the blood vessel walls.

Classification of LDL, Total, and HDL Cholesterol (mg/dl)

LDL cholesterol*

<100	Optimal
100–129	Near or above optimal
130–159	Borderline high
160–189	High
≥190	Very high

Total cholesterol

<200	Desirable
200–239	Borderline high
≥240	High

HDL cholesterol

<40	Low
≥60	High

*In 2004, the Adult Treatment Panel III issued a recommendation for people at highest risk for CHD (smokers with heart disease or patients whose blood pressure is not well controlled, for example) to lower LDL cholesterol to 70.
Source: Expert Panel on Detection, Evaluation, and Treatment of High Blood Cholesterol in Adults. (2001). Executive summary of the third report of the National Cholesterol Education Program (NCEP) expert panel on detection, evaluation, and treatment of high blood cholesterol in adults (Adult Treatment Panel III). *Journal of the American Medical Association, 285*:2486–2497.
Grundy, S. M., Cleeman, J. I., Merz, N. B., Brewer, H. B. Jr., Clark, L. T., Hunninghake, D. B., Pasternak, R. C., Smith, S. C., & Stone, N. J. (2004). Implications of recent clinical trials for the National Cholesterol Education Program Adult Treatment Panel III Guidelines. *Circulation, 110*:227–239.

It is firmly established that the level of bad cholesterol, or LDL, is of major importance in the development of atherosclerosis and coronary artery disease (Expert Panel, 2001). As the level of LDL rises, the risk of coronary artery disease and atherosclerosis rises because LDL is related to the formation and growth of plaques.

The level of good cholesterol, or HDL, is very important too. As the level of HDL rises, the risk of coronary artery disease and atherosclerosis falls. (Table 12-3 lists the classification levels for HDL and LDL.) High HDL levels are the key to why premenopausal women, in general, do not experience heart attacks at as young an age as men; the female sex hormone estrogen raises women's HDL levels by about 20%. Results of research show that postmenopausal women who take 1 gram of calcium daily increase their HDL levels by 7% (Reid et al., 2002). As noted in Table 12-3, desirable levels of HDL cholesterol are above 40 mg/dl.

The protective mechanism of HDL is not fully understood at this time. A primary component of HDL called apolipoprotein A-I (apoA-I) has been shown to reverse atherosclerosis and is therefore a potentially powerful treatment for vascular diseases. The Diversity in Health essay on page 327 describes how a mutant form of this cholesterol-lowering protein found in a certain Italian family (apoA-I [Milano]) protects them against vascular disease. ApoA-1 (Milano) has a more effective cholesterol-removing function than apoA-1 and may therefore prove to be a more effective treatment (Chiesa & Sartori, 2003).

Triglycerides, which are plasma lipids different from cholesterol, are also important in cardiovascular health. When the body does not immediately use all the nutrients consumed, it converts them to triglycerides and transports them to fat cells for storage. Excess triglycerides in the plasma are linked to CAD in some people. Additionally, researchers have linked high levels of triglycerides to an increased risk of stroke (Tanne et al., 2001). A normal, fasting triglyceride level is less than 150 mg/dl.

Cigarette Smoking

Smoking cigarettes significantly increases the risk of heart attack and stroke. Cigarette smokers are more than five times as likely to develop cardiovascular disease than are nonsmokers. In addition, smoking interacts with other risk factors, multiplying its negative health effects. Smoking is directly responsible for as many as 20% of deaths from cardiovascular diseases (AHA, 2002). Even more alarming is that cigarette smoking is directly responsible for the majority of heart disease in women under the age of 50 (U.S. Department of Health and Human Services [USDHHS], 2001). These figures show that premenopausal women, who are generally protected from heart attacks by estrogen, raise their risk of heart disease significantly when they smoke.

Research results show that cigarette smokers tend to have reduced HDL levels, increased LDL levels, and increased levels of blood clotting factors (Nakanishi et al., 2000; Imamura et al., 2001; USDHHS, 2004b). In addition, evidence suggests that compounds in cigarette smoke enter the bloodstream and may damage blood vessel linings directly, leading to the formation of plaques (USDHHS, 2004b). Chewing tobacco is a significant CVD risk factor also, but cigar and pipe smoking appear to be less important because cigar and pipe smokers are less likely than cigarette smokers to inhale the smoke (AHA, 2005a).

Passive smoking, breathing in other people's smoke, has also been identified as an important risk factor for cardiovascular disease. The AHA estimates that approximately 40,000 people die each year from heart and blood vessel disease caused by passive smoking (AHA, 2005a). Results of research show a harmful effect of passive smoking on the circulation of blood within the heart tissue itself (Otsuka et al., 2001).

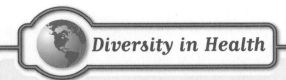

The Italian Gene: A Hope for Reversing Atherosclerosis?

The University of Milan's Dr. Cesare Sirtori could hardly believe it: Thirty-eight members of one Italian family had no atherosclerosis. If that was not surprising enough, many of them smoked cigarettes and ate high amounts of fat in their diets. What was protecting them from developing plaques in their blood vessels? The answer to that question is a mutation in the gene that directs the production of a cholesterol-lowering protein.

We all have this cholesterol-lowering protein in our bodies: apolipoprotein A-I (apoA-I). ApoA-I is a primary component of high-density lipoprotein (HDL), so-called good cholesterol. HDL helps bring excess cholesterol to the liver for transport out of the body. (Researchers do not fully understand the exact mechanism of this action.) In women, estrogen increases the body's production of apoA-I, and is thought to be one reason that premenopausal women have a greater protection than men of the same age from the development of atherosclerosis and heart attacks.

Apolipoprotein A-I (Milano) (apoA-IM) is a mutant apoA-I protein produced by the mutated Italian gene. The change in the molecular structure of apoA-IM from the nonmutant form makes this HDL molecule more stable and alters its properties so that it works even better than its normal counterpart. Those who carry the apoA-IM gene—the members of the Italian family that Sirtori studied—are protected against vascular disease.

Researchers have been able to make apoA-IM in the laboratory. They have used this synthetic molecule in animal models to study its potential as a treatment to reverse atherosclerosis and cardiovascular disease. Results showed a rapid regression of atherosclerosis in the treated animals. Similar studies have been performed with humans and have shown similar results. Scientists are currently conducting larger clinical trials. If successful, scientists and generations of one Italian family will have made a medical breakthrough in slowing the death rate from the United States' number one killer.

Sirtori, C. R., Calabresi, L., & Franceschini, G. (1999). Recombinant apolipoproteins for the treatment of vascular diseases. *Atherosclerosis, 142*:29–40.

Nissen, S. E., Tsunoda, T., Tuzcu, E. M., Schoenhagen, P., Cooper, C. J., Yasin, M., Eaton, G. M., Lauer, M. A., Sheldon, W. S., Grines, C. L., Halpern, S., Crone, T., Blankenship, J. C., & Kerensky, R. (2003). Effect of recombinant ApoA-1 Milano on coronary atherosclerosis in patients with acute coronary syndromes: A randomized controlled trial. *Journal of the American Medical Association, 290*:2292–2300.

High Blood Pressure

Blood pressure becomes elevated during periods of excitement or exertion; however, in healthy individuals it returns to normal levels when the activity stops. **Hypertension**, persistently high arterial blood pressure, is a major risk factor for heart attack and the most important risk factor for stroke. Data show that 90% of middle-aged and older Americans are likely to develop hypertension over their remaining lifetimes (Vasan et al., 2002).

The cause of most cases of high blood pressure is unknown. It has been shown, however, that hypertension may have a genetic link; it runs in families. There are also racial genetic links in hypertension. African Americans and Latinos are more likely to have hypertension than whites and, as a result, suffer strokes at an earlier age and with greater severity. Nongenetic, modifiable factors that contribute to hypertension are obesity, lack of physical activity, cigarette smoking, stress, and eating excessive amounts of salt. Other identifiable causes of hypertension include sleep apnea, drugs, chronic kidney disease, and thyroid or parathyroid disease (Chobanian et al., 2003).

You may know your blood pressure reading, such as 120/75 mm Hg (millimeters of mercury). The first (higher) number is the **systolic pressure**, which is the pressure exerted by the blood on the artery walls when the left ventricle contracts. The second (lower) number is the **diastolic pressure**, which is the pressure exerted by the blood on the artery walls when the left ventricle relaxes. The units, mm Hg, refer to the force

hypertension persistently high arterial blood pressure.

systolic pressure (sis-TOL-ik) the higher number in the blood pressure reading, which is the pressure exerted by the blood on the artery walls when the left ventricle contracts.

diastolic pressure (DIE-as-TOL-ik) the lower number in the blood pressure reading, which is the pressure exerted by the blood on the artery walls when the left ventricle relaxes.

needed to push a column of mercury to a particular height, such as 120 mm or 75 mm. The normal blood pressure level for people over 18 is less than 120/80 mm Hg. *Prehypertension* is indicated by a systolic blood pressure between 120 and 139 mm Hg, or a diastolic pressure between 80 and 89 mm Hg. *Stage 1 hypertension* is indicated by a systolic reading between 140 and 159, or a diastolic reading of 90 to 99. *Stage 2 hypertension* is indicated by a systolic reading of 160 or more, or a diastolic reading of 100 or more (Chobanian et al., 2003).

Persistently high arterial blood pressure contributes to the development of atherosclerosis in two ways. First, high blood pressure may injure the lining of artery walls, triggering plaque formation. In addition, the increased pressure enhances the amount of lipid added to plaques, especially if serum LDL cholesterol levels are elevated.

Physical Inactivity

Within the past two decades, physical inactivity has been shown to be a major risk factor for developing cardiovascular disease. Physically inactive people are about twice as likely as active people to develop coronary artery disease.

The 1996 Surgeon General's report on physical activity and health recommended that persons of all ages obtain "a minimum of 30 minutes of physical activity of moderate intensity (e.g., brisk walking) on most, if not all, days of the week" (USDHHS, 1996). However, as a group, Americans are relatively sedentary; more than 50% of American adults do not get enough physical activity to provide health benefits, and 26% are not active at all during leisure time (USDHHS, 2004a).

In addition to its direct cardiovascular benefits, routine exercise helps alleviate stress, reduce body weight, and control diabetes—other CVD risk factors. (Chapter 11 discusses the importance of a physically active lifestyle to health.)

Obesity

Most medical researchers agree that obesity increases the risk of cardiovascular disease. If you are obese, you nearly double your risk of CAD. Being mildly overweight also increases your risk. Studies show a strong positive association between weight and heart disease in both men and women. Are you within the desirable weight range for your age and height? Do you have a body mass index (BMI) of less than 25? See Chapter 10 for an explanation of BMI and for a BMI graph.

Diabetes Mellitus

Diabetes mellitus is a group of diseases in which glucose is not metabolized properly. Affected individuals are at a higher risk of developing cardiovascular disease because of their elevated blood glucose levels, which damage heart muscle, small coronary vessels, and major arteries. Therefore, atherosclerosis occurs more frequently and at an earlier age in diabetic patients, particularly women. Unfortunately, people with diabetes mellitus are about five times as likely to develop cardiovascular disease as are persons without this disease.

Anxiety

As mentioned previously, stress can result in spasms of the coronary arteries, which can contribute to angina attacks. In addition, research studies link anxiety disorders (such as phobias and panic disorders; see Chapter 2) to an increased risk of fatal CAD and particularly to sudden, fatal heart attacks in men (Jiang et al., 1996; Harter et al., 2003; Katerndahl, 2004). Persons with anxiety disorders are from two to six times as likely to die from a heart attack as persons without anxiety disorders. Current studies are investigating the impact of stress on cardiovascular health in women.

Elevated C-Reactive Protein

Results of recent research show that elevated blood levels of C-reactive protein (CRP) can be a positive risk factor for coronary artery disease (Pai et al., 2004). C-reactive protein is produced by the liver during acute inflammation. Inflammation may be present at the site of plaques in CAD, but it may also be present in other diseases such as rheumatoid arthritis. Therefore, it is not a test specific to CAD. In addition, a low CRP value does not mean that inflammation is absent.

Healthy Living Practices

- If any of your male first-degree relatives had a heart attack before age 55, or female first-degree relatives before age 65, you may be genetically predisposed to heart disease. See your health care practitioner for an evaluation and advice.
- If you are a healthy adult, you should have your serum cholesterol level and HDL level measured once every 5 years.

Maintaining Cardiovascular Health

Table 12-4 presents a summary of recommendations to help you maintain cardiovascular health and lower your risk of cardiovascular disease. As you can see, there are many factors to consider. You cannot control heredity, gender, and age. However, you can stop smoking, exercise regularly, lose weight, eat less fat, learn to relax, and reduce your salt intake. Results of a large-scale study, which included more than 350,000 participants, reconfirm that making these lifestyle changes enhances cardiovascular health and the life span. In the study, persons with favorable levels of cholesterol and blood pressure who did not smoke and did not have diabetes or heart abnormalities lived from 5.8 to 9.5 years longer than those who had elevated cholesterol or blood pressure levels, or smoked (Stampfer et al., 1999).

Emotional stress contributes to hypertension and the incidence of angina attacks (Carels et al., 1999). Chapter 3, "Stress and Its Management," describes stress management skills and coping strategies that may help you lower your risk of stress-related hypertension and angina.

If you have diabetes mellitus, work with your health care practitioner to develop a diabetes management plan that is specific for you; diabetics who conscientiously manage their disease and their blood sugar level lower their risk of cardiovascular disease.

Getting regular medical checkups (the frequency of which should be determined by your health care practitioner) can help you assess your CVD risk factors. Your health care practitioner may recommend other steps to lower CVD risks. The following sections describe actions that health care practitioners often recommend for reducing CVD risk and maintaining cardiovascular health.

Smoking Cessation

If you smoke, stop now. If you do not smoke, avoid breathing in secondhand (other people's) smoke. Approximately 115,000 cardiovascular deaths could be avoided each year if people did not smoke cigarettes. Studies suggest that the smoker who quits cuts his or her elevated risk of CAD in half only 1 year after quitting. Within 15 years, the elevated risk of a former smoker declines to the level of a nonsmoker (AHA, 2005b). The risk of stroke reverts to that of nonsmokers 2 to 5 years after quitting (National Stroke Association, 1999). The more cigarettes a person smokes and the earlier a person started to smoke are factors that lengthen recovery time. In addition, the risk of cardiovascular disease increases as the number of cigarettes smoked increases. Therefore, smoke fewer

Table 12-4	How to Reduce Your Risk of Cardiovascular Disease

Get regular medical checkups.

Do not smoke cigarettes.

Manage diabetes mellitus properly.

Exercise regularly.

Maintain an intake of dietary cholesterol of less than 300 mg per day.

Maintain an intake of dietary fat of less than 30% of daily calories.

Maintain an intake of saturated fats of less than 10% of daily calories.

Eat foods rich in soluble fiber, such as fruits, beans, and oats.

Eat a diet rich in fruits, vegetables, and low-fat dairy products.

Maintain an appropriate weight for your height.

Limit alcohol consumption to 1 drink per day for women and 2 drinks per day for men.

Maintain salt intake at less than $1\frac{1}{4}$ teaspoons or 2,400 mg of sodium per day.

Reduce your stress level.

cigarettes if you cannot quit. Smoking "low-yield" (low tar and nicotine) cigarettes does not appear to reduce CVD risk.

Weight Control

If your BMI is 25 or more, then losing weight will reduce your risk of cardiovascular disease. Chapter 10, "Body Weight and Its Management," presents background and suggestions for weight management. In general, a regular exercise program coupled with a low-calorie diet will reduce body fat. Weight reduction lowers total blood cholesterol levels, raises HDL levels, and lowers LDL levels. It also helps maintain proper blood glucose levels.

Exercise

In the late 1980s, a review of 43 studies about the relationship between physical activity and the risk of CAD and atherosclerosis was conducted (Powell et al., 1987). Two-thirds of these studies documented a substantial inverse relationship between physical activity and risk for these two related diseases: As the level of physical activity rose, the risk of CAD and atherosclerosis declined and vice versa. These findings have been upheld by more recent studies (USDHHS, 2004a). Research results also show that exercise is associated with a decreased risk of stroke in men (Lee et al., 1999).

Exercise has been shown to lower blood pressure and boost HDL levels. The American Heart Association recommends that healthy people perform any moderate-to vigorous-intensity aerobic activity, such as brisk walking, hiking, stair-climbing, jogging, bicycling, and swimming, for at least 30 minutes on most days of the week at 50% to 75% of their maximum heart rate. (Aerobic activities are those that raise the heart rate for a sustained period of time.) The AHA notes that regular physical activity for longer periods or at greater

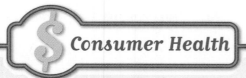

Consumer Health

Vitamin Pills for a Healthier Heart?

Vitamins A, C, E, B_6, B_{12}, folate, and the non-nutrient beta-carotene . . . what do they have to do with cardiovascular health? Should you be rushing to the store for vitamin supplements to keep your blood vessels healthy?

Vitamins play many roles in cardiovascular health. For example, our bodies use vitamins B_6, B_{12}, and folate in the metabolism of amino acids, including the essential amino acid methionine. In the process of metabolizing methionine, cells produce homocysteine (ho-mo-SIS-tih-een), another amino acid. High blood levels of this amino acid can damage artery walls and encourage the formation of blood clots and plaques. However, if the cells have enough folate, B_6, and B_{12}, then methionine is metabolized normally and the blood level of homocysteine does not rise.

Methionine intake also affects homocysteine levels. In general, the more methionine people eat, the higher their blood levels of homocysteine. Diets rich in animal protein contain high amounts of methionine and may elevate blood homocysteine levels. Conversely, diets rich in plant protein may lower homocysteine levels, because plant foods are relatively low in methionine yet rich in folate and vitamin B_6.

Other factors also influence homocysteine blood levels. Smoking cigarettes, drinking coffee, and a sedentary lifestyle are all associated with decreased B_6 activity, and therefore higher homocysteine levels. The use of oral contraceptives and hormone replacement therapy lower homocysteine blood levels in women. Homocysteine levels also depend on age, gender, kidney function, genetics, and general health.

So do you need to take vitamin pills to lower your blood homocysteine levels? The answer is not simple, and only your health care practitioner can tell you for sure. If you show evidence of B_6 or B_{12} deficiency (more likely in elderly than in younger populations) or evidence of folate deficiency (more likely in younger than in elderly populations), your health care practitioner may suggest testing. Also, if you are experiencing kidney failure, are on a special metabolic diet, have cancer, or have a strong family history of heart attack, stroke, or abnormal blood clotting, your physician may recommend that your homocysteine levels be checked. The determination of homocysteine levels is complex, and interpretation of the finding is not simple.

So what about vitamins A, C, E, and beta-carotene? (Beta-carotene is a yellow pigment in plants that the body converts to vitamin A.) As discussed in Chapter 9, vitamins E and C and beta-carotene are antioxidants, substances that can protect cells by preventing or reducing the formation of free radicals. Studies have consistently shown that the more antioxidants a population consumes in its food, the lower the rate of cardiovascular disease. But what about vitamin supplements? Randomized controlled trials of antioxidant supplementation show mixed results. In fact, supplementation with beta-carotene was found to increase lung cancer and coronary artery disease in smokers. However, recent research results suggest a reduced incidence of major CAD events at high supplemental vitamin C intakes. The risk reductions at high vitamin E intakes appear small.

So . . . should you take vitamin pills to reduce your risk of CVD? Only your physician can advise you properly, since the answer depends on the status of various facets of your health, family history, and lifestyle. The best advice at this time is to get your vitamins in the food you eat—be sure to have at least five servings of fruits and vegetables every day, including dark, leafy greens and members of the cabbage family. Consult your health care practitioner to determine if you might also need to take vitamin pills to have a healthier heart and blood vessels.

Sources: Knekt, P., Pereira, M. A., O'Reilly, E. J., Augustsson, K., Fraser, G. E., Goldbourt, U., Heitmann, B. L., Hallmans, G., Liu, S., Pietinen, P., Spiegelman, D., Stevens, J., Virtamo, J., Willett, W. C., Rimm, E. B., & Ascherio, A. (2004). Antioxidant vitamins and coronary heart disease risk: A pooled analysis of 9 cohorts. *American Journal of Clinical Nutrition, 80*:1508–1520.
Havranek, E. P. (1999). Primary prevention of CHD: Nine ways to reduce risk. *American Family Physician, 59*:1455–1463.
Kiningham, R. (1999). The value of antioxidant vitamin supplements. *American Family Physician, 60*:742–743.
Langman, L. J., & Cole, D. (1999). Homocysteine: Cholesterol of the 90s? *Clinica Chimica Acta, 286*:63–80.

intensity will likely provide greater health benefits. Even moderate-intensity activities, such as slow walking, gardening, housework, and recreational activities, can have some long-term health benefits when performed daily, and can help lower the risk of cardiovascular disease.

Lowering Blood Pressure

Nearly one of every three American adults has hypertension. In 90% to 95% of cases, hypertension can be controlled. Doing so reduces the risk of both stroke and heart attack. The American Heart Association recommends having your blood pressure checked every 2 years and more often if it is high.

To lower blood pressure, the AHA suggests decreasing sodium intake to a maximum of 2,400 mg per day, which is about 1 teaspoon of salt. Nutritionists suggest checking the amount of sodium that you consume in prepackaged, processed foods and not salting your food. The sodium in salt causes the body to retain fluids and may contribute to hypertension in some people.

Dietary factors in addition to sodium affect blood pressure. The DASH diet (Dietary Approaches to Stop Hypertension) has been shown to lower blood pressure in diverse subgroups of the U.S. population. This diet is low in total and saturated fat compared to a more typical U.S. diet, and is rich in fruits, vegetables, and low-fat dairy foods. Researchers also studied decreased sodium intake with both the DASH diet and the typical U.S. diet. Data show highly significant decreases in blood pressure with either diet. Researchers conclude that the DASH diet plus reduced sodium intake is effective in controlling blood pressure (Vollmer et al., 2001).

The blood pressure of overweight individuals often drops when they lose weight. If you are overweight and have high blood pressure, weight reduction is the most important action you can take to lower your blood pressure and risk of CVD. Regular aerobic exercise lowers blood pressure (Whelton et al., 2002) and will also help control weight. Reducing the intake of dietary saturated fat and cholesterol will promote overall cardiovascular health and will also help reduce caloric intake, which is important for weight control.

The heavy consumption of alcoholic beverages has also been shown to lead to high blood pressure, increasing the risk of heart attack, stroke, and death from CAD. Limiting consumption to 1 oz. of alcohol (ethanol) per day (two drinks or fewer) for men and 0.5 oz (one drink) for women may help lower blood pressure and may reduce your risk of cardiovascular disease. One ounce of ethanol is equivalent to 2 oz. of 100-proof whiskey, 8 to 10 oz. of wine (the alcohol content in wines varies), or two 12-oz. cans of beer.

If none of these lifestyle changes lowers the blood pressure sufficiently, hypertension can be treated with a wide array of antihypertensive drugs. These drugs are not suitable or appropriate for all hypertensive individuals, but may be essential therapy for many.

Reducing Blood Cholesterol

Pioneering experiments were conducted in the 1950s and 1960s regarding the effect of diet on serum cholesterol levels. These early experiments pointed out that, in general, animal fats raised the blood cholesterol level, and vegetable oils (with the exception of the tropical oils) lowered them. Therefore, dietary recommendations included eating less animal fat and eating more vegetable oils. Since that time, further experimentation has revealed that the cholesterol-lowering effects of vegetable oils were overestimated. In addition, eating certain types of margarine to reduce your intake of animal fat, cholesterol, and saturated fats from butter is not a good idea. Margarines contain trans fatty acids, compounds that may be associated with a risk of heart attack (Clifton et al., 2004; Ascherio et al., 1999). Trans fatty acids are formed as hydrogen atoms are added to the unsaturated fats in vegetable oil to harden it. Stick margarines contain more trans fatty acids than tub or liquid margarines.

In general, today's guidelines recommend diets low in total fat, saturated fat, and cholesterol to reduce the blood cholesterol level, raise the "good" cholesterol (HDL) level, and lower the "bad" cholesterol (LDL) level. Additionally, omega-3 fatty acids, which are found in certain fish such as salmon, tuna, cod, and sole, appear to lower the risk of CAD and stroke (Hu et al., 2002). The American Heart Association suggests that individuals should adjust their total fat intake to meet their caloric needs. People who are overweight or obese should limit their overall fat intake to less than 30% of their daily intake of calories. In addition, the AHA recommends that healthy Americans over age 2 should limit their saturated fat intake (primarily animal fats and tropical oils) to less than 10%. (Chapter 9 describes the types of fats in foods. Table 9-5 lists a variety of foods and their percentages of saturated fatty acids.)

To achieve a diet low in cholesterol, restrict your cholesterol intake to 300 mg per day. (One large egg, for example, has slightly over 200 mg, and a quarter-pound

Figure 12-12 **Foods High in Soluble Fiber.** Soluble fiber helps lower the cholesterol level by binding to cholesterol-containing compounds in the digestive system and carrying them out of the body. The foods shown here include wheat bread, oatmeal, broccoli, navel oranges, red kidney beans, avocado, pitted prunes, and canned beans.

cheeseburger has slightly over 100 mg. Table 9-6 lists a variety of foods and their cholesterol content.) Studies show that, on average, people can achieve a 10% reduction in cholesterol levels by following these dietary guidelines. Each 1% reduction in the blood cholesterol level reduces the risk of CAD by 2% to 3%, so a 10% reduction reduces your risk of CAD by 20% to 30%. If you are at high risk for cardiovascular disease, your physician will likely place you on a diet that has cholesterol and other fat intake recommendations different from those mentioned here, which are for the general population (Expert Panel, 2001).

Eating whole grains (Liu et al., 1999) and foods rich in soluble fiber (such as fruits, beans, oats, and barley) can help reduce your blood cholesterol level (Figure 12-12). Soluble fiber helps reduce blood cholesterol because it binds to cholesterol-containing compounds in the digestive system, carrying them out of the body. Research data indicate, however, that eating more than 35 g of dietary fiber a day may be unwise since fiber may bind to minerals in the diet also, removing them from the body. (Thirty-five grams of fiber is the equivalent of 14 apples, or 14 raw whole carrots, or nearly 2 cups of uncooked oats.)

If eating a heart-healthy diet and exercising regularly do not significantly reduce elevated blood cholesterol levels, cholesterol-lowering medications called "statins" are available by prescription. Some studies show that, on average, 20% reductions in the cholesterol level are achieved with drug therapy. Research results have shown that statins are safe, reduce CAD deaths, and appear to reduce the risk of stroke (Corsini, 2004; Ansell et al., 1999; Steinberg & Gotto, 1999).

Aspirin Therapy

A treatment to reduce the risk of cardiovascular disease that has gained attention in recent years is long-term use of low-dose aspirin. An analysis of research data revealed that the benefit of aspirin therapy increases with increasing cardiovascular risk (Hayden et al., 2002). Since aspirin can have damaging effects on the gastrointestinal system and reduces the blood's ability to clot, long-term aspirin therapy should be undertaken only on the advice of a physician.

Hormone Replacement Therapy

Until 2002, hormone replacement therapy was often recommended for the prevention of CVD in post-menopausal women. Hormone replacement therapy (HRT) is the use of estrogen plus progestin in women who no longer produce these hormones. Results of research from the Women's Health Initiative (WHI) study on the risks and benefits of HRT reversed this recommendation. The researchers concluded that estrogen plus progestin therapy should not be begun or continued in postmenopausal women for the prevention of CVD because it does not help prevent CVD or inhibit its progression in this population. Additionally, WHI researchers concluded that the overall health risks for serious diseases exceeded the benefits in healthy American postmenopausal women. The study did not include all diseases and conditions, such as gallbladder disease, diabetes, and cognitive function (Writing Group for the WHI Investigators, 2002). Therefore, before any woman chooses HRT, she should weigh the risks and benefits in her particular situation and consult her physician.

Healthy Living Practices

- One of the most important things you can do to lower your risk of coronary artery disease and stroke is to reduce your modifiable risk factors.

- If you smoke cigarettes, quitting will significantly reduce your risk of cardiovascular disease.

- Researchers estimate that you will reduce your risk of heart attack from 35% to 55% if you maintain a healthy body weight.

- You can lower your risk of heart attack 35% to 55% by maintaining an active lifestyle that includes regular aerobic exercise.

- To lower your blood pressure, engage in regular aerobic exercise, lose weight if you are overweight, limit your alcohol consumption to 1 oz. of ethanol per day for men and 0.5 oz. per day for women, and limit your daily sodium intake to 2,400 mg.

- To reduce your total cholesterol level, raise your HDL level, and lower your LDL level, eat no more than 30% of your daily intake of calories from fat and no more than 10% from saturated fat. Also, eat foods rich in soluble fiber, such as fruits, beans, and oats.

Across
THE LIFESPAN

Cardiovascular Health

The American Heart Association estimates that approximately 35,000 babies are born each year with a variety of heart and blood vessel structural abnormalities—about 35 types are recognized. Many congenital defects (those present at birth) can now be diagnosed before birth with the use of echocardiography, or ultrasound of the heart. Sound waves are directed through the heart of the fetus; as they pass through different types of tissues (such as heart muscle and blood), they are reflected, or echoed, producing an image of the movements of the heart structures. This technique can also be used with infants, children, and adults. Such early diagnostic techniques have helped surgeons correct infants' cardiovascular defects within the first few weeks of life. This approach helps avoid complications from cardiovascular defects in older children and adults. Presently about 1 million Americans have congenital heart defects.

Cardiovascular disease due to atherosclerosis is a process that has been shown to begin in childhood. Habits of diet and lifestyle develop at an early age and often continue into adulthood, affecting this disease process. Data from the Bogalusa Heart Study (Nicklas et al., 2001), a long-term study of CVD in the community of Bogalusa, Louisiana, show that the average diet of children and adolescents consists of 14% of their total daily calories from protein, 50% from carbohydrate, and 36% from fat. Such diets do not meet the recommendations of the American Heart Association and can lead to the development of atherosclerosis and obesity, both risk factors for coronary artery disease and stroke. It is estimated that more than one-third of American youths aged 19 and younger have blood cholesterol levels of 170 mg/dl or higher, which corresponds to 200 mg/dl in adults.

In the Bogalusa study, school breakfasts and lunches had a major impact on the diets of children, providing approximately half of the day's total caloric intake and about 49% of daily total fat intake—too high a proportion. Many school lunch programs have reduced their percentages of total fat, saturated fat, and sodium. In addition, several innovative "heart-healthy" school lunch programs such as Healthy Edge, Lunch Power, and Heart Smart have been developed in schools across the nation.

Until recently, medical experts used medication to treat elderly patients with high overall blood cholesterol levels. Data from current studies suggest that high cholesterol levels in the elderly do not place them at higher risk for heart attack or stroke. In fact, long-term low cholesterol levels may increase the risk of death in the elderly (Schatz et al., 2001). Nevertheless, research results show that it is important to lower elevated LDL cholesterol levels in the elderly to reduce their cardiovascular risk (Davidson et al., 2003).

The results of studies show that high blood pressure should be treated in all elderly patients because lower blood pressure in old age, as in middle age, is associated with better rates of survival (Hansson, 2001).

This article focuses on claims that manufacturers make on food labels. Explain why you think this article is a reliable or an unreliable source of information. Use the model for analyzing health information to guide your thinking; the main points of the model are noted below. The model is fully explained on pages 13–15.

1. Which statements are verifiable facts, and which are unverified statements or value claims?
2. What are the credentials of the author? Does his or her background and education qualify him or her as an expert in this area?
3. What might be the motives and biases of the author? State reasons for your answers.
4. Which information is relevant to the issue or main points of the article? Which information is irrelevant?
5. Is the source reliable? Does it have a reputation for publishing misinformation?
6. Does the article attack the credibility of conventional scientists or medical authorities?

Revealing *Trans* Fats

Scientific evidence shows that consumption of saturated fat, *trans* fat, and dietary cholesterol raises low-density lipoprotein (LDL), or "bad" cholesterol, levels, which increases the risk of coronary heart disease (CHD). According to the National Heart, Lung, and Blood Institute of the National Institutes of Health, more than 12.5 million Americans have CHD, and more than 500,000 die each year. That makes CHD one of the leading causes of death in the United States.

The Food and Drug Administration has required that saturated fat and dietary cholesterol be listed on food labels since 1993. Starting Jan. 1, 2006, listing of *trans* fat will be required as well. With *trans* fat added to the Nutrition Facts panel, you will know for the first time how much of all three—saturated fat, *trans* fat, and cholesterol—are in the foods you choose. Identifying saturated fat, *trans* fat, and cholesterol on the food label gives you information you need to make food choices that help reduce the risk of CHD. This revised label will be of particular interest to people concerned about high blood cholesterol and heart disease.

However, everyone should be aware of the risk posed by consuming too much saturated fat, *trans* fat, and cholesterol. But what is *trans* fat, and how can you limit the amount of this fat in your diet?

What Is *Trans* Fat?

Basically, *trans* fat is made when manufacturers add hydrogen to vegetable oil—a process called hydrogenation. Hydrogenation increases the shelf life and flavor stability of foods containing these fats.

Trans fat can be found in vegetable shortenings, some margarines, crackers, cookies, snack foods, and other foods made with or fried in partially hydrogenated oils. Unlike other fats, the majority of *trans* fat is formed when food manufacturers turn liquid oils into solid fats like shortening and hard margarine. A small amount of *trans* fat is found naturally, primarily in dairy products, some meat, and other animal-based foods.

Trans fat, like saturated fat and dietary cholesterol, raises the LDL cholesterol that increases your risk for CHD. Americans consume on average 4 to 5 times as much saturated fat as *trans* fat in their diets.

Although saturated fat is the main dietary culprit that raises LDL, *trans* fat and dietary cholesterol also contribute significantly.

Are All Fats the Same?

Simply put: No. Fat is a major source of energy for the body and aids in the absorption of vitamins A, D, E, and K and carotenoids. Both animal- and plant-derived food products contain fat, and when eaten in moderation, fat is important for proper growth, development, and maintenance of good health. As a food ingredient, fat provides taste, consistency, and stability and helps you feel full. In addition, parents should be aware that fats are an especially important source of calories and nutrients for infants and toddlers (up to 2 years of age), who have the highest energy needs per unit of body weight of any age group.

While unsaturated fats (monounsaturated and polyunsaturated) are beneficial when consumed in moderation, saturated and *trans* fats are not. Saturated fat and *trans* fat raise LDL cholesterol levels in the blood. Dietary cholesterol also contributes to heart disease. Therefore, it is advisable to choose foods low in saturated fat, *trans* fat, and cholesterol as part of a healthful diet.

What Can You Do About Saturated Fat, *Trans* Fat, and Cholesterol?

When comparing foods, look at the Nutrition Facts panel, and choose the food with the lower amounts of saturated fat, *trans* fat, and cholesterol. Health experts recommend that you keep your intake of saturated fat, *trans* fat, and cholesterol as low as possible while consuming a nutritionally adequate diet. However, these experts recognize that eliminating these three components entirely from your diet is not practical because they are unavoidable in ordinary diets.

Where Can You Find *Trans* Fat on the Food Label?

Although some food products already have *trans* fat on the label, food manufacturers have until January 2006 to list it on all their products.

You will find *trans* fat listed on the Nutrition Facts panel directly under the line for saturated fat.

How Do Your Choices Stack Up?

With the addition of *trans* fat to the Nutrition Facts panel, you can review your food choices and see how they stack up. The accompanying table illustrates total fat, saturated fat, *trans* fat, and cholesterol content per serving for selected food products.

Don't assume similar products are the same. Be sure to check the Nutrition Facts panel because even similar foods can vary in calories, ingredients, nutrients, and the size and number of servings in a package. Even if you continue to buy the same brand of a product, check the Nutrition Facts panel frequently because ingredients can change at any time.

Total Fat, Saturated Fat, *Trans* Fat, and Cholesterol Content Per Serving*

Product	Common Serving Size	Total Fat (g)	Sat. Fat (g)	%DV for Sat. Fat	*Trans* Fat (g)	Combined Sat. and *Trans* Fat (g)	Chol. (mg)	%DV for Chol.
French fried potatoes± (fast food)	Medium (147 g)	27	7	35%	8	15	0	0%
Butter**	1 tbsp	11	7	35%	0	7	30	10%
Margarine, stick†	1 tbsp	11	2	10%	3	5	0	0%
Margarine, tub†	1 tbsp	7	1	5%	0.5	1.5	0	0%
Mayonnaise†† (soybean oil)	1 tbsp	11	1.5	8%	0	1.5	5	2%
Shortening±	1 tbsp	13	3.5	18%	4	7.5	0	0%
Potato chips±	Small bag (42.5 g)	11	2	10%	3	5	0	0%
Milk, whole±	1 cup	7	4.5	23%	0	4.5	35	12%
Milk, skim†	1 cup	0	0	0%	0	0	5	2%
Doughnut±	1	18	4.5	23%	5	9.5	25	8%
Cookies± (cream filled)	3 (30 g)	6	1	5%	2	3	0	0%
Candy Bar±	1 (40 g)	10	4	20%	3	7	<5	1%
Cake, pound±	1 slice (80 g)	16	3.5	18%	4.5	8	0	0%

*Nutrient values rounded based on FDA's nutrition labeling regulations.
** Butter values from FDA Table of *Trans* Values, 1/30/95.
† Values derived from 2002 USDA National Nutrient Database for Standard Reference, Release 15.
†† Prerelease values derived from 2003 USDA National Nutrient Database for Standard Reference, Release 16.
± 1995 USDA Composition Data.

How Can You Use the Label to Make Heart-Healthy Food Choices?

The Nutrition Facts panel can help you choose foods lower in saturated fat, *trans* fat, and cholesterol. Compare similar foods and choose the food with the lower combined saturated and *trans* fats and the lower amount of cholesterol.

Although the updated Nutrition Facts panel will list the amount of *trans* fat in a product, it will not show a Percent Daily Value (%DV). While scientific reports have confirmed the relationship between *trans* fat and an increased risk of CHD, none has provided a reference value for *trans* fat or any other information that the FDA believes is sufficient to establish a Daily Value or a %DV.

There is, however, a %DV shown for saturated fat and cholesterol. To choose foods low in saturated fat and cholesterol, use the general rule of thumb that 5 percent of the Daily Value or less is low and 20 percent or more is high.

You can also use the %DV to make dietary trade-offs with other foods throughout the day. You don't have to give up a favorite food to eat a healthy diet. When a food you like is high in saturated fat or cholesterol, balance it with foods that are low in saturated fat and cholesterol at other times of the day.

Do Dietary Supplements Contain *Trans* Fat?

Would it surprise you to know that some dietary supplements contain *trans* fat from partially hydrogenated vegetable oil as well as saturated fat or cholesterol? It's true. As a result of the FDA's new label requirement, if a dietary supplement contains a reportable amount of *trans* or saturated fat, which is 0.5 gram or more, dietary supplement manufacturers must list the amounts on the Supplement Facts panel. Some dietary supplements that may contain saturated fat, *trans* fat, and cholesterol include energy and nutrition bars.

Fat Tips

Here are some practical tips you can use every day to keep your consumption of saturated fat, *trans* fat, and cholesterol low while consuming a nutritionally adequate diet.

- Check the Nutrition Facts panel to compare foods because the serving sizes are generally consistent in similar types of foods. Choose foods lower in saturated fat, *trans* fat, and cholesterol. For saturated fat and cholesterol, keep in mind that 5 percent of the Daily Value (%DV) or less is low and 20 percent or more is high. (There is no %DV for *trans* fat.)

- Choose alternative fats. Replace saturated and *trans* fats in your diet with monounsaturated and polyunsaturated fats. These fats do not raise LDL cholesterol levels and have health benefits when eaten in moderation. Sources of monounsaturated fats include olive and canola oils.

- Sources of polyunsaturated fats include soybean oil, corn oil, sunflower oil and foods like nuts and fish.

- Choose vegetable oils (except coconut and palm kernel oils) and soft margarines (liquid, tub, or spray) more often because the amounts of saturated fat, *trans* fat, and cholesterol are lower than the amounts in solid shortenings, hard margarines, and animal fats, including butter.

- Consider fish. Most fish are lower in saturated fat than meat. Some fish, such as mackerel, sardines, and salmon, contain omega-3 fatty acids, which are being studied to determine if they offer protection against heart disease.

- Choose lean meats, such as poultry without the skin and not fried, and lean beef and pork, not fried, with visible fat trimmed.

- Ask before you order when eating out. A good tip to remember is to ask which fats are being used in the preparation of your food when eating or ordering out.

- Watch calories. Don't be fooled! Fats are high in calories. All sources of fat contain 9 calories per gram, making fat the most concentrated source of calories. By comparison, carbohydrates and protein have only 4 calories per gram.

To keep your intake of saturated fat, *trans* fat, and cholesterol low:

- Look at the Nutrition Facts panel when comparing products. Choose foods low in the combined amount of saturated fat and *trans* fat and low in cholesterol as part of a nutritionally adequate diet.

- Substitute alternative fats that are higher in mono- and polyunsaturated fats like olive oil, canola oil, soybean oil, corn oil, and sunflower oil.

Highlights of the Final Rule on *Trans* Fat

- Manufacturers of conventional foods and some dietary supplements will be required to list *trans* fat on a separate line, immediately under saturated fat on the nutrition label.

- Food manufacturers have until Jan. 1, 2006, to list *trans* fat on the nutrition label. The phase-in period minimizes the need for multiple labeling changes, allows small businesses to use current label inventories, and provides economic savings.

- FDA's regulatory chemical definition for *trans* fatty acids is all unsaturated fatty acids that contain one or more isolated (i.e., nonconjugated) double bonds in a *trans* configuration. Under the agency's definition, conjugated linoleic acid would be excluded from the definition of *trans* fat.

- Dietary supplement manufacturers must also list *trans* fat on the Supplement Facts panel when their products contain reportable amounts (0.5 gram or more) of *trans* fat. Examples of dietary supplements with *trans* fat are energy and nutrition bars.

Source: Food and Drug Administration. (2003, September–October). *FDA Consumer*. Retrieved January 15, 2005, from http://www.fda.gov/fdac/features/2003/503_fats.html.

CHAPTER REVIEW

Summary

The leading cause of death in the United States is a noninfectious disease: coronary artery disease (CAD). In CAD, the arteries that supply blood to the heart become blocked, restricting blood flow. CAD is only one disease of the cardiovascular system; hypertension, stroke, and rheumatic heart disease are three other prominent cardiovascular diseases. Atherosclerosis is an important cardiovascular disease process that is an underlying cause of CAD and stroke.

The cardiovascular system includes the heart and blood vessels. The heart, a muscular fist-sized organ, pumps blood to the body. The blood performs many functions, such as bringing nutrients and oxygen to the tissues and removing wastes, including the waste gas carbon dioxide. Blood vessels called arteries bring blood away from the heart; veins return blood to the heart. Microscopic vessels called capillaries join the two and allow the exchange of nutrients, gases, and wastes at the tissues.

Fatty deposits develop in arteries as part of a disease called atherosclerosis. Atherosclerosis occurs most frequently in the arteries supplying blood to the heart, brain, and legs. In coronary artery disease, the coronary arteries, which supply the heart muscle with blood, become blocked by fatty deposits, a blood clot, or both. When the heart is deprived of the blood (and therefore the oxygen) that it needs, chest pain (angina pectoris) or a heart attack results. A physician usually performs diagnostic tests to assess the degree and location of blockage. Medication can help widen blood vessels and reduce symptoms.

During a heart attack, part of the heart muscle dies. As the muscle dies, it may trigger electrical activity that causes the ventricles to stop beating properly, possibly resulting in heart failure and death. A heart attack victim needs immediate medical care.

A stroke occurs when arteries that supply blood to the brain become blocked by fatty deposits or by a blood clot. A stroke may cause a loss or dimming of vision, difficulty in speaking or understanding speech, headache, dizziness, unsteadiness, and even death.

The major risk factors for developing cardiovascular disease are family history, elevated blood cholesterol, cigarette smoking, high blood pressure, physical inactivity, obesity, diabetes mellitus, and stress. Behaviors that may lower the risk of cardiovascular disease are stopping smoking, controlling weight, exercising, lowering the blood pressure, reducing the blood cholesterol level, managing diabetes mellitus to stabilize the blood glucose level, and coping effectively with stress.

Infants may be born with a wide variety of heart and blood vessel structural abnormalities. Many of these congenital defects can now be diagnosed before birth and treated during the first few weeks of life.

Cardiovascular disease due to atherosclerosis may begin in childhood. American children are still consuming diets that promote cardiovascular disease. Healthy school meal programs can help change this fact, and education can promote healthy lifestyles.

Recent data suggest that physicians should treat high LDL blood cholesterol levels and high blood pressure in the elderly.

Applying What You Have Learned

1. If a family member experienced a transient ischemic attack, how would you recognize it? What would you do? What long-term action might this family member take to avoid the onset of a stroke? `Analysis`

2. Analyze your lifestyle to determine which modifiable risk factors are raising your probability of developing cardiovascular disease. List these risk factors. `Analysis`

3. Using the list you developed by answering question 2, describe how you could modify your behavior to lower your risk of developing cardiovascular disease. `Synthesis`

4. List all of your risk factors for developing cardiovascular disease, both those you can change and those you cannot. Using the information from answer 3, evaluate your course of action. Which changes do you realistically expect to make and which do you expect not to make? Give rationales for your answers. If you follow this plan, do you think that you will substantially reduce your risk of developing CVD? Why or why not? `Evaluation`

Key

`Analysis`	breaking down information into component parts.
`Synthesis`	putting together information from different sources.
`Evaluation`	making informed decisions.

Reflecting on Your Health

1. If you are a parent or plan to be a parent some day, what are you doing (or will you do) to encourage your child's heart-healthy lifestyle?

2. If you are a cigarette smoker, do you think your risk for cardiovascular disease is affected by your habit? After learning about the effects of smoking on cardiovascular health, are you willing to quit? If not, discuss the reasons behind your answer and explain why you are willing to risk your health to continue smoking. If you are a nonsmoker, list the situations in which you regularly breathe second-hand smoke. Reflect on what you believe to be your increased risk of cardiovascular disease because of your exposure. What can you do to lessen your exposure?

3. Do you feel confident that you would be able to recognize when another person is having a stroke, TIA, or heart attack and help them? Why or why not? If not, what do you think you need to do to be prepared better to handle such an emergency?

4. Rate your lifestyle on a scale of 1 to 10, with 1 being an extremely heart-unhealthy lifestyle and 10 being an extremely heart-healthy lifestyle. Why did you rate your lifestyle as you did? Based on what you read in this chapter, what changes can you make to move closer to a 10 if you're not already there?

5. Do you think medical researchers are able to assess accurately the factors that are detrimental or helpful to cardiovascular health? Why do you feel this way? How do you think your attitudes concerning medical research affect your behavior? Have your attitudes about medical research and cardiovascular health changed since reading this chapter? Why or why not?

References

American Heart Association. (2002). *2002 Heart and stroke statistical update.* Dallas, TX: American Heart Association.

American Heart Association. (2005a). *Cigarette smoking and cardiovascular disease: AHA scientific position.*

American Heart Association. (2005b). *Heart disease and stroke statistics— 2005 update.* Dallas, TX: American Heart Association.

Ansell, B. J., Watson, K. E., & Fogelman, A. M. (1999). An evidence-based assessment of the NCEP adult treatment panel II guidelines. *Journal of the American Medical Association, 282*:2051–2057.

Ascherio, A., Katan, M. B., Zock, P. L., Stampher, M. J., & Willett, W. C. (1999). Trans fatty acids and coronary heart disease. *New England Journal of Medicine, 340*:1994–1998.

Berenson, G. S., Srinivasan, S. R., Bao, W., Newman, W. P., 3rd, Tracy, R. E., & Wattigney, W. A. (1998). Association between multiple cardiovascular risk factors and atherosclerosis in children and young adults: The Bogalusa Heart Study. *New England Journal of Medicine, 338*:1650–1656.

Brox, J., Bjørnstad, E., Olaussen, K., Østerud, B., Almdahl, S., & Løchen, M. L. (2002). Blood lipids, fatty acids, diet and lifestyle parameters in adolescents from a region in northern Norway with a high mortality from coronary heart disease. *European Journal of Clinical Nutrition, 56*:694–700.

Carels, R. A., Sherwood, A., Babyak, M., Gullette, E. C., Colemen, R. E., Waugh, R., Jiang, W., & Blumenthal, J. A. (1999). Emotional responsivity and transient myocardial ischemia. *Journal of Consulting and Clinical Psychology, 67*:605–610.

Carpentier, P. H., Maricq, H. R., Biro, C., Poncot-Makinen, C. O., & Franco, A. (2004). Prevalence, risk factors, and clinical patterns of chronic venous disorders of lower limbs: A population-based study in France. *Journal of Vascular Surgery, 40*:650–659.

Chiesa, G., & Sirtori, C. R. (2003). Recombinant apolipoprotein A-1 (Milano): A novel agent for the induction of regression of atherosclerotic plaques. *Annals of Medicine, 35*:267–273.

Chobanian, A. V., Bakris, G. L., Black, H. R., Cushman, W. C., Green, L. A., Izzo, J. L., Jones, D. W., Materson, B. J., Oparil, S., Wright, J. T., Jr., Roccella, E. J., & the National High Blood Pressure Education Program Coordinating Committee. (2003). The seventh report of the Joint National Committee on Prevention, Detection, Evaluation, and Treatment of High Blood Pressure: The JNC7 report. *Journal of the American Medical Association, 289*:2560–2572.

Clifton, P. M., Keogh, J. B., & Noakes, M. (2004). Trans fatty acids in adipose tissue and the food supply are associated with myocardial infarction. *Journal of Nutrition, 134*:874–879.

Corsini, A. (2004). The use of statins in optimizing reduction of cardiovascular risk: Focus on fluvastatin. *International Journal of Clinical Practice, 58*:494–503.

Davidson, M. H., Kurlandsky, S. B., Kleinpell, R. M., & Maki, K. C. (2003). Lipid management and the elderly. *Preventive Cardiology, 6*(3):128–133.

Expert Panel on Detection, Evaluation, and Treatment of High Blood Cholesterol in Adults. (2001). Executive summary of the third report of the National Cholesterol Education Program (NCEP) expert panel on detection, evaluation, and treatment of high blood cholesterol in adults (Adult Treatment Panel III). *Journal of the American Medical Association, 285*:2486–2497.

Felberg, R. A., Okon, N. J., El-Mitwalli, A., Burgin, W. S., Grotta, J. C., & Alexandrov, A. V. (2002). Early dramatic recovery during intravenous tissue plasminogen activator infusion: Clinical pattern and outcome in acute middle cerebral artery stroke. *Stroke, 33*:1301–1307.

Frazier, O. H., Tuzun, E., Eichstadt, H., Boyce, S. W., Lansing, A. M., March, R. J., Sartori, M., & Kadipasaoglu, K. A. (2004). Transmyocardial laser revascularization as an adjunct to coronary artery bypass grafting: A randomized, multicenter study with 4-year follow-up. *Texas Heart Institute Journal, 31*:231–239.

Galli, M., Zerboni, S., Politi, A., Llambro, M., Bonatti, R., Molteni, S., & Ferrari, G. (1999). Percutaneous transmyocardial revascularization with holmium laser in patients with refractory angina: A pilot feasibility study. *Giornale Italiano di Cardiologia, 29*:1020–1026.

Hansson, L. (2001). How far should we lower blood pressure in the elderly? *Cardiovascular Drugs & Therapy, 15*:275–279.

Harter, M. C., Conway, K. P., & Merikangas, K. R. (2003). Associations between anxiety disorders and physical illness. *European Archives of Psychiatry and Clinical Neuroscience, 253*:313–320.

Hayden, M., Pignone, M., Phillips, C., & Mulrow, C. (2002). Aspirin for the primary prevention of cardiovascular events: A summary of the evidence for the U.S. Preventive Services Task Force. *Annals of Internal Medicine, 136*:161–172.

Hu, F. B., Bronner, L., Willett, W. C., Stampfer, M. J., Rexrode, K. M., Altert, C. M., Hunter, D., & Manson, J. E. (2002). Fish and omega-3 fatty acid intake and risk of coronary heart disease in women. *Journal of the American Medical Association, 287*:1815–1821.

Imamura, H., Miyamoto, N., Uchida, K., Teshima, K., Masuda, Y., & Kobata, D. (2001). Cigarette smoking, blood pressure and serum lipids and lipoproteins in middle-aged women. *Journal of Physiological Anthropology & Applied Human Science, 20*:1–6.

Jawien, A. (2003). The influence of environmental factors in chronic venous insufficiency. *Angiology, 54*(Suppl 1):S19–S31.

Jiang, W., Babyak, M., Krantz, D. S., Waugh, R. A., Coleman, R. E., Hanson, M. M., Frid, D. J., McNulty, S., Morris, J. J., O'Connor, C. M., & Blumenthal, J. A. (1996). Mental stress-induced myocardial ischemia and cardiac events. *Journal of the American Medical Association, 275*:1651–1656.

Katerndahl, D. (2004). Panic plaques: Panic disorder and coronary artery disease in patients with chest pain. *Journal of the American Board of Family Practice, 17*:114–126.

Kohn, M., & Jacobson, M. S. (2004). Cholesterol (and cardiovascular risk) in adolescence. *Current Opinions in Pediatrics, 16*:357–362.

Korkola, S., Lachapelle, K., & Chiu, R. C. (1999). Exploring the scientific basis of surgery: Transmyocardial revascularization. *Journal of the Formosan Medical Association, 98*:301–308.

Kroeger, K., Ose, C., Rudofsky, G., Roesener, J., & Hirche, H. (2003). Risk factors for varicose veins. *International Angiology, 23*:29–34.

Krost, W. S. (2004). Cardiogenic shock. *Emergency Medical Services, 33*(9):69–73, 78.

Lee, A. J., Evans, C. J., Allan, P. L., Ruckley, C. V., & Fowkes, F. G. (2003). Lifestyle factors and the risk of varicose veins: Edinburgh Vein Study. *Journal of Clinical Epidemiology, 56*:171–179.

Lee, I. M., Hennekens, C. H., Berger, K., Buring, J. E., & Manson, J. E. (1999). Exercise and risk of stroke in male physicians. *Stroke, 30*:1–6.

Liu, S., Stampfer, M. J., Hu, F. B., Giovannucci, E., Rimm, E., Manson, J. E., Hennekens, C. H., & Eillett, W. C. (1999). Whole-grain consumption and risk of coronary heart disease: Results from the Nurses' Health Study. *American Journal of Clinical Nutrition, 70*:412–419.

McGill, H. C., Jr., & McMahan, C. A. (1998). Determinants of atherosclerosis in the young: Pathobiological Determinants of Atherosclerosis in Youth (PDAY) research group [Review]. *American Journal of Cardiology, 82*(10B):30T–36T.

McDaniel, D. H., Ash, K., Lord, J., Newman, J., Adrian, R. M., & Sukowski, M. (1999). Laser therapy of spider leg veins: Clinical evaluation of a new long pulsed alexandrite laser. *Dermatologic Surgery, 25*:52–8.

Nakanishi, N., Tatara, K., Nakamura, K., & Suzuki, K. (2000). Association of lifestyle with serum lipid levels: A study of middle-aged Japanese men. *Journal of Epidemiology, 10*:216–225.

National Center for Health Statistics. (2004). *Health, United States, 2004 with chartbook on trends in the health of Americans.* Washington, DC: U.S. Government Printing Office.

National Stroke Association. (1999). Prevention of a first stroke: A review of guidelines and a multidisciplinary consensus statement from the National Stroke Association. *Journal of the American Medical Association, 281*:1112–1120.

Nicklas, T. A., Elkasabany, A., Srinivasan, S. R., & Berenson, G. (2001). Trends in nutrient intake of 10-year-old children over two decades (1973–1994): The Bogalusa Heart Study. *American Journal of Epidemiology, 153*:969–977.

Oalmann, M. C., Strong, J. P., Tracy, R. E., & Malcom, G. T. (1997). Atherosclerosis in youth: Are hypertension and other coronary heart disease risk factors already at work? *Pediatric Nephrology, 11*:99–107.

Otsuka, R., Watanabe, H., Hirata, K., Tokai, K., Muro, T., Yoshiyama, M., Takeuchi, K., & Yoshikawa, J. (2001). Acute effects of passive smoking on the coronary circulation in healthy young adults. *Journal of the American Medical Association, 286*:436–441.

Pai, J. K., Pischon, T., Ma, J., Manson, J. E., Hankinson, S. E., Joshipura, K., Curhan, G. C., Rifai, N., Cannuscio, C. C., Stampfer, M. J., Rimm, E. B. (2004). Inflammatory markers and the risk of coronary heart disease in men and women. *New England Journal of Medicine, 351*:2599–2610.

Powell, K., Thompson, P., Caspersoen, C., & Kendrick, J. (1987). Physical activity and the incidence of coronary heart disease. *Annual Review of Public Health, 8*:253–287.

Reid, I. R., Mason, B., Horne, A., Ames, R., Clearwater, J., Bava, U., Orr-Walker, B., Wu, F., Evans, M. C., & Gamble, G. D. (2002). Effects of calcium supplementation on serum lipid concentrations in normal older women: A randomized controlled trial. *American Journal of Medicine, 112*:343–347.

Rogers, C. D. (2004). Optimal stent design for drug delivery. *Reviews in Cardiovascular Medicine, 5*(Suppl 2):S9–S15.

Schatz, I. J., Masaki, K., Yano, K., Chen, R., Rodriguez, B. L., & Curb, J. D. (2001). Cholesterol and all-cause mortality in elderly people from the Honolulu Heart Program: A cohort study. *Lancet, 358*:351–355.

Smalley, S. E., Wittler, R. R., & Oliverson, R. H. (2004). Adolescent assessment of cardiovascular heart disease risk factor attitudes and habits. *Journal of Adolescent Health, 35*:374–379.

Spertus, J. A., Jones, P. G., Coen, M., Garg, M., Bliven, B., O'Keefe, J., March, R. J., & Horvath, K. (2001). Transmyocardial CO_2 laser revascularization improves symptoms, function, and quality of life: 12-month results from a randomized controlled trial. *American Journal of Medicine, 111*:341–348.

Stampfer, J., Stamler, R., Meaton, J. D., Wentworth, D., Daviglus, M. L., Garside, D., Dyer, A. R., Liu, K., Greenland, P. (1999). Low risk-factor profile and long-term cardiovascular and noncardiovascular mortality and life expectancy. *Journal of the American Medical Association, 282*:2012–2018.

Steinberg, D., & Gotto, A. M., Jr. (1999). Preventing coronary artery disease by lowering cholesterol levels: Fifty years from bench to bedside. *Journal of the American Medical Association, 282*:2043–2050.

Steptoe, A., Wardle, J., Cui, W., Bellisle, F., Zotti, A., Baranyai, R., & Sanderman, R. (2002). Trends in smoking, diet, physical exercise, and attitudes toward health in European university students from 13 countries, 1990–2000. *Preventive Medicine, 35*:97–104.

Tanne, D., Koren-Morag, N., Graff, E., & Goldbourt, U. (2001). Blood lipids and first-ever ischemic stroke/transient ischemic attack in the Benzafibrate Infarction Prevention (BIP) Registry: High triglycerides constitute an independent risk factor. *Circulation, 104*:2892–2897.

U.S. Department of Health and Human Services. (1996). *Physical activity and health: A report of the Surgeon General.* Atlanta, GA: U.S. Departments of Health and Human Services, Centers for Disease Control and Prevention, National Center for Chronic Disease Prevention and Health Promotion.

U.S. Department of Health and Human Services. (2001). *Women and smoking: A report of the Surgeon General.* Atlanta, GA: U.S. Departments of Health and Human Services, Centers for Disease Control and Prevention, National Center for Chronic Disease Prevention and Health Promotion.

U.S. Department of Health and Human Services. (2004a). *Physical activity and good nutrition: Essential element to prevent chronic diseases and obesity 2004.* Atlanta, GA: Centers for Disease Control and Prevention, National Center for Chronic Disease Prevention and Health Promotion.

U.S. Department of Health and Human Services. (2004b). *The health consequences of smoking: A report of the Surgeon General.* Atlanta, GA: Centers for Disease Control and Prevention, National Center for Chronic Disease Prevention and Health Promotion, Office on Smoking and Health.

Van den Oever, R., Hepp, B., Debbaut, B., & Simon, I. (1998). Socio-economic impact of chronic venous insufficiency: An underestimated public health problem. *International Angiology, 17*:161–167.

Vasan, R. S., Beiser, A., Seshadri, S., Larson, M. G., Kannel, W. B., D'Agostino, R. B., & Levy, D. (2002). Residual lifetime risk for developing hypertension in middle-aged women and men: The Framingham Heart Study. *Journal of the American Medical Association, 287*:1003–1010.

Vollmer, W. M., Sacks, F. M., Ard, J., Appel, L. J., Bray, G. A., Simons-Morton, D. G., Conlin, P. R., Svetkey, L. P., Erlinger, T. P., Moore, T. J., & Karanja, N. (2001). Effects of diet and sodium intake on blood pressure: Subgroup analysis of the DASH-Sodium Trial. *Annals of Internal Medicine, 135*:1019–1028.

Whelton, S. P., Chin, A., Xin, S., & He, J. (2002). Effect of aerobic exercise on blood pressure: A meta-analysis of randomized, controlled trials. *Annals of Internal Medicine, 136*:493–503.

Writing Group for the Women's Health Initiative Investigators. (2002). Risks and benefits of estrogen plus progestin in healthy postmenopausal women: Principal results from the Women's Health Initiative randomized controlled trial. *Journal of the American Medical Association, 288*:321–333.

Yarnell, J. W. G., Patterson, C. C., Thomas, H. F., & Sweetnam, P. M. (2000). Comparison of weight in middle age, weight at 18 years, and weight change between, in predicting subsequent 14 year mortality and coronary events: Caerphilly Prospective Study. *Journal of Epidemiology and Community Health, 54*:344–348.

What You'll Learn

Chapter Overview

What is cancer?

How cancers develop and spread

How physicians detect cancer

How cancer is treated

Which cancers are the most prevalent in the United States

How you can reduce your risk of cancer

Diversity in Health

Stomach Cancer: Variation in Mortality Among Countries

Consumer Health

Alternative Cancer Therapies

Managing Your Health

Summary of ACS Recommendations for Early Detection | Testicular Self-Examination | Reducing Your Risk for Cancer | Cancer's Seven Warning Signs

Across
THE LIFESPAN

Cancer

Student Workbook

Self-Assessment: Torabi Cancer Prevention Behavior Scale

Changing Health Habits: Modifying Behavior to Reduce Cancer Risk

Do You Know?

· *What the most prevalent cancer is for your age group?*

· *What you can do to lower your risk of cancer?*

· *Which cancers are on the rise?*

Cancer

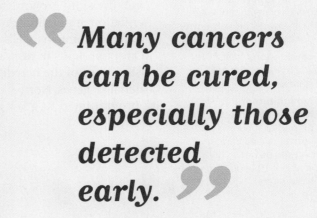

"**B**y winning the Tour, you stick in the minds and hearts of the cycling public. You can win every classic and the world championship, but the Tour is everything. It's a global event."

These words were uttered to newspaper reporters by Lance Armstrong, only the second American ever to win the Tour de France. On that clear sunny day in July of 1999, he won more than this most rigorous and prestigious three-week cycling race, however. He showed the world that he had truly won his battle with testicular cancer—a battle that had nearly cost him not only his career but also his life. The photo shows the champion nearing the end of the grueling course, which took competitors over the Alps and Pyrenees Mountains and into five countries bordering France. Armstrong is wearing a yellow jersey, the race's symbol of overall leadership. He went on to become a seven-time Tour de France champion, winning the Tour also in 2000, 2001, 2002, 2003, 2004, and 2005.

Although it is still the nation's second biggest killer (cardiovascular disease is the first), cancer is not an automatic death sentence. Armstrong and other cancer survivors, such as former major league baseball pitcher Dave Dravecky and pro football Hall of Famer Len Dawson, are living testimony to that fact. Many cancers can be cured, especially those detected early. Even cancers in advanced stages, as was Armstrong's, may respond to therapies available today.

Cancer researchers are making discoveries daily that help win the war against cancer. For example, Canadian researchers Anil Srivastava and Nancy Kreiger (2000) discovered that teenage boys who exercise regularly and men who have physically demanding jobs in their 20s may be more likely to develop testicular cancer than less active teenage boys and young men. Although the mechanism for this increased risk is unknown, Srivastava and Kreiger speculate that exercise affects the levels of male hormones, which may somehow increase risk of the cancer. Although more research is needed to formulate recommendations regarding exercise and testicular cancer risk in these age groups, a tremendous body of research is already available that provides guidelines to help people avoid

> *Many cancers can be cured, especially those detected early.*

cancer. However, avoiding cancer is a primary health goal, and there are many actions people can take to lessen their risk of developing certain cancers. We discuss such preventive measures throughout this chapter.

What Is Cancer?

People often talk about cancer as if it were a single disease. However, cancer is many diseases. Lung cancer, for example, is a very different disease from leukemia (cancer of the blood) or skin cancer. Although different, all cancers have common characteristics: Their cells exhibit abnormal growth, division, and differentiation. Differentiation is the process by which cells develop into certain types, such as liver cells or muscle cells. In addition, cancer cells have the potential to **metastasize**, or spread from where they develop to another part of the body.

Cells are the building blocks of all organisms; they are the smallest unit of living material. In any multicelled organism such as humans, cells divide and differentiate as an individual grows and develops, and when its tissues need repair. The timing and events of cell division, growth, and differentiation are highly controlled by regulatory proteins. Cells make regulatory proteins in response to the instructions of the hereditary material, or genes. Normal cells are programmed to grow and divide, and to stop growing and dividing at appropriate times.

Unlike normal cells, cancer cells do not stop growing and dividing at appropriate times. Additionally, cancer cells do not differentiate normally and tend to spread. These cells may form masses called **malignant tumors** that invade body tissues and interfere with the normal functioning of tissues and organs. Tumors often cause pain as they invade nerves or press on nerves. Why do cancer cells behave differently from noncancer cells? The answer lies in the genetic material in the cell.

How Cancers Develop and Spread

Cancer develops only in cells that have **mutations**, that is, damaged genes. Mutations can be inherited or can occur from exposure to low-dose radiation, drugs, or toxic chemicals. Infection with certain viruses can also cause changes in genes. Excluding inheritance, then, cancer is determined largely by environmental factors, including components of lifestyle. Lifestyle factors play a major role in cancer prevention.

Genes and Cancer Development

Oncogenes are "on" switches that speed cell growth. Successive mutations to the hereditary material of particular body cells produce oncogenes. **Tumor-suppressor genes** are "off" switches that slow cell growth. If tumor-suppressor genes mutate or are lost from the hereditary makeup of a cell, they will no longer restrict cell growth.

metastasize (meh-TAS-tah-size) the ability of cancer cells to spread from where they develop to another part of the body.

malignant tumors (mah-LIG-nant) masses of cancer cells that invade body tissues and interfere with the normal functioning of tissues and organs.

mutations (myou-TAY-shunz) changes in genes or chromosomes; damaged genes.

oncogenes (ONG-ko-geenz) tumor genes that manufacture altered proteins that speed cell growth and decrease the level of cell differentiation.

tumor-suppressor genes pieces of hereditary material that slow cell growth; anti-onco-genes.

carcinogens (kar-SIN-oh-jenz) cancer-causing substances.

benign tumors (be-NINE) encapsulated masses of abnormal cells that remain in one location and do not invade surrounding tissues.

(a)

(b)

Figure 13-1 **A Comparison of Dysplastic and Normal Cells.** (a) Dysplastic cells. These cells (stained differently from those in [b]) are irregular in size and the appearance of their nuclei. (b) Normal cells. These cells are all approximately the same size and have nuclei that look similar.

The activation of oncogenes and deactivation of tumor-suppressor genes (and, therefore, the development of cancer) is a multistage process. In other words, successive genetic changes must take place for a normal cell to change into a cancer cell. These changes take place over time as various environmental factors affect cells and cause mutations. Therefore, the chances of developing cancer generally increase with age and with exposure to cancer-causing substances, or **carcinogens**. Of course, many factors determine an individual's risk for developing cancers. These factors, which we will discuss throughout this chapter, modify this generalization.

Cells that begin to grow abnormally, although not yet cancer cells, may form growths called **benign tumors**. Surrounded by a fibrous capsule, benign tumors remain in one location; they do not invade surrounding tissues. Usually these growths are not life threatening unless their presence interferes with a vital function. For example, a benign brain tumor may be life threatening if it compresses blood vessels serving a vital center in the brain. In most cases benign tumors can be removed completely by surgery.

Some benign tumor cells exhibit traits that are characteristic of the development of cancer cells. These cells are said to exhibit dysplasia. Notice that the dysplastic cells in Figure 13-1a vary in size, shape, and the appearance of their nuclei. They are not differentiating properly into a specific type of cell. The normal cells, however, are somewhat regular in these same characteristics (Figure 13-1b). Dysplastic cells have the potential to develop into cancer cells.

Metastasis

One of the characteristics of cancer cells is their ability to spread, or metastasize, from where they initially developed to other places in the body. Cells with the ability to metastasize are *malignant*. As a cancer develops, metastasis does not take place immediately. As cancer cells grow and divide, they often form a malignant tumor. At this stage the cancer is in situ (in place), because it has not invaded other tissues. However, these localized cancer cells begin to secrete chemicals that destroy the substances that hold the surrounding tissues together. When this occurs, cancer cells enter blood and lymph vessels and travel to other parts of the body. Cancerous cells can move out of the blood vessels at a distant location, enter the tissues there, and divide to form new masses of malignant cells. Figure 13-2 shows this process of cancer cell division and metastasis. Once metastasis occurs, the cancer becomes much more difficult to control.

Figure 13-2 **How Cancer Cells Multiply and Spread.** Cancer cells secrete chemicals that destroy the substances holding tissues together. As these tissues break down, cancer cells move from their original site, enter the blood and lymph, and travel to other parts of the body.

Tumor in bronchial epithelium.

Connective tissue

Capillary

(a)

Cells break through base of epithelium to invade capillary.

(b)

Cells travel through bloodstream and may eventually adhere to the capillary wall in the liver or other organ.* The cells then move out of the capillary.

Cells multiply to form metastasis of the liver.

*Less than 1 in 1,000 survive to form metastases.

(c)

(d)

Figure 13-3 **Cancer Death Rates, 1930–2000.** (a) Male. (b) Female. Source: *Cancer facts and figures 2004.* Copyright © American Cancer Society, 2004. www.cancer.org. Reprinted with permission.

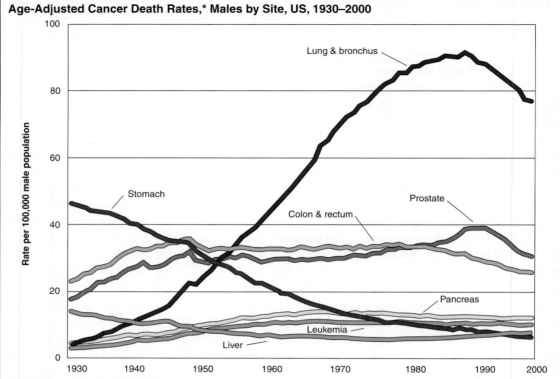

Age-Adjusted Cancer Death Rates,* Males by Site, US, 1930–2000

*Per 100,000, age-adjusted to the 2000 US standard population.
Note: Due to changes in ICD coding, numerator information has changed over time. Rates for cancers of the liver, lung and bronchus, and colon and rectum are affected by these coding changes.
Source: US Mortality Public Use Data Tapes 1960–2000, US Mortality Volumes 1930–1959,
National Center for Health Statistics, Centers for Disease Control and Prevention, 2003.

(a)

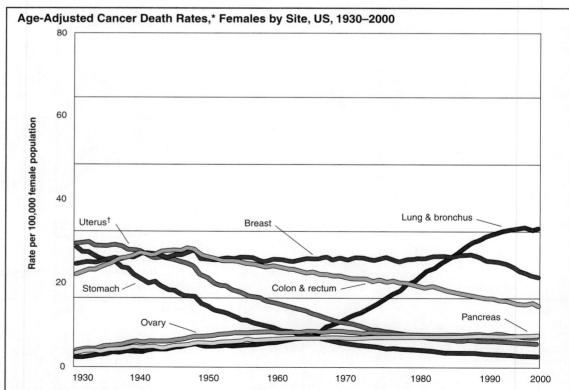

Age-Adjusted Cancer Death Rates,* Females by Site, US, 1930–2000

*Per 100,000, age-adjusted to the 2000 US standard population. †Uterus cancer death rates are for uterine cervix and uterine corpus combined.
Note: Due to changes in ICD coding, numerator information has changed over time. Rates for cancers of the liver, lung and bronchus, colon and rectum, and ovary are affected by these coding changes.

Source: US Mortality Public Use Data Tapes 1960–2000, US Mortality Volumes 1930–1959,
National Center for Health Statistics, Centers for Disease Control and Prevention, 2003.

(b)

Cancers are named according to the type of tissue from which they develop. **Carcinomas** (which comprise most adult cancers) arise from epithelial tissue, which lines and covers internal and external body surfaces. Lung, oral, stomach, skin, breast, colon, and ovarian cancers are carcinomas. **Sarcomas** are cancers that arise from connective or muscle tissue. **Leukemias** are cancers of the blood and related cells. **Lymphomas** are cancers of the lymphatic system, the network of vessels and nodes that transports and filters tissue fluid. Cancers of the nervous system have a variety of names.

Figure 13-3 shows death rates (the number of persons dying per year per 100,000 people) of various cancers in the United States. Overall cancer death rates and incidence rates decreased from 1995 through 2001. Continued declines for overall cancer death rates and for many of the top cancers (see Figure 13-3) reflect progress in the prevention, early detection, and treatment of cancer (Jemal et al., 2004).

■ Cancer Detection

Cancer screening is an examination to detect malignancies in a person who has no symptoms. The American Cancer Society (ACS) recommends the screening procedures listed in the Managing Your Health box on page 348. Some screening procedures are expensive, invasive (that is, they require entering a body cavity or interrupting normal body functions), or both. Most such procedures are not performed unless a person is in a high-risk category for a particular cancer, or if symptoms indicate that a particular cancer may be present.

Cancer screening or detection methods vary depending on the location of the possible cancer. Superficial cancers, such as cancers of the skin and oral cavity, can be detected by visual examination. Some cancers in internal areas can be detected by collecting cells for microscopic examination. This process is possible, for example, for detecting cancer of the cervix and of the esophagus. Some cancers, such as colon cancer and stomach cancer, can be detected by fiberoptic examination. To see these internal areas of the body, the physician inserts a flexible tube called a fiberscope into the area to be examined. The fiberscope contains bundles of specially coated glass or plastic fibers that transmit an image from the lighted end of the scope to an eyepiece.

Other cancers that grow embedded in tissues, such as breast cancer and lung cancer, can be detected by x rays. CT scans and MRI can also be used to detect deeply embedded cancers, such as brain cancer. CT scans, or computed tomography, are x rays of thin sections of the body that the computer constructs into three-dimensional images (Figure 13-4). MRI, or magnetic resonance imaging, uses magnetic fields and radio waves instead of x rays. As in CT scans, a computer constructs three-dimensional images of internal tissues. Ultrasound, an imaging technique that uses sound waves, is used occasionally to detect cancerous growths. (See page 104 for a more thorough description of ultrasound.)

The 5-year survival rate is the percentage of persons who are alive 5 years after their cancer is diagnosed, whether they are disease-free, under treatment, or

carcinomas (KAR-si-NO-mahz) cancers that arise from epithelial tissues.

sarcomas (sar-KO-mahz) cancers that arise from connective or muscle tissue.

leukemias (lew-KEY-me-ahz) cancers of the blood and related cells.

lymphomas (lim-FOE-mahz) cancers of the lymphatic system.

cancer screening an examination to detect malignancies in a person who has no symptoms.

(a)

(b)

Figure 13-4 **(a) CT and (b) MRI Scans of the Brain.** Both have color added to visualize structures better. The outer skull, underlying fat, and brain tissues can be seen clearly in both. The MRI more clearly shows the convolutions of the brain.

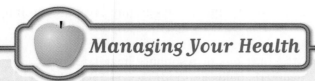

Summary of American Cancer Society Recommendations for the Early Detection of Cancer in Asymptomatic People

Site	Recommendation
Breast	Women 40 and older should have an annual mammogram and an annual clinical breast examination (CBE) by a health care professional. Women ages 20 to 39 should have a CBE by a health care professional every 3 years. Breast self-exam (BSE) by women over 20 is optional.
Colon and rectum	Over age 50, men and women should follow one of the examination schedules below:* · A fecal occult blood (FOBT) test or a fecal immunochemical test (FIT) every year, or · A flexible sigmoidoscopy (FSIG) every 5 years, or · Annual FOBT test or FIT and flexible sigmoidoscopy every 5 years.† · A double-contrast barium enema every 5 to 10 years. · A colonoscopy every 10 years.
Prostate	The PSA test and the digital rectal examination should be offered annually, along with information on potential risks and benefits, to men over 50 who have a life expectancy of at least 10 years. Men at high risk (African American men and men with a strong family history of one or more first-degree relatives diagnosed with prostate cancer at an early age—younger than 65) should begin testing at age 45.
Uterus	**Cervix:** All women 3 years after their first vaginal intercourse but no later than age 21 should have an annual conventional Pap test or biannual liquid-based Pap test. After three or more consecutive satisfactory examinations with normal findings in women over 30, the Pap test may be performed every 2 to 3 years. Discuss the matter with your physician. Women over 70 may choose to stop screening after three normal Pap smears in a row within the past 10 years. Women should discuss the need for a pelvic exam with their health care practitioners. **Endometrium:** The American Cancer Society recommends that women at menopause should be informed about the risks and symptoms of endometrial cancer, and strongly encouraged to report any unexpected bleeding or spotting to their physicians. Annual screening for endometrial cancer with endometrial biopsy beginning at age 35 should be offered to women with or at risk for hereditary nonpolyposis colon cancer (HNPCC). These women, and women at menopause who are at increased risk (those with a history of estrogen therapy or tamoxifen, late menopause, having no children, infertility or failure to ovulate, obesity, diabetes, or high blood pressure) should also be informed about the potential benefits, risks, and limitations of early endometrial cancer detection.
Cancer-related checkup	Persons over 20 should have a physical exam (including examinations for cancers of the thyroid, testicles, mouth, ovaries, skin, and lymph nodes) and health counseling (including counseling about tobacco, sun exposure, diet and nutrition, risk factors, sexual practices, and environmental and occupational exposures) on the occasion of a periodic health exam.

*A digital rectal exam should be done at the same time as sigmoidoscopy, colonoscopy, or double-contrast barium enema.
† Yearly FOBT or FIT plus flexible sigmoidoscopy every 5 years is preferred over either option alone.

in remission (having a partial or complete disappearance of the signs and symptoms of the cancer). Table 13-1 shows the 5-year survival rate for cancers discussed in this chapter.

■ Cancer Treatment

The principal forms of cancer treatment are surgery, radiation, and chemotherapy. Newer modes of treatment are biomodulation (immunotherapy), photodynamic therapy, antiangiogenesis therapy, and bone marrow and peripheral blood stem cell transplants. In the past, physicians referred to a cancer as "cured" if the patient survived for 5 years with no sign of the cancer returning. This is no longer the case, however, because some cancers grow after extended periods and others recur after they seem to have been eliminated. Today, the term *cure* means that all traces of a localized tumor have been removed from the body and the former cancer patient has the same life expectancy as a person who never had cancer.

Table 13-1	Five-Year Relative Survival Rates* by Stage at Diagnosis, 1992–1999			
Site	All Stages %	Local %	Regional %	Distant %
Breast (female)	86.6	97.0	78.7	23.3
Colon & rectum	62.3	90.1	65.5	9.2
Esophagus	14.0	29.1	13.1	2.2
Kidney	62.6	89.9	60.0	9.1
Larynx	64.7	82.6	47.9	20.0
Liver	6.9	16.3	6.0	1.9
Lung & bronchus	14.9	48.7	16.0	2.1
Melanoma	89.6	96.7	60.1	13.8
Oral cavity	57.2	82.1	47.9	26.1
Ovary	53.0	94.7	72.0	30.7
Pancreas	4.4	16.6	6.8	1.6
Prostate†	97.5	100.0	—	34.0
Stomach	22.5	59.0	21.7	2.5
Testis	95.5	99.1	95.0	73.1
Thyroid	95.8	99.3	95.5	59.9
Urinary bladder	81.8	94.4	48.2	5.8
Uterine cervix	71.3	92.2	50.9	16.5
Uterine corpus	84.4	96.2	64.7	26.0

*Rates are adjusted for normal life expectancy and are based on cases diagnosed from 1992 to 1999, followed through 2000.
†The rate for local stage represents local and regional stages combined.
Local: An invasive malignant cancer confined entirely to the organ of origin.
Regional: A malignant cancer that (1) has extended beyond the limits of the organ of origin directly into surrounding organs or tissues; (2) involves regional lymph nodes by way of lymphatic system; or (3) has both regional extension and involvement of regional lymph nodes.
Distant: A malignant cancer that has spread to parts of the body remote from the primary tumor either by direct extension or by discontinuous metastasis to distant organs, tissues, or via the lymphatic system to distant lymph nodes.
Data Source: Surveillance, Epidemiology, and End Results Program, 1973–2000, Division of Cancer Control and Population Sciences, National Cancer Institute, Bethesda, MD.
Source: *Cancer facts and figures 2004.* Copyright © American Cancer Society, 2004. www.cancer.org. Reprinted with permission.

Surgery

Most cancer cures are accomplished by surgery. During surgery, physicians remove a localized cancer by cutting it away from noncancerous tissue. Microscopic extensions of cancerous tissue may not be easy to detect during surgical procedures, so a physician usually removes tissue beyond the obvious cancer to increase the probability that all the cancerous tissue is removed. Although surgery is often a life-saving treatment, one drawback is that removal of healthy tissue with unhealthy tissue may impair the body's functioning or cause disfigurement.

Radiation

Radiation is also used to treat localized cancers, either alone or in conjunction with surgery. Radiation is energy or particles emitted from the nucleus of an atom. The energy of any high-dose radiation interferes with the molecular structures of cells, killing them. Healthy cells recover more quickly and easily from radiation treatment than do cancer cells, so the healthy tissue surrounding a cancer usually survives while the cancer dies. For this reason, a physician may recommend radiation over surgery in particular instances. Preserving healthy tissue surrounding a cancer is extremely important, especially with cancers such as laryngeal cancer (cancer of the voice box), in which it may mean the difference between a patient's retaining or losing the ability to speak. Physicians also choose radiation over surgery for treatment of cancers that respond well to radiation therapy, such as cervical cancer, prostate cancer, and Hodgkin's disease. Additionally, physicians often use radiation treatment with elderly patients because their chances of recovering from it may be higher than that of recovering from surgery.

High-dose x-ray and gamma-ray irradiation are widely used today. Patients may undergo one of two methods of radiation treatment. One method is to focus a beam of radiation on the cancerous tissue from an outside source. The machine delivering the beam of radiation rotates around the patient while continually targeting the tumor, so that various areas of healthy tissue receive minimal doses of radiation but the tumor receives high doses. Another method is to implant tiny radioactive "beads" in the cancerous tissue for a specific time and then remove them. With either approach, cancer patients usually undergo numerous treatments over a 5- to 8-week period.

Figure 13-5 shows a highly effective treatment against cancer called *proton therapy.* In this treatment, a patient's cancer is bombarded with a stream of positively charged subatomic particles called protons.

At high doses, proton irradiation kills cells, as does any type of high-dose radiation. Proton radiation, however, can be focused more precisely on the cancer than can other forms of radiation. Therefore, a higher dose of radiation can be used with less radiation affecting surrounding cells. However, proton therapy is still not in widespread use because it is about three times as costly as traditional radiation therapies, and few treatment facilities in the United States offer proton irradiation.

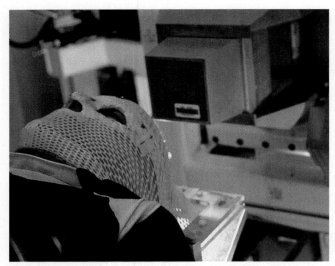

Proton Therapy. This patient at the Proton Treatment Center at Loma Linda University is ready to receive proton therapy to treat cancer of the eye. The mask immobilizes the head to ensure that the beam will hit its target.

Chemotherapy

Chemotherapy is the use of anticancer drugs to inhibit cancer cell reproduction or to destroy cancer cells. Chemotherapy is used most often when cancer has spread to various regions of the body. As with radiation therapy, chemotherapy may be used in conjunction with surgery. In certain cases, physicians combine all three approaches to cancer treatment.

biomodulation
manipulation of the body's immune system to rid the body of cancer.

Radiation and chemotherapy treatments also kill and damage healthy cells and may cause serious side effects such as severe nausea and hair loss. In addition, these treatments do not always destroy cancers completely because their doses are not high enough to do so. Doses sufficiently high to kill all cancer cells often cause too much damage to normal tissue. Also, certain tumors are drug resistant or develop drug resistance during therapy.

Biomodulation/Immunotherapy

A new breed of cancer treatment has emerged in the war against cancer: the manipulation of the body's own immune system to rid the body of its cancer. The umbrella term for these relatively new and often experimental methods is **biomodulation** (biological response modification), or immunotherapy. It includes the use of gene therapy techniques.

Gene therapy is the introduction of hereditary material into cells to treat a specific disorder or condition. A key factor in the body's capability to mount its defense is its ability to recognize an intruder as foreign. Like other foreign substances, cancer cells are marked as intruders because they contain proteins called antigens that are not normally found in the body. However, tumor cells appear to contain antigens that evoke only a weak response from the immune system. As a result, the immune system has difficulty detecting and identifying malignant tumors, so it does a poor job destroying these abnormal cells.

What kinds of things do biomodulators do to help the body ward off cancer? Injecting tumor antigens into the patient's bloodstream can increase the numbers of tumor-fighting immune system cells in the body (Linehan et al., 1999). This procedure is similar to the way in which a vaccine works to boost the body's immune response against an infectious disease. For this reason, such cancer-fighting products are called *cancer vaccines*. However, cancer vaccines are given to patients who already have cancers to help rid them of their diseases. They are not given to cancer-free persons to prevent cancer. At this time, cancer vaccines for prostate, colorectal, lung, and breast cancers, and for malignant melanoma are in clinical trials.

Examples of other biomodulators are drugs that decrease the suppressor mechanisms of the immune system, thus increasing the host's immune response. Another approach is to augment the patient's immune system by bone marrow transplants (tissue that produces immune system cells) or transfusions of particular immune system cells. Other biomodulators are chemicals that act on tumor cells by making them more recognizable by the body or more susceptible to dying as a result of immune system processes.

Photodynamic Therapy

In photodynamic therapy, a chemical called a photosensitizer, which is administered to the patient, reacts with a special type of light, killing tumor cells. The treatment is specific to tumors because they take up the photosensitizer better than do normal tissues, and physicians target the light at the tumors. Therefore, this type of treatment does not significantly damage normal tissues. Death of the tumor results from the interaction of the light and the chemical.

The use of photodynamic therapy in the treatment of benign and malignant tumors has increased dramatically over the past 10 years and is used in many countries for the treatment of cancers of the lung, bladder, cervix, and esophagus (Ackroyd et al., 2001). It also shows promise for use with pancreatic cancer.

Antiangiogenesis Therapy

The word *angiogenesis* means "blood vessel" (*angio-*) "beginning" (*genesis*). Thus, angiogenesis is the growth of new blood vessels. *Antiangiogenesis* (ant-eye-an-gee-oh-JEN-uh-sis) therapy is the use of drugs or other substances to stop cancerous tumors from developing new blood vessels. Tumors need their own blood supplies to grow; without blood bringing them oxygen and nutrients and removing wastes, cancerous tumors shrink to about the size of the head of a pin.

In general, antiangiogenesis drugs have mild side effects, because they work only to inhibit the growth of new blood vessels and do not kill normal body cells. In addition, cancers do not appear to develop resistance to these drugs. However, antiangiogenesis drugs cannot be given to pregnant women or to women who might become pregnant, because their antiangiogenesis properties could affect a developing fetus. In addition, antiangiogenesis drugs cannot be used when a patient has surgery, because the body must repair the blood vessel damage that results. Persons with damaged blood vessels (such as those with heart disease or stroke) may not be able to take antiangiogenesis drugs as well.

Bone Marrow and Peripheral Blood Stem Cell Transplants

Stem cells are undifferentiated cells whose daughter cells can develop into a variety of cell types. Bone marrow cells are a type of stem cell that continually give rise to a variety of types of blood cells. Peripheral blood (blood in the bloodstream) can be used as a source of blood stem cells too, but donors must be treated with growth factors (hormonelike substances) a few days before the donation, which causes their stem cells to grow and enter their bloodstream. Their harvested blood is processed by a machine that separates out the stem cells; the rest of the blood is returned to the donor.

Bone marrow and peripheral blood stem cell transplants are used in two primary ways in cancer treatment: (1) to resupply the bone marrow when it has been destroyed by chemotherapy or radiation, or (2) to supply healthy stem cells to a person who has cancer of the blood-forming tissue, such as leukemia. In the first situation, a patient's own stem cells are harvested before chemotherapy or radiation, and the stem cells are given back to the patient after the treatment. In the second instance, the stem cells come not from the patient but from a healthy donor whose tissue type best matches the patient. The healthy stem cells are transplanted into the patient, and these cells produce healthy blood cells.

Patients receive stem cell transplants (whether the stem cells are their own or those of a donor) in a process much like a blood transfusion. The stem cells take up residence in the bone marrow, grow, and send out new blood cells.

However, even as scientists discover new ways to treat the nation's number two killer, prevention and early detection are still the best ways to live a healthy, long, cancer-free life.

■ Prevalent Cancers in the United States

Over decades of research, scientists have learned what causes certain cancers. In some cases, scientists are unsure of the cause but know which factors are related to cancer development. These factors, which, when present, increase the chances that a person will develop a particular cancer, are called risk factors. Although heredity influences cancer risk, it explains only a fraction of all cancers and variations in cancer risk. Behavioral factors such as cigarette smoking, dietary patterns, physical activity, and weight control, however, *substantially* affect the risk of developing cancer (ACS, 2004b).

This chapter organizes the discussion of cancers according to factors that appear to be significant in the development of particular cancers, most of which are prevalent in the United States. Advanced age is a significant risk factor for most cancers except certain childhood cancers, testicular cancer, cervical cancer, and, in part, breast cancer.

Before reading this section, fill out the Cancer Prevention Behavior Scale in the student workbook to determine if your behaviors are healthy with respect to cancer prevention.

Cancers Caused by or Related to Tobacco

In 2004, U.S. Surgeon General Richard Carmona issued a report on smoking and health that listed tobacco smoking as a cause of various cancers. Table 13-2 lists these cancers. Thirty percent of all cancer deaths, including 87% of lung cancer deaths, can be attributed to tobacco (ACS, 2004b).

This section explores the first seven cancers in Table 13-2 because they are all caused primarily by this preventable risk. Stomach cancer and cancer of the cervix are discussed in other sections of this chapter because their primary causes relate to factors other than tobacco use.

Lung Cancer Looking at Table 13-3, you can see that lung cancer is the leading cause of cancer deaths in both men and women in the United States. Death rates

Table 13-2 Cancers Caused by Cigarette Smoking

Bladder

Esophagus

Kidney

Larynx (voice box)

Acute myeloid leukemia

Lung

Mouth and throat

Pancreas

Stomach

Cervix

Source: U.S. Department of Health and Human Services. (2004). *The health consequences of smoking: A report of the Surgeon General.* Washington, DC: U.S. Government Printing Office.

due to lung cancer have risen dramatically in men since the 1940s through the 1980s and in women since the 1960s through the 1980s (see Figure 13-3). These increases are due primarily to increases in the percentage of the population who smoked tobacco in the decades prior to the 1960s. Lung cancer, like most cancers, takes years to develop, so a rise in lung cancer death rates occurs decades after a rise in the percentage of the population who smoke.

Evidence suggests that women are more susceptible than men to developing lung cancer caused by tobacco use. Results of research show that a gene called GRPR, which is linked to the abnormal growth of lung cells, is much more active in women than in men. Located on the X chromosome, a piece of hereditary material that determines gender, the GRPR gene is turned on more frequently in women nonsmokers than in men nonsmokers, and is activated earlier in women than in men in response to cigarette smoke. The presence of two copies of the GRPR gene in women, one

Table 13-3 Leading Sites of New Cancer Cases and Death by Gender, U.S., 2004 Estimates*

Cancer Cases by Site and Sex		Cancer Deaths by Site and Sex	
Male	Female	Male	Female
Prostate 230,110 (33%)	Breast 215,990 (32%)	Lung and bronchus 91,930 (32%)	Lung and bronchus 68,510 (25%)
Lung and bronchus 93,110 (13%)	Lung and bronchus 80,660 (12%)	Prostate 29,500 (10%)	Breast 40,110 (15%)
Colon and rectum 73,620 (11%)	Colon and rectum 73,320 (11%)	Colon and rectum 28,320 (10%)	Colon and rectum 28,410 (10%)
Urinary bladder 44,640 (6%)	Uterine corpus 40,320 (6%)	Pancreas 15,440 (5%)	Ovary 16,090 (6%)
Melanoma of the skin 29,900 (4%)	Ovary 25,580 (4%)	Leukemia 12,990 (5%)	Pancreas 15,830 (6%)
Non-Hodgkin's lymphoma 28,850 (4%)	Non-Hodgkin's lymphoma 25,520 (4%)	Non-Hodgkin's lymphoma 10,390 (4%)	Leukemia 10,310 (4%)
Kidney 22,080 (3%)	Melanoma of the skin 25,200 (4%)	Esophagus 10,250 (4%)	Non-Hodgkin's lymphoma 9,020 (3%)
Leukemia 19,020 (3%)	Thyroid 17,640 (3%)	Liver 9,450 (3%)	Uterine corpus 7,090 (3%)
Oral cavity 18,550 (3%)	Pancreas 16,120 (2%)	Urinary bladder 8,780 (3%)	Multiple myeloma 5,640 (2%)
Pancreas 15,740 (2%)	Urinary bladder 15,600 (2%)	Kidney 7,870 (3%)	Brain 5,490 (2%)
All sites 699,560 (100%)	All sites 668,470 (100%)	All sites 290,890 (100%)	All sites 272,810 (100%)

*Excludes basal and squamous cell skin cancers and in situ carcinoma except urinary bladder.
Note: Percentages may not total 100% due to rounding.
Source: *Cancer facts and figures 2004.* Copyright © American Cancer Society, 2004. www.cancer.org. Reprinted with permission.

CRITICAL THINKING

The article "Big Tobacco Targets College Students" focuses on tobacco-sponsored events and their effect on smoking in college students. Explain why you think this article is a reliable or an unreliable source of information. Use the model for analyzing health information to guide your thinking; the main points of the model are noted below. The model is explained fully on pages 13–15.

1. Which statements are verifiable facts, and which are unverified statements or value claims?

2. What are the credentials of the author? If this information is available, does his or her background and education qualify the author as an expert in this area?

3. What might be the motives and biases of the author? State the reasons for your answers.

4. Which information is relevant to the issue or main points of the article? Which information is irrelevant?

5. Is the source reliable? Does it have a reputation for publishing misinformation?

6. Does the article attack the credibility of conventional scientists or medical authorities?

Based on your analysis, do you think this article is a reliable source of health-related information? Explain why or why not.

Big Tobacco Targets College Students

Tobacco companies have aimed their marketing dollars at college students, hosting parties in nightclubs and on college campuses as a cover to distribute free cigarettes and encourage youth smoking, a Harvard School of Public Health study has found.

Researchers polled students in 119 U.S. colleges and learned that tobacco-sponsored events were attended by up to 27 percent of 18- to 24-year-old students at all but one of the schools.

In all, 8.5 percent of students reported they had attended a tobacco industry-sponsored event.

"I was surprised that these parties existed," said Dr. Nancy Rigotti, head of the study and director of the Tobacco Research and Treatment Center of Massachusetts General Hospital.

"The industry is targeting young adults through these bar and club promotions. I think that colleges need to be aware that this is happening on their campuses or near them."

Study results also show that cigarette promotions of this type had the strongest effect on those who had entered college as nonsmokers. Of the students polled who did not smoke regularly before age 19, 23.7 percent who became smokers had attended tobacco-sponsored events.

Debra Rachman, co-chairwoman of the American Cancer Society's Relay For Life event in Peabody, was disappointed to hear the study results.

"It's just disturbing that now they have kind of pushed the high school kids to the side and are going after the college kids," Rachman said of the tobacco companies.

Shoppers at Downtown Crossing in Boston yesterday agreed.

"That goes back to Joe Camel when they were marketing to kids, so that's no surprise," said Colette Twigg, 43, of Falmouth, Maine. "A kid in college, even though they're 18, is still very impressionable."

"It shows that their mission is to get children addicted and to make lifetime clients. That's unfortunate," said Emerson College graduate Meredith Cohen, 22, of Brighton.

Alternative Cancer Therapies

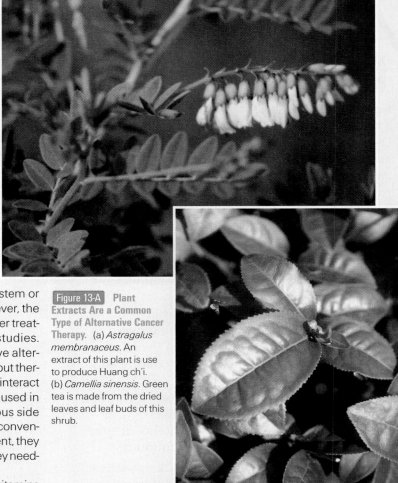

(a)

Modern medicine has its limitations; not every condition can be prevented, managed, or cured. It is not surprising, therefore, that some individuals who are diagnosed with incurable conditions seek help from anyone who offers a cure. Cancer patients who seek alternative therapies also hope to find a "softer" treatment with fewer side effects. Many want to use a holistic approach or take charge of their health when conventional medicine offers no more options. When faced with a potentially life-threatening illness such as cancer, most people feel the need to do everything possible to survive.

Most users of alternative cancer therapies expect their treatments to boost their immune system or slow the progression of or cure their cancer. However, the effectiveness of most alternative therapies in cancer treatment has not been established in scientific studies. Additionally, cancer patients erroneously perceive alternative therapies as safe because they are "natural," but therapies such as herbal and vitamin supplements may interact in dangerous ways with drugs or therapies being used in conventional cancer treatment. Many have serious side effects of their own. And if cancer patients delay conventional treatment in favor of unconventional treatment, they may diminish their chances of survival, spend money needlessly, and lower their quality of life.

Herbal therapies, plant extracts, and therapeutic vitamins are the most common alternative therapies in cancer treatment today, and up to 45% of cancer patients use some form of alternative treatment. A few of the more popular of these therapies are discussed on the next page. The greatest danger with the use of substances not controlled by the Food and Drug Administration (FDA) in cancer treatment is the risk of contamination, misidentification, or substitution with a harmful substance because of lack of quality control.

If you or someone you know is thinking about using alternative therapies for cancer treatment, remember that it is important to evaluate all evidence about these methods carefully and make decisions with a qualified health care provider. At the least, informing the health care provider about other therapies being used can help avoid adverse drug interactions. Also, in evaluating therapies, remember that any remedy used by a large number of people will, by chance, be used by a long-term survivor. In many cases, the patient used conventional treatments as well as alternative ones. However, the alternative method often gets the credit even though there is no evidence to show that it played a role in the patient's long-term survival.

Figure 13-A Plant Extracts Are a Common Type of Alternative Cancer Therapy. (a) *Astragalus membranaceus*. An extract of this plant is use to produce Huang chʻi. (b) *Camellia sinensis*. Green tea is made from the dried leaves and leaf buds of this shrub.

(b)

Sources: Fernandez, C. V., Stutzer, C. A., MacWilliam, L., & Fryer, C. (1998). Alternative and complementary therapy use in pediatric oncology patients in British Columbia: Prevalence and reasons for use and nonuse. *Journal of Clinical Oncology, 16*:1270–1286.

Kaegi, E. on behalf of the Task Force on Alternative Therapies of the Canadian Cancer Research Initiative. (1998). Unconventional therapies for cancer 1: Essiac. *Canadian Medical Association Journal, 158*:897–902.

Kaegi, E. on behalf of the Task Force on Alternative Therapies of the Canadian Cancer Research Initiative. (1998). Unconventional therapies for cancer 2: Green tea. *Canadian Medical Association Journal, 158*:1033–1035.

Kaegi, E. on behalf of the Task Force on Alternative Therapies of the Canadian Cancer Research Initiative. (1998). Unconventional therapies for cancer 5: Vitamins A, C, and E. *Canadian Medical Association Journal, 158*:1483–1488.

Ottenweller, J., Putt, K., Blumenthal, F. J., Dhawale, S., & Dhawale, S. W. (2004). Inhibition of prostate cancer-cell proliferation by Essiac. *Journal of Alternative and Complementary Medicine, 10*:687–691.

Spaulding-Albright, N. (1997). A review of some herbal and related products commonly used in cancer patients. *Journal of the American Dietetic Association, 97*(S2):S208–S215.

Verhoef, M. J., Hagen, N., Pelletier, G., & Forsyth, P. (1999). Alternative therapy use in neurologic disease: Use in brain tumor patients. *Neurology, 52*:617–622.

Alternative Therapy	What Is It?	Claims and Research Studies	Possible Side Effects
Huang ch'i	Extract from the plant *Astragalus membranaceus* (Figure 13-A)	*Claims:* Stimulation of the immune system. *Studies:* Results of a University of Texas study show that it may boost immune system function. It may also reduce the side effects of chemotherapy.	Can trigger low blood pressure. May induce dizziness and fatigue. Too much may suppress the immune system.
Essiac	Herbal tea. Mixture of four herbs: burdock root, Indian rhubarb, sheep sorrel, and slippery elm	*Claims:* Strengthens immune system, improves appetite, relieves pain, may reduce tumor size. *Studies:* Results are contradictory. Some studies show no activity in reducing the size of animal tumors, while others show some inhibition of tumor cell growth and enhancement of the immune response.	Nausea, vomiting, diarrhea
Green tea	Tea made from the steamed and then dried leaves and leaf buds of the shrub *Camellia sinensis* (Figure 13-B). (Black tea is prepared from the fermented leaves of this plant.)	*Claims:* Results of a variety of studies suggest that regular consumption moderately decreases the risk of cancer, especially cancers of the upper digestive tract. Therefore, use as a treatment is being studied. *Studies:* Results are contradictory. Some researchers think green tea may play a role in delaying metastasis.	High caffeine content may cause nervousness, insomnia, and irregularities in heart rate. Moderate consumption appears safe.
Vitamins A (or beta-carotene), C, and E	Vitamin "cocktail" taken in megadoses	*Claims:* Combination of these vitamins improves general well-being, strengthens immune system, and may delay the development and progression of serious disease. *Studies:* Some animal studies have shown the ability of vitamin A and beta-carotene to enhance the immune response, to retard tumor growth, and to decrease the size of established tumors. In laboratory experiments, vitamin C has been shown to inhibit tumor growth. Results of some studies also suggest that vitamin C may kill tumor cells and may enhance the effects of some cancer drugs. Very little research has been conducted on the role of vitamin E in cancer treatment. At this time, there is not enough evidence for physicians to recommend that cancer patients take vitamin supplements.	Vitamin A: Headache, irritability, drowsiness, dizziness, itchiness. Megadoses may cause liver damage. Taking beta-carotene, which is transformed into vitamin A in the body, is safer than taking vitamin A. Vitamin C: Generally well tolerated. Megadoses may cause stomach irritation, heartburn, nausea, vomiting, drowsiness, headaches, rash, and abnormalities in iron metabolism. Vitamin E: Toxicity in adults appears to be low. High levels can adversely affect the absorption of vitamins A and K. Long-term megadoses may cause nausea, diarrhea, and blurred vision.

on each of their two X chromosomes, may be a factor in their increased susceptibility to tobacco-induced lung cancer (Shriver et al., 2000). Men have only one X chromosome, along with a Y chromosome.

Incidence rates of lung cancer in both sexes have begun to stabilize, and to drop slightly in males (see Figure 13-3). This stabilization reflects the beginning of a predicted decline in incidence rates due to the steady decline in cigarette smoking in the U.S. population since 1964. In that year, U.S. Surgeon General Luther Terry issued a report that linked cigarette smoking with the development of lung cancer and other diseases (U.S. Public Health Service, 1964). In 1999 the American Cancer Society set goals for 2015 of a 25% reduction in cancer incidence and a 50% reduction in cancer mortality rates, to which they still adhered in 2004 (ACS, 2004b).

Signs and Symptoms In the early stages of disease, the signs and symptoms of lung cancer may be hard to detect. Cigarette smokers often have chronic cough, chronic bronchitis, or excess sputum (saliva and mucus) production (see Chapter 8). Tumors growing in the bronchioles (small airways in the lungs) also cause a cough and sputum production; they may also cause blood to appear in the sputum as they disrupt airway tissues. A lung cancer victim may also wheeze when breathing if the airways become substantially narrowed by tumor growth. In addition, the air sacs in that part of the lung may collapse and cease to function; infection may develop. The patient may experience pain in the chest, shoulder, and arm if the cancer spreads to the chest wall and affects certain nerves there.

Physicians use chest x rays, analyses of the types of cells in the sputum, and fiberoptic examination of the bronchial passageways to assist in their diagnoses.

Risk Factors and Prevention Malignant growths develop in the lungs and airways in many persons as they inhale cancer-causing substances such as tobacco smoke over long periods of time.

The risk of lung cancer rises proportionately with the number of cigarettes (or cigars or pipes) a person smokes per day, the number of years a person smokes, and how deeply he or she inhales. Persons who smoke low-tar cigarettes have a lower risk of lung cancer than those who smoke high-tar cigarettes (USDHHS, 2004). (Smoking "low-yield" cigarettes does not lower cardiovascular disease risk; see Chapter 12.) Likewise, those who smoke filter-tipped cigarettes have a lower risk of lung cancer than those who smoke unfiltered

passive smoking the inhalation, by nonsmokers, of tobacco smoke in the air.

asbestos (as-BES-tose) a fiberlike mineral found in rocks that, when inhaled, can cause lung cancer or other lung conditions.

cigarettes. However, male cigarette smokers, on average, are 20 times more likely to develop lung cancer than are nonsmokers (ACS, 2004a). Additionally, results of research show that people who smoke filter-tipped or "low-yield" cigarettes are at increased risk for developing deep lung tumors because, when smoking, they inhale more deeply and forcefully than people who smoke non-filter-tipped or "regular-yield" cigarettes (USDHHS, 1999b).

If you are a smoker (of any age), giving up cigarette smoking will slowly lower your risk of developing lung cancer, several other cancers, and cardiovascular disease as well. Your risk of developing lung cancer will never return to that of a lifetime nonsmoker (USDHHS, 2004). (However, your risk of developing cardiovascular disease will lower considerably in only 1 year, and return to that of a nonsmoker in 3 to 15 years, depending on how much and how long you smoked.)

Scientists have been unable to show that lung cancer is inherited. Nonetheless, correlational studies show that relatives of lung cancer patients have a higher risk of developing lung cancer if they smoke than do smokers with no relatives who have lung cancer. Scientists speculate that relatives of lung cancer patients may inherit a defect in their cells' ability to resist genetic damage by the carcinogens in cigarette smoke.

In the early 1970s medical researchers began investigating the effects of **passive smoking** on the development of lung cancer. Passive smoking is the inhalation by nonsmokers of environmental tobacco smoke (ETS) present in the air from others who smoke. Environmental tobacco smoke has been associated with a 35% to 50% increase in lung cancer risk. Recent reviews of past studies, however, suggest that the scientific evidence does not uphold the assertion that passive smoking significantly raises the risk of lung cancer in nonsmokers (Adlkofer, 2001; Nilsson, 2001).

Substances other than those in tobacco smoke have also been linked to lung cancer and are listed in Table 13-4. Only people in certain occupations encounter most of these substances. Two substances significantly associated with the development of lung cancer and often encountered in the environment are asbestos and radon.

Asbestos is a fiberlike mineral found in rocks that resists damage by fire or other natural processes. Because of these properties, asbestos has been used in the manufacture of a variety of products and is used in the construction, shipbuilding, and railroad industries. People in these industries as well as those who mine asbestos

Table 13-4 Documented Occupational Lung Carcinogens

Substance	Occupational Exposures
Arsenic	Smelters, pesticide manufacturers
Asbestos	Miners, millers, insulators, railroad, and shipyard workers
Beryllium	Workers in electronic industries and for aerospace and nuclear reactor parts manufacturers
Chloromethyl ethers	Ion-exchange resin manufacturers
Chromium	Chromate and pigment manufacturers
Hydrocarbons	Coal gas workers, roofers
Mustard gas	Poison gas manufacturers
Nickel	Refiners
Radiation (radon)	Miners of uranium and other ores

Source: Frank, A. L. (1989). Epidemiology of lung cancer. In J. Roth, J. Ructersall, & T. Weisenburger (Eds.). *Thoracic surgery.* Philadelphia: W. B. Saunders Co., p. 6. Reprinted with permission.

are at risk of developing lung cancer if they inhale asbestos particles. Additionally, the effects of inhaling asbestos particles multiplies the effects of smoking tobacco and therefore greatly increases risk. Chapter 16 discusses asbestos in greater detail.

Exposure to **radon gas** also appears to multiply the carcinogenic effect of tobacco smoke (USDHHS, 1999a). Radon gas is colorless and odorless, and is produced as the radioactive element uranium decays, emitting subatomic particles and energy. When inhaled, radon can cause mutations in cells because it is radioactive also. Radon is present in the rocks and soils in many areas in the United States (Figure 13-6). People who live in these regions may be exposed to radon gas if it leaks through cracks in basement walls

and collects in their homes. Home radon detectors can ascertain the presence of this gas. If radon is present, specialists in radon abatement can advise a homeowner on procedures to prevent this gas from leaking into and accumulating in the house.

Treatment Physicians treat lung cancer with surgery, radiation, and chemotherapy. Surgeons often remove the lobe of the cancerous lung. They may combine therapies if the cancer has spread, using radiation or chemotherapy with surgery.

Cancers of the Larynx, Oral Cavity, and Esophagus

Although these cancers are not as prevalent as others, they have preventable causes: tobacco use, which includes the use of cigarettes, cigars, pipes, and smokeless (chewing) tobacco of all types; and excessive alcohol consumption. Heavy consumption of alcohol is often a causal factor in cancers of the esophagus and liver, but if a heavy drinker is also a smoker, the effects of both substances multiply the risk of developing cancer of the larynx, oral cavity, and esophagus.

Cancers of the larynx, or voice box, are usually detected early if they involve the vocal cords because the voice quickly becomes hoarse. However, cancers of the larynx that do not involve the vocal cords are more difficult to discover early. Their symptoms may include a sore throat, difficulty in swallowing, or a visible lump in the neck.

The esophagus is the tube that carries food and drink from the mouth to the stomach. Difficulty swallowing is also a symptom of esophageal cancer. In addi-

radon gas
a colorless, odorless, radioactive gas present in the rocks and soils in many areas in the United States that, when inhaled, can cause mutations in cells.

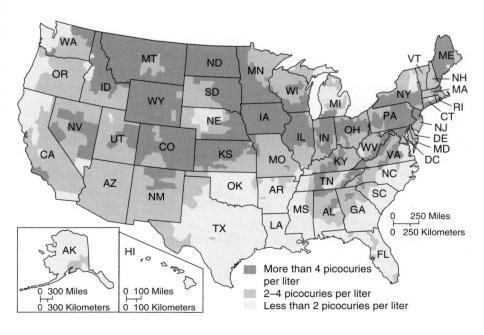

Figure 13-6 Areas of the United States in Which Radon Gas Is Most Prevalent.

More than 4 picocuries per liter
2–4 picocuries per liter
Less than 2 picocuries per liter

Figure 13-7 **Tongue Cancer.** This close-up of a cancer patient's mouth shows a malignant tumor on the edge of the tongue. This type of cancer spreads rapidly. The survival rate is low. Tongue cancer may be related to smoking cigarettes or to the use of smokeless tobacco.

tion, people who have recurrent heartburn or a burning sensation while swallowing should be checked for possible esophageal carcinoma.

In oral cancer, malignant or benign growths are often visible (Figure 13-7). Malignancies may appear as sores that bleed easily and do not heal, red or white patches that do not go away, or thickened areas of tissue. Oral cancer metastasizes relatively quickly; approximately 50% of cases are diagnosed in advanced stages. To detect oral cancer early, persons over the age of 50 should have complete oral examinations as part of their annual physical checkups. Dentists should routinely screen all of their patients for oral cancer.

Cancers of the Kidney and Bladder The kidneys and bladder are organs of the urinary system, yet tobacco smoking is a causal factor in cancers of these organs. These organs come in contact with inhaled carcinogens in tobacco smoke (or other inhaled carcinogens) after they enter the bloodstream at the lungs. The kidneys filter the carcinogens into the urine, which exposes the kidneys and bladder to these substances before urination.

Most signs and symptoms of kidney and bladder cancer are the same as those of several other conditions, so experiencing any of them is not a sure sign of cancer. One such sign of both cancers is blood in the urine. Frequent, urgent, or difficult urination is also a sign of bladder cancer. Additional signs and symptoms of kidney cancer include a fever of unknown origin, weight loss, and anemia (a decrease in the hemoglobin in the blood).

Most people who get bladder or kidney cancer are men over 50 years of age who are heavy smokers. Cigarette smokers have 2 to 10 times the risk of developing bladder or kidney cancer as do nonsmokers. As with lung cancer, the risk increases with the number of cigarettes smoked per day and the number of years a person has been a smoker. People lessen their risk when they decrease the number of cigarettes they smoke or stop smoking. Obesity is another known risk factor for kidney cancer (Jemal et al., 2004).

Cancer of the Pancreas A long, slender gland, the pancreas lies near the stomach. As an accessory organ of the digestive system, the pancreas secretes digestive enzymes that enter the small intestine by means of a duct. As an endocrine gland, the pancreas secretes the hormones insulin and glucagon, which help regulate blood levels of glucose.

Pancreatic cancer is a particularly deadly form of cancer, striking men and women fairly equally. The fourth most common cause of cancer death in men and fifth in women (see Table 13-3), pancreatic cancer is often called a silent cancer because the early symptoms, which include nausea, vomiting, and weakness, are vague and nonspecific. The more specific signs and symptoms of pancreatic cancer—jaundice (yellowing of the eyeballs and skin), pain, and weight loss—do not occur until the disease is advanced and then may be confused with many other diseases, such as gallbladder or liver disease.

The risk of pancreatic cancer increases after age 50; most cases occur in persons aged 65 to 79 years. The incidence of pancreatic cancer for smokers is more than twice as high as for nonsmokers. Other persons at risk for developing pancreatic cancer are chemists and those in occupations that involve close exposure to gasoline and dry cleaning agents. Inhaled carcinogens appear to reach the pancreas via the bloodstream. Risk also appears to increase with obesity, physical inactivity, chronic inflammation of the pancreas, diabetes, and cirrhosis of the liver. In addition, rates of pancreatic cancer are higher in countries whose populations eat diets high in fat (ACS, 2004a).

Only 4% of people who have pancreatic cancer survive beyond 5 years, and only 1% of people with pancreatic cancer are cured. Late detection and metastasis reduce survival. For the rare patients who discover their cancer in its early stages, surgery is a primary treatment that may lead to a cure and long-term relief of symptoms. Occasionally, radiation therapy and anticancer drugs are used.

Acute Myeloid Leukemia Acute myeloid leukemia (AML) affects blood-producing cells in the bone marrow. In AML, white blood cells that combat bacterial infection (neutrophils) are primarily affected, but occasionally red blood cells or platelets are affected as well. These cells do not differentiate properly from stem cells in the bone marrow (see page 351) resulting in fewer than normal numbers of these cells in the bloodstream. AML is a serious disease and is likely fatal if not treated. Chemotherapy and stem cell transplantation are standard treatments.

The primary known causes of AML are exposure to benzene and ionizing radiation. Cigarette smoke contains benzene and substances that emit ionizing radiation, along with other substances thought to cause AML. Data from human and experimental animal studies show a causal relationship between smoking and acute myeloid leukemia. The risk for AML increases with the number of cigarettes smoked and with the duration of smoking (USDHHS, 2004).

Cancers Related to Diet

Research results suggest that about one-third of the cancer deaths that occur annually in the United States are due to nutrition and physical activity factors, including obesity. For Americans who do not use tobacco, dietary choices and physical activity are *the most important* modifiable determinants of cancer risk (ACS, 2004b). Along with adopting a physically active lifestyle and maintaining a healthful weight, the American Cancer Society recommends eating a variety of healthful foods, with an emphasis on plant sources. Table 13-5 lists the ACS's dietary recommendations.

As you can see from Table 13-5, diet has both a positive and a negative effect on the development of cancer. There are dietary components that raise the risk of certain cancers and others that lower the risk of certain cancers. One cancer strongly related to diet is stomach cancer. The other cancer related to diet—colorectal cancer—can be affected significantly by one's heredity. Other cancers, such as breast cancer, have risk factors related to diet but are related to other risk factors as well.

Table 13-5 | **Dietary Recommendations for Reducing Cancer Risk**

- Eat five or more servings of fruits and vegetables per day.
- Eat whole-grain foods rather than processed (refined) grain foods.
- Limit consumption of red meats, processed meats, and high-fat foods.
- Choose foods that help maintain a healthy weight, including foods with little added sugars.

Source: Adapted from American Cancer Society. (2004). *Cancer facts and figures, 2004.* Atlanta, GA: Author.

Cancer of the Stomach The incidence of and mortality from stomach cancer has declined dramatically over the past 60 to 70 years in the United States. In the early part of the twentieth century, stomach cancer, not lung cancer, was the number one cancer killer of Americans. (See the Diversity in Health essay on page 360–361 for an explanation of this decline.)

Stomach cancer is another of the silent cancers because no signs and symptoms appear early in its course. As the disease progresses, a person may experience mild stomach discomfort with gas pains or vague sensations of fullness. Suspecting minor digestive problems, a person with these symptoms may take antacid tablets, and the symptoms disappear. As the cancer continues to grow, the malignancy causes more severe pain that is less responsive to antacids. The stomach cancer victim may then experience a decreased appetite, a feeling of fullness after just beginning to eat, pain on eating, nausea and vomiting, weight loss, excessive burping, and weakness.

The risk of stomach cancer increases with age and doubles each decade over the age of 55. However, the primary risk factors for cancer of the stomach are dietary factors. Diets high in salt-cured, nitrate-cured, or smoked food increase the risk of stomach cancer. Cigarette smoking and consuming large quantities of alcoholic beverages are also risk factors. The Diversity in Health essay discusses the risk factors for stomach cancer in greater detail.

Stomach cancer is easily diagnosed with barium studies. During this procedure, the patient swallows a milky fluid called barium sulfate. As this material reaches the stomach, a series of x rays are taken that show the movement of this fluid through the stomach, while visualizing obstructions and other growths. Additionally, physicians often obtain stomach cells by the use of a fiberoptic tube, which can be fitted with instruments

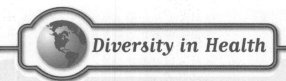

Stomach Cancer: Variation in Mortality Among Countries

More Americans died of stomach cancer in 1930 than of any other type of cancer. In the United States, the death rate due to this cancer has fallen dramatically since then (see Figure 13-3). However, stomach cancer is still the number two cancer killer worldwide. (Lung cancer is number one.) Why has the death rate from this cancer fallen in the United States? Why is this cancer so prevalent in other parts of the world?

As scientists studied worldwide patterns of mortality from stomach cancer, they noticed high mortality rates in Central and South American countries such as Brazil, Chile, Colombia, Costa Rica, and Venezuela. They also noticed large differences in death rates from stomach cancer in some of these countries. In Colombia, for example, death rates from this disease differ dramatically in populations living in the mountains compared with populations living along the coast. A similar situation exists in Central and Eastern European countries. There are high mortality rates from stomach cancer in these countries; however, the death rates between countries and within countries in this part of the world vary. In addition, as you can see in Figure 13-B, Japan, China, and the Russian Federation have extremely high mortality rates from stomach cancer. Why are some countries' rates of death due to stomach cancer dramatically higher than others? (You can research incidence and mortality rates for various cancers in countries around the world at http://www-dep.iarc.fr/.)

Scientists have determined that differences in worldwide stomach cancer death rates are related to diet and environment rather than to race or country of origin. Likewise, the reduction in stomach cancer deaths in the United States is due primarily to these factors.

Regarding diet, methods of food processing and preservation affect the incidence of stomach cancer. In the early 1900s in the United States, methods of food processing and preservation changed dramatically. By mid-century, refrigeration and freezing replaced salting, pickling, and smoking as the primary methods of food preservation. Scientists have since discovered that the regular consumption of highly salted foods (including pickled foods) increases the risk of developing stomach cancer. Foods that are smoke-cured, charbroiled, or grilled contain high quantities of polycyclic aromatic hydrocarbons (PAHs), which are carcinogenic and mutagenic. These compounds are also found in cigarette smoke and air pollution, since they are the products of the incomplete combustion of fossil fuels such as charcoal and gasoline. Although many Americans enjoy eating grilled foods, their consumption of smoked, salted, and pickled foods has decreased since the early 1900s, reducing Americans' risk of developing and dying from stomach cancer. However, peoples of various cultures still use salting and smoking to preserve meats and pickling to preserve vegetables, thereby increasing their risk of stomach cancer.

Another dietary factor with an environmental link plays a role in the development of this disease. Ingesting nitrosamines, which are found in nitrite-cured foods (such as bacon, cold cuts, and some hot dogs) and in water supplies in some parts of the world (such as Colombia and South America), appears to increase the risk of stomach cancer. Nitrosamines are also found in cigarette smoke. Additionally, chemical reactions that occur in the stomach produce nitrosamines from other compounds. For example, substances in certain fish consumed in Japan and in fava beans consumed in Colombia are converted in the stomach to nitrosamines.

Eating fruits and vegetables appears to inhibit the reactions in the stomach that form nitrosamines. In addition, they

---

for such procedures. If a tumor is found, a **biopsy**, or small piece of tissue, is taken of the growth so that the cells can be studied and the diagnosis confirmed. In the United States, stomach cancer is no longer a major killer; therefore, routine screening is not performed as it is in high-risk populations such as Japan. Thus, most stomach cancers are not diagnosed early in the United States. If found early, however, stomach cancers are treated with surgery to remove the tumor. Chemotherapy is also used to treat stomach cancer; many stomach cancers respond well to this treatment.

biopsy
(BI-op-see) a small piece of tissue that is taken from a growth so that the cells can be studied and a diagnosis confirmed.

Cancer of the Colon and Rectum The **colon**, or large intestine, is an organ of the digestive system that reabsorbs water and certain chemicals from waste materials (feces). Bacteria in the colon decompose materials that the human body cannot digest. The **rectum** is the lower part of the large intestine; it terminates at the anus.

Cancer of the colon and rectum, jointly referred to as *colorectal cancer,* is the third most deadly cancer in the United States (see Table 13-3). The signs and symptoms of colorectal cancer depend on the location of the tumor. A person may have no symptoms or few symptoms at first. Some persons first experience vague or crampy abdominal pain that may be mistaken for an appear to protect the stomach from the effects of carcinogens. Populations who consume large quantities of fruit and vegetables generally have a low risk of stomach cancer. Recent studies have confirmed that taking high-dose beta-carotene pills does not lower the risk of any cancer and appears to raise the risk of lung cancer in smokers.

In addition to dietary factors, infection with the bacterium *Helicobacter pylori* has been found to be associated with the development of stomach cancer. *H. pylori*, which also increases the risk of digestive system ulcers, is highly prevalent in Asian countries. Persons with *H. pylori* can be treated with antibiotics to eradicate the stomach infection. Although killing this microorganism is an effective treatment for ulcers, it results in only a slowing of the precancerous process and does not prevent all stomach cancers.

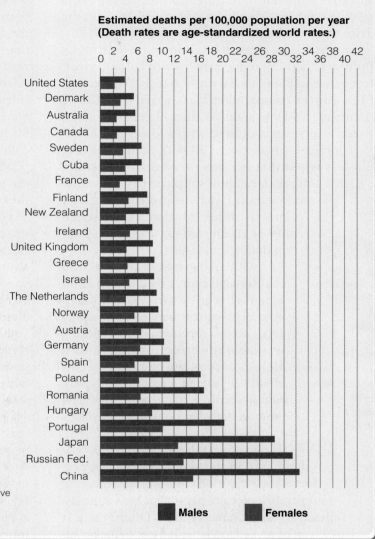

Estimated deaths per 100,000 population per year (Death rates are age-standardized world rates.)

Figure 13-B Estimated Rates from Stomach Cancer around the World, 2002. Data: The GLOBOCAN 2002 database. Unit of Descriptive Epidemiology at the International Agency for Research on Cancer. Available at http://www-dep.iarc.fr/.

ulcer. Other indications may be a change in bowel habits, such as constipation alternating with diarrhea. Blood may be visible in the stool (feces) or, on screening, a person may have a positive occult (hidden) blood test. As the cancer worsens, a person with colorectal cancer may have a complete obstruction of the colon that requires emergency surgery.

The primary risk factors for developing colorectal cancer are advanced age, heredity, personal or family history of colorectal polyps (small growths) or inflammatory bowel disease, physical inactivity, obesity, a diet high in fat and/or red meat, an inadequate intake of fruits and vegetables, smoking cigarettes, and hav-

ing more than one alcoholic drink per day (ACS, 2004a).

Beginning at age 40, both men and women are at increased risk for developing colorectal cancer; this risk doubles with each decade after age 50 and peaks at about age 70. People who have hereditary conditions in which they tend to grow numerous (sometimes hundreds) of polyps in their gastrointestinal tracts have very high incidences of colorectal malignancies. In addition, people who have a first-degree relative (parent or sibling) with colon cancer are three to five times more

colon
the large intestine.

rectum
the lower part of the large intestine.

likely to develop colorectal cancer than are people with no such family history of this disease.

Recently, aspirin has been found to have a protective effect in both men and women against colorectal cancer, reducing the risk by about 40% to 50% (Giovannucci, 1999). However, chronic aspirin use can cause stomach irritation and bleeding, so this preventive therapy should be undertaken only on the advice of one's physician.

Research results consistently show that high levels of physical activity reduce the risk of colon cancer. Most active individuals have a 40% to 50% lower risk of this cancer compared to least active individuals (Hardman, 2001). In addition, diets high in vegetables and fruits are associated with a lower risk of colorectal cancer (ACS, 2004b). Some data also suggest that hormone replacement therapy, folic acid, calcium supplements, selenium, and vitamin E may be protective against colorectal cancer. However, more research must be conducted to support the present data (ACS, 2004a).

As with all cancers, early detection of colorectal cancer usually results in a high chance of survival. Although colorectal cancer may have no easily recognizable early symptoms, tests are available to screen for this cancer. Common tests are the fecal occult blood test, digital rectal examination, sigmoidoscopy, and colonoscopy. A less common test is the double-contrast barium enema.

The **fecal occult blood test** detects hidden blood in the stool. The patient performs the simple test at home by smearing stool onto a piece of paper that has been sensitized to detect occult blood. Often, the test papers can be mailed to a laboratory or to the physician for interpretation. This test will not detect all colorectal cancers, however, because not all colorectal cancers bleed. Also, positive tests may indicate conditions other than colorectal cancer. Feasibility studies are currently being conducted on an early detection fecal test that identifies genetic markers from cells that initiate colorectal tumors (Traverso et al., 2002).

To perform the **digital rectal exam**, a physician uses a gloved finger to feel the rectum for abnormal growths. This test, however, detects only 10% of colorectal cancers. **Sigmoidoscopy** can detect up to 50% of colorectal cancers. It is a procedure in which the physician views the lower portion of the colon (the sigmoid [S-shaped] colon) with a flexible fiberoptic tube. Persons at high

fecal occult blood test (FEE-kle ok-KULT) home test that detects hidden blood in the stool.

digital rectal exam a test in which a physician uses a gloved finger to feel the rectum or the prostate for abnormal growths.

sigmoidoscopy (SIG-moid-OS-ko-pee) a procedure in which a physician views the lower portion of the colon via a flexible fiberoptic tube.

colonoscopy (KO-lon-OS-ko-pee) a procedure in which a physician views the entire length of the colon using a flexible fiberoptic tube.

risk for colorectal cancer are often screened with a similar procedure called a **colonoscopy**, during which the fiberoptic tube is threaded through the length of the colon. The sigmoidoscope or colonoscope can also be used to remove or biopsy polyps or other growths.

The double-contrast barium enema is an x-ray examination of the colon when it is filled with a barium solution. Additional x rays are taken after the patient expels the solution. The barium provides a contrast medium that helps visualize polyps or other growths. Study results showed colonoscopy to be a more effective screening tool for colon cancer than the barium enema (Fletcher, 2000; Winawer et al., 2000). See the Managing Your Health box on page 348 for the American Cancer Society's screening guidelines for early detection of colorectal cancer.

When colorectal cancer is detected early, surgery is the primary treatment. Physicians often use chemotherapy and radiation therapy after surgery to kill any metastasized cancer that was not detected or removed by surgery. If surgery is not possible, a physician may treat the cancer with chemotherapy or radiation therapy alone.

Cancers Related to Hormone Function

Breast Cancer From the late 1940s until 1985 in the United States, breast cancer was the number one cancer killer of women. Lung cancer then usurped the top position, but only because its death rate rose. The mortality rate from breast cancer in women has remained stable for decades, but its incidence increased about 4% per year between 1980 and 1987 and by 0.5% per year between 1987 and 1998 (ACS, 2001). The rapid increase between 1980 and 1987 is due largely to more widespread use of screening techniques such as mammography, which will be discussed shortly. Breast cancer is unusual in men, but it does occur.

Signs and Symptoms The signs and symptoms of breast cancer involve changes in the breast tissue, including lumps in the breast; dimpling, thickening, discoloration, irritation, or scaling of the breast skin; tenderness of the nipple or nipple discharge; and swelling or distortion of the breast. Pain is not usually a sign of breast cancer; most breast cancers are painless in their early development. Breast pain is usually due to cyclic hormonal changes and related breast swelling.

Risk Factors and Prevention Approximately 5% of breast cancers are due to heredity. Women with first-degree relatives (mothers, sisters, daughters) who have breast cancer are at increased risk for developing the disease. In 1994 an American team of researchers identified the exact location of one gene thought to be responsible: a tumor-suppressor gene called BRCA1 (Jenks, 1994).

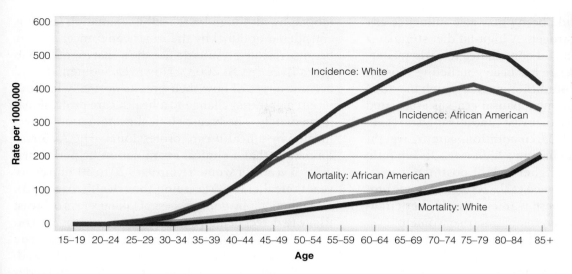

Figure 13-8 Female Breast Cancer: Age-Specific Incidence and Death Rates, by Race, United States, 1996–2000. Source: American Cancer Society. (2003). Breast cancer facts and figures, 2003–2004. Atlanta, GA: American Cancer Society.

Data sources: *Incidence*—Surveillance, Epidemiology, and End Results Program, 1973–2000, Division of Cancer Control and Population Science, National Cancer Institute, 2003. *Deaths*—National Center for Health Statistics, Centers for Disease Control and Prevention, 2003.

Inheriting a defective copy of this gene puts a woman at high risk for developing breast cancer and may also influence her risk for ovarian cancer. The BRCA1 gene is thought to account for about half the inherited cases of breast cancer.

The following year, a British team identified the approximate location of a second breast cancer gene, BRCA2, which is responsible for male breast cancers as well as most of the rest of inherited female breast cancers (Wooster et al., 1995). This gene does not appear to influence ovarian cancer risk, unlike the BRCA1 gene. In 2002, British and Dutch scientists found another tumor-suppressor gene that may be responsible for up to 1% of breast cancers in women and 9% in men. When mutated, the CHEK2 gene increases the risk of breast cancer in persons not already carrying BRCA1 or BRCA2 mutations (CHEK2-Breast Cancer Consortium, 2002). Genetic testing is now available for people whose family history suggests that they carry the BRCA1 or other harmful genes.

Another major risk factor for the development of breast cancer in women is age. Breast cancer is rare in women younger than 20, but the incidence begins to climb throughout the 20s, rises dramatically during the 30s through the mid-70s, and then drops significantly (Figure 13-8). Ninety-four percent of new cases and 96% of breast cancer deaths reported during the period from 1996 to 2000 occurred in women aged 40 and older. Incidence and death rates from breast cancer are generally highest among white and African American women (ACS, 2003).

In addition to age and heredity, a third major group of breast cancer risk factors appears to be those that increase a woman's cumulative exposure to ovarian hormones, particularly estrogen. Evidence suggests that having a high number of menstrual cycles is a breast cancer risk factor. For example, early menarche (younger than age 12) and late menopause (older than age 55) are risk factors for breast cancer. Also, women who have not borne children (therefore did not have their cycles interrupted) are at a higher risk than those who have (ACS, 2003).

A recent reanalysis of worldwide data regarding the relationship between breast cancer risk and use of combination oral contraceptives shows that breast cancer risk is slightly elevated in women currently taking oral contraceptives and remains slightly elevated until about 10 years after they discontinue oral contraceptive use (Westhoff, 1999; ACS, 2003).

Additionally, results from the Women's Health Initiative (WHI) study, the first randomized controlled trial to quantify the degree of risk for breast cancer on postmenopausal women taking hormone replacement therapy (HRT), show that HRT raises breast cancer risk. In the study, combined estrogen plus progestin HRT raised breast cancer risk 26% during the first 5 years of use and 53% for more than 5 years of use (Writing Group for the Women's Health Initiative Investigators, 2002).

Drugs have been developed that prevent bone loss and reduce blood cholesterol in postmenopausal women but do not raise their risk of breast cancer. These drugs are called selective estrogen receptor modulators, or SERMs. An example of a SERM that is now available in the United States is raloxifene (Genazzani & Gambacciani, 1999).

A high-fat diet and obesity may also influence circulating levels of estrogen. A high-fat diet stimulates estrogen production and contributes to early menarche. Although evidence has been conflicting (Bosetti et al., 2002), recent studies show that a high intake of animal fat during premenopausal years is associated with an increased risk of breast cancer (Bingham et al., 2003; Cho et al., 2003). In addition, gaining weight over the lifetime and having a high waist-to-hip ratio is associated with a higher risk of postmenopausal breast cancer (Friedenreich et al., 2002). Fat tissue produces estrogen, so obese women have higher circulating levels of estrogen than nonobese women.

Some breast cancer risk factors such as heredity, age, and exposure to estrogen are impossible or difficult to control. However, physical activity appears to be a modifiable risk factor for breast cancer. That is, breast cancer risk appears to be reduced by regular physical activity. The optimal type, intensity, frequency, and duration of exercise as a breast cancer preventive measure have not yet been firmly established (McTiernan, 2000; Thune & Furberg, 2001). Longer duration appears to provide the most benefit, however, and the activity need not be strenuous (McTiernan et al., 2003). Medical researchers think that one reason for the risk reduction may be that exercise modifies a woman's menstrual cycle, possibly lengthening the cycle and altering the production of ovarian hormones such as estrogen (Hoffman-Goetz et al., 1998).

In addition to exercising regularly, a woman can lower her risk of breast cancer by not drinking alcoholic beverages. The intake of three or more alcoholic drinks per week increases a woman's risk of developing breast cancer. Women who drink alcohol while taking estrogen replacement therapy may as much as triple their blood levels of the hormone (Ginsburg, 1999; Ginsburg et al., 1997). Therefore, a woman should consult her physician for advice on balancing the benefit of drinking a few glasses of wine per week to reduce her risk of cardiovascular disease against the increased risk of breast cancer.

Women who live in Western countries (North America and Northern Europe) have five to six times the risk of developing breast cancer as women who live in Asia and Africa. Evidence suggests that this association is not genetic but is connected to lifestyle or environmental factors that have yet to be discovered. Approximately 75% of women diagnosed with breast cancer have no identifiable risk factors other than that they are from a Western culture.

Early Detection Three methods are generally used to detect breast cancer as early as possible: the breast self-examination, the breast clinical examination, and mammography, although breast self-examination (BSE) is considered optional by the American Cancer Society because research results do not show that monthly BSE saves lives (ACS, 2003). However, women should become aware of how their breasts normally feel and report any breast change to a health care professional immediately. The breast clinical examination is performed by a health care professional. The ACS recommends that a clinical examination be performed every 3 years for women from ages 20 to 39, and every year thereafter (see Managing Your Health, page 348).

Mammography is the process of taking x rays of breast tissue to detect benign and malignant growths. As you can see in Figure 13-9, each breast is placed over a plate containing x-ray film, and the tissue is compressed. The ACS recommends that women aged 40 and older have a mammogram every year. Women at high risk for breast cancer, such as those with a strong family history of the disease, should consult their physicians regarding the need for mammograms on a different schedule (e.g., at an earlier age, or more often).

Figure 13-9 **Mammography.** Each breast is placed on a platform, and the tissue is compressed while the x ray is taken.

If screening reveals a suspicious mass in the breast tissue, a physician usually performs a biopsy. To perform this procedure, a physician inserts a fine needle into the mass and withdraws cells. An individual trained to detect cancer studies the cells to determine if the growth is malignant. Fine-needle biopsy is relatively painless and is about 90% accurate.

Treatment Data suggest that a **lumpectomy**, surgical removal of the tumor, followed by breast irradiation is appropriate therapy for women with a breast tumor measuring 4 cm (about $1\frac{1}{2}$ in.) or less in diameter. The surgeon also removes a layer of normal tissue surrounding the tumor so that it is less likely that cancer tissue is left in the breast. The physician removes some lymph nodes under the nearby armpit to determine if the cancer has spread. Six or seven weeks of radiation therapy typically follows lumpectomy. Data show that lumpectomy is as effective as **total mastectomy** (removal of the entire breast and involved lymph nodes) in patients with tumors of this size (ACS, 2001).

Women with breast malignancies larger than 4 cm may need more aggressive surgery. In a **radical mastectomy**, the surgeon removes the entire breast and underlying muscle as well as the underarm lymph nodes and fat. In a **modified radical mastectomy**, underlying muscle is not removed. However, these procedures are performed much less often than in the past because lumpectomy followed by radiation therapy has been so successful in curing breast cancers (ACS, 2001).

Today hormonal therapy is often used to treat advanced breast cancer. The primary drug used is tamoxifen (Kotwall, 1999), an antiestrogen. It counteracts the effects of estrogen on breast cancers that depend on estrogen for their growth. It has few serious side effects compared to other anticancer drugs and positively affects approximately one-third of patients for whom it is prescribed.

Chemotherapy is also used to treat breast cancer (sometimes in conjunction with tamoxifen), but many anticancer drugs have serious side effects and breast cancer is only moderately sensitive to such agents. However, in recent years new compounds have been discovered that have demonstrated good antitumor activity in breast cancer treatment. These drugs are called taxanes. The drug taxol was the first of this group to be discovered. (Taxol is found in the bark of the Pacific yew tree [*Taxus brevifolia*].) Taxane drugs play a significant role in breast cancer therapy (Hudis, 1999).

Endometrial Cancer The endometrium is the lining of the uterus, the organ in which a fetus develops until birth (see Chapter 5). Endometrial cancer most often occurs in postmenopausal women; only 15% to 25% of endometrial cancers occur in premenopausal women. The primary symptom of this cancer is abnormal uterine bleeding. Premenopausal women usually experience symptoms of irregular, heavy, or prolonged uterine bleeding during menstrual periods or bleeding between periods. Postmenopausal women experience uterine bleeding although they no longer have menstrual periods.

Most endometrial cancer is usually diagnosed at an early stage because of postmenopausal bleeding. The Pap test for cervical cancer does not detect cancer in the body of the uterus. (This test will be discussed shortly.) However, if the physician suspects that a patient has endometrial cancer, he or she usually performs an endometrial biopsy, in which a sample of tissue is removed from the endometrium and examined microscopically.

Although the cause of endometrial cancer is unknown, it is associated with prolonged exposure to estrogen. Therefore, the risk factors for endometrial cancer are similar to those for breast cancer: early menarche, late menopause, not bearing children, and delaying pregnancy. Research results suggest that estrogen replacement therapy without the accompanying ovarian hormone progesterone (unopposed ERT) is a risk factor as well. Using oral contraceptives that combine estrogen and progesterone appears to decrease the risk of endometrial cancer. Additionally, women who are more than 50 pounds overweight, especially postmenopausal women, have a tenfold greater risk for developing endometrial cancer than women who are not overweight.

Most women diagnosed with endometrial cancer undergo total hysterectomy: removal of the uterus, fallopian tubes, and ovaries. Additionally, certain types of radiation therapy are sometimes used after surgery. The outlook for survival after treatment for endometrial cancer is good: About 90% of patients with endometrial cancer survive their disease.

Cancers Related to Viral Infection: Cervical Cancer

Certain viruses are implicated in the development of a variety of cancers; Table 13-6 lists these viruses and the cancers to which they are related. However, viruses alone do not appear to cause cancer. Scientists think that interactions between these viruses and other agents, or co-carcinogens, result in the development of cancer. For example, the high incidence of liver cancer

lumpectomy
(lum-PECK-toe-me) surgical removal of a breast tumor, including a layer of surrounding tissue.

total mastectomy
(mas-TEK-toe-me) surgical removal of a breast and involved lymph nodes for the treatment of breast cancer.

radical mastectomy
surgical removal of a breast, underlying muscle, and underarm fat and lymph nodes as a treatment for breast cancer.

Table 13-6

Table 13-6 Viruses and Cancers to Which They Are Related

Virus	Cancer Type
Hepatitis B virus (HBV)	Primary liver cancer
Human T-cell lymphotropic/ leukemia virus (HTLV)	Adult T-cell lymphoma/ leukemia
Cytomegalovirus (CMV)	Kaposi's sarcoma
Human papillomavirus (HPV)	Cervical cancer, penile cancer
Epstein-Barr virus (EBV)	Burkitt's lymphoma, nasopharyngeal cancer

in certain regions of Africa and Asia appears to be caused by interactions between the hepatitis B virus and aflatoxins. Aflatoxins are a group of carcinogens produced by a mold that grows on improperly stored peanuts and grains. Many people in these regions eat these moldy foods.

The virally related cancer most prevalent in the United States is cervical cancer. Since 1960 the incidence of cervical cancer has declined by 63%, primarily because of the widespread routine use of the **Papanicolaou test (Pap test)** to screen women for cervical cancer. To perform the Pap test, a physician or other specially trained health care professional takes a sample of cells from the cervical canal. These cells are examined under a microscope.

Papanicolaou test (Pap test) (PAP-eh-nik-eh-LOUW) a screening procedure for cervical cancer in which cells from the cervical canal are removed and then smeared on a glass slide for microscopic examination.

Most women who are diagnosed with cervical cancer have no symptoms; their cancers are discovered at an early stage during their annual gynecologic examination and Pap test. If undiagnosed, the cancer may cause symptoms of abnormal vaginal bleeding (the most common symptom), pelvic pressure or pain, and/or a foul-smelling vaginal discharge.

Cervical cancer most often develops in young women, generally between the ages of 20 and 40 years, peaking at approximately age 30. If untreated, cervical cancer can invade surrounding tissues and metastasize. Having regular screening tests can reduce the risk of developing invasive cancer of the cervix.

A causal association exists between human papilloma virus (HPV) and cervical cancer. HPV is transmitted by infected men to their female partners during sexual intercourse, and vice versa. Therefore, the greater the number of male sexual partners a woman has over time, the greater are her chances of becoming infected with HPV. If a woman is monogamous but her male sex partner is not, her risk rises because he is more likely to become infected than if he were monogamous. Also, women who had their first sexual intercourse before age 17 are at increased risk because they are more likely to have a greater number of sexual partners over time than those women who became sexually active at an older age.

At low risk for cervical cancer are women who are celibate, such as Roman Catholic nuns, or who are monogamous with a monogamous partner over many years. Sexually active women with multiple partners or with nonmonogamous partners can lower their risk by using male or female condoms to protect themselves against infection with HPV.

Scientists are studying possible HPV co-carcinogens. The most documented co-carcinogen is tobacco smoke. Women who are infected with HPV and who smoke cigarettes are more likely to develop cervical cancer; the carcinogens of tobacco smoke affect the cervix by passing out of the blood and into the cervical mucus. Additionally, oral contraceptives have been shown to confer an increased risk for cervical cancer in HPV-infected women. Conflicting data exist regarding herpes simplex virus type II (HSV-II) as a co-carcinogen. (See Chapter 14 for more information concerning HPV and herpes viruses.)

The American Cancer Society recommends that all women should have annual conventional Pap tests or biannual liquid-based Pap tests 3 years after their first vaginal intercourse but no later than age 21. The ACS suggests that after three consecutive normal Pap tests, women over 30 may have this test performed every 2 to 3 years or at the discretion of their physicians.

If the Pap test shows that cervical cancer may be present, a physician usually performs a *colposcopy*. Using a specially designed microscope, the physician examines the cervix. If the physician observes abnormal cervical tissue during this procedure, he or she usually performs a biopsy to confirm the diagnosis.

Physicians treat dysplasia or cervical cancers in situ with surgery, electrocoagulation, cryotherapy, and carbon dioxide (CO_2) laser surgery. Laser energy destroys the tissue. Cryotherapy is the use of extreme cold to destroy cells. Usually solid carbon dioxide or liquid nitrogen is applied briefly to the abnormal tissue with a sterile cotton-tipped applicator. A blister forms and the tissue dies. Electrocoagulation kills the tissue through intense heat by electric current.

With invasive cervical cancers, surgeons may perform a simple hysterectomy (removal of just the uterus) or a total hysterectomy (removal of the uterus and ovaries). With certain cervical cancers, radiation is the treatment of choice. Detected early, cervical cancer is highly survivable.

Cancers Related to Ultraviolet Radiation: Skin Cancers

Lying on the beach or on a tanning bed to develop a tanned "healthy" look is anything but healthy! When skin tans it is a sign of skin damage. Certain skin cells produce a pigment called *melanin* to protect the skin from the damaging rays of the sun. Melanin is a built-in sun protector for dark-skinned people and is produced in response to sun damage in light-skinned people. In addition to causing the skin to wrinkle and age prematurely, the ultraviolet (UV) radiation in sunlight can result in the development of skin cancer. In fact, UV light exposure is the most important factor (other than heredity and age) that influences the development of skin cancer.

There are three types of ultraviolet radiation: UVA, UVB, and UVC. All three types are harmful and have the potential to cause skin cancer. Claims by tanning parlors that using only UVB rays will protect you from the effects of UV radiation are false. This type of ultraviolet radiation is associated with sunburn and skin cancer formation, as is UVA radiation. UVA radiation is also strongly associated with premature aging effects. Artificial UV sources, such as sun lamps and tanning beds, may also generate UVC rays. UVC radiation is a highly potent cancer-causing radiation. Although a danger from artificial sources, these rays are filtered out by the Earth's atmosphere and pose little danger from environmental sources.

There are three main types of skin cancer: basal cell carcinoma, squamous cell carcinoma, and malignant melanoma. Approximately 60% of skin cancers are basal cell carcinomas and approximately 30% are squamous cell carcinomas. Although malignant melanoma makes up less than 10% of skin cancers, this fast-growing, metastasizing cancer results in the most deaths. Malignant melanoma spreads quickly via the blood and lymph. Death is usually due to either respiratory failure or to brain or spinal cord complications. Table 13-7 lists steps for preventing skin cancer.

Basal cell carcinoma, the most common cancer of the skin, often affects persons older than 40 years of age. A slow-growing cancer that rarely metastasizes, basal cell carcinoma frequently develops on portions of the skin exposed to the sun: the face, head, neck, and arms. Lesions may look like moles or chronic pimples with pearl-like borders. They often become crusty and scaly and may ulcerate and bleed Figure 13-10a. Basal cell carcinoma tumors are usually removed by surgery and cryotherapy, freezing with liquid nitrogen. The cure rate for basal cell carcinoma is high.

Squamous cell carcinoma is the second most common skin cancer in light-skinned persons; it develops in the same sun-exposed areas as does basal cell carcinoma. However, dark-skinned people *can* develop this type of cancer, not from sunlight exposure, but from exposure to noxious chemicals and high levels of x rays, as well as from trauma (burns and chronic ulcers). The skin lesions of squamous cell carcinoma look flat, red, scaling, and may be slightly elevated Figure 13-10b. These tumors are removed by the same methods as basal cell carcinoma.

Both basal and squamous cell carcinomas develop from prolonged, repeated exposures to the sun. At risk are persons who are outdoors much of the time, such as construction workers, farmers, and people who regularly sunbathe.

Malignant melanoma is a deadly skin cancer. It is the most frequent cancer in women aged 25 to 29 and is the second most frequent cancer in women aged 30 to 34. (Breast cancer is the most frequent cancer of this age group.) Half of all melanoma victims are younger than 50.

During the 1970s, the incidence rate of melanoma increased about 6% per year. Since 1981, however, the rate of increase has slowed to a little less than 3% per year. The risk for developing malignant melanoma and other skin cancers is higher the closer a person lives to the equator because of the increasing intensity of UV rays. Additionally, fair-skinned people are at greater risk than those who have darker skin. Incidence rates are more than 10 times higher in whites

basal cell carcinoma (BAY-sl) the most common cancer of the skin, which frequently develops on portions of the skin exposed to the sun.

squamous cell carcinoma (SKWAY-muss) a common form of skin cancer that develops from exposure to noxious chemicals and high levels of x rays, as well as from trauma.

malignant melanoma (MEL-ah-NO-mah) a deadly form of skin cancer that develops most often in persons who have been exposed to the sun in short, intense sessions, have had severe sunburn and extensive sun exposure in childhood, or have first-degree relatives who had the disease.

Table 13-7	Steps to Reduce the Risk of Melanoma and Other Skin Cancers

- Do not use tanning beds.
- Avoid exposure to the sun (particularly sunbathing), especially between 10 A.M. and 4 P.M. when UV radiation is highest.
- When in the sun, wear sunglasses that block at least 99% of UVA and UVB radiation. Larger glasses and wraparounds provide the best protection.
- When in the sun, wear wide-brimmed hats and clothing that covers as much as possible of the arms, legs, and torso.
- Use sunscreens with a sun protection factor (SPF) of 15 or higher regularly on sun-exposed skin.

(a)

Figure 13-10 **Skin Cancers.**
(a) This basal cell carcinoma is on the cheek of a man. It is a raised lesion with central depressions that bleed and crust over. (b) Squamous cell carcinoma looks like a red rounded mass or a flat sore as shown in the photo. (c) Lesions of malignant melanoma are characterized by irregular borders with red, white, blue, or blue-black spots. Some portions may be raised.

(b)

(c)

than in African Americans (ACS, 2004a). At highest risk are persons with light blue eyes, very light hair, and skin that burns easily and freckles rather than tans. Malignant melanoma develops more often in persons who are exposed to the sun in short intense sessions, such as persons who work indoors and then vacation in a sunny climate. Severe sunburn and extensive sun exposure in childhood also increase the risk for developing malignant melanoma in adulthood. Additionally, first-degree relatives of people with melanoma have a two- to eightfold increase in their

risk of developing this cancer. Individuals who have two or more relatives with a history of melanoma may be at substantially higher risk.

Malignant melanoma can develop on any skin surface as well as in the eye and on mucous membranes. In men, the trunk is the most common site; in women, the legs are a common site. If you are in a high-risk group for skin cancer, especially melanoma, examine your skin regularly. Early detection is key to curing this disease. Typically, melanoma tumors are asymmetrical, have irregular borders, multiple colors (such as blue, black, red, or gray), and have a diameter greater than a pencil eraser Figure 13-10c. An easy way to remember these signs is ABCD: asymmetry, border, color, and diameter.

A *Healthy People 2010* goal is to increase to at least 75% the proportion of persons aged 18 or older who use at least one of the following protective measures: limit sun exposure, use sunscreens and protective clothing when exposed to sunlight, and avoid artificial sources of UV light. Baseline data from the *Healthy People 2010* report (USDHHS, 2000) show, however, that this goal is far from being realized. Only 28% of U.S. adults reported that they limited their exposure to the sun, 31% said that they used sunscreen routinely, and 24% noted that they wore protective clothing. Forty-seven percent regularly used at least one protective measure. Nevertheless, the *Healthy People 2010* progress review of 2002 projected that the melanoma objective would be met by 2010—2.5 melanoma cancer deaths per 100,000, down 11% from 2.8 deaths per 100,000 in 1998.

Cancers with Unknown Causes

Prostate Cancer The prostate is a walnut-sized accessory sex organ in men. It lies beneath the bladder, surrounding the urethra, and secretes part of the seminal fluid. (See Chapter 5 for more information on this gland.)

Prostate cancer is the most prevalent cancer in men, and the second most prevalent cause of cancer deaths in men (see Table 13-3). (Lung cancer is the most prevalent cause of cancer death in men.) The signs and symptoms of prostate cancer mimic those of benign prostatic hypertrophy (BPH) and other noncancerous conditions of the prostate (see page 126). Therefore, experiencing symptoms that include uneven flow of urine while urinating, incomplete emptying of the bladder, reduced urine flow, and urinating more frequently at night does not necessarily mean a man has prostate cancer. However, serious signs and symptoms that are more likely to be related to prostate cancer are pain in the floor of the pelvis, sudden development of impotence, and presence of blood in the urine.

Men living in Western countries are more likely to develop prostate cancer. Scientists suspect that a high-fat diet, which is characteristic of the Western world, may contribute to the development of prostate cancer (ACS, 2004a). Race also plays a role in one's risk of this disease. African Americans have about a 30% higher risk than that of Caucasians, while Native American men and Asians living in the United States have the lowest incidence. Men with certain occupations also have higher rates of prostate cancer: loggers, chemists, farmers, textile workers, painters, and rubber tire workers. However, researchers are unsure which factors related to working in these environments influence the development of this disease.

Advanced age and heredity are also strong risk factors for prostate cancer. This disease is rare in men younger than 45 years, but its incidence rises as men age. More than 70% of prostate cancers are diagnosed in men 65 years or older (ACS, 2004a). Also, if a man's father or brother had prostate cancer, he may have as much as an 11-fold increase in risk and may be stricken before age 50.

Scientists have been unsuccessful in determining the cause of or other risk factors for prostate cancer. Obesity and a diet high in fat may also be risk factors (ACS, 2004a). The results of studies strongly suggest that vitamin A may lessen the risk of developing prostate cancer. The body converts beta-carotene found in abundance in leafy dark green vegetables, and yellow/orange fruits and vegetables, into vitamin A. Also, a particular pigment in tomatoes called lycopene appears to have a protective effect.

For early detection of prostate cancer, the American Cancer Society and the American Urological Association recommend that all men older than 50 have an annual digital rectal exam and annual prostate specific antigen (PSA) test. During the digital rectal exam, a physician inserts a gloved finger into the rectum to feel the prostate gland (see page 126). The PSA is a blood test that detects a protein secreted by the prostate. If the protein concentration in the blood is elevated, it indicates that the prostate may be abnormal but not necessarily cancerous, and should be checked further. Chapter 5 describes methods of screening the prostate.

Physicians may treat localized prostate cancer by surgically removing the prostate. However, this treatment can result in impotence, incontinence, and other complications. New surgical techniques with fewer side effects have been developed, leading to a resurgence of prostate surgery as a treatment. Advanced prostate cancer is sometimes treated with drug/hormone therapy or by removal of the testicles to reduce male sex hormone levels, which may influence the progression of this cancer. Medical researchers are currently experimenting with implanting tiny radioactive particles in the prostate to destroy the cancer, and with using cryotherapy to destroy the gland.

Prostate cancer is, in many cases, a slow-growing cancer. Data show that about 95% of prostate cancer patients ultimately die with prostate cancer rather than of it. Therefore, studies are being conducted to determine if treating prostate cancers makes a difference in patient survival rates. Because the side effects of prostate cancer treatment can be quite serious, physicians carefully consider "watchful waiting" as the treatment of choice for this cancer (ACS, 2004a).

Testicular Cancer The testicles, or testes, are the organs in which sperm develop and are located in the scrotal sac beneath the penis. Cancer of the testicles is a rare and highly curable cancer. Only 1% of cancers in men occur in the testicles.

The signs and symptoms of testicular cancer are a painless, swollen testis and a sensation of heaviness or aching in the testis. Men who perform testicular self-examination might feel a small lump in one testis.

Youth is a risk factor for testicular cancer. Additionally, research results show that teenage boys who exercise regularly and those with physically demanding jobs in their 20s may be more likely to develop testicular cancer than less active boys and young men (Srivastava & Kreiger, 2000). This cancer strikes primarily teenagers and men between the ages of 15 and 35. Its incidence declines steadily after age 40. Another risk factor for testicular cancer is the failure of one or both of the testicles to descend into the scrotum by age 6 years. As with breast and prostate cancer, testicular cancer occurs most frequently in Western countries. Its incidence is lowest in Asia and Africa. Caucasian males are at highest risk, Latino males are at less risk, and African American men are at least risk.

To detect testicular cancer early, the American Cancer Society recommends that men perform a **testicular self-examination (TSE)** once a month after a warm bath or shower (see the Managing Your Health box). The heat relaxes the scrotal skin, making tumors easier to

testicular self-examination (TSE) (tes-TIK-you-lar) a self-screening test that males can perform to detect cancer of the testicles.

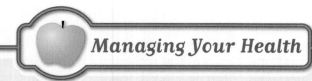
Testicular Self-Examination

A simple procedure called testicular self-exam (TSE) can increase the chances of finding a tumor early. Men should perform TSE once a month—after a warm bath or shower. The heat causes the scrotal skin to relax, making it easier to find anything unusual. TSE is simple and only takes a few minutes.

- Examine each testicle gently with both hands. The index and middle fingers should be placed underneath the testicle while the thumbs are placed on the top. Roll the testicle gently between the thumbs and fingers. One testicle may be larger than the other. This is normal.
- The epididymis is a cordlike structure on the top and back of the testicle that stores and transports the sperm. Do not confuse the epididymis with an abnormal lump.

- Feel for any abnormal lumps—about the size of a pea—on the front or the side of the testicle. These lumps are usually painless.

If you do find a lump, contact your doctor right away. The lump may be due to an infection, and a doctor can decide the proper treatment. If the lump is not an infection, it is likely to be cancer. Remember that testicular cancer is highly curable, especially when detected and treated early. Testicular cancer almost always occurs in only one testicle, and the other testicle is all that is needed for full sexual function.

Routine testicular self-exams are important, but they cannot substitute for a doctor's examination. Your doctor should examine your testicles when you have a physical exam. You also can ask your doctor to check the way you do TSE.

Source: National Cancer Institute (NIH Publication No. 93-2636).

---

detect. If detected and treated early, testicular cancer is one of the most curable cancers. Chemotherapy is most often used; radiation and surgery are also used in some cases.

Ovarian Cancer The ovaries are female organs in which eggs mature and are ovulated each month. Ovaries also produce the female sex hormones estrogen and progesterone. Cancer of the ovaries is difficult to detect, especially in its early stages when most women have no symptoms. However, as the cancer progresses and the ovarian tumor enlarges, many women develop symptoms such as frequent urination or bloating and pressure in the abdomen. Thus, advanced ovarian cancer is confused frequently with other urinary and gastrointestinal tract disorders. Additionally, postmenopausal women may experience vaginal bleeding, while premenopausal women may have irregular or heavy menses.

Eighty-five to 90% of ovarian cancers develop in postmenopausal women; only 10% to 15% are diagnosed in premenopausal patients. The median age for developing ovarian cancer is 60 to 65 years. Other than advanced age, the risk factors for ovarian cancer are similar to those of breast and endometrial cancer: early menarche, late menopause, and not bearing children. The links between these risk factors and ovarian cancer, however, are not as well defined as they are in breast

and endometrial cancer. Additional risk factors are living in a Western country and being obese (ACS, 2004a).

Research shows that the use of oral contraceptives that contain both estrogen and progesterone lower a woman's risk of developing ovarian cancer. Most studies show that for each year a woman uses oral contraceptives, her risk of ovarian cancer decreases by 40% to 50% (LaVecchia & Franceschi, 1999). Estrogen replacement therapy without progesterone increases a woman's risk of this cancer (ACS, 2004a).

The cause of ovarian cancer is unknown. Hereditary factors seem to play a role in only 3% to 4% of ovarian malignancies. Even though the risk factors mentioned previously have been defined, almost all cases of ovarian cancer seem to arise in patients for whom there is no apparent risk factor or genetic predisposition.

A reliable means of detecting ovarian cancer in its early stages has not yet been developed. There is a blood test for ovarian cancer, but it detects only 50% of ovarian cancers. During a pelvic examination, a physician feels a woman's ovaries in an attempt to detect abnormal growths. Almost three-fourths of patients have advanced disease by the time it is diagnosed.

If a physician suspects that a woman has ovarian cancer, a reliable diagnosis may be possible only through surgery. Ultrasound techniques (see page 104) are also used occasionally to confirm the diagnosis of ovarian cancer. Treatment for ovarian cancer involves removal of the cancerous ovary and chemotherapy. Radiation is occasionally used.

Healthy Living Practices

- To lower your risk of developing lung cancer, do not smoke cigarettes, avoid inhaling airborne asbestos fibers, and avoid exposure to radon gas.
- If you are exposed to lung carcinogens at your place of work, explore ways to avoid future exposure.
- To prevent the development of larynx, mouth, and esophagus cancers, avoid smoking and chewing tobacco, and excessive drinking of alcoholic beverages.
- Have a complete oral examination annually for early cancer detection.
- To lower your risk of developing cancer of the bladder and kidney, avoid smoking cigarettes.
- To lower your risk of pancreatic cancer, avoid smoking cigarettes and inhaling chemical fumes.
- To lower your risk of developing stomach cancer, avoid eating salt-cured, nitrate-cured, or smoked foods. Also avoid smoking cigarettes and drinking excessive amounts of alcoholic beverages.
- To reduce your risk of developing colorectal cancer, follow the American Cancer Society's screening guidelines.
- If you are female, you can reduce your risk of breast cancer by exercising and avoiding alcoholic beverages.
- To detect breast cancer in its early stages, follow the ACS guidelines for breast clinical examination and mammography.
- If you are female, you can reduce your risk of developing endometrial cancer by losing weight if you are overweight, and by controlling diabetes mellitus if you have this disease.
- Discuss the impact of estrogen replacement therapy on the development of endometrial cancer with your health care provider if you are considering or are taking this medication.

- If you are female and older than 40 years, have annual pelvic examinations for early detection of endometrial cancer.
- If you are a sexually active woman with multiple partners or with nonmonogamous partners, you can lower your risk of cervical cancer by using male or female condoms to protect yourself against HPV.
- All women can lower their risk of cervical cancer by avoiding cigarette smoking.
- If you have been sexually active and are age 21 or older, the American Cancer Society recommends that you have annual Pap tests to screen for cervical cancer. See the ACS guidelines for detailed recommendations.
- To protect against skin cancer, stay out of the sun and wear sunscreen when outdoors.
- Detect melanoma early by checking your skin for growths that exhibit these warning signs: asymmetry, irregular border, multiple colors, and large diameter.
- If you are male and older than 50, talk to your health care provider about annual digital rectal exams and PSA tests for the early detection of prostate cancer.
- If you are male, perform a testicular self-examination once every month to detect this cancer early.

■ Reducing Your Risk for Cancer

You cannot change some of your cancer risk factors: heredity, age, ethnicity, lifelong exposure to naturally produced estrogen (in women), and the nondescent of testes (in male children). However, you can avoid many risk factors, thereby reducing your risk of developing one or more cancers. The Managing Your Health box entitled "Reducing Your Risk for Cancer" lists modifiable cancer risks and actions you can take to lower your risk.

A summary of the American Cancer Society's recommendations for the early detection of cancer is listed in the Managing Your Health box on page 348. Finally, the Managing Your Health box on page 373 lists cancer's seven warning signs. In addition to being aware of these signs, you can learn the more detailed early warning signs for the various cancers described in this chapter. If you have concerns about your risk of developing cancer, discuss them with your health care provider. Early detection and treatment are critical to winning the war against cancer.

Cancer

Most cancers arise in people older than 50 years, and the risk continues to rise as people grow older. The only cancers described in this chapter that are prevalent in young adults are malignant melanoma, testicular cancer, cervical cancer, and breast cancer. Additionally, only 1% of cancers occur in children. However, cancer is the most frequent cause of death from disease in American children older than 1 year of age. The most prevalent cancers of children up to 5 years old are listed in Table 13-8 .

Adult cancers rarely occur in children. These cancers are largely related to the effects of cancer-causing agents acting on cells over a lifetime, while children's cancers seem more often related to genetic factors.

Although pediatric cancers usually grow more rapidly than adult cancers, they are, in general, more responsive to anticancer drugs than are adult cancers. For this reason chemotherapy is the treatment of choice for most childhood cancers, while surgery and radiation are the primary treatments for adult cancers. Effective cancer chemotherapy has produced a remarkable decline in childhood deaths due to cancer over the past 25 years.

Table 13-8	The Most Prevalent Cancers of Children up to Age 5
Leukemia (cancer of the blood)	
Central nervous system cancers	
Lymphomas (cancer of the lymph nodes)	
Nervous system tumors (often in adrenal glands)	
Wilms' tumor (cancer of the kidney)	
Bone cancer	
Retinoblastoma (cancer of the eye)	
Liver cancer	

Managing Your Health

Reducing Your Risk for Cancer

DO'S

- Eat a diet low in red meats, especially high-fat and processed meats.
- Eat a variety of fruits and vegetables daily.
- Follow the American Cancer Society's recommendations for screening tests to detect cancer in its early stages.
- Men should perform monthly testicular self-examinations.
- Know the warning signs of cancer and see your health care provider immediately if you detect any of them.
- Sexually active women with multiple partners or with nonmonogamous partners should use male or female condoms during sexual intercourse to protect themselves against infection with human papillomavirus.
- Maintain a healthy weight.
- Women should consult their health care providers regarding the use of oral contraceptives and estrogen replacement therapy with respect to cancer prevention and risk.
- Exercise most days of the week.
- When in the sun, wear wide-brimmed hats and sunglasses that block UV radiation.
- Wear sunscreen on sun-exposed skin.

DON'TS

- Don't smoke cigarettes. If you can't quit, cut down.
- Avoid breathing environmental tobacco smoke.
- Don't chew tobacco products.
- Don't drink excessive amounts of alcoholic beverages.
- Women should avoid drinking alcoholic beverages to reduce the risk of breast cancer.
- Avoid unnecessary exposure to ionizing radiation, such as x rays and ultraviolet light.
- Don't lie in the sun or in tanning beds.
- Avoid direct sun exposure between 10 A.M. and 4 P.M.
- Avoid exposure to toxic chemicals, such as certain occupational carcinogens.
- Avoid inhaling chemical fumes, such as gasoline fumes.
- Avoid breathing asbestos dust and radon gas.
- Avoid eating salt-cured, nitrate-cured, or smoked foods.

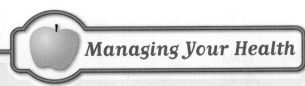

Cancer's Seven Warning Signs

You can remember the following signs easily by knowing that they are a CAUTION— these signs do not necessarily mean you have cancer but that you should see your health care provider to evaluate the sign.

Change in bowel or bladder habits
A sore that does not heal
Unusual bleeding or discharge
Thickening or lump in breast or elsewhere
Indigestion or difficulty in swallowing
Obvious change in a wart or mole
Nagging cough or hoarseness

CHAPTER REVIEW

Summary

Cancer is a variety of diseases that have common characteristics: Their cells exhibit abnormal growth, division, and differentiation and have the potential to spread from where they develop. These cells form masses called malignant tumors that interfere with normal body processes.

Cancer develops in cells that have damaged or mutated genes. Mutations can be inherited or can occur from exposure to low-dose radiation, drugs, toxic chemicals, or certain viruses. Successive genetic changes must take place for a normal cell to change into a cancer cell. Therefore, the probability of developing cancer generally increases with age and with exposure to cancer-causing substances.

This chapter organizes the discussion of cancers according to factors that appear to be most significant in their development. Advanced age is a risk factor for most cancers; heredity is a significant risk factor in some cancers.

Cancers caused by tobacco use are lung, larynx, oral cavity, esophageal, kidney, bladder, pancreatic, stomach, acute myeloid leukemia, and cervical cancer. To lower the risk of developing any of these cancers, avoid smoking and chewing tobacco products. Additionally, avoid drinking excessive amounts of alcoholic beverages to lower the risk of developing larynx, oral, and esophageal cancer. Have a complete oral examination annually for early cancer detection in this area.

Diet accounts for a significant number of cancers, and has both a positive and a negative effect on the development of cancer. A primary risk factor in the development of stomach cancer is eating salt-cured, nitrate-cured, or smoked foods. To lower the risk of developing this cancer, avoid eating these foods. To reduce the risk of developing colorectal cancer, avoid having more than one alcoholic drink per day and eat a diet high in vegetables and fruits. People older than 50 years of age should have a fecal occult blood test annually and a sigmoidoscopy every 5 years. Refer to the ACS recommendations for more details.

The cancers related to hormone function are breast cancer and endometrial cancer. These cancers are associated significantly with prolonged exposure to estrogen. Risk factors associated with these cancers are early menarche, late menopause, not bearing children, and delaying pregnancy. Exercising helps reduce breast cancer risk in women. Avoiding alcoholic beverages also reduces the risk. For early cancer detection, women aged 20 to 39 years should have a breast clinical examination every 3 years, and every year at age 40 and after. Women aged 40 and older should have a mammography every year. For early detection of endometrial cancer, women at menopause should report any unexpected bleeding or spotting to their physician.

Certain viruses are implicated in the development of a variety of cancers. The virally related cancer most prevalent in the United States is cervical cancer. The virus implicated in this disease, human papilloma virus (HPV), is transmitted by infected men to their female partners during sexual intercourse, and vice versa. Sexually active women with multiple partners or with nonmonogamous partners can lower their risk of cervical cancer by using male or female condoms to protect themselves against HPV. Women can also lower their risk by avoiding cigarette smoking.

The ultraviolet radiation in sunlight is the most important factor that influences the development of cancer of the skin. There are three main types of skin cancer: basal cell carcinoma, squamous cell carcinoma, and malignant melanoma. Malignant melanoma results in the most deaths of these cancers because it is a fast-growing metastatic cancer. Light-skinned, fair-haired Caucasians are a high-risk group for developing skin cancer. To protect against skin cancer, stay out of the sun and wear sunscreen when outdoors. Detect melanoma early by checking your skin for growths exhibiting these warning signs: asymmetry, irregular border, multiple colors, and large diameter.

Cancers with unknown causes include prostate cancer, testicular cancer, and ovarian cancer. The risk factors for prostate cancer are age and heredity. For early detection of this cancer, men older than 50 should have annual digital rectal exams and prostate specific antigen blood tests. Men between the ages of 15 and 35 are at the highest risk for testicular cancer. For early detection of this disease, all males older than 15 should perform monthly testicular self-examinations. Ovarian cancer is primarily a disease of postmenopausal women.

Childhood cancers, although rare, are the most frequent cause of death from disease in American children older than 1 year. Children develop cancers due to hereditary or developmental reasons. Occasionally environmental agents are the cause. Treatment for childhood cancers is highly effective.

Applying What You Have Learned

1. Imagine that you or a female friend had an annual Pap test. The report from the lab stated that cells exhibiting dysplasia were seen in the smear. What does this statement mean? How would these cells look different from normal cells? What would be your or your friend's next course of action? `Application`

2. List three cancer risk factors over which a person has no control. Suppose that at least one of them was a risk factor for you. List this hypothetical (or real) factor and the cancer(s) related to this risk. What might you do regarding cancer prevention if you are aware of this (these) factor(s)? `Application`

3. Your good friend is a heavy drinker, eats lots of spicy food, and experiences heartburn regularly. He takes antacids, but recently they have not helped. He also tells you that he seems to have some difficulty swallowing but he's not quite sure. He thinks it's "all in his head." What would you advise your friend to do? Might cancer be causing his problems? If so, which type? Which symptoms lead you to this conclusion? `Application`

4. List two dietary factors related to the development of cancer and two dietary factors related to low-

ering the risk of cancer. Name the cancers to which these dietary factors relate. Now list, as best you can remember, the foods you ate for the past two days. What is your intake of the types of foods related to cancer development and prevention? Based on this analysis, should you make changes in your diet to lower your risk of certain cancers? `Evaluation`

5. With respect to the cancers discussed in this chapter, which cancer(s) are you at least risk for developing? Why? Which cancers are you at highest risk for developing? Why? `Synthesis`

6. Referring to your answer to question 5, what can you do to lower your risk of developing the cancers for which you are at high risk? State rationales for each suggestion. Why will these lifestyle changes lower your risk? `Evaluation`

Key

`Application`   using information in a new situation.

`Synthesis`   putting together information from different sources.

`Evaluation`   making informed decisions.

Reflecting on Your Health

1. In what ways have your attitudes about cancer changed since reading this chapter?

2. Were you aware of all the ACS recommendations for the early detection of cancer prior to reading this chapter? If you were not, which recommendations were new to you? Will you follow these recommendations? Why or why not? If you were aware of all the ACS recommendations, do you follow those recommendations for your sex and age group? Why or why not?

3. Do you know anyone who has or has had cancer, or have you read stories written by cancer patients

about their disease? What did you learn about cancer from them that affected your life?

4. The highest score one could attain on the Torabi Cancer Prevention Behavior Scale (see the self-assessments in the student workbook) is 150. Take the assessment and compare your score to 150. The closer your score is to 150, the healthier your behavior is regarding cancer prevention. Does your score match your self-perception of your behavior? Did the self-assessment identify behaviors you should change? If so, discuss what you might do to change those behaviors.

References

Ackroyd, R., Kelty, C., Brown, N., & Reed, M. (2001). The history of photodetection and photodynamic therapy. *Photochemistry and Photobiology, 74*: 656–669.

Adlkofer, F. (2001). Lung cancer due to passive smoking—a review. *International Archives of Occupational & Environmental Health, 74*:231–241.

American Cancer Society. (2001). *Breast cancer facts and figures 2001–2002.* Atlanta, GA: American Cancer Society.

American Cancer Society. (2003). *Breast cancer facts and figures, 2003–2004.* Atlanta, GA: Author.

American Cancer Society. (2004a). *Cancer facts and figures, 2004.* Atlanta, GA: Author.

American Cancer Society. (2004b). *Cancer prevention and early detection facts and figures, 2004.* Atlanta, GA: Author.

Bingham, S. A., Luben, R., Welch, A., Wareham, N., Khaw, K., & Day, N. (2003). Are imprecise methods obscuring a relation between fat and breast cancer? *Lancet, 362*:212–214.

Bosetti, C., Altieri, A., & La Vecchia, C. (2002). Diet and environmental carcinogenesis in breast/gynaecological cancers. *Current Opinion in Obstetrics & Gynecology, 14*:13–18.

CHEK2-Breast Cancer Consortium. (2002). Low-penetrance susceptibility to breast cancer due to CHEK2*1100delC in noncarriers of BRCA1 or BRCA2 mutations. *Nature Genetics, 31*:55–59.

Cho, E., Spiegelman, D., Hunter, D. J., Chen, W. Y., Stampfer, M. J., Colditz, G. A., & Willett, W. C. (2003). Premenopausal fat intake and risk of breast cancer. *Journal of the National Cancer Institute, 95*:1079–1085.

Fletcher, R. H. (2000). The end of barium enemas? *New England Journal of Medicine, 342*:1823–1824.

Friedenreich, C. M., Courneya, K. S., & Bryant, H. E. (2002). Case-control study of anthropometric measures and breast cancer risk. *International Journal of Cancer, 99*:445–452.

Genazzani, A. R., & Gambacciani, M. (1999). Hormone replacement therapy: The perspectives for the 21st century. *Maturitas, 32*:11–17.

Ginsburg, E. S. (1999). Estrogen, alcohol, and breast cancer risk. *Journal of Steroid Biochemistry & Molecular Biology, 69*:299–306.

Ginsburg, E. S., Mello, N. K., Mendelson, J. H., Barbieri, R. L., Teoh, S. K., Rothman, M., Gao, X., & Sholar, J. W. (1997). Effects of alcohol ingestion on estrogens in postmenopausal women. *Journal of the American Medical Association, 276*(21):1747–1752.

Giovannucci, E. (1999). The prevention of colorectal cancer by aspirin use. *Biomedicine & Pharmacotherapy, 53*:303–308.

Hardman, A. E. (2001). Physical activity and cancer risk. *Proceedings of the Nutrition Society, 60*:107–113.

Hoffman-Goetz, L., Apter, D., Demark-Wahnefried, W., Goran, M. I., McTiernan, A., & Reichman, M. E. (1998). Possible mechanisms mediating an association between physical activity and breast cancer. *Cancer, 83*(3 Suppl.):621–628.

Hudis, C. A. (1999). The current state of adjuvent therapy for breast cancer: Focus on paclitaxel. *Seminars in Oncology, 26* (1 Suppl. 2):1–5.

Jemal, A., Clegg, L. X., Ward, E., Ries, L. A. G., Wu, X., Jamison, P. M., Wingo, P. A., Howe, H. L., Anderson, R. N., & Edwards, B. K. (2004). Annual report to the nation on the status of cancer, 1975–2001, with a special feature regarding survival. *Cancer, 101*(1):3–27.

Jenks, S. (1994). Breast cancer gene found. *Journal of the National Cancer Institute, 86*:1444–1445.

Kotwall, C. A. (1999). Breast cancer treatment and chemoprevention. *Canadian Family Physician, 45*:1917–1924.

LaVecchia, C., & Franceschi, S. (1999). Oral contraceptives and ovarian cancer. *European Journal of Cancer Prevention, 8*:297–304.

Linehan, D. C., Bowne, W. B., & Lewis, J. J. (1999). Immunotherapeutic approaches to sarcoma. *Seminars in Surgical Oncology, 17*:72–77.

McTiernan, A. (2000). Physical activity and the prevention of breast cancer. *Medscape Women's Health, 5*(5):E1.

McTiernan, A., Kooperberg, C., White, E., Wilcox, S., Coates, R., Adams-Campbell, L. L., Woods, N., & Ockene, J. (2003). Recreational physical activity and the risk of breast cancer in postmenopausal women: The Women's Health Initiative Cohort Study. *Journal of the American Medical Association, 290*:1331–1336.

Nilsson, R. (2001). Environmental tobacco smoke revisited: The reliability of the data used for risk assessment. *Risk Analysis, 21*:737–760.

Shriver, S. P., Boordeau, H. A., Gubish, C. T., Tirpak, D. L., Gaither Davis, A. L., Luketich, J. D., & Siegfried, J. M. (2000). Sex-specific expression of gastrin-releasing peptide receptor: Relationship to smoking history and risk of lung cancer. *Journal of the National Cancer Institute, 92*:24–33.

Srivastava, A., & Krieger, N. (2000). Relation of physical activity to risk of testicular cancer. *American Journal of Epidemiology, 15*:78–87.

Thune, I., & Furberg, A. S. (2001). Physical activity and cancer risk: Dose-response and cancer, all sites and site-specific. *Medicine & Science in Sports & Exercise, 33*(6 suppl.):S530–550.

Traverso, G., Shuber, A., Levin, B., Johnson, C., Olsson, L., Schoetz, D. J., Hamilton, S. R., Boynton, K., Kinzler, K. W., & Vogelstein, B. (2002). Detection of *APC* mutations in fecal DNA from patients with colorectal tumors. *New England Journal of Medicine, 346*:311–320.

U.S. Department of Health and Human Services. (1999a). Radon testing in households with a residential smoker—United States, 1993–1994. *Morbidity and Mortality Weekly Report, 48*:683–686.

U.S. Department of Health and Human Services. (1999b). Tobacco use—United States, 1900–1999. *Morbidity and Mortality Weekly Report, 48*:986–993.

U.S. Department of Health and Human Services. (2000). *Healthy People 2010.* Washington, DC: U.S. Government Printing Office.

U.S. Department of Health and Human Services. (2004) *The health consequences of smoking: A report of the Surgeon General.* Washington, DC: U.S. Government Printing Office.

U.S. Public Health Service. (1964). *Smoking and health: Report of the advisory committee to the Surgeon General of the Public Health Service.* (PHS Publication No. 1103). Atlanta, GA: U.S. Department of Health, Education, and Welfare, Public Health Service, CDC.

Westhoff, C. L. (1999). Breast cancer risk: Perception versus reality. *Contraception, 59*(1 suppl.):25S–28S.

Winawer, S. J., Stewart, E. T., Zauber, A. G., Bond, J. H., Ansel, H., Waye, J. D., Hall, D., Hamlin, A., Schapiro, M., O'Brien, M. J., Sternberg, S. S., & Gottlieb, L. S. (2000). A comparison of colonoscopy and double-contrast barium enema for surveillance after polypectomy. *New England Journal of Medicine, 342*:1766–1772.

Wooster, R., Bignell, G., Sancaster, J., Swift, S., Seal, S., Mangion, J., Collins, N., Gregory, S., Gumbs, C., & Micklem, G. (1995). Identification of the breast cancer susceptibility gene BRCA2. *Nature, 378*(6559):789–792.

Writing Group for the Women's Health Initiative Investigators. (2002). Risks and benefits of estrogen plus progestin in healthy postmenopausal women: Principal results from the Women's Health Initiatives randomized controlled trial. *Journal of the American Medical Association, 288*:321–333.

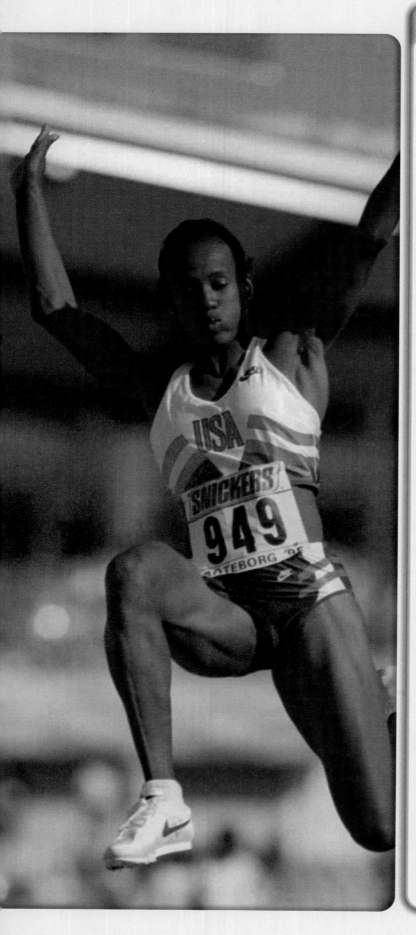

Chapter Overview

Causes of noninfectious diseases

Symptoms of and treatments for noninfectious diseases

Trends in infectious diseases since 1900

How the chain of infection works

How nonspecific and specific immunity work

How to protect yourself against infectious disease

Symptoms of sexually transmitted infections

Treatments and prevention methods for sexually transmitted infections

Diversity in Health
Sickle Cell Disease: Why Does This Deleterious Gene Persist?

Consumer Health
Over-the-Counter Cold Medications: Do They Help?

Managing Your Health
Eliminating or Reducing Your Risk of HIV Infection and Other STIs

Across
THE LIFESPAN

Infectious and Noninfectious Diseases

Student Workbook

Self-Assessment: STI Attitude Scale

Changing Health Habits: Reducing Your Risk of Contracting an STI

Do You Know?

· *How to protect yourself from sexually transmitted infections?*

· *If over-the-counter cold remedies really work?*

· *Which types of diseases you can catch and which you cannot?*

Infection, Immunity, and Noninfectious Disease

Jackie Joyner-Kersee: Olympian gold, silver, and bronze medalist. Some consider Joyner-Kersee the greatest woman athlete ever. At this writing, she is the heptathlon world record holder and the American record holder in the long jump. She has won six Olympic medals, more than any woman in track and field history. Joyner-Kersee officially retired from track and field in 2001.

In late 2004, Joyner-Kersee was honored by USA Track & Field, the national governing body for track and field, long-distance running, and race walking in the United States. They cited Joyner-Kersee's breaking of her own women's heptathlon world record at the 1988 Olympic Games as the ninth greatest moment in U.S. track and field history in the last 25 years. Clearly, exercise-induced asthma has not deterred this outstanding athlete from making her indelible mark in the world of sports, nor has it deterred other athletes.

Exercise-induced asthma is a condition in which the airways narrow after sustained exertion, making it more difficult than usual for a person to breathe. What triggers this problem is the cooling and reheating of the airways as a person exercises. As exercise begins, a person begins to breathe deeply and rapidly. During this deep and rapid inhalation, more air is moistened and warmed in the respiratory passageways than before exercise began, which draws moisture and heat from the airways. After a person is warmed up, the breathing rate falls, and the airways return to their normal temperature. Health scientists do not know how airway cooling and reheating triggers asthma attacks.

Asthma is one of a variety of noninfectious diseases. **Diseases** are processes that affect the proper functioning of the body and are usually accompanied by characteristic signs and symptoms. **Infectious diseases**, such as colds or the flu, are caused by **pathogens**, which are agents of infection: bacteria, rickettsias, viruses, fungi, protozoans, and parasitic worms. (Infectious diseases are discussed later in this chapter.) **Noninfectious diseases** are caused by abnormalities in the hereditary material (genetic diseases), interactions between heredity and environmental

" Exercise-induced asthma has not deterred this outstanding athlete from making her indelible mark in the world of sports . . . "

factors (especially those related to lifestyle, such as asthma), or environmental factors alone, as in repetitive-use injuries or lead poisoning (see Chapter 16, "Environmental Health").

Noninfectious Diseases

Genetic Diseases

There are two types of genetic diseases: inherited diseases and diseases caused by errors when gametes (sex cells) are formed. **Inherited diseases** are transmitted solely by gene transfer from parents to offspring. They occur more frequently among close relatives than in the general population and show patterns in their transmission. For example, an inherited disease may strike only males, or there may be no male-to-male transmission of the disease.

Inherited diseases are caused by disorders of the hereditary material, or genes. Genes carry information about every aspect of an organism and may carry normal instructions in one person and defective instructions in another. A defective gene in the sex cells of an individual can be passed on to a child unless the person dies before reaching reproductive age.

Defective genes arise through mutation. A **mutation** is a change in a gene or a chromosome. Mutations in eggs and sperm can occur for no apparent reason or from exposure to a variety of environmental sources. One source is ionizing radiation such as x rays, which is the reason the dentist places a protective lead shield over your pelvic area when taking x rays of your teeth. Another source of damage to genes is drugs such as lysergic acid diethylamide (lysergide, LSD) or marijuana (*Cannabis sativa*). Chapter 7 describes these drugs and their effects on the body in more detail. Toxic chemicals are a third source of genetic damage. (Poisoning, another effect

of toxic chemicals, is discussed in Chapter 16.) People often come into contact with toxic chemicals in the workplace and do not realize the danger because they feel no ill effects.

Three hereditary diseases that are common in the United States are sickle cell disease, cystic fibrosis, and Duchenne muscular dystrophy. The Diversity in Health essay "Sickle Cell Disease: Why Does This Deleterious Gene Persist?" discusses this hereditary disease, which is common among African Americans.

Cystic fibrosis (CF) is the most common lethal genetic disease in the Caucasian population. (It seldom affects African Americans, Asians, or Jews.) Cystic fibrosis affects the glands that secrete mucus and sweat. In CF patients, the sweat glands produce an abnormally salty secretion and the mucous glands produce an exceptionally thick and sticky secretion that builds up and plugs the ducts of glands and other passageways. Although the pancreas (an organ that secretes digestive juices) is often seriously affected, lung disease accounts for most of the illness and nearly all deaths from CF. Multiple disorders of the lungs arise when mucus blocks the airways. Infections result and breathing becomes impaired. Today a person with CF can expect to live only about 24 years.

Duchenne muscular dystrophy (DMD) is the most common type of muscular dystrophy (*dys* means "abnormal"; *trophy* means "growth"). DMD is a disease in which the muscles gradually weaken and degenerate. It occurs in about 1 in 3,500 to 4,000 newborn males and kills an average of 2 boys per day, usually striking before the age of 6 years. These children are usually slow to walk and talk. Their thigh and pelvic muscles gradually deteriorate, resulting in unsteadiness in standing, walking, climbing stairs, and getting up from a seated position. As the muscles of the shoulder, trunk, and back weaken, the child's spine begins to curve and the posture becomes swayback. This abnormal body posture interferes with the functioning of internal organs, especially the lungs. Although heart problems sometimes cause sudden death in DMD patients, these children and young adults usually die in their teens or 20s of respiratory infections or respiratory failure when the diaphragm (a sheetlike muscle that forms the floor of the chest cavity and that is essential to breathing) becomes affected.

As mentioned previously, the second category of genetic diseases or disorders is caused by errors in cell division that can occur when gametes, or sex cells, are produced in the ovaries or testes. Sometimes eggs or sperm are made that have too many or too few chromosomes; some gametes may be formed in which parts

(a)

(b)

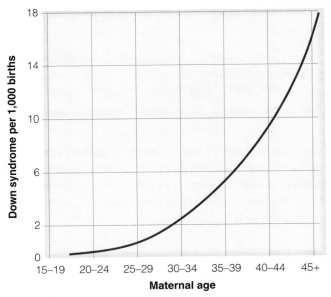

Figure 14-1 **Down Syndrome.** (a) This girl has Down syndrome. She exhibits the stocky build, short hands, and flattened facial features characteristic of this genetic condition. (b) Down syndrome is called *trisomy 21* because it is caused by the presence of an extra 21st chromosome, as shown in the karyotype, the array of chromosomes in a cell. In addition, Down syndrome individuals experience delays in physical and intellectual development. Although some Down syndrome individuals function in the low average range of intellectual capability, the majority function in the mild to moderate range of mental retardation.

of chromosomes have been lost, gained, or moved to new positions. If conception takes place with a gamete that has a severe defect, the usual result is a spontaneous abortion. However, some genetic defects result in a fertilized egg that is capable of developing into a full-term baby. The child may be born with structural or functional problems, or both.

Down syndrome, which affects approximately 1 in 700 to 800 newborns, is a common genetic disorder caused by improper cell division in gametes. Cell division problems occur more often in eggs than in sperm because men produce new sperm throughout their lives, while women are born with all the potential eggs they will ever have. Therefore, a woman's eggs age as she ages. Each month, a single egg reaches maturity. During this maturation process, a division of the potential egg takes place. The division may result in an error in the number of chromosomes in the mature egg. The majority of Down syndrome children have three number 21 chromosomes instead of the usual pair (Figure 14-1). For this reason Down syndrome is also called *trisomy 21*. As the graph in Figure 14-2 shows, the risk of bearing a child with Down syndrome or another chromosomal abnormality rises dramatically after

Figure 14-2 **The Effect of Maternal Age on the Incidence of Down Syndrome.** As maternal age increases, the age of a woman's eggs also increases and genetic abnormalities become more common. The graph shows that the incidence of Down syndrome rises significantly as maternal age increases beyond 30 years.

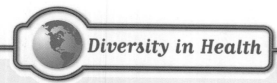

Sickle Cell Disease: Why Does This Deleterious Gene Persist?

Sickle cell disease is one of the most common genetic disorders among African Americans, having arisen in their African ancestors. It has also been observed in people whose ancestors came from the Mediterranean basin, the Indian subcontinent, the Caribbean, and parts of Central and South America (particularly Brazil). The sickle cell gene has persisted in these populations—even though the disease eventually kills its victims—because of a curious interaction between this disease and another disease prevalent in these regions. Today, an estimated 70,000 Americans of African American and Hispanic origins have the disease, and approximately 2.5 million carry the trait.

Sickle cell disease gets its name from the curved (sickle) shape of the red blood cells of individuals with this disease (Figure 14-A). Anemia, or a low number of red blood cells, results from the short life of these abnormal cells. An error in the gene that codes for hemoglobin, the oxygen-carrying molecule in red blood cells, is responsible for the signs and symptoms of sickle cell disease.

These sickle-shaped cells cause pain when they become trapped in the small blood vessels of the body. This condition results in oxygen depletion to the tissues surrounding the blocked vessels, which damages tissues and causes infections. Most sickle cell patients die in their 40s or 50s from conditions such as stroke, infection, kidney failure, or congestive heart failure.

To have sickle cell disease, a person must inherit two defective hemoglobin genes—one from each parent. A person who inherits a single defective gene is a carrier and is

Figure 14-A **Normal and Sickled Red Blood Cells.** The red blood cells to the left have a normal, rounded shape. Those to the right have the curved shape of sickle cell disease, which results in their becoming trapped in the small blood vessels of the body.

said to have *sickle cell trait*. This gene is quite prevalent in the populations mentioned previously. For example, 1 in 400 African American newborns has sickle cell disease and 1 in 12 has sickle cell trait. People with sickle cell trait do not have sickle cell disease, but they do have something in common with sufferers of sickle cell disease—resistance to malaria.

Those with the sickle cell gene have a survival advantage in regions of the world in which malaria is prevalent. The map in Figure 14-B shows where malaria is widespread; notice from the listing of affected populations in the first paragraph that sickle cell disease is prevalent in these areas as well. Although many of these peoples have since migrated from these areas, this ancestral gene persists in their populations.

How does a defective hemoglobin gene protect against malaria? In sickle cell trait, red blood cells sickle under a variety of conditions, such as when the oxygen tension is low (at high altitudes, for example) and if these cells become acidic. Results of research show that infection of the red

---

the maternal age of 30. Therefore, various screening methods have been developed to detect whether a fetus is affected with trisomy 21 or other chromosomal problems. Prenatal diagnosis is discussed in Chapter 5 on pages 104 to 105.

Diseases Caused by an Interaction of Genes and the Environment

During the development of certain noninfectious diseases, there is often an interplay between genetic and environmental factors. Environmental factors may include substances to which an individual is exposed, such as air pollution, or may relate to a person's lifestyle,

such as maintaining a high-fat diet or exercising very little or not at all. Genetic factors can predispose a person to a disease; that is, a person may contract a particular disease more readily or easily than other people in the general population exposed to the same environmental factors. For example, persons with asthma may have genetic factors that influence the functioning of their airways. They may also live in environments in which cigarette smoke and air pollution are present. These factors may lead to a chronic inflammatory state in their airways and result in asthma. However, other people with no genetic link to the disease may remain disease-free while living in the same environments.

blood cells by malaria parasites causes the infected cells to become acidic due to the metabolism of the parasite. This change induces the red blood cells to sickle, which interrupts multiplication of the parasite. The spleen, an organ that destroys worn-out red blood cells, traps the sickled cells. Under these conditions, the parasites die and malaria does not develop. For populations who live in regions where malaria is prevalent, the sickle cell gene persists because people who harbor the gene are more likely to live to reproductive age than those who do not have the gene and die from malaria. Therefore, this "deleterious" gene is beneficial to those with sickle cell trait living in malaria-infested areas and is passed from generation to generation. Unfortunately, some offspring inherit sickle cell disease and not simply sickle cell trait.

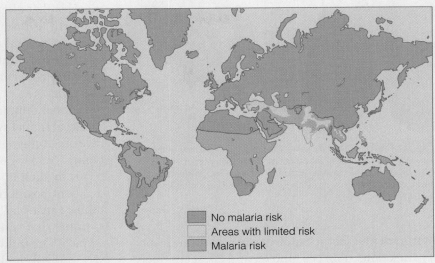

No malaria risk
Areas with limited risk
Malaria risk

Figure 14-B **Areas of the World in Which Malaria Is Prevalent.** Malaria is a serious infectious desease in the tropical and subtropical regions of the world. Sickle cell disease is prevalent in these regions as well.

Health care providers alleviate symptoms by administering painkillers and blood transfusions. Penicillin is given to children aged 1 to 5 years to ward off infection. But a breakthrough in treatment may increase the quality and duration of life for sickle cell sufferers. In February 1995, the National Heart, Blood, and Lung Institute released the results of an extensive study showing that the drug hydroxyurea reduces the frequency of pain, hospital admissions, and life-threatening complications by about 50% (Marwick, 1995). In 1998, bone marrow stem cell transplantation was used for the first time to treat sickle cell disease (Associated Press, 1999). Bone marrow stem cells

are undifferentiated cells that give rise to all types of blood cells. In October 2004, the U.S. House of Representatives passed the Sickle Cell Treatment Act to help treat and expand services for patients with the blood disorder. At this writing, the bill needed to be approved by the Senate before being signed into law by the president.

Couples can be screened to detect if they are carriers of the trait to help them in their family-planning decisions. Eventually, medical experts may discover a way to weed out this life-threatening gene in populations no longer living in malaria-prone areas.

Asthma, ulcers, diabetes mellitus, migraine headaches, cardiovascular disease, and cancer are common diseases that have both genetic and environmental causes. Ulcers are sores in the lining of the esophagus, stomach, or duodenum. They are discussed on page 59 of Chapter 3. Diabetes mellitus is a group of diseases in which a person does not metabolize carbohydrates properly. Diabetes is discussed in Chapter 9 on pages 229 to 230. Migraine headaches are thought to be an inherited disorder that can be triggered by a variety of environmental factors. Migraines are discussed on page 60 of Chapter 3. The nation's number one killers—cardiovascular disease and cancer—are discussed in separate chapters (Chapters 12 and 13,

respectively) because they affect the nation's health so significantly.

Asthma, the most common chronic illness in childhood, is a disease of the airways. The bronchioles of asthmatics narrow in response to certain stimuli much more easily than do the bronchioles of nonasthmatics. (*Bronchioles* are air passageways, about the diameter of a pencil lead, that lead to the air sacs of the lungs [Figure 14-3]). When these airways become narrowed, air flow to and from the lungs is blocked. As a result, asthmatic people have trouble breathing and begin to wheeze, which people refer to as having an *asthma attack*.

asthma
(AZ-mah) a common, chronic, childhood illness characterized by sensitive airways.

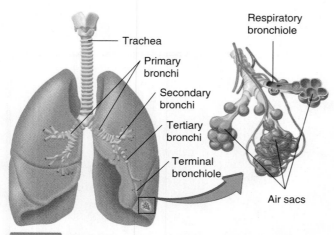

Figure 14-3 **The Respiratory System.** The bronchioles are the narrow air passageways that branch from the bronchi and lead to the air sacs of the lungs. The bronchioles are covered with muscle tissue that constricts during asthma attacks, narrowing these passageways and making it difficult to breathe.

Labels in figure: Trachea; Primary bronchi; Secondary bronchi; Tertiary bronchi; Terminal bronchiole; Respiratory bronchiole; Air sacs

Environmental factors such as air pollution, respiratory infections, tobacco smoke, and allergens such as dust mites often trigger asthma attacks. (Dust mites are microscopic organisms that live in carpets, mattresses, pillows, and curtains.) As mentioned in the opening paragraphs of this chapter, exercise may also stimulate asthma attacks. Breathing warm, moist air is best for the athlete with exercise-induced asthma. For example, swimming in a warm pool will usually cause fewer problems than snow skiing. Also, warming up before exercise reduces the likelihood of an exercise-induced asthma attack. With other types of asthma, the key to management is discovering what stimulates attacks and avoiding these factors. For example, if a trigger is house dust mites, exposure can be reduced by not using carpeting or draperies, and washing bedding often in hot water. Medication is another important tool for asthma management.

carpal tunnel syndrome numbness, pain, or pins-and-needles sensations in either of the hands that extends down the fingers, resulting from improper alignment of the wrist while engaging in repetitive-use activities.

Noninfectious Conditions with Environmental or Unknown Causes

Many conditions are caused by exposure to various substances in the environment. In general, environmental factors that are the sole cause of disease are toxic chemicals (see Chapter 16, "Environmental Health"). Not only are toxic chemicals present in the home, workplace, and environment, they are used and abused in ways that seriously affect health. The adverse effects of drug and alcohol abuse are described in Chapters 7 and 8, respectively. The toxic chemi-

cals found in tobacco products are discussed in Chapter 8.

A few noninfectious conditions are caused by the ways in which people use their bodies. Temporomandibular disorder, characterized by pain in the jaw and chewing muscles that often results from grinding or clenching the teeth, is discussed in Chapter 3. **Carpal tunnel syndrome**, a painful condition of the hands and fingers, results from improper positioning of the wrist while engaging in repetitive activities that use the hands, wrists, and arms. Ten percent of the population experiences occasional symptoms of this syndrome.

Carpal tunnel syndrome is usually the result of repetitive use. Activities such as using power tools frequently, typing for a long time, and playing piano or guitar often result in such injuries because people hold the wrist in a bent position rather than holding it straight. The injury causes inflammation and a buildup of fluid in a tunnel that runs through the bones of the wrist, or carpals. The fluid presses on the nerve and blood vessels in the tunnel. Other conditions such as arthritis, diabetes, and pregnancy may also contribute to pressure in the carpal tunnel. To help avoid injury when typing for a long time, place your computer keyboard at elbow height and keep your wrists unbent as shown in Figure 14-4. Use wrist rests and arm rests only when you are resting, not when you are typing.

Labels in figure: Display at eye level or slightly below; 18 to 28 inches; Soft incoming light; Keyboard at elbow height; Thigh parallel to floor; Feet flat on floor or foot rest

Figure 14-4 **The Proper Sitting Position for Typing at the Computer.** The screen should be at eye level or slightly lower. The keyboard should be at elbow height, the forearms parallel to the floor, the back supported, the thighs parallel to the floor, and the feet flat on the floor or foot rest.

- The risk of chromosomal abnormalities in a woman's eggs increases significantly after her thirtieth birthday. Therefore, if you and your partner are considering a pregnancy at or beyond this age, consult your health care provider for advice regarding options to increase your chances of having a healthy infant.
- If you have asthma, learn your asthma triggers and avoid them. If you have exercise-induced asthma, consider restricting your activity on cold days or when the pollen count or air pollution levels are high.
- Abusing drugs, or living and working under toxic conditions, can damage the hereditary material of your cells, particularly the sex cells. Therefore, to protect your health and possibly that of your offspring, avoid exposure to toxic substances.
- Carpal tunnel syndrome often results from bending the wrists while engaging in a repetitive activity such as typing, using hand tools, or engaging in various household chores. To help prevent repetitive-use injury, always keep your wrists unbent while engaging in such activities.

Trends in Infectious Disease

In 1900 the three leading causes of death were infectious diseases: pneumonia, tuberculosis, and enteritis (inflammation of the intestine, causing severe diarrhea) (Centers for Disease Control and Prevention [CDC], 1999). Since that time, the United States (and other industrialized countries) has made achievements in public health that have changed this picture dramatically. Early in the twentieth century, U.S. departments of public health were established, whose activities provided for clean drinking water, uncontaminated food, and proper sewage disposal and treatment. These actions have reduced the transmission of pathogens tremendously. *Antibiotics,* which are medications that kill bacteria, and *vaccines,* which are preparations that boost the immune system to help it ward off infection from specific pathogens, combat infection as well. Additionally, new treatments for certain viral illnesses such as influenza have been developed. As a result, after a century, the three leading causes of death in

2002 were no longer infectious diseases, but were non-infectious diseases: heart disease, cancer, and stroke. The only infectious diseases in the "top ten" were pneumonia and influenza, together ranked as the seventh leading cause of death (Kochanek & Smith, 2004).

Although infectious diseases are not significant contributors to death in the United States at this time, the worldwide picture is much different. Infectious diseases are the leading cause of death in the world. At least 30 new diseases have emerged in the past 25 years, including HIV infection, Ebola viral hemorrhagic fever, and a new strain of hepatitis—hepatitis C. Additionally, many bacterial diseases once easily cured with antibiotics are appearing as incurable diseases, resistant to the variety of antibiotics available at this time. "Old" diseases that once seemed under control, such as diphtheria and tuberculosis, are making a comeback as well.

We are living in an age when international travel is commonplace, making transmission of infection a worldwide concern, not just a concern in our own country, state, or city. The resistance of many strains of bacteria to antibiotics and the reemergence of serious diseases once thought conquered makes complacency to infection a dangerous attitude. In this time of increasing illness and death from infectious disease in the global community, it is important to understand how infectious diseases are transmitted and how pathogens interact with the body. This knowledge is key to avoiding infection and staying healthy.

host in reference to disease, an organism that supports the growth of a pathogen; the third, and last, link in the chain of infection.

transmission in reference to disease, the means by which a pathogen gets to a host; the second link in the chain of infection.

chain of infection the relationship among the factors important in the development of infectious diseases: the pathogen, transmission, and the host.

The Chain of Infection

Infection results from the interaction between a pathogen (also called an agent of infection) and a **host**, the organism that supports the growth of the pathogen. The pathogen is considered the first link in the chain of infection. The host is the third and last link. Joining these two links is **transmission**, the route by which the pathogen gets to the host. Figure 14-5 depicts the **chain of infection**, the relationship among the factors important in the development of infectious diseases.

The First Link: Pathogens

The severity of an infectious disease depends on a variety of factors:

- the type of pathogen (such as a bacterium or virus),

Figure 14-5 The Chain of Infection. Infection is the invasion of the body by disease-causing organisms, or pathogens. Infection results when the pathogen (the first link in the chain) is transmitted (the second link) to a host (the third link). The host is the organism that supports the growth of the pathogen.

Agent of infection

Host

Transmission

- its *virulence* (how easily it causes disease),
- its ability to multiply and spread within the body,
- its ability to combat the defense mechanisms of the body, and
- the body's reaction to this invader.

This chapter first describes pathogens that cause infectious diseases. A later section focuses on the host's defense mechanisms.

Bacteria and Rickettsias Bacteria produce infections such as strep throat, bacterial pneumonia, food poisoning, and infected cuts. These organisms are unicellular and microscopic, with a simple cell structure.

When bacteria enter the body, they adhere to the surfaces of host cells and grow and multiply there. Some bacteria penetrate deeply into the tissues (moving between body cells). Many pathogenic bacteria produce one or more chemicals that aid their invasion. A few types of bacteria produce toxins, or poisons, that cause diseases such as certain types of food poisoning.

Rickettsias are bacteria-like organisms that live *within* host cells. These organisms cause diseases such as typhus, which is transmitted by lice, and Rocky Mountain spotted fever, which is transmitted by ticks.

Viruses Viruses cause many diseases with which you are familiar: the common cold, influenza (the flu), mumps, measles (Figure 14-6), chicken pox, hepatitis, and **acquired immunodeficiency syndrome (AIDS)**. Viruses are very

bacteria unicellular, microscopic organisms with a simple cell structure; some are pathogenic to humans and produce infections such as strep throat, bacterial pneumonia, food poisoning, and infected cuts.

virus hereditary material surrounded by a coat of protein; some viruses are pathogenic to humans and produce infections such as the common cold, influenza, mumps, measles, chicken pox, hepatitis, and AIDS.

acquired immuno-deficiency syndrome (AIDS) a set of certain diseases and conditions that results from infection by the human immunodeficiency virus (HIV).

different from bacteria, and, in fact, are very different from *any* organism: They do not have a cellular structure. Since the basis of life is the cell, viruses are not considered living organisms. They are simply hereditary material surrounded by a coat of protein.

Like bacteria, viruses cause disease by adhering to host cells, but unlike bacteria, viruses enter the cells of the body and use those cells to make more virus particles. The new virus particles break open the infected cell, killing it, and are then ready to infect additional body cells. The death of body cells causes many of the signs and symptoms of viral disease.

Certain types of viruses invade cells but enter a *latent state* during which time infective virus particles are not produced. Although no signs or symptoms of the viral infection are apparent, latency may cause changes in a cell that lead to cancer (see Chapter 13). In many instances, the latent viral hereditary material can become reactivated and replicate once again, causing disease.

Figure 14-6 Child with the Typical Rash of Measles. This highly contagious viral disease is characterized by a spreading rash. The rash consists of small, red spots; some of the spots may be raised.

Some infections are characterized by a cycling of latent and actively replicating periods, such as the sexually transmitted infection (STI) genital herpes. During the usual course of this disease (see pages 403–405), a person suffers active episodes when he or she can transmit this disease to others. The infection then subsides (latency) only to reappear at another time, often triggered by stress or other factors.

Fungi You have probably heard of, or may have experienced, yeast infections or athlete's foot (Figure 14-7), which is a type of ringworm (a fungal infection of the skin, hair, or nails). These diseases are caused by **fungi**, more commonly known as molds and yeasts. Fungi cannot make their own food and, therefore, grow on a wide range of organisms that they use as food sources, such as rotting logs, spoiling fruit, and the human body. Most human fungal infections, with the exception of yeast infections, are caused by molds.

Medical researchers know less about how fungi cause disease in humans than they know about the other agents of infection. However, fungi appear to invade humans in much the same way as do bacteria. Humans have a high degree of resistance to fungi, which may explain why humans become infected with fungi less often than with bacteria or viruses. Fungi are considered *opportunistic* organisms; that is, they invade the human body when the host has another disease or condition that diminishes its ability to combat fungal infection. People with diabetes or AIDS, for example, are more likely to contract fungal infections than people with no underlying illness.

Other Types of Pathogens Two additional groups of organisms cause infections in humans: *protozoans* and *worms*. Protozoans cause diseases such as malaria (a tropical disease transmitted by mosquitoes) and trichomonas urogenital infections, or "trich" infections. All protozoans that cause infectious diseases in humans are single-celled organisms, but they differ from one another in the ways they cause disease.

The other group of infectious organisms are the parasitic worms: certain types of roundworms, flatworms (tapeworms), and flukes. Tapeworms are contracted by eating infected pork or beef; these worms live in the intestines, producing digestive disturbances. Adult roundworms also inhabit the intestinal tract and cause digestive disorders; they enter the body in various ways depending on the species of worm. Flukes differ in that they can inhabit the intestine, the liver, the lungs, or the veins depending on the species; they are contracted from water infected with human feces and are not prevalent in the United States.

One other group of organisms important to mention is the *arthropods*. Certain species of this group live on or in the skin of humans, a condition usually referred to as *infestation* rather than infection. Arthropods are organisms such as lice, fleas, mites, and ticks. Some STIs are caused by certain lice and mites (see pages 411–412). Ticks only occasionally infest humans but may transmit other pathogens to humans, as can mosquitoes, lice, and flies.

The Second Link: Transmission

Some infectious diseases are passed from person to person and others are not. Those that are spread from person to person, such as colds, flu, strep throat, and STIs, are **communicable** diseases. Diseases that are *not* transmitted from person to person, including both infectious and noninfectious diseases, are **noncommunicable**.

Noncommunicable Infectious Diseases Noncommunicable infectious diseases can be caused in various ways: by the growth of bacteria that normally inhabit the body, the ingestion of poisons produced by some bacteria, or infection with pathogens from environmental or animal sources.

Many species of bacteria normally reside on and in the human body. However, these beneficial bacteria can cause occasional problems. For example, *Staphylococcus* bacteria normally present on the skin can multiply and cause skin infections, especially in persons with chronic diseases such as diabetes.

Noncommunicable infections can also be caused by the ingestion of *toxins*, or poisons, produced by some bacteria. Staphylococcal food poisoning

fungi
(FUN-jeye)
cellular organisms that cannot make their own food; some are pathogenic to humans and produce infections such as athlete's foot, ringworm, and yeast infections. *Fungus* is the singular term.

communicable
(ka-Myoo-ni-kah-bl)
transmissible from person to person.

noncommunicable
not transmissible from person to person.

(formerly called ptomaine poisoning), for example, is caused by taking in a toxin that certain staphylococcal bacteria produce when they grow on foods. Dairy products and poultry are the foods most commonly contaminated with staphylococcal bacteria from their animal sources or from infected food handlers. The staphylococcal bacteria grow well in high-protein, high-carbohydrate foods. Most often, staphylococcal food poisoning occurs when people eat foods such as potato salad, chicken salad, custard, or cream pies that have not been refrigerated properly after preparation. Picnics are a common time of infection because such foods are left out under warm conditions for long periods of time, which allows the bacteria to grow and produce toxin. Because the bacteria grow on the food and not in the body, this type of noncommunicable infection is more properly called *intoxication* (poisoning) rather than infection. Staphylococcal food poisoning should not be confused with *Salmonella* food infection, in which the bacteria are taken in with food and multiply in the small intestine.

Botulism is another type of food poisoning, caused by a powerful toxin produced by the bacterium *Clostridium botulinum.* This organism most often grows in improperly home-canned, low-acid foods such as green beans and green peppers. Boiling home-canned foods for 10 to 15 minutes inactivates the toxin. (Infants can contract botulism from raw honey [see Chapter 9].)

A third type of noncommunicable infection is caused by pathogens that infect people via environmental or animal sources. Legionnaire's disease, caused by the bacterium *Legionella pneumophila,* is an infectious disease contracted from an environmental source. Under favorable conditions, this pathogen can grow in and be dispersed by any apparatus that provides a water aerosol or mist, such as air conditioners, whirlpool

spas, humidifiers, decorative fountains, showerheads, and water faucets. When this water mist is inhaled, these microbes lodge in the lungs and multiply, producing a pneumonia-like disease that includes high fever, cough, chest pain, and diarrhea. This disease is quite serious; 5% to 30% of its victims die. To reduce the growth of this organism and protect yourself against infection, periodically clean and thoroughly disinfect mist-creating items, such as those mentioned previously, and maintain an appropriate concentration of chlorine in home spas.

Lyme disease is an example of a noncommunicable infection contracted from an animal source. Named for the small community of Lyme, Connecticut, where the disease was first recognized in 1975, this bacterial disease is transmitted by ticks that infest animals such as white-footed mice and white-tailed deer. The ticks ingest the bacterial pathogen that causes Lyme disease from infected animals. When a tick harboring this bacterium bites a human, it injects the bacterium into the bloodstream. Usually a painless but large rash (sometimes looking like a "bull's-eye") appears at the site of the bite from a few days to one month after being bitten (Figure 14-8). This rash is generally accompanied by severe headaches, fatigue, chills, and fever. If the disease is not treated with antibiotics at this early stage, it may develop into severe inflammation of the heart muscle or nervous system weeks to months later. Within two years, if untreated, arthritic attacks develop (inflammation of the joints) that can become chronic.

In the United States, Lyme disease is found primarily in the northeast, the mid-Atlantic (Virginia and North Carolina area), and the upper midwest. It has also been reported in several areas in northwestern California. Deer ticks favor a moist, shaded environment, particularly areas of woods, brush, or tall grass. If you are walking, gardening, or engaging in other activities in the areas described above and in which deer and mice live (and therefore deer ticks), wear long pants and a long-sleeved shirt. Tuck your pant legs into your socks or boots. Spray insect repellent containing at least 30% DEET on your clothing and exposed skin. (Do not spray it on your face. Spray it on your hands and pat that on your face. Use products with no more than 10% DEET on children.) Check yourself carefully for ticks, removing any you find with tweezers. Another way to protect yourself is by immunization. A Lyme disease vaccine was introduced in 1999, but the manufacturer withdrew the vaccine from the market in 2002, citing poor sales.

Communicable Infectious Diseases Communicable diseases are transmitted from person to person by direct or indirect contact, by means of a common vehicle,

Figure 14-8 **The "Classic" Rash That Develops at the Site of a Tick Bite in Lyme Disease.** Not everyone who contracts Lyme disease will develop this type of rash.

through the air, and by means of vectors such as mosquitoes.

Some infectious diseases, such as STIs, are passed from person to person by close physical (direct) contact. In the case of STIs, of course, the close contact is usually sexual intercourse but may involve genital contact without intercourse. Other diseases such as colds and the flu are often transmitted by direct contact also, such as shaking hands. These diseases can also be transmitted indirectly by means of an object, such as a shared drinking glass, or through close contact with droplets sneezed or coughed by a person. Strep throat and measles are spread in this way.

Frequently, a source contaminated with pathogens from humans may transmit an infectious disease to many people. Examples of common sources of infection are a blood supply contaminated with human immunodeficiency virus, food contaminated with the hepatitis virus by an infected food handler, and water contaminated by the feces of a person infected with typhoid fever. A variety of infectious diseases are transmitted via food or water.

Some communicable diseases can be transmitted from infected persons to noninfected persons through the air on microscopic water droplets or on dust particles. Certain disease-causing organisms of the respiratory tract, such as the bacterium that causes tuberculosis, can be transmitted in this way, propelled into the air when an infected person coughs or sneezes.

Other communicable diseases are spread indirectly by means of vectors. A *vector* is an organism (other than a human) that transmits a pathogen from one person to another. Usually a part of the life cycle of the pathogen takes place in or on the vector. For example, the malaria organism is a protozoan that carries out part of its life cycle in humans and another part in the gut of *Anopheles* mosquitoes. When a mosquito bites an infected person, it ingests blood that contains the protozoan. After the organism undergoes sexual reproduction in the mosquito, its progeny can infect new hosts when the mosquito bites them.

The Third Link: The Host

Why do you remain healthy sometimes, yet get sick at other times? How did you avoid getting the cold that everyone else seems to have? Why didn't your husband come down with the flu like the rest of the family? So far we've seen that some of the answers to these questions have to do with the pathogen and certain of its characteristics, such as its virulence. Transmission may also mean the difference between infection and health. Persons exposed frequently to pathogens are likely to become infected more often than those exposed less

frequently. The other answers to these questions have to do with your body's resistance to the invading microbe.

As described in Chapter 3, stress can be one factor that reduces your resistance to infection. High-intensity or exhaustive exercise, such as running more than 60 miles per week or for 3 or more hours per session, also suppresses the immune system. Moderate exercise, however, such as running fewer than 20 miles per week or walking for 45 minutes per day for 5 days per week, stimulates the immune system. Exercising when you are sick lowers the body's defenses.

Race and age affect an individual's resistance or susceptibility to certain diseases. Africans or people with African ancestry, for example, have a higher resistance to tropical diseases such as malaria and yellow fever than do non-Africans. Asians are more resistant to the sexually transmitted infection syphilis than are non-Asians. Children are more likely to contract certain "childhood" infectious diseases such as measles and chicken pox, while the elderly are more susceptible to pneumonia and influenza. And, as mentioned earlier, people with other diseases, such as AIDS, diabetes, and cancer, have weakened defense mechanisms.

Your body has two main types of defenses against infectious agents: mechanisms of nonspecific resistance, which are a variety of defenses that combat any foreign invader, and the immune system, which is a specific defense system that combats the particular invading pathogen. The following sections describe these two major defense mechanisms.

Healthy Living Practices

- Refrigerate cold starchy and protein-rich foods and cold foods made with dairy products or poultry immediately after preparation. At picnics, keep these foods chilled until it is time to eat.
- Boil all low-acid home-canned foods before eating or avoid eating home-canned foods.
- Periodically clean and thoroughly disinfect mist-creating items such as humidifiers and maintain an appropriate concentration of chlorine in home spas.
- Avoid close contact with people who have communicable diseases.
- Do not share drinking glasses and eating utensils with others.

- Do not share hypodermic needles with others because they may be contaminated with pathogens such as the hepatitis B virus or the AIDS virus.

- Use a condom when engaging in sex unless you are in a long-term, mutually monogamous relationship with an uninfected partner. Infectious bodily secretions can be passed from one partner to another during sexual activity.

- Use insect repellents formulated to repel ticks and flying insects that may be carriers of disease-producing organisms.

- Do not drink the water when traveling in developing countries. Also avoid raw fruits, vegetables, and salads because they may have been washed with contaminated water.

- Avoid the following hazardous foods when traveling in developing countries: uncooked or poorly cooked beef, pork, fish, and seafood and unpasteurized milk and other local dairy products.

- Avoid stress; high levels of stress reduce your resistance to infection.

- Avoid high-intensity or exhaustive exercise because it reduces your resistance to infection.

- Engage in moderate exercise to boost the immune system.

Immunity

Immunity is protection from disease, particularly infectious disease. You have two types of immunity: nonspecific and specific. **Nonspecific immunity** comprises a variety of defense mechanisms that combat any type of damage to the body, including the invasion of infectious agents. **Specific immunity** is carried out by the immune system. The **immune system** recognizes and combats pathogens and other foreign cells (such as cancer cells or tissue transplants) with cells and proteins that are specific for particular invaders. The immune system is discussed later in this chapter.

immunity (im-MYOU-nih-tea) resistance to disease.

nonspecific immunity a variety of defense mechanisms that combat any type of damage to the body, including the invasion of infectious agents.

specific immunity defense mechanism carried out by the immune system.

Nonspecific Immunity

Pathogens can enter the body at sites called **portals of entry** (Figure 14-9). The mucous membranes lining the respiratory, digestive, urinary, and reproductive sys-

tems are all portals of entry. Whether due to a cut, insect bite, burn, or injection, broken skin is a portal of entry. The placenta may be a portal of entry for a fetus, which may become infected with pathogens (mostly viruses) from an infected mother. Unbroken skin is a portal of entry only for some fungi and the larvae of certain parasitic worms.

The Skin and Mucous Membranes The skin provides a *mechanical barrier* to pathogens. The hardened cells at the surface of the skin provide a waterproof barrier that most infective agents cannot penetrate. In addition, acidic skin oils and sweat help make the skin an inhospitable environment for most organisms.

Body openings, such as the eyes, and tubes that open to the outside, such as the digestive and respiratory tracts, are lined with tissue called *mucous membranes*. Most mucous membranes have a thin layer of cells that produces a sticky, viscous secretion called mucus. Mucus keeps the membrane moist and traps foreign particles and organisms.

Another defense mechanism that works with the mucous membranes is *cilia*. These short, hairlike structures project from the surfaces of the cells lining the upper respiratory tract. As they beat in wavelike fashion, they move mucus that contains trapped foreign material such as dust and bacteria up toward the back of the mouth where it can be swallowed, keeping it

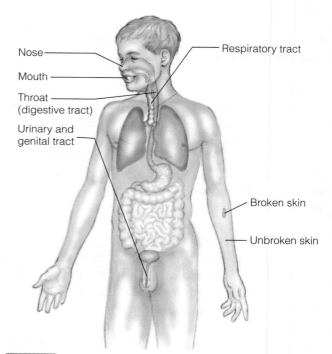

Nose
Mouth
Throat (digestive tract)
Urinary and genital tract
Respiratory tract
Broken skin
Unbroken skin

Figure 14-9 **Portals of Entry of the Human Body.** Portals of entry are areas of the body where pathogens can intrude: the skin and mucous membranes lining the respiratory, digestive, urinary, and reproductive systems; the placenta; broken skin; and unbroken skin (only for some fungi and the larvae of certain parasitic worms).

away from lower respiratory structures, especially the lungs.

Other tissues have a *chemical defense* mechanism. The lacrimal glands (located above the upper, outer corners of the eyes) produce tears that wash away foreign material on the eyes and also contain a chemical called *lysozyme* that kills certain bacteria. Lysozyme is also found in saliva. Another structure that provides a nonspecific chemical defense is the stomach. Stomach acid kills most of the microorganisms ingested with food.

White Blood Cells and Phagocytosis   Another nonspecific line of defense is the action of certain white blood cells, or **leukocytes**, that ingest foreign cells and debris, such as the dirt or dead cells in a cut. This process is **phagocytosis** (literally, *phago*, "eating," and *cyto*, "cell") and is shown in Figure 14-10. Two types of leukocytes—the neutrophils and the macrophages—are important phagocytes in the human body. Other white blood cells called *lymphocytes* help protect the body against infection and are part of the immune system.

The Lymphatic System   The lymphatic system, another key player in nonspecific immunity, is composed of vessels and nodes through which tissue fluid, or **lymph**, flows. Pictured in Figure 14-11, the lymphatic system also consists of lymphocytes and three lymphatic organs: the tonsils, the spleen, and the thymus (which is only active until puberty). The lymphatic system removes microorganisms and other foreign substances from the tissue fluid, the fluid surrounding the cells that is derived from the blood.

Lymph nodes are located at many points along the lymphatic vessels. Lymphatic vessels enter and exit each lymph node, which is a mesh of tissue containing lymphocytes and macrophages. The nodes cleanse tissue fluid by trapping microorganisms and other foreign substances in their weblike structures; macrophages in the nodes phagocytize this material.

The tonsils are large groups of lymph nodes located at the back of the oral cavity; they rid the nose and mouth area of bacteria and other debris. The spleen, located in the upper left corner of the abdominal cavity (see Figure 14-11), not only performs the function of a lymph node but also destroys worn-out red blood cells and stores red blood cells to provide an emergency supply in the case of severe loss. The thymus, located just above the heart at the midline of the chest, is the place where the lymphocytes destined to be T cells

immune system   a collection of cells and organs of the body that recognizes and combats pathogens and other foreign substances with cells and proteins that are specific for particular invaders. The immune system has two branches: antibody-mediated immunity and cell-mediated immunity.

portal of entry   site on or in the body at which pathogens enter.

leukocytes   (LEWK-oh-sites) white blood cells; active in both specific and nonspecific defenses of the body.

phagocytosis   (FAG-oh-site-OH-sis) the process of white blood cells ingesting foreign cells and debris, such as the dirt or dead cells in a cut.

lymph   (limf) tissue fluid.

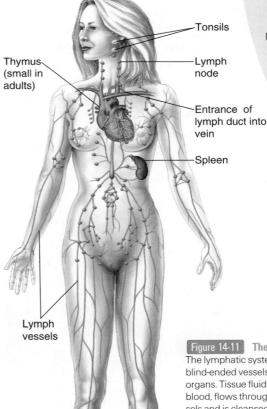

Tonsils

Thymus (small in adults)

Lymph node

Entrance of lymph duct into vein

Spleen

Lymph vessels

Figure 14-11   **The Lymphatic System.** The lymphatic system is made up of blind-ended vessels, nodes, and a few organs. Tissue fluid, derived from the blood, flows through the lymphatic vessels and is cleansed of debris and microorganisms by white blood cells that reside in the nodes. The fluid eventually returns to the blood.

Figure 14-10   **White Blood Cell Ingesting Bacteria.**   This is a highly magnified, colorized photo of a white blood cell called a macrophage (yellow/orange). Macrophages are the scavengers of the body, and protect it by "eating" bacteria and other foreign material. The bacteria (green) it is ingesting cause tuberculosis in humans.

mature during fetal life and early childhood (see "Specific Immunity"). (These T cells then reside in the lymphatic tissue and will produce new T cells when the thymus is no longer active.)

Inflammation Can you remember the last time you got a splinter or a cut? If so, you can probably remember (quite well!) your body's response. The inflammatory response is a series of events that takes place when the body is harmed by occurrences such as bacterial or viral invasion (infection), cuts, chemical damage, and burns. This response can be *local,* as in the case of getting a splinter in your finger, or *systemic* (affecting the whole body), as in the case of contracting a cold. Inflammation involves a variety of defense mechanisms that isolate and destroy the pathogens or other injurious agents and then remove the foreign materials and damaged cells so the body can repair itself.

The presence of infectious agents or damage to the body triggers the inflammatory response. As a result, many chemicals are released. Some of these chemicals, such as histamine, cause an increase of blood flow to the affected area, which brings phagocytes and other white blood cells to ingest microorganisms and debris—pieces of a splinter, for example. In addition, other chemicals stimulate phagocytes to move to the affected area, where they leave the blood and enter the damaged tissues. Yet other chemicals allow the surrounding blood vessel walls to leak, permitting phagocytes, certain blood-clotting factors, and other chemicals that enhance the inflammatory response to enter the tissues. The blood-clotting factors wall off the infected area, which prevents the spread of the infection. Figure 14-12 illustrates the inflammatory process.

The signs of local inflammation are redness, heat, swelling, pain, and a loss of function. The redness, heat, and swelling are results of increased blood flow to the affected area, including movement of fluids into surrounding tissues. Pain results as nerves are stimulated by the swelling and the chemicals released during inflammation. The pain, tissue damage, and swelling may contribute to a temporary loss of function of the affected body part.

Systemic inflammation occurs when you have a widespread infection such as a cold, the flu, strep throat, or pneumonia. Systemic inflammation has the same signs as local inflammation, but additional processes occur that result in more significant signs. The red bone marrow, located in the ends of certain bones, produces and releases large numbers of white blood cells. In addition, invading microorganisms and white blood cells release chemicals that affect the body's temperature-regulating system in the brain, resulting in a fever.

A *fever* is a rise in the internal body temperature from the human average of about 98.6°F. A fever lower than 104°F helps the body fight infection by enhancing phagocytosis and inhibiting the growth of certain microorganisms. However, a prolonged fever of 104°F, or a fever higher than 104°F, is dangerous because it can destroy proteins in the body. Other signs of systemic inflammation are fatigue, aches, and weakness.

The inflammatory process continues until the pathogens are killed or inactivated, or other injurious agents are walled off from the rest of the body and no longer pose a threat. Phagocytes ingest cellular debris and other organic material as the tissues recover from the infection.

Natural Killer Cells Natural killer cells are specialized white blood cells that attack cancer cells and body cells invaded by viruses. Natural killer cells secrete a chemical that pokes holes in the membranes of these two types of cells, destroying them. The response of natural killer cells to viral infections or developing cancer cells is quick, providing the body with protection until the immune system takes over (see "Specific Immunity").

Interferons Released from virally infected cells, **interferons** are proteins that protect uninfected cells from viral invasion. Interferons stimulate these cells to produce a protein that breaks down the hereditary material of the virus. When the damaged viruses enter cells they are unable to replicate and the viral infection is eventually halted. Interferons enhance the activity of the phagocytes as well as the action of other, more specific, immune system responses. In this role, interferons enhance the body's ability to fight invasions from most disease-causing agents, not just viruses.

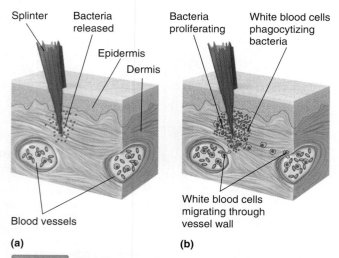

Splinter Bacteria released Bacteria proliferating White blood cells phagocytizing bacteria

Epidermis

Dermis

Blood vessels

White blood cells migrating through vessel wall

(a) (b)

Figure 14-12 **The Inflammatory Process.** (a) A splinter damages the skin, thrusting bacteria deep into the wound. Injured cells release chemicals such as histamine that cause the blood vessels to widen, bringing more blood to the area. (b) White blood cells squeeze through vessel walls and migrate to the bacteria, where they phagocytize them. Blood clots and connective tissue wall off the area.

Specific Immunity

Specific immunity is a function of the immune system. The immune system is made up of cells residing in tissues scattered throughout the body. These cells are able to react to specific pathogens and foreign molecules.

The immune system has two branches: *antibody-mediated immunity* and *cell-mediated immunity,* which will be discussed shortly. Each branch works slightly differently to attack foreign invaders and stop an infection. The immune system also has a memory: cells that react quickly to subsequent attacks by an invader.

Antigens: The Triggers of Specifc Immunity **Antigens** are usually foreign, or "non-self" proteins. Sometimes, entire infectious agents act as antigens. In other instances, parts of pathogens or the poisons they may secrete act as antigens. Noninfectious agents such as plant pollens, blood transfusions, or tissue transplants are antigenic, although the response to these antigens may differ from person to person. Unfortunately, the body sometimes perceives its own cells as foreign, attacking them and causing localized and systemic reactions, as in the case of **autoimmune diseases** such as *rheumatoid arthritis*. In this disease, the reactions include inflammation and deformity of the joints. The following sections describe how the immune system reacts to antigens that enter the body.

Antibody-Mediated Immunity The antibody-mediated portion of the immune system reacts to *extracellular* antigens, that is, antigens that reside outside of body cells, such as most bacteria and any toxins they produce. **Antibodies** are proteins that interact in a lock-and-key fashion with antigens. When they bind with an antigen, antibodies interfere with the normal functioning of the antigen. Antigen–antibody binding also stimulates the inflammatory response and promotes phagocytosis of the antigen.

The workhorses of antibody-mediated immunity (the cells that produce antibodies) are specialized white blood cells called *B lymphocytes,* or **B cells**. Each B cell has receptors on its membrane that bind to a specific antigen. When a foreign antigen enters the body, B cells bind to it. After stimulation by lymphocytes called helper T cells, the B cells reproduce in large numbers and become plasma cells, which produce antibodies. Figure 14-13 illustrates the antibody-mediated immune response.

Some of the stimulated B cells do not differentiate into plasma cells. These cells circulate as *memory B cells,* which respond more rapidly and forcefully whenever the antigen is encountered in the future. Memory cells confer immunity (resistance) to a disease. Many infections stimulate lifelong immunity (measles and chicken pox, for example); others, such as diphtheria, confer immunity for only a few years. Unfortunately, not all infectious agents stimulate the formation of memory cells, so no immunity is produced as a result of their infection. Examples of such infections are strep throat and gonorrhea (an STI).

Cell-Mediated Immunity The cell-mediated portion of the immune system reacts to *intracellular* antigens; that is, antigens that reside inside our body cells, such as viruses, fungi, a few types of bacteria, and parasites. It also acts against foreign tissues such as organ transplants and controls the growth of tumor cells.

Lymphocytes called **T cells** function in cell-mediated immunity. T cells reside in lymphoid tissues and in the

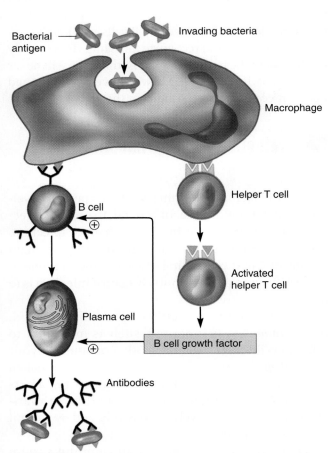

Figure 14-13 **The Antibody-Mediated Immune Response.** White blood cells called macrophages ingest invading microbes and display their antigenic parts. Helper T cells and B cells specific to the antigens attach to them, which activates both types of cells. The helper T cells produce a chemical that stimulates the growth of the B cells. These B cells, now called plasma cells, secrete proteins called antibodies. Antibodies attach to and promote the death of the invading microbes.

interferons (IN-ter-FEAR-onz) proteins produced by the body during a viral infection that protect uninfected cells from viral invasion.

antigens (AN-tih-jenz) proteins that are foreign or recognized as "non-self" by the body.

autoimmune diseases diseases in which the body perceives its own cells as foreign, attacking them and causing localized and systemic (whole body) reactions.

antibodies proteins that interact in a lock-and-key fashion with antigens, interfering with the normal functioning of the antigen.

B cells specialized white blood cells (lymphocytes) that function in antibody-mediated immunity and produce antibodies.

T cells specialized white blood cells (lymphocytes) that function in cell-mediated immunity; there are four types of T cells.

bloodstream with the B cells. The body contains thousands of different T cells. Upon binding to antigens, T cells reproduce and differentiate into four types: cytotoxic T cells, helper T cells, suppressor T cells, and memory T cells.

Cytotoxic T cells destroy invading intracellular pathogens (primarily viruses) by secreting chemicals that break apart infected host cells. By destroying host cells, the cytotoxic T cells take away what a virus or any other intracellular infective agent needs to reproduce or replicate. Cytotoxic T cells destroy non-self tissue transplants or tumorous growths in much the same way (Figure 14-14).

Helper T cells and *suppressor T cells* regulate the activities of both branches of the immune system. Helper T cells secrete various chemicals that enhance the activity of cytotoxic T cells and suppressor T cells and attract phagocytes to the area. Some helper T cells secrete chemicals that enhance the development and reproduction of B cells.

When the infection has subsided, suppressor T cells shut down the immune system. Although these cells inhibit the activity of various immune system cells, they increase in number more slowly than do other T cells. Therefore, suppressor T cells shut down the immune response only after it has successfully done its job.

A group of stimulated T cells circulates as *memory T cells*. Like memory B cells, memory T cells respond rapidly and forcefully during subsequent encounters with antigens, resulting in immunity to a disease.

acquired immunity specific resistance to infection that is not inherited but develops during a person's lifetime.

vaccine a preparation of a killed or weakened pathogen or its antigenic parts to be administered to a person to induce immunity and thereby prevent infectious disease.

Interactions Between Specific and Nonspecific Immunity

The mechanisms of nonspecific and specific defense work together to prevent infection or combat infection once it occurs. For example, the intact skin, mucous membranes, and chemicals in body fluids are effective barriers against viral invasion. However, if viruses gain entry to the body, macrophages phagocytize them before they can enter body cells. Activated helper T cells secrete chemicals that stimulate the B cells to become antibody-producing cells.

If some of the virus particles enter body cells in spite of these defenses, the infected cells produce interferons, which protect uninfected cells. Natural killer cells poke holes in the infected cells, killing them, thus destroying the virus's host. After binding to infected cells, cytotoxic T cells reproduce, developing large populations specific for this viral infection. As armies of cytotoxic T cells break apart infected cells, the freed viruses are phagocytized by macrophages and inactivated by antibodies. Usually this complex process stops the viral infection. The memory B cells and T cells continue to circulate, and recognize this same virus quickly if it re-enters the body. Most likely, the virus will never again cause infection, for it will have been stopped before it could gain a foothold in the cells.

■ Protection Against Infectious Diseases

A variety of factors determine whether a person develops an infectious disease. In general, to prevent infectious disease, you must break the chain of infection. This chapter offers many tips on breaking the chain of infection and preventing disease. However, one of the best ways to protect yourself against infection is to increase your resistance.

Specific immunity is either inborn or acquired. *Inborn immunity* is inherited, such as immunity to infectious diseases that attack other organisms (your cat or dog, for example) but not humans. **Acquired immunity** is not inherited; it develops during a person's lifetime. Acquired immunity develops in a variety of ways: either actively or passively, and by natural or artificial means.

Active acquired immunity is an immune system response developed as a result of contact with a pathogen, which includes development of memory B cells or T cells. Contact with the pathogen can occur naturally, during day-to-day life. It can also occur artificially, by a **vaccine** prepared from a killed or

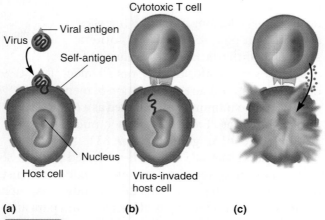

(a)   **(b)**   **(c)**

Cytotoxic T cell

Viral antigen

Virus

Self-antigen

Nucleus

Host cell

Virus-invaded host cell

Figure 14-14 **The Cell-Mediated Immune Response.** Cytotoxic T cells are key to the cell-mediated immune response. Here, whole T cells, not just antibodies, attach to cells infected with viruses, to cancer cells, or to tissue transplants. The T cell then secretes chemicals that destroy the host cell before the virus can enter the nucleus and begin to replicate.

weakened pathogen or its antigenic parts. Depending on how the vaccine is prepared, it may have long- or short-term effects. That is why people need booster vaccinations every few years against some infectious diseases.

Children develop active acquired immunity to many serious childhood diseases by being vaccinated according to a schedule recommended by the American Academy of Pediatrics and the American Academy of Family Physicians. The Web site of this textbook contains a link to the current childhood immunization schedule. Prior to travel to foreign countries, immunization of adults and children leads to active acquired immunity to diseases not generally found in the United States. If you are traveling outside the United States, consult your physician 4 to 6 weeks prior to your trip for the required and recommended immunizations. A link provided on the Web site to this textbook gives the most recent health information for travel to various areas of the world and a list of vaccinations necessary for those areas. (For both, see "Content Links" for Chapter 14.)

Passive acquired immunity is conferred when a person is given antibodies. Passive immunity can be acquired naturally when antibodies from a mother cross the placenta and enter the bloodstream of a developing fetus. After birth, a breast-fed infant passively acquires antibodies from its mother's milk. These antibodies help a newborn resist disease for the first month of life until its own immune system becomes functional. Passive immunity can also be acquired artificially, when a person receives an injection of antibodies after exposure to a serious infection (such as hepatitis A or rabies) or a lethal poison (such as certain snake venoms).

Drugs That Combat Infection

Once a person has an infection like the common cold, what can he or she do to combat it? Most often, getting rest and drinking sufficient fluids helps the body as it mounts its defense. (Sometimes over-the-counter cold medications can help relieve symptoms. See "Over-the-Counter Cold Medications: Do They Help?") For other infections, the individual can obtain specific recommendations from health care professionals who are trained to diagnose and treat the illness. These medical practitioners often prescribe medicines to inhibit the growth of or inactivate the infectious agent.

Antibiotics are a group of chemicals that kill bacteria or inhibit their growth. Antibiotics work by attacking parts of bacterial cells or bacterial processes that differ from human cells. When taking an antibiotic, it is important to finish the medication your physician prescribed, even though your symptoms may be gone prior to that time. All the bacteria may not have been killed, and the infection could return.

Antibiotics do nothing to combat viral infections and may kill some of the body's normal bacterial inhabitants. These bacteria control the growth of troublesome microorganisms; when they are gone, it is easier for unwanted disease-causing bacteria to multiply and cause a secondary bacterial infection. Therefore, taking antibiotics when they are unnecessary can be harmful. Furthermore, the unnecessary use of antibiotics provides additional opportunities for antibiotic-resistant strains of bacteria to develop.

antibiotics (AN-tie-by-OT-iks) a group of chemicals that kill bacteria or inhibit their growth.

Various topical antibiotics (those applied to the skin, such as bacitracin) are available without prescription to treat or prevent minor skin infections. Over-the-counter topical antifungal drugs are also available to treat fungal infections of the skin, such as athlete's foot and ringworm, and vaginal yeast infections. Antifungal drugs that must be taken orally for more serious fungal infections require a prescription.

Progress in the production of effective antiviral drugs has been slow because viruses reside inside the body's cells. Therefore, a drug must inactivate the virus without harming its host. A few antiviral drugs treat infections caused by the herpes virus (such as genital herpes, cold sores, and chicken pox) and others treat diseases associated with AIDS. Antiviral medications have been developed to control influenza (flu) infection (Sintchenko & Dwyer, 1999).

Specific medications have also been developed to treat protozoal diseases such as malaria, amebic dysentery, and trichomoniasis. Likewise, prescription medicines are available to treat infestations of worms such as tapeworms and pinworms.

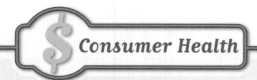
Over-the-Counter Cold Medications: Do They Help?

Every year Americans spend millions of dollars on over-the-counter (nonprescription) cold and cough remedies. Thousands of products on the market purport to relieve your aches, fever, coughs, and congestion. But do these medications help?

Dr. Nancy Hutton of the Johns Hopkins School of Medicine in Baltimore answers no when it comes to cold remedies helping children. Dr. Hutton conducted a study with 96 5-year-olds suffering from colds. She divided the children into three groups. One group received an antihistamine-decongestant product, a second group received a placebo (pill with no active ingredients), and the third group received nothing. Two days later, half the children in each group reported feeling better—those taking "cold remedies" did as well as those taking the placebo or nothing (Hutton et al., 1991).

What about the use of these remedies with adults? Decongestants may make you feel less stuffed up, but you may feel worse when you stop taking the medicine due to rebound congestion—the blood vessels may swell beyond their original swollen state when the medication wears off. You may choose to treat your dripping nose and sneezing with an antihistamine, but these products may be effective only against allergy, not cold, symptoms. Cough suppressants may help you cough less, but you need to expel the buildup of thick mucus to keep your airways clear. Expectorants can help thin the mucus and facilitate its removal from the airways as you cough. Drinking lots of water gives the same result. Cough drops may help keep a dry throat lubricated but may upset your stomach. Sucking on hard candy may be just as lubricating. You can spray your sore throat with an anesthetic, but gargling with warm salty water several times a day can also relieve the soreness.

Sorting out the pros and cons of taking cold remedies can be made easier by becoming more informed. Physicians generally recommend that you simply drink plenty of fluids (without alcohol or caffeine), get lots of rest, and take one of the medications listed below for fever and aches.

The following information lists each cold symptom along with its over-the-counter (OTC) remedies approved by the federal Food and Drug Administration (FDA). Precautions for the drugs are also noted. Don't let the sometimes long

and difficult-to-pronounce names bother you; just match the names to those on the list of active ingredients of particular products. As with all OTC medications, follow the directions for taking the product and the recommended dosage on the packaging. (The Consumer Health feature on page 179 explains OTC package labels.) If you suffer an unexpected or severe side effect, discontinue taking the medication and contact your physician. Do not drink alcoholic beverages while you are taking medications. Ask your pharmacist or physician which medications can be taken together—drugs can interact with one another.

Note: The authors are not promoting the use of OTC remedies but are presenting information for educational purposes only. Consult your physician for advice on taking medication.

Minor Aches, Pains, and Fever

Pain and fever relievers (also called analgesics) are products such as aspirin, acetaminophen, ibuprofen, and naproxen sodium. Each works just about as well as the others.

Precautions: Don't give children aspirin when they have a cold or other viral infection. Except under a doctor's instruction, none of these drugs should be taken for more than 10 days by adults or more than 5 days by children to relieve pain, and not more than 3 days to relieve fever. Overdoses of acetaminophen can cause severe liver damage and even death. Aspirin can irritate the gastric lining and cause gastrointestinal bleeding. In addition, aspirin interferes with blood clotting and can cause allergic reactions.

Sore Throat

Anesthetics in spray or lozenge (cough drop) form will inhibit all sensations from the throat, including temperature and pressure sensations as well as pain sensations. However, using analgesics (mentioned above) may help with the pain without affecting the other sensations. Benzocaine, benzyl alcohol, dyclonine hydrochloride, hexylresorcinol, phenol preparations, and phenolate sodium are FDA-approved medications found in anesthetic sprays and lozenges.

Precautions: Never give children younger than age 2 throat lozenges because they can choke on them. Many of these drugs have restrictions regarding their use with children; read directions carefully.

Dry Coughs

Cough suppressors (also called antitussives) inhibit coughing with dry coughs that produce no mucus-like discharge.

Drugs that affect the cough center in the brain are codeine and dextromethorphan. In some states, the purchaser of a codeine cough product must sign a special register. In other states, these products can be obtained only with a doctor's prescription. Other types of cough suppressors act on the throat and bronchial tubes to lessen pain, relax the involuntary muscles involved in coughing, and/or thin out the mucus in the throat. Two common cough suppressors of this type are camphor and peppermint oil (menthol). Both are found in topical ointments to rub on the neck and chest or in liquids to put in vaporizers; these active ingredients are breathed in as they vaporize with body heat or in a steam vaporizer. Menthol and dextromethorphan are the only active ingredients found in throat lozenges (cough drops) that appear to be effective.

Precautions: Codeine is a narcotic and is addictive in large quantities; the potential for abuse exists. The effectiveness of camphor and menthol in rubs and inhalants is still under question by the FDA. Do not take cough suppressants for more than one week; see your physician if the cough lasts beyond this time. People with chronic lung disorders such as emphysema who need to clear their airways should not take cough suppressants.

Wet (Secretion-Laden) Coughs

Expectorants thin the secretions, allowing them to be coughed up and removed from the airways. A variety of expectorant products have been on the market for decades with conditional FDA approval. Recent studies suggest, however, that only one expectorant, guaifenesin (glycerol guaiacolate), is safe and effective, so the others have been (or will be) taken off the market.

Precautions: Do not give this drug to children younger than 2 years unless instructed by your physician.

Congestion

Nasal decongestants narrow, or constrict, the blood vessels of the nasal lining that become swollen during a cold. As these vessels swell, the nasal passageways become narrowed, impeding air flow.

The FDA-approved active ingredients in inhalants (from inhalers or steam vaporizers) are desoxyephedrine-L and propylhexedrine. Camphor and menthol are conditionally approved; their effectiveness is in question.

The FDA-approved active ingredients in medications applied directly to the nasal mucosa, such as nasal drops, sprays, and jellies, are ephedrine preparations, naphazoline hydrochloride, oxymetazoline hydrochloride, phenylephrine hydrochloride, and xylometazoline. Bornyl acetate, cedar-leaf oil, menthol, and phenylpropranolamine preparations are conditionally approved.

The FDA-approved active ingredients in oral (pill) medications are phenylephrine hydrochloride and pseudoephedrine preparations. Ephedrine preparations and phenylpropanolamine preparations are conditionally approved.

Precautions: Decongestants can cause rebound congestion. Medications placed directly in the nasal area are more likely to have this effect than oral medications. However, oral medications affect the entire body, whereas nasal preparations do not. To reduce the possibility of rebound congestion, take the lowest dose of the decongestant for no more than 3 days. The topical medication naphazoline hydrochloride should not be used by children younger than 12 and can be habit-forming. Phenylephrine hydrochloride (topical or oral) and pseudoephedrine preparations should not be used by people who take drugs prescribed for severe depression or high blood pressure containing monoamine oxidase (MAO) inhibitors because the decongestants may interact with these drugs, seriously affecting the heart.

Runny Nose

Antihistamines are supposed to dry up cold secretions, but their usefulness with colds is questionable. Antihistamines are allergy medications and work by counteracting the effects of histamines. Histamines promote the manufacture of fluids by tissues, but histamines are not released during a cold. Because antihistamines cause drowsiness, a cold-sufferer may want to take them at night as a sleep aid. (Sleep aids are antihistamines.) Of the many antihistamines, most formerly prescription medications, the following are currently approved by the FDA: brompheniramine maleate, chlorcyclizine hydrochloride, chlorpheniramine maleate, dexbrompheniramine maleate, diphenhydramine hydrochloride, doxylamine succinate, phenidramine tartrate, pheniramine maleate, pyrilamine maleate, thonzylamine hydrochloride, and triprolidine hydrochloride. The one conditionally approved antihistamine is phenyltoloxamine dihydrogen citrate.

Precautions: Pregnant or nursing women should not take doxylamine succinate because of its questionable link to birth defects and adverse effects on infants.

- If you contract an infection, consult a health care professional for specific recommendations on treating it.
- If you contract a systemic infection such as a cold or the flu, rest and drink sufficient fluids to help your body mount its defense.
- If a health care professional prescribes medication for you to combat an infection, follow all instructions and take the prescribed amount of medication.

A high score on this assessment indicates a predisposition toward high-risk STI behavior. A low score indicates a predisposition toward low-risk STI behavior. This chapter will help you develop low-risk behaviors.

- To protect yourself and others against the transmission of sexually transmitted infections, use latex condoms during sexual intercourse.

■ Sexually Transmitted Infections

Sexually transmitted infections (STIs), which are also called sexually transmitted diseases (STDs), are spread from person to person by the intimate contact that occurs during sexual activity, primarily sexual intercourse. In general, the pathogens that cause STIs are passed from the sores, secretions, or tissues of an infected individual's reproductive system to the mucous membranes or broken skin of the reproductive system and surrounding tissue of another. (As you read the rest of this chapter please refer to Figure 5-1, which shows the male reproductive organs, and Figure 5-3, which shows the female reproductive organs.)

Contracting a sexually transmitted infection is more likely when other STIs are present. For example, infection with the herpes simplex virus (HSV) or with syphilis has been shown to increase the risk of human immunodeficiency virus (HIV) transmission by as much as 10- to 100-fold for a single act of intercourse. Both HSV and syphilis cause sores on the genitals, which apparently facilitate the transfer of the human immunodeficiency virus.

Most pathogens that cause STIs cannot survive long (or at all) outside the human body. Therefore, most STIs cannot be contracted by genital contact with contaminated toilet seats or bed linens. Most STIs are passed directly from one person to another.

Some sexually transmitted infections are caused by yeasts, protozoans, mites (organisms closely related to spiders), and lice (organisms closely related to fleas). Most STIs are caused by bacteria and viruses.

Before you read more of this chapter, complete the STI Attitude Scale self-assessment in the student workbook.

sexually transmitted infection (STI) infection spread from person to person by intimate sexual contact, primarily sexual intercourse.

hepatitis B a serious infectious disease of the liver transmitted via blood or blood products.

■ Sexually Transmitted Infections Caused by Viruses

Sexually transmitted infections caused by viruses are extremely serious because they cannot be cured. Certain medications ease the discomfort of viral STI symptoms, but virus particles remain in the tissues and can cause recurrent symptoms. Also, the virus can be passed continually from chronically infected individuals to others during sexual activity.

In addition to causing STIs, three sexually transmitted viruses have been implicated in the development of particular cancers: HIV, human papillomavirus (HPV), and **hepatitis B virus (HBV)**. Therefore, contracting any one of these viruses not only results in an incurable infectious disease but also increases the risk of developing particular types of cancers. HPV is discussed on page 366. HBV causes a serious inflammation of the liver and can result in liver cancer. Although hepatitis is caused by a variety of hepatitis viruses (such as A, B, C, and D), hepatitis B virus is the one most commonly transmitted by sexual contact. Although hepatitis B is a serious and long-term disease, people can recover from it.

Human immunodeficiency virus is the most serious viral sexually transmitted pathogen. HIV infection not only raises the risk of developing the cancer Kaposi's sarcoma, but also the virus attacks the immune system, disabling the body's defenses. Eventually the immune system of an HIV-infected individual becomes so weakened that he or she succumbs to an array of illnesses (the syndrome known as AIDS) that lead to death.

Human Immunodeficiency Virus

As of January 1995, AIDS became the leading cause of death among all Americans aged 25 to 44. By 1996 death rates from AIDS began to decline, and by

Figure 14-15 Leading Causes of Death for Men (a) and Women (b) Aged 25 through 44, United States, 1987–2001. When the data for males and females are combined, they show that AIDS was the leading cause of death in this age group in 1995. By 1996, this was no longer the case. Source: National Center for Health Statistics, National Vital Statistics System. U.S. Department of Health and Human Services.

Note: For comparison with data for 1999-2000, data for 1987-1998 were modified to account for ICD-10 instead of ICD-9 rules.

Note: For comparison with data for 1999-2000, data for 1987-1998 were modified to account for ICD-10 instead of ICD-9 rules.

1998 AIDS had dropped to the fifth leading cause of death in this age group. However, as Figure 14-15 shows, the death rate from AIDS is higher for men than it is for women. This higher death rate reflects the fact that 70% of new HIV infections each year in the United States occur among men. In this country, the AIDS epidemic still primarily affects men who have sex with men (National Institutes of Health [NIH], 2004).

Since AIDS was first recognized in the early 1980s, the number of known deaths in all age groups in the United States increased annually, until the decline in 1996 through 1998. Deaths have since leveled off (Figure 14-16). The number of cases reported increased steadily until its dramatic increase in 1993. Much of the 1993 increase is due to a change in the definition of AIDS, which broadened the list of conditions reportable as AIDS and included measures of immune

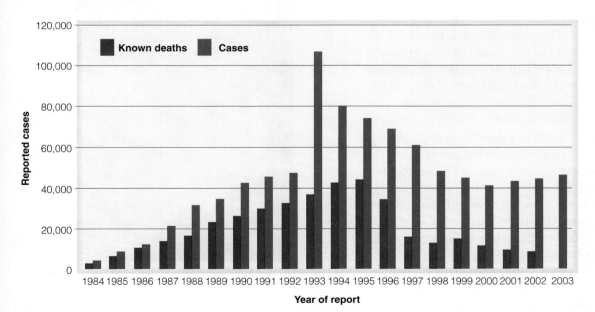

Year of report

Notes: Includes Guam, Puerto Rico, the U.S. Pacific Islands, and the U.S. Virgin Islands.

Figure 14-16 Reported Cases and Known Deaths from AIDS, United States, 1984–2002. The extreme rise in reported cases in 1993 is due to a change in the definition of AIDS, which broadened the list of conditions reportable as AIDS and included measures of immune system function. Source: National Center for Health Statistics, National Vital Statistics System. U.S. Dept. of Health and Human Services, Centers for Disease Control and Prevention.

system function. Since 1993 the number of AIDS cases reported has declined steadily through 2000. This decrease reflects, in part, the waning effect of the 1993 definition change.

Globally, HIV infection is a widespread epidemic disease. Almost 38 million people are living with HIV. In 2003, almost 5 million people became newly infected (United Nations Programme on HIV/AIDS [UNAIDS], 2004). Ninety percent of people infected with HIV live in developing countries, where death rates from AIDS have not fallen as they have in industrialized countries. In industrialized countries such as the United States, costly treatment regimens have allowed HIV-infected people to manage their disease better and live longer. By 2002, prices for HIV drugs sold to poor countries had fallen dramatically. Thus, treatment is becoming available to a greater proportion of the worldwide populace (UNAIDS, 2004).

The Progression of the Disease: HIV Infection and AIDS

Although medical researchers realized in 1981 that AIDS was a new disease, its cause (infection with human immunodeficiency virus) was not discovered until 1983. AIDS is a *syndrome,* a set of signs and symptoms occurring together. Being infected with HIV does not mean that a person has AIDS; infection *leads* to AIDS. Current data suggest that all infected individuals will develop AIDS eventually because HIV infection results in a continuous, prolonged, and ongoing disease process that still cannot be cured.

Approximately 1 to 3 weeks after becoming infected with HIV, most people (about 90%) experience a brief flulike illness. This illness lasts for 1 to 2 weeks and includes such symptoms as fever, sore throat, headache, rash, and general weakness and discomfort. During this stage of infection, people usually do not know that they are infected with HIV and think that they have a particularly bad case of the flu. After learning of their infection, many people remember this flulike illness and realize that it marks the time shortly after their infection.

When this initial illness subsides, the HIV-infected person seems to be healthy, but is in the *asymptomatic phase* of HIV disease, which usually lasts about 8 to 10 years. (*Asymptomatic* means that no disease symptoms are apparent.) This time varies widely among individuals; it can be as short as a few months or longer than 12 years. During this time, many HIV-infected individuals do not realize that they are infected and may pass the virus on to others.

Although people with asymptomatic HIV infection may feel well, the virus is actively killing helper T cells in their bodies. Gradually, the number of helper T cells declines.

Although various laboratory tests can detect abnormalities in infected asymptomatic patients, these persons remain relatively symptom-free until they enter the *symptomatic phase* of HIV disease. The symptomatic phase usually begins when helper T cells have declined to about 500 cells (or fewer) per cubic millimeter of blood (500 cells/mm³). The normal level is 800 to 1,200 helper T cells/mm³. When the T cell count drops to 500/mm³, the body begins to have trouble warding off infections that a normal, healthy body resists. These infections are called *opportunistic infections* because they are caused by organisms that normally cannot produce infections except in people with lowered resistance.

During this phase of disease, the HIV-infected individual experiences a tremendous array of signs and symptoms. Some of these are nonspecific; that is, they are not in response to any opportunistic infection. These nonspecific signs and symptoms include fever, night sweats, headache, and fatigue. Chronic diarrhea usually occurs as opportunistic organisms infect the digestive system. Also, the HIV-infected individual often contracts minor oral infections such as thrush, caused by the yeast *Candida albicans* (KAN-de-dah AL-bih-kanz) (Figure 14-17). These symptoms and infections of the symptomatic phase are not usually life threatening, but the infected individual has trouble maintaining the normal pace of his or her lifestyle.

Figure 14-17 **Thrush, or Oral Candidiasis.** This oral infection is caused by the yeast *Candida albicans* and is a common infection of the symptomatic stage of HIV infection. It can also occur in persons taking broad-spectrum drugs or medications that suppress the immune system. Infants can acquire the disease during birth from mothers with vaginal candidiasis.

As the helper T cell count declines further to about 200/mm³, the rate of contracting serious opportunistic diseases increases. Common infections at this stage include *Pneumocystis carinii* pneumonia (a fungal infection of the lungs), *Cryptococcus* meningitis (a fungal infection of the coverings that surround the brain), toxoplasmosis (a protozoal infection of the brain, heart, and/or lungs), Kaposi's sarcoma (a type of cancer; Figure 14-18), and cytomegalovirus retinitis (a viral infection of the retina). A condition called *wasting syndrome* can also occur at this stage, which includes a marked loss of weight and a decrease in physical stamina, appetite, and mental activity. A person with HIV infection is usually diagnosed as having AIDS when the helper T cell count falls below 200/mm³ and one of these conditions (or another condition typical of this stage) is present.

On average, people diagnosed with AIDS live for about 2 years. Again, the amount of time varies tremendously from individual to individual. But as the T cell count falls below 50/mm³, the risk of death increases dramatically.

Figure 14-18 **Kaposi's Sarcoma.** Named after an Austrian dermatologist, this cancer is a serious opportunistic disease of the HIV-infected person. It begins in the skin and metastasizes to the lymph nodes and body organs.

How HIV Is Transmitted Human immunodeficiency virus is transmitted in three ways: sexual contact with an infected person; exposure to infected blood or blood products; and placental transfer during fetal development, during labor and delivery, and during breastfeeding. These transmission routes are related in that, with the exception of breastfeeding, they all require the blood of the uninfected person to come into direct contact (or close contact, as in the case of placental transfer) with the blood, semen, or vaginal secretions of an infected person.

In 2004, approximately 60% of the men in the United States with HIV/AIDS contracted the infection through homosexual sex. However, heterosexual men and women become infected with HIV also. Approximately 75% of the women in the United States with HIV/AIDS contracted the disease through heterosexual sex (NIH, 2004). Sexual behaviors that carry risk of HIV infection are unprotected anal intercourse between men, and unprotected anal or vaginal intercourse between a man and a woman. However, any sexual behavior that results in the contact of infected blood, semen, or vaginal secretions with the blood of an uninfected individual is risky because it may result in HIV transmission. Since minor abrasions or tears in the skin and mucous membranes of the genitals often occur during sex without partners being aware of it, such contact may take place much more readily than might be thought. Another primary route of HIV transmission is the sharing of contaminated needles and syringes among injecting drug abusers. (Chapter 7 describes drug abuse in detail.)

Some children and adults with AIDS acquired the disease by receiving contaminated blood during blood transfusions. These incidents occurred before blood banks instituted HIV antibody testing. In addition, the staff at U.S. blood banks use new, sterile needles and syringes with each person who donates blood, so that donating blood never has been a risk and is not a risk now.

Most children with AIDs contracted it before or at birth from their infected mothers. However, not all infants of HIV-infected mothers are born with HIV disease. Various maternal factors influence whether the fetus becomes infected, such as the mother's stage of HIV infection. Data suggest that pregnant women who take zidovudine (AZT) during pregnancy decrease the chances of HIV being transmitted to their fetuses (Cooper et al., 1996). Evidence also suggests that transmission is possible through breastmilk, so HIV-infected mothers should not breastfeed their babies.

How HIV Is Not Transmitted There is no need to worry about contracting HIV disease if you work, go to school, and come into casual contact with a person who is infected with HIV. People in certain professions, such as health professionals and police officers, are at some risk of HIV infection because they may come into contact with HIV-infected blood. The results of numerous studies show that HIV is not transmitted by sharing such things as telephones or drinking fountains. Likewise, living with an HIV-infected person and sharing personal items such as combs, towels, eating utensils, and dishes do not transmit the virus.

Although HIV has been detected in saliva, it does not appear to be transmitted by kissing. A protein in the saliva attaches to the surfaces of certain white blood cells and prevents their infection with HIV. The oral cavity is rarely a site of HIV transmission (Shugars, 1999). However, evidence suggests that HIV transmission can take place through oral sex, from penis to mouth and vagina to mouth. Transmission from mouth to penis is less likely (Edwards & Crane, 1998).

Certain insects are known to transmit pathogens from human to human. Thus, some persons worry about contracting HIV disease from insect bites. Research data indicate that transmission of the virus by mosquitoes or other insects does not occur (CDC, 2003).

Protecting Yourself against HIV Infection The primary means of protecting yourself against becoming infected with HIV is not to engage in any behavior that puts your blood in contact with the blood, semen, or vaginal secretions of an infected person. Abstaining from sex with infected individuals will eliminate that particular risk of HIV infection. Engaging in sex in a mutually monogamous relationship in which neither partner is infected also eliminates that risk. HIV testing before engaging in sex will assure both of you that there is no risk of contracting the disease. Of course, both of you must *remain* monogamous throughout your relationship.

Unfortunately, you may not know if a potential sexual partner is infected; also, the partner may be unaware of his or her own infection. Therefore, to reduce your risk of HIV infection, reduce your number of sexual partners. Table 14-1 lists the characteristics of high-risk partners. Avoid casual sexual encounters (having sex with people you do not know well) so that you have time to evaluate whether potential partners have any of these characteristics.

Always use a latex condom or a polyurethane vaginal pouch (female condom) during each act of sexual intercourse. Both types of condoms provide a barrier between you and the body fluids of another. Never use a male condom and a female condom at the same time. The two materials may tear as they rub against one

Table 14-1	People at High Risk for HIV Infection (United States)
Injecting drug users	
People who have had sex with injecting drug users	
Homosexual or bisexual men	
Women who have had sex with bisexual men	
People who received blood transfusions between 1978 and 1985	
People with hemophilia	
People who have another STI, particularly syphilis or herpes	
Women from countries where heterosexual transmission is common (Latin America, the Caribbean, and Africa)	

another and the condoms may not stay in place. Also, do not use contraceptives that contain the spermicide nonoxynol-9. Some contraceptives containing this chemical might increase the risk of transmission of HIV and other STIs (CDC, 2002). (See pages 117–119 for more detailed information on the use of condoms.)

Another risk factor for HIV infection is drug abuse of both injecting and noninjecting drugs. Eliminate this risk by abstaining from using drugs. Injecting drug abusers are primarily at risk because HIV-contaminated needles transmit the virus to anyone who shares the contaminated needles. Noninjecting drug abusers are also at an increased risk of contracting HIV because drug abusers engage in risky sexual behaviors while under the influence of drugs.

If you use drugs, you can reduce your risk of HIV infection by never sharing needles or syringes. If you do share needles and syringes, cleaning this equipment with bleach and then rinsing it with water will reduce your risk of infection. Do not have sex while under the influence of drugs.

In summary, medical researchers have discovered the ways in which HIV is transmitted and the ways in which it is not. This information was used to develop the lists shown in the Managing Your Health box "Eliminating or Reducing Your Risk of HIV Infection and Other STIs." One list summarizes the behaviors that virtually eliminate your risk of HIV infection and the other summarizes the behaviors that reduce your risk.

Treatment of HIV Infection There is no cure for HIV infection and AIDS. Thus far, attempts to develop an effective vaccine to protect against HIV infection have been unsuccessful.

Researchers are continually working on ways to treat HIV infection by boosting the immune system, inactivating the virus, or protecting immune system cells

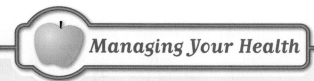

Managing Your Health

Eliminating or Reducing Your Risk of HIV Infection and Other STIs

How to Eliminate Your Risk of Becoming Infected with HIV or Other STIs

Abstain from sex. If that is not an option:

- Do not have sex with HIV-infected individuals or those infected with any STI.
- Engage in sex only in a monogamous relationship in which it is certain that neither partner is infected.
- Abstain from using drugs.

Note: People in certain professions, such as health care workers and police officers, have additional risks of infection due to the nature of their work. Such risks are not eliminated by these practices. These people can become infected with hepatitis B virus or HIV if their blood mixes with the blood or bodily secretions of an infected person.

How to Reduce Your Risk of Becoming Infected with HIV or Other STIs

- Reduce your number of sexual partners.
- Avoid having sex with high-risk partners.
- Avoid having sex with people you do not know well.
- Avoid having sex while under the influence of drugs, including alcohol.
- Use a new latex condom during each act of sexual intercourse.
- Never share needles or syringes.

---

from infection. All approved anti-HIV drugs interfere with viral replication (copying). However, the virus becomes immune to the drugs quite quickly as it mutates. Therefore, combinations of drugs appear to work best to retard HIV.

At this time, AIDS researchers consider a drug regimen referred to as HAART (highly active antiretroviral therapy) to be the most effective. HAART combines three or more HIV drugs, including the newest class of anti-HIV drugs, *fusion inhibitors*. As their name suggests, these drugs are designed to prevent HIV from fusing with host cells so that the virus cannot inject these cells with its genetic material.

Antiretroviral drugs have unpleasant side effects, which make it difficult for an AIDS patient to take the medications on the prescribed schedule. When doses are missed, drug-resistant strains of HIV often emerge, making the medication much less effective or not effective at all. Therefore, physicians are suggesting that patients not take these drug cocktails until absolutely necessary, since an AIDS patient must take the drugs on a regular basis for the rest of his or her life (Pereira & Paridaen, 2004).

Another promising area of research in the treatment of AIDS is *gene therapy*. In this approach, the HIV-infected cells of an AIDS patient are replaced with cells engineered to resist virus replication. The results of clinical trials suggest that this approach may be useful, but many obstacles remain (Yang, 2004).

Genital Herpes

Genital herpes is another STI that many people fear contracting because it is painful and incurable. When asked, "Do you worry about contracting an STI?" one health student responded:

I am really worried about getting herpes. Once you have it, you can't get rid of it. That's scary!

The herpes "scare" began in the United States in the 1970s, and the incidence of this disease has been on the rise since then, as Figure 14-19 shows. Since genital herpes is not a disease that must be reported to the CDC, epidemiologists (medical researchers who study such topics as the spread of disease) can only estimate its prevalence. (Reportable STIs are AIDS, gonorrhea, hepatitis B, lymphogranuloma venereum, syphilis, chlamydia, and chancroid, a disease that is rare in most parts of the United States and is not discussed in this chapter.) The CDC estimates that at least 1 million people are diagnosed with genital herpes each year in the United States, and that approximately 45 million Americans are infected with the virus (CDC, 2000).

genital herpes
an STI caused by the herpes simplex virus that results in sores in the genital and anal areas.

Like all STIs, genital herpes is contracted through sexual intercourse with an infected individual. However, herpes infections are caused by two herpesviruses, a fact that increases the ways in which this disease is

Figure 14-19 **Genital Herpes Simplex Virus Infections—Initial Visits to Physicians' Offices, United States, 1966–2003.** Source: Centers for Disease Control and Prevention.

Visits (in thousands)

transmitted. Herpes infections are caused by *herpes simplex virus type 1 (HSV-1)*, which causes sores primarily on the mouth and lips (cold sores), and *herpes simplex virus type 2 (HSV-2)*, which usually causes sores in the genital and anal areas. Each viral type, however, is capable of infecting *both* oral and genital areas. Therefore, a person who has cold sores can infect his or her partner's genital area during oral sex. Likewise, a person who has genital herpes can infect a partner's oral area during oral sex.

The virus first infects the skin cells in the immediate area of contact and spreads to surrounding cells. During an incubation period (the time between exposure to the pathogen and the onset of symptoms) that lasts about a week, the virus begins to replicate and destroy skin cells. The patient may experience irritation at these sites of infection prior to the eruption of skin lesions. These first lesions appear as groups of tiny, raised, solid bumps that turn clear or yellowish and become filled with fluid. These blisters eventually break open, oozing fluid containing viruses, and then develop into painful sores. The sores turn gray, crust over, and heal usually in 5 to 10 days. With this initial infection, the patient often experiences a headache, fever, weakness, and muscle pain.

Herpes simplex virus usually infects the labia, vagina, and cervix in women and the penis in males, but it can also infect tissues in the genital/anal area that are not protected by a condom. Therefore, the use of latex condoms can only *reduce* the risk of herpes transmission; it does not eliminate the risk for neighboring tissues. Follow the practices outlined in the section "Protecting Yourself Against STIs" (pages 412–413).

Transmission of the herpesvirus occurs when the infected tissues of a person who is shedding virus come in contact with the mucous membranes or with small cracks in the skin in the genital or anal areas of another. A person sheds virus when the virus is present in the skin cells, usually just prior to the appearance of sores and when they first appear. Often, a person shedding virus is unaware of this danger; he or she may have no symptoms of disease at the time. The sexual partners of a person shedding virus may not see sores or other indications that their partner is infected.

When the sores heal, the herpes infection is not cured—the virus is establishing itself in the nervous system for life. The virus particles enter the nerve endings in the area of infection and move up these nerves until they are close to the base of the spinal cord. There, the virus particles lie dormant. During the dormant phase, the infected person shows no signs or symptoms of herpes, and is not shedding the virus.

From time to time, the virus becomes reactivated. Researchers are unsure about the exact mechanisms of reactivation, but infected individuals appear to have triggers that initiate a recurrence of infection. Common triggers are stress, lack of sleep, and menstruation. During a recurrence, the virus descends along the nerves close to the areas of original infection. No symptoms may be present, but the person sheds virus and can infect others during this time. Often, skin lesions appear, but these sores are not usually as painful nor do they last as long as during the initial infection. Most individuals experience five to eight recurrences per year. However, treatment with the drug acyclovir reduces the recurrence rate dramatically. Some persons have no recurrences for as long as 2 years.

Herpesvirus can also infect newborns as they pass through the cervical opening and vagina of a mother with an active infection. Infected newborns may die or suffer damage to their nervous systems. In cases of active maternal infection, cesarean section (delivering the baby surgically, by cutting through the abdominal wall and the uterus) is often recommended.

Genital Warts

Genital warts (*Condylomata acuminata*) are not painful, unlike the sores of herpes infection, but some of the viruses that cause this STI are associated with the development of cervical cancer. This association with cancer and the possible transmission of this disease to the respiratory tract of infants during birth are the gravest concerns of this disease.

Warts are noncancerous skin tumors, masses of cells that result from uncontrolled cell growth. All warts are called *papillomas* and are caused by the *human papillomavirus* (PAP-ih-LOW-mah-vigh-rus) (*HPV*). However, there are over 60 types of papillomaviruses (named HPV-1, HPV-2, and so on); each affects only certain areas of the body.

More than 20 types of HPV can infect the genital tract, but visible genital warts are usually caused by HPV-6 and HPV-11. These viruses cause warts particularly in the cervical, vaginal, and vulvar areas in women and various parts of the penis in men. They can also infect the urethra and anal areas in both sexes (Figure 14-20). The HPV types that infect the genital area but do not result in the growth of warts cause tissue changes that a health care provider usually can see by using special techniques. Some of these viruses, particularly HPV-16 and HPV-18, are associated with cancer of the cervix and less often with cancer of the vulva

Figure 14-20 *Condylomata acuminata* (Genital Warts). These warts are growing around the anus of a man, nearly obscuring that opening.

and penis. The American Cancer Society recommends that women have regular Papanicolaou tests (Pap smears) to detect atypical, precancerous, or cancerous cells within the cervix (see page 348 for specific recommendations) and that men consider having any abnormal tissue growth in the genital area microscopically examined for the presence of cancer.

Health care professionals are not required to report cases of genital warts to the CDC, so only estimates of prevalence are available, as shown in Figure 14-21 . More Americans have herpes than genital warts. The incidence of warts fell from 1987 to 1997 but has been rising since then. In 2003 the

genital warts
an STI caused by the human papillomavirus that results in noncancerous skin tumors of the genital area.

Visits (in thousands)

Figure 14-21 Human Papillomavirus (Genital Warts)—Initial Visits to Physicians' Offices, United States, 1966–2003.
Source: Centers for Disease Control and Prevention.

number of initial visits to physicians' offices for genital warts was slightly higher than for herpes.

To avoid infection with this cancer-causing virus, follow the precautions in "Protecting Yourself Against STIs." Remember, however, that HPV, like genital herpes, can infect genital and anal tissue that is not protected by a condom. Additionally, because skin-to-skin contact can transmit HPV, infection can occur even if anal or vaginal intercourse does not take place. Transmission is also possible during oral sex, so that a person with genital HPV could infect the lips, tongue, or palate of an uninfected sexual partner. Adults as well as infants can develop warts on the larynx, or voice box, if the virus is breathed in. Furthermore, infants may acquire such infections from an infected mother during the birth process.

Although genital warts may go away on their own, the virus particles may remain in the tissue, and can reactivate and infect others. These warts may also persist, grow larger, and spread. The removal of genital warts involves applying medications to the skin that break down the wart tissue, freezing them with liquid nitrogen, cauterizing (burning) them, or treating them with carbon dioxide lasers. Treatment for hard-to-remove warts involves the injection of the antiviral agent alpha-interferon directly into the tumorous growths.

If you contract genital warts, you may want to discuss the benefits and drawbacks of various treatments with your health care provider. Many treatments are far more painful than the warts, interferon treatments can be costly, and medical researchers are unsure whether treatment to remove warts reduces the risk of transmission. Efforts to develop a vaccine to protect against HPV infection or to use in its treatment have proved fruitless, primarily because the virus is extremely difficult to culture in the laboratory.

syphilis
(SIF-ih-lis) an STI that can progress from skin sores to more generalized symptoms (e.g., weight loss and muscle pain) to life-threatening, tissue-destroying skin abnormalities.

gonorrhea (GON-ah-REE-ah) an STI characterized by infection of the urethra in men and the cervix in women, usually resulting in a thick discharge from the penis or vagina.

Healthy Living Practices

- To virtually eliminate your risk of contracting HIV infection, do not have sex with infected persons or share needles and syringes.
- To reduce your risk of contracting HIV, use a new latex condom with each act of sexual intercourse.

Sexually Transmitted Infections Caused by Bacteria

In contrast to viral STIs, bacterial STIs can be cured. Nevertheless, bacterial infections can be quite serious. If not treated, or not treated promptly and properly, bacterial STIs can damage the reproductive system, possibly resulting in infertility. Some diseases such as syphilis can cause even more devastating health effects. Therefore, it is crucial to seek medical attention immediately if you suspect that you are infected and to refrain from sex to avoid transmitting the disease to others.

Syphilis

For centuries, **syphilis**, a serious STI caused by the bacterium *Treponema pallidum* (TREP-oh-NEE-mah PAL-ih-dum), has been a dreaded disease. Historically, the infection rate of syphilis reached a peak in the United States at the end of World War II. Physicians were soon able to demonstrate the effectiveness of the antibiotic penicillin against the syphilis bacterium. Although syphilis is not as prevalent as it once was, its incidence increased in the late 1980s, but has since declined as Figure 14-22 shows. Despite the overall decline, syphilis remains an important problem in the South, and in some urban areas in other regions of the country (CDC, 2004).

An individual can contract syphilis by having sex with a person who has skin lesions (sores) caused by *T. pallidum*. These bacteria enter the body through a break in the skin of an uninfected person. Some syphilis bacteria remain in the skin at the site of entry, where a dime-sized sore called a chancre forms. Some of these bacteria move to the lymph nodes.

The incubation period for syphilis is about 3 weeks. The first sign of the disease is a chancre, which is characteristic of the first stage of syphilis, *primary syphilis*. Most often this sore appears in the genital or anal areas, but it can occur on the lips, tongue, breast, or fingers. The chancre first appears as a dull, red, flat spot, but becomes raised and then ulcerates. Figure 14-23 is a photograph of a chancre on the penis. Although it looks as though it would be extremely painful, a chancre does not hurt. If untreated, a chancre usually heals in 3 to 6 weeks. During that time, however, *T. pallidum* is multiplying in the body; the disease is not gone.

After the chancre heals, the signs and symptoms of *secondary syphilis* appear. These symptoms are systemic because the bloodstream has distributed the bacteria to most of the tissues. Common symptoms of secondary syphilis are sore throat, weakness, headache, weight loss, fever, and muscle pain. In some patients,

Figure 14-22 Primary and Secondary Syphilis—Reported Rates, United States, 1970–2003. Source: Centers for Disease Control and Prevention.

wartlike growths develop in moist areas of the body such as the genital region and under the arms. Most persons develop a rash that covers the body—even the soles of the feet. Although the appearance of this rash varies from person to person, it is often scaly.

When the symptoms of secondary syphilis subside, the infected person is said to be in *latent syphilis*. He or she has no outward signs of disease but is still infected. This stage may last a lifetime, or the infected individual may enter *tertiary syphilis*. During the tertiary stage of infection, tissue-destroying lesions called *gummas* develop. Gummas not only affect the skin but can destroy any type of tissue in the body—even bones. This stage of syphilis is, therefore, often disfiguring. If the tissues of the heart, major blood vessels, or brain are destroyed, paralysis and death can result.

Since the introduction of antibiotics, few people with syphilis in the United States reach this stage of the disease. Most people are given antibiotics for various infectious diseases over a period of years; even if they are

not treated specifically for syphilis, the administration of penicillin for any reason will kill *T. pallidum*. Nevertheless, approximately 100 people each year die in the United States as a result of untreated tertiary syphilis.

Unfortunately, the syphilis bacterium can cross the placenta during pregnancy, infecting the fetus. Infants infected with *T. pallidum* are born with a wide variety of serious conditions, such as bone deformities, low birth weight, lung damage, brain damage, deafness, and blindness. In addition, the infant can be infected during birth or after birth by coming into contact with the mother's lesions.

Gonorrhea

Despite the fact that the incidence of gonorrhea declined dramatically between 1975 and 1996, and then remained relatively stable through 2003, it still has not reached the level set by the *Healthy People 2010* report, as shown in **Figure 14-24**. In 2003, the age group with the highest prevalence of gonorrhea infection was young women aged 15 to 24 years and young men aged 20 to 24 years (CDC, 2004). This is worrisome to health officials because gonorrhea can cause irreversible damage to the reproductive tract.

Gonorrhea is caused by tiny, spherical bacteria called *Neisseria gonorrhoeae* (neye-SEE-ree-ah GON-ah-REE-ah) that enter the body via the mucous membranes. The bacteria infect primarily the urethra in men and the cervix in women. Therefore, condoms are an excellent measure to prevent gonorrhea because they protect these areas well.

The incubation period of gonorrhea is from 2 to 8 days. In men, infection with gonorrhea bacteria usually causes urethritis, an inflammation of the urethra,

Figure 14-23 A Syphilitic Chancre of the Penis. These painless sores can occur on the genital or anal areas, lips, tongue, breast, or fingers. They are characteristic of the first stage of syphilis.

Figure 14-24
Figure 14-24 Gonorrhea—Reported Rates, United States, 1970–2003.
Source: Centers for Disease Control and Prevention.

Rate (per 100,00 population)

Note: The Healthy People 2010 target for gonorrhea is 19.0 cases per 100,000 population.

the tube through which urine exits the body. Urethritis is also commonly known as a urinary tract infection (UTI). A UTI caused by the gonorrhea bacterium results in a pus-containing discharge from the urethra (Figure 14-25). (Pus is a thick fluid made up of tissue fluid, white blood cells, dead microorganisms, and dead body cells.) The infected male then experiences painful urination and an urgency to urinate. Most men seek attention quickly because of these symptoms, but if untreated, within several weeks to several months their body's natural defenses will suppress the infection. Until an infection is suppressed, however, a man can spread it to his sexual partners.

Figure 14-25 Pus-Containing Discharge from the Penis as a Result of Gonorrhea.

Gonorrhea infection in females may cause urethritis, but it more commonly causes inflammation of the cervix and uterus, resulting in a pus-containing vaginal discharge, uterine bleeding, and abnormally long and heavy menstrual periods. A woman also experiences the symptoms of urethritis if the urethra is infected.

The bacteria can infect the prostate, epididymis, and seminal vesicles in males. Although infection of these male reproductive structures is rare, it does occur and can result in sterility. Women are more prone to widespread infection of the reproductive tract than are men. Infection of the uterine (fallopian) tubes or other female reproductive organs is called *pelvic inflammatory disease (PID)*.

Gonorrhea is the most common cause of PID, which develops in approximately 10% to 20% of women infected with gonorrhea. PID is a serious, painful condition. Its symptoms are lower abdominal pain, pain during sexual intercourse, abnormal menstrual periods, bleeding between periods, and sometimes fever. Often, the uterine tubes become constricted from infection, resulting in sterility or in ectopic pregnancy. An *ectopic pregnancy* occurs when a fertilized egg implants outside of the uterus, most often in a uterine tube (see Figure 5-7). Ectopic pregnancies are extremely serious situations. Abscesses (collections of pus) on the pelvic organs are also complications of PID and may require a hysterectomy, an operation to remove some or all of a woman's reproductive organs.

Another complication of gonorrhea is that the eyes of newborns can become infected with N. *gonorrhoeae* during birth if the mother is infected. If untreated, blindness may occur. For this reason, the eyes of all newborns in the United States are treated with antibiotic ointment or silver nitrate immediately after birth.

Gonorrhea can be treated with a variety of antibiotics. In recent years, many antibiotic-resistant strains of bacteria have emerged, sometimes making treatment difficult. However, laboratory testing of the particular strain can determine the most effective antibiotic to administer. Although gonorrhea is curable, reinfections are possible.

Chlamydial Infections

Chlamydia trachomatis (klah-MID-dee-ah trah-ko-MA-tiss) causes **chlamydial infections**, which are similar to gonorrhea. The bacteria that cause both STIs infect mucous membranes in the genital area, primarily infecting the urethra in males and the urethra and cervix in females. The symptoms of both infections are similar, and both organisms can travel throughout the reproductive tract to spread infection. Both can cause PID in women. One difference is that the incubation period for gonorrhea is from 2 to 8 days, and that of chlamydial infections is from 2 to 3 weeks.

Chlamydia is one of the most prevalent STIs in the United States and its rate is increasing, as Figure 14-26 shows. One reason for its prevalence is that infection with the organism causes only mild symptoms in most infected men and no symptoms in approximately 70% of infected women. Therefore, many infected people transmit the disease unknowingly to their sexual partners. Complicating the situation, until recently, was the lack of a suitable laboratory test to detect this bacterium. So diagnosing chlamydial infections in persons with very mild, or no symptoms has been extremely difficult. This disease is important to diag-

nose, however, because women with silent chlamydial infections are at a high risk for developing more serious illness such as PID, and they can transmit the infection to their children during birth. Men rarely develop serious disease from *C. trachomatis* infection, but men with undiagnosed infection continue to transmit the organism to women.

The symptoms of chlamydial infection in men are painful urination and a whitish or clear discharge from the urethra. The amount of discharge and the level of pain are usually much milder than with gonorrheal infections, so men tend to wait longer to seek treatment than with gonorrheal infections. Occasionally, *C. trachomatis* travels to other parts of the male reproductive tract and causes epididymitis, an inflammation of the epididymides, tubules located on the back of the testes in which sperm mature. This bacterium also infects the rectum in people who engage in anal sex.

chlamydial infection (klah-MID-dee-ahl) an STI that results in gonorrhea-like symptoms.

From 15% to 25% of women develop urethritis when they are infected with *C. trachomatis*. Most often, the main site of female infection is the cervix, and a vaginal discharge may occur.

One of the most serious consequences of infection with chlamydia is pelvic inflammatory disease; it causes approximately one-third of all cases of PID. No matter which organism causes it, PID has similar symptoms and can result in sterility or ectopic pregnancy, even though chlamydia causes less painful infection than other organisms such as *N. gonorrhoeae*.

Babies born to mothers with chlamydial infections not only can develop serious eye infections but their lungs can become infected as well. Chlamydial pneumonia in a newborn can cause long-term damage

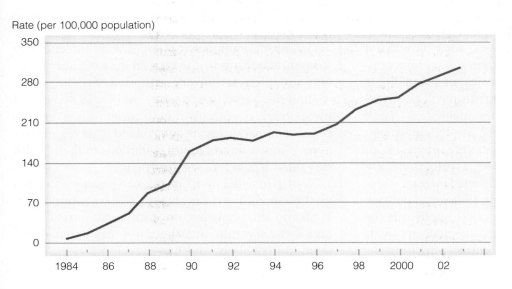

Rate (per 100,000 population)

Figure 14-26 **Chlamydia—Reported Rates, United States, 1984–2003.**
Source: Centers for Disease Control and Prevention.

to the lungs, which affects lung function throughout childhood.

Chlamydia trachomatis infections are treated with various antibiotics. The CDC suggests using latex condoms to reduce the risk of contracting chlamydial infections and following suggestions such as those in the section entitled "Protecting Yourself Against STIs."

■ Other Sexually Transmitted Infections

Organisms other than bacteria and viruses also cause sexually transmitted infections. The itch mite (a close relative of spiders) and the pubic louse (a close relative of fleas) cause sexually transmitted *infestations,* conditions in which these organisms live on the skin in the genital area. A yeast, *Candida albicans,* causes an infection of the genital tract, primarily in women, that can be acquired sexually or in nonsexual ways. *Trichomonas vaginalis,* a protozoan (a single-celled organism much more complex than a bacterium), causes an infection of the lower genital tract of both men and women.

Trichomonas vaginalis Infections

As the name of this organism implies, **T. vaginalis infections** (trichomoniasis) are more of a problem for women than for men. Women are 20 times more likely to contract trichomoniasis than are men. The reason for higher infection rates in women is that *T. vaginalis* lives on the surface tissues of the reproductive tract, such as the walls of the vagina, and uses glucose (a sugar) as a principal nutrient. This nutrient is more abundant in the reproductive tract of women than men. However, *Trichomonas* does not grow well in acidic conditions, which is the normal environment of the vagina (and of the male urethra). If the acid environment of the vagina changes, such as when a woman has another genital infection, is taking antibiotics, or when she is pregnant, the organism will grow easily if she becomes infected.

An estimated 12% to 15% of women in the United States are infected with *Trichomonas.* These infections are almost always contracted by having sexual intercourse with an infected partner. (Men do become infected, but usually the infection goes away quickly without treatment.) It is possible to contract a *Trichomonas*

infection from contaminated objects such as toilet seats, but such transmission is rare.

The symptoms of this STI in men are that of a mild infection of the urethra: mildly painful urination and urgency to urinate. The symptoms in women are more extensive and serious: an abnormal, bad-smelling vaginal discharge, which may be thin and foamy, along with itching, burning, swelling, redness, and tenderness of the vulva. These symptoms vary in their severity among patients. *Trichomonas* infections are treated with a specific drug that kills the organism.

Yeast Infections

Yeast infections (candidiasis) are common among women; medical researchers estimate that 75% of women experience at least one yeast infection during their childbearing years. Yeast infections are acquired in a variety of ways, including sexual intercourse.

Candida albicans is the organism most commonly responsible (85% to 95% of the time) for yeast infections. (These infections are *not* caused by the yeasts used to make certain baked products or beer.) These organisms are thought to be always present in the genital-anal area (as are a variety of bacteria) because they are present in fecal material. The bacteria that normally inhabit the vagina in high numbers keep yeast and other bacteria from growing because they produce acids and outcompete other organisms for nutrients and space. However, under certain conditions, yeast may grow in the vagina.

Yeast may begin to grow and produce a vaginal infection during antibiotic use or pregnancy. Women who have poorly controlled diabetes or other STIs are also prone to yeast infections. Yeast grow best under warm and moist conditions, so clothing that is tight and poorly ventilated in the crotch may also contribute to the development of yeast infections. All these factors change the vaginal environment, allowing the yeast to grow.

The most common symptom of yeast infections in women is itching in the genital area. Other symptoms are soreness, burning, irritation, swelling, and a vaginal discharge that is white and looks somewhat like cottage cheese. Although numerous over-the-counter preparations are available to treat yeast infections, women should report symptoms to their health care providers before self-treatment.

Women infected with *Candida* can pass the infection to their male partners during sexual intercourse. Typically, the penis becomes infected; parts of this organ, the scrotum, and the groin may become irritated and swollen, and may develop a rash, white

T. vaginalis infection an STI caused by a protozoan, resulting in infection of the urethra in men and of the urethra and walls of the vagina in women.

yeast infection a condition in which the fungus *Candida albicans* grows in the vagina or on the penis; also known as candidiasis or moniliasis.

pubic louse a close relative of fleas that causes sexually transmitted infestation; also called crabs.

The Pubic Louse. This color-enhanced scanning electron microscope image shows two pubic lice, one adult and one juvenile, magnified about 40 times. They are hanging from pubic hair by their massive, crablike claws.

patches, or both. Infected men may also experience the symptoms of a mild urethritis.

Pubic Lice

Phthirus pubis (THIR-us PEW-bis) is a **pubic louse,** often called a crab louse because it has crablike claws (Figure 14-27). Therefore, infestation with pubic lice is often referred to as "having crabs." Pubic lice are closely related to head lice, but are not found in the scalp or on head hair. Crab lice can also attach to underarm hair and eyelashes, and occasionally infest these body areas.

Pubic lice are transmitted primarily by sexual contact and are rarely spread via contaminated toilet seats and bed linens, although these routes of infestation are possible. They move from the pubic hairs of an infected individual to a partner when the genital areas touch. The lice then anchor themselves by grasping pubic hairs. For nourishment, pubic lice pierce the host's skin with their mouthparts and suck the blood of their host. When a person contracts pubic lice, he or she may notice tiny droplets of blood on the underwear before the symptoms of itching, swelling, redness, and irritation begin.

Pubic lice also reproduce in the pubic area. Female lice lay their eggs and then glue them to pubic hairs, where they eventually hatch and mature. Unless the infestation is treated, the lice will continue to reproduce and infest their host.

Both nonprescription and prescription medications are available to treat infestations of pubic lice, but a health care provider should be consulted to confirm the diagnosis. Bed linens and clothing should be washed in hot water and dried to kill any eggs or lice. Sexual partners must also be treated at the same time, as with all STIs, so that reinfestation (or reinfection) does not occur.

scabies (SKAY-beez) an infestation of the pubic area in which a spiderlike organism burrows into the skin and lays eggs there.

Scabies

Scabies (*Sarcoptes scabiei*) (sar-COP-tees SKAY-bee-ee) produce infestations of the pubic area similar to those of the pubic louse. These spiderlike organisms (often called *itch mites*) burrow into the skin and lay eggs there. Therefore, one sign of infestation with scabies is thin, red lines or bumps in the skin, which result from burrowing and egg laying. In addition to the pubic region, these organisms infest other areas of the body (Figure 14-28).

The Distribution of Scabies Skin Lesions. The red dotted areas show where infestation usually occurs. The areas without dots are rarely affected.

Itch mites are transmitted by prolonged, close, personal contact, including sexual intercourse. However, if one member of a family becomes infested, the infestation can spread to other family members via infected bed linens, towels, or other household items. Outbreaks also occur in institutional settings such as hospitals and nursing homes. Scabies is treated with prescription medications that are applied to the skin and sometimes with accompanying oral medications.

■ Protecting Yourself Against STIs

The first step in protecting yourself against sexually transmitted infections is to realize that STIs can strike anyone who is sexually active. Regardless of your age, gender, ethnicity, or socioeconomic status, if you are sexually active you can contract an STI.

The Managing Your Health box on page 403 lists behaviors that will help protect you from infection with HIV and other STIs. Of course, you may choose to abstain from sexual activity and drug use, which virtually eliminates your risk of contracting a sexually transmitted infection. If you choose not to abstain from sex, having sex with noninfected individuals also eliminates your risk. How do you know if your partner is infected?

The best way to know if you are having sex with an uninfected partner is to be in a *long-term,* monogamous relationship in which you and your partner have been tested for STIs. A monogamous relationship is one in which a person has only one mate or partner at any one time. Unfortunately, monogamy is not foolproof. You must be absolutely certain that your partner is not having sex with anyone else. Consider the comment by a health student when asked, "Do you know someone who has a sexually transmitted infection? What was their reaction when they found out?":

> A married friend of mine went to the doctor right away after she suspected she had a sexually transmitted infection. The doctor said she had herpes. She was so upset with her husband; she . . . later divorced him.

Apparently, this "monogamous" relationship was one-sided. It obviously did not eliminate this woman's risk of contracting an STI. Also, don't equate *serial monogamy* with elimination of risk. Having sex with only one person for a short period and then having sex only with a new partner, and so on, does not eliminate your risk of contracting a sexually transmitted infection.

Because it is difficult to eliminate your risk of contracting an STI (or to be certain that you have no risk), it is prudent to adhere to behaviors that reduce your chances of becoming infected.

Limiting your number of sexual partners statistically reduces your chances of contracting any STI. With regard to the partners you have, you will lower your risk if you delay having sex with people until you know them well enough to assess their risk as sexual partners. Although you may question your partner about his or her previous sexual experiences, history of STIs, and drug use habits, be aware that people often conceal this information. Avoid having sex with individuals who consistently have sex with multiple partners. Also avoid having sex with individuals who are in the high-risk categories listed in Table 14-1. If you choose to have sex with a person in one or more of these categories, avoid penetrating activities: anal, vaginal, and oral sex. Also, do not use contraceptives that contain nonoxynol-9, which might increase the risk of transmission of STIs.

If you use drugs, you are putting yourself in jeopardy of contracting an STI. To avoid contracting STIs, never share needles and syringes if you are an injecting drug user, and never have sex while under the influence of drugs or alcohol. While under the influence, you are more likely to engage in sexually risky and dangerous behaviors.

The most effective strategy to prevent HIV and other STIs is to refrain from sexual intercourse with infected partners. The second most effective strategy is to use latex condoms during sexual activity. According to the CDC, condom use substantially reduces the risk for contracting the following STIs: gonorrhea, HSV infection, syphilis, HIV infection, hepatitis B, and chlamydial infection. By reducing the risk of gonorrheal and chlamydial infections in women, condoms also reduce their risk of contracting pelvic inflammatory disease.

Although the use of synthetic condoms will reduce your risk of becoming infected, they do not provide a guarantee against transmission because they may tear or slip (although with proper use, this is unlikely) and they do not cover the entire genital area. Condoms made of natural membranes such as sheep intestine are not effective barriers. HIV and other sexually transmitted viruses can penetrate this type of condom, so use latex ones. When using latex condoms, however, do not use oil-based lubricants such as petroleum jelly, mineral oil, vegetable oils, massage oils, and body lotions, which can weaken the latex. Apply only water-based lubricants such as K-Y Jelly.

Another practice to avoid is storing condoms in hot cars or wallets for extended periods of time; keep them in a cool, dry place and out of direct sunlight. Do not use them after the expiration date, or if the packaging on condom shows signs of damage or deterioration, such as brittleness, stickiness, or discoloration.

It is important to use condoms consistently (a new one for each act of intercourse) and properly for them to be effective in reducing your risk against STIs. As you use a condom, handle it carefully, being sure not to damage it with your fingernails, teeth, or other sharp objects. Figure 5-18 and the accompanying text show and describe the correct procedure for putting on a male condom.

Female polyurethane condoms are also available. Laboratory tests show that viruses such as HIV cannot pass through the polyurethane. However, there have been few studies conducted regarding STI transmission during use, and no clinical trials to compare the differences in disease transmission between male and female condoms (Langenberg, 2004).

The female condom is a plastic sheath that covers the cervix much like a diaphragm, lines the vagina, and covers the labia. The same precautions and care regarding the use of male condoms should be followed when using female condoms. Figure 5-19 and the accompanying text show and describe the correct procedure for using a female condom.

Healthy Living Practices

- If you are sexually active, you are at risk for contracting sexually transmitted infections. You can virtually eliminate your risk by abstaining from sex, or by engaging in sex only within a mutually monogamous relationship in which you and your partner are free of disease.

- You can reduce your risk by limiting your number of sexual partners, never sharing needles and syringes during drug use, and not engaging in sex while under the influence of alcohol or drugs.

- Another way to reduce your STI risk is by using synthetic condoms for each act of sexual intercourse. If you choose not to use condoms, you can reduce STI risk by having both yourself and your partner screened for STIs before engaging in sex.

Infectious and Noninfectious Diseases

Noninfectious diseases and conditions that are present at birth are termed *birth defects*. Some birth defects are caused by environmental influences such as fetal exposure to *teratogens*—drugs, alcohol, viruses, or other substances that directly damage the tissues of the embryo (during weeks 3 to 8 of pregnancy) or fetus (during week 9 of pregnancy through birth). Table 5-1 lists some teratogens known to cause birth defects. Chapter 7 describes problems that can occur during prenatal development when a pregnant woman takes drugs. Chapter 8 discusses fetal alcohol syndrome. Dietary deficiencies during pregnancy can also cause birth defects.

Metabolic diseases are also types of birth defects. An infant born with a metabolic disease lacks an enzyme necessary for normal metabolism. Such problems are genetic and result in an infant's cells being unable to make a necessary body compound. Sometimes abnormal substances are made that build up in the blood and urine; these substances can damage tissues in the body such as the liver, brain, and kidney.

Most metabolic diseases are rare; two of the more well-known are Tay-Sachs disease and phenylketonuria. In Tay-Sachs disease, which occurs predominantly among Ashkenazi Jews (the descendants of Jews who settled in Eastern and Central Europe), certain fat-like molecules accumulate in the brain and other tissues, retarding development and causing death by the age of 3 to 4 years. In phenylketonuria (PKU), cells are unable to convert the amino acid phenylalanine to other needed compounds. Phenylalanine and related chemicals build up in the blood and damage tissues, causing mental retardation. Because the ill effects of this disease can be avoided by restricting the amount of phenylalanine in the diet, most newborn infants are tested for this disorder.

Although many genetic diseases claim the lives of infants and children, genetic disorders persist in those children who survive to become adolescents or young adults. Down syndrome, cystic fibrosis, and Duchenne muscular dystrophy are all noninfectious diseases, mentioned on pages 380 and 382, that affect children. The hope for curing these and other genetic diseases is *gene therapy,* in which corrected copies of defective genes are inserted into the hereditary material of infected individuals. A preventive measure is *genetic counseling,* in which prospective parents seek advice regarding the probability that they will have a child with particular genetic disorders. Couples can use this information to make family planning decisions (see the Managing Your Health essay "Genetic Counseling and Prenatal Diagnosis" in Chapter 5).

Most genetic diseases strike early in life. However, one disease, Huntington's chorea (also called Huntington's disease), does not become evident until approximately age 40. By this time, victims may have already passed on the genes for this disease to their children. In Huntington's chorea, the patient makes involuntary, purposeless, rapid motions such as flexing and extending the fingers or raising and lowering the shoulders. (*Chorea* refers to involuntary muscle twitching.) The mental faculties of the person also deteriorate. Fifteen years or so after the onset of the disease, the patient dies. Although there is no cure or effective treatment for this disease, certain medications can relieve or lessen some of the symptoms. Genetic testing is available so that young adults who have affected parents can learn whether they carry the lethal gene. The gene is dominant, which means that if you inherit one gene from either parent, you will develop this disease. This information allows people at risk for this disease to make informed reproductive choices.

Other than heart disease, cancer, and stroke, which are discussed in Chapters 12 and 13, one of the most well-known noninfectious diseases of the elderly is Alzheimer's disease. This disease has a strong genetic link and is discussed on pages 434 to 435 in Chapter 15.

Infectious diseases also have a variety of effects across the life span. As life begins, infection can do harm. Viral infections can be dangerous to a pregnant woman because many viruses can cross the placenta, the organ through which the fetus absorbs nutrients and excretes wastes. Certain viruses, such as the German measles virus, can cause birth defects, including deafness, heart defects, and mental retardation. Other viruses, such as the human immunodeficiency virus (HIV), can infect the fetus, resulting in an infected newborn. Most bacteria cannot cross the placenta, but if bacteria infect the birth canal at the time of delivery, the baby can become infected as it passes through, as in the case of gonorrhea (see pages 408 to 409).

In the past, certain bacterial diseases (e.g., diphtheria and whooping cough) and viral diseases (e.g., measles, mumps, and German measles) were common childhood infectious diseases in the United States. However, vaccines for these diseases have been developed, and children are immunized routinely in the United States according to a schedule. Occasionally, outbreaks of these diseases occur in people who are not immunized, but such events are rare. However, these childhood diseases are still prevalent in developing countries.

Other than contracting common infections such as colds and the flu, sexually active adolescents, teens, and young adults are at highest risk for contracting STIs because they frequently have unprotected intercourse and are biologically more susceptible to infection. For example, the rate of chlamydial infections is highest among females aged 15 to 24 years. Gonorrhea is highest among 20- to 24-year-olds. (CDC, 2004).

The one nonsexually transmitted infectious disease prevalent in adolescents and young adults is infectious mononucleosis. "Mono" primarily strikes young adults ranging in age from 15 to 25 years (although some suggest this age range extends from 10 to 35).

Infectious mononucleosis has been nicknamed the "kissing disease" because it is spread via infectious saliva. However, it is also contracted by inhaling infectious droplets sneezed or coughed into the air by an infected person or by drinking from an infected person's glass. This disease is usually not serious, but the Epstein-Barr (EB) virus (a herpesvirus), which causes mononucleosis, has been associated with the subsequent development of two forms of cancers: Burkitt lymphoma in certain African populations and nasopharyngeal (nose and throat) carcinoma in Asian populations. Furthermore, infection with EB virus can cause a prolonged period of exhaustion, lasting up to 2 to 3 months. Rest is the primary treatment.

The most common symptoms of infectious mononucleosis are a sore throat; low-grade, long-term fever; swollen lymph nodes and spleen (which may result in pain in the upper left side of the abdomen); fatigue; and weakness. However, the symptoms can vary and may include a rash, headache, or nausea. Previously difficult to diagnose in some cases, health care practitioners can now test for mono in their offices.

Infections are a major cause of illness and death among the elderly; respiratory infections are the fourth and fifth leading causes of death in this group. Bacterial pneumonia and influenza, for example, together have over 100 times the fatality rate for persons over 65 than for those between the ages of 25 and 44 (Kochanek & Smith, 2004).

The elderly are more susceptible to infections and have a more difficult time recovering from them than younger persons for a variety of reasons. The cell-mediated component of the immune system functions less well as people age. Also, the respiratory tract changes during the aging process, resulting in decreased elasticity of the lungs and a diminished cough reflex, making elderly people more susceptible to respiratory infections. Other organ systems may also experience structural and degenerative changes that predispose elderly persons to infection. Many elderly people have chronic diseases too, which lower their organs' functional reserves and contribute to their decreased resistance to infection. However, older adults and the elderly are in a low-risk category for contracting STIs because they usually have fewer sexual partners than younger people.

Analyzing
Health-Related Information

The following article was written for high school students to inform them about the dangers of body piercing and tattooing. Explain why you think this article is a reliable or an unreliable source of information. Use the model for analyzing health information to guide your thinking; the main points of the model are noted after the article. The model is fully explained on pages 13–15.

1. Which statements are verifiable facts, and which are unverified statements or value claims?

2. What are the credentials of the person who wrote the article? Do her background and education qualify her as an expert in the topic area? Is it difficult to tell if the author has specific health expertise?

3. What might be the motives and biases of the author? State the reasons for your answer.

4. What is the main point of the article? Which information is relevant to the issue or main point? Which information is irrelevant?

5. Is the source reliable, or does it have a reputation for publishing misinformation? Does the article present both the pros and cons of body piercing and tattooing?

6. Does the article attack the credibility of conventional scientists or medical authorities?

Based on your analysis, do you think that this article is a reliable source of health-related information? Summarize your reasons for coming to this conclusion.

Getting the FACTS About Body Piercing

by Katie Sharp

Jackie, Carmen, and Lisa sat at their usual table in the cafeteria. Carmen and Lisa mentioned they were going shopping on Saturday for new earrings.

"I wish I had pierced ears," Jackie said.

"You're probably the only girl at school who doesn't," Lisa teased.

"Even most of the boys have theirs pierced," laughed Carmen.

Jackie laughed, but she really was envious. She had asked her parents time and time again, but they just didn't like the idea of pierced ears. They did, however, agree to consider it for her 16th birthday, which was only two months away.

That night she decided to bring it up again.

"Mom, Dad, do you remember saying that you would think about letting me get my ears pierced for my 16th birthday? Well, can I?"

Jackie's mom spoke first. *"Have you looked into what it means to have pierced ears? You know, what's involved and what the risks are?"*

Jackie thought for a moment before answering. *"Not really."*

"I'll tell you what," Jackie's dad said, "you do some research on the risks of piercing your ears and report back to us what you find. If, based on what you learn, you still want to go ahead with it, you may get them pierced."

Here's what Jackie learned.

Today, it is not uncommon to see people of all ages with pierced ears, as well as other body parts. And decorating the body goes beyond piercing. Body tattoos are showing up on more people—in more places. But just because tattooing and body piercing are trendy, that doesn't necessarily mean they are safe. Knowledge about these processes is very important before jumping onto the body-piercing bandwagon.

Body-Piercing Precautions

Piercing any part of the body can be risky, especially if precautions are not taken. The biggest danger is that of transmitting diseases, such as hepatitis. Another complication is infection of the earlobe.

If you plan to have your ears pierced, it's best to leave the job to health professionals. This helps to ensure sterile conditions and correct placement of the holes. Piercing can be done with a sterile needle or with a device that punctures the earlobe while inserting the post of a sterilized earring. Using other objects or piercing the cartilage of the ear is not recommended, as this can lead to infection.

Once the ears are pierced, caring for them is very important. The newly inserted stud must be rotated or moved frequently to keep it from sticking. Many physicians recommend the ears be swabbed on a regular basis with alcohol or an antibiotic ointment. This keeps the ears clean and bacteria-free. It usually takes four to eight weeks for the ears to heal. Once healed, it's best to wear earrings with posts or wires made of gold, silver, platinum, or stainless steel. Earrings made of other materials may cause severe reactions, which include pain, swelling, and infection. Alcohol treatment should be continued to keep ear lobes clean, and earrings should be removed each evening before going to bed.

If you're not careful and don't keep up with the care routine, problems can arise. Elongated holes may result from earrings that are too heavy, and lobe injuries may occur when hoop earrings or longer earrings get caught on other objects. To help minimize these complications, avoid these types of earrings, or wear them for only limited amounts of time.

Skin Paintings Can Be Dangerous

Jackie found out a lot about tattooing, too. And while she had no desire to get a tattoo herself, she knew some people who had one—and she was curious.

Tattooing, a technique of marking the skin with colors, is not new. Some people view tattoos as works of art. Others see them as identifying with a group or as being different.

Permanent tattoos are applied with a machine that pierces the skin with needles. Tattooing is illegal in seven (U.S.) states and heavily regulated in others, mostly because in the past many tattoo parlors were known to operate without concern for the health and safety of their customers. Today a major health concern of tattooing is the spread of hepatitis B and HIV, the virus that causes AIDS. While there are no documented cases of someone contracting HIV as a result of getting a tattoo, the threat is still there.

To help prevent the spread of disease, professional organizations for tattoo artists now recommend certain procedures that they say all professional tattooists should follow. Some of these organizations even hold classes for tattooists to teach them cleanliness and sterilization techniques. They say that anyone considering a tattoo should ask the tattooist whether he or she has taken the class and ask to see the certificate of completion.

Getting a tattoo can be a painful experience. A small tattoo can take up to an hour to complete. Once a tattoo is finished, proper care is essential until the area has healed. Some complications include adverse reactions to the dyes used, which is rare, and infection. Infection typically can be avoided with proper care.

Although tattoos are meant to be permanent, there are methods for removing them but they are costly and can be painful.

Jackie reported her findings to her parents. They discussed what would be expected of her in the care of her ears. Jackie made an appointment with her physician—and guess what she got for her birthday?

CHAPTER REVIEW

Summary

Noninfectious diseases are processes that affect the proper functioning of the body, are usually accompanied by characteristic signs and symptoms, and are not caused by pathogens. Rather, abnormalities in the hereditary material, factors in the environment, or an interaction of the two cause noninfectious diseases.

Genetic factors are the sole cause of some noninfectious diseases; such genetic diseases are inherited or are caused by mistakes during cell division when gametes are formed. Inherited diseases are caused by disorders of the hereditary material, or genes. Two inherited diseases that are prevalent in the United States are cystic fibrosis and Duchenne muscular dystrophy. Down syndrome is a genetic disease caused by errors during gamete formation.

Some diseases are caused by an interaction of genetic and environmental factors. Genetic factors can predispose a person to a disease. Diseases having both genetic and environmental causes include asthma, ulcers, diabetes mellitus, and migraine headaches.

Some noninfectious conditions have environmental or unknown causes. Many of these conditions are discussed in Chapter 16, "Environmental Health." A few noninfectious conditions are caused by improperly performing certain activities. Carpal tunnel syndrome, for example, is a painful condition of the hands and fingers that results from improper positioning of the wrist while engaging in repetitive activities that use the hands, wrists, and arms.

Birth defects are noninfectious conditions present at birth that affect either the body's structures or how it functions. Anatomical defects can be caused by genetic or environmental factors or a combination of both. Metabolic defects are genetic and affect a person throughout life. Alzheimer's disease, which is discussed in Chapter 15, is a prominent noninfectious disease of the elderly.

Infectious diseases affect the proper functioning of the body, are usually accompanied by characteristic signs and symptoms, and are caused by disease-producing (pathogenic) bacteria, viruses, fungi, protozoans, or worms. Some infectious diseases are communicable; that is, they are spread from person to person either directly or by means of an intermediary organism called a vector. Other infectious diseases are noncommunicable; they are caused by organisms such as bacteria that normally (and usually harmlessly) reside on a person's body, by the ingestion of toxins produced by pathogens, or by pathogens from environmental or animal sources.

The severity of a disease's symptoms depends on a variety of factors: the type of organism; its virulence; the manner in which it enters, multiplies, and spreads in or on the body; the chemicals it produces, if any; its ability to combat the defense mechanisms of the body; and the body's reaction to the invading microbe.

Two primary causes of infectious diseases are bacteria and viruses. Bacteria, microscopic organisms that have a simple cell structure, cause disease by first adhering to the surfaces of cells. Some penetrate more deeply into tissues, and many bacteria produce chemicals that break down the connections between cells, aiding their invasion. Viruses are noncellular, nonliving, protein-coated pieces of hereditary material. They cause infection by adhering to cells also, but then enter cells and use them to make more viruses, killing the cells in the process.

The human body has two main types of immunity, or defense against disease: nonspecific and specific immunity. Nonspecific immunity combats any foreign invader. Mechanisms of nonspecific immunity include the skin and mucous membranes, white blood cells and their phagocytic properties, the lymphatic system, the inflammatory response, natural killer cells, and interferons.

Specific immunity combats each specific invading pathogen and is carried out by the immune system. The immune system has two branches: antibody-mediated immunity and cell-mediated immunity. Antibody-mediated immunity reacts to antigens (foreign proteins) that reside outside of the body cells, such as most bacteria and the toxic products they produce. Cell-mediated immunity reacts to antigens that reside inside body cells, such as viruses, fungi, a few types of bacteria, and parasites. It also acts against foreign (non-self) tissues such as transplanted organs and controls the growth of tumor cells.

Immunity is either inborn or acquired. Inborn immunity is inherited, such as immunity to infectious diseases that attack other organisms but not humans. Acquired immunity develops during a person's lifetime. Immunity is acquired either actively or passively, and by natural or artificial means.

Many drugs have been developed to combat infection. Antibiotics kill or inhibit the growth of bacteria and are in wide use. Antiviral drugs are limited in availability and scope. Specific medications have been developed to treat protozoal diseases and infections caused by worms.

Sexually transmitted infections (STIs) are infectious diseases spread from one person to another during sexual activity, primarily sexual intercourse. Most pathogens that cause STIs can survive for only a short time outside of the body; therefore transmission of these diseases from objects, such as toilet seats, is either impossible or rare, depending on the STI. Sexually transmitted infections are caused primarily by viruses and bacteria, but some infections and infestations are caused by yeast, protozoans, mites, and lice. The transmission of STIs is often facilitated in persons infected with other STIs.

Sexually transmitted infections caused by viruses are incurable although the body may clear itself of some human papillomavirus (HPV) infections. In addition to causing STIs, three sexually transmitted viruses have been implicated in the development of particular cancers: human immunodeficiency virus (HIV), HPV, and hepatitis B virus (HBV).

The most serious viral STI is HIV infection because it not only raises the risk of developing a particular type of cancer, but also the virus attacks the immune system, disabling the body's defenses. Eventually the immune system of an HIV-infected individual becomes so weakened that he or she succumbs to an array of illnesses that lead to death. This stage in HIV infection is called acquired immunodeficiency syndrome (AIDS). The best ways to protect yourself against contracting this deadly disease or any STI are to refrain from having sex with infected individuals, reduce your number of sexual partners, avoid sex with high-risk partners, and use a latex condom with each act of sexual intercourse.

Sexually transmitted infections caused by bacteria are curable with antibiotics. Three prevalent bacterial STIs are syphilis, gonorrhea, and chlamydial infections.

One protozoan, *Trichomonas vaginalis*, causes a sexually transmitted infection primarily in women. The yeast *Candida albicans* may cause troublesome, itchy infections in women that can be transmitted sexually. The crab louse, *Phthirus pubis*, and itch mite, *Sarcoptes scabiei*, both can cause sexually transmitted infestations of the genital area.

Adolescents and young adults are in the highest-risk age category for contracting sexually transmitted infections. Infants are at risk of infection from infected mothers. Middle-aged and older people are less likely to contract sexually transmitted infections because they are less likely to have multiple sex partners. However, anyone who practices high-risk behaviors or who has sex with an infected person can contract a sexually transmitted infection.

Applying What You Have Learned

1. Based on the information in this chapter, describe two ways (other than picking your relatives!) in which you can lower your or your unborn children's risk of contracting noninfectious diseases. **Analysis**

2. The human immunodeficiency virus (HIV) attacks helper T cells. Why is this attack so devastating to the body's ability to resist disease? **Application**

3. Think about the last infectious disease you contracted. Outline what you think might have been the chain of infection for this disease. Could you have done anything to break the chain of infection and avoid becoming infected? **Analysis**

4. Analyze your behaviors regarding your risk for contracting STIs. What can you do to lower your risk of contracting a sexually transmitted infection? **Analysis**

5. A man develops a sore on his genitals but is too busy to go to his health care provider. The sore heals, so he decides that he "got better" on his own. State two reasons why his reasoning is faulty and dangerous. With which STI(s) might this man be infected? Support your answer with evidence. **Synthesis**

6. State a behavior or behaviors that you could adopt or change to help you become more resistant to infection in general. How would this behavioral change increase your resistance to infection? **Evaluation**

Key

Application	using information in a new situation.
Analysis	breaking down information into component parts.
Synthesis	putting together information from different sources.
Evaluation	making informed decisions.

Reflecting on Your Health

1. Think back to a time when you dated a person you'd only recently met. What did you do to be sure that you would not catch an STI from this person? What did you do to reduce your risk of infection? After reading this chapter, would you behave any differently now to protect yourself? Why or why not? If so, what would you do differently?

2. When you have a common communicable infectious disease like a cold or the flu, do you do anything to protect others, like members of your family, from catching your illness? If so, what? Would you do anything differently after reading this chapter? If so, what?

3. Have you ever traveled outside the United States? If so, to what countries did you travel? Think back to your trip and describe what you did before departing to protect yourself from infection. What did you do to protect yourself while you were there? Has reading this chapter alerted you to additional steps you should take to protect yourself from infection? If so, what? If you have never traveled outside of the country, pick a country to which you would like to travel and explain what steps you would take before you left to protect yourself from infection. What steps would you take while you were there?

4. Do any hereditary diseases run in your family? If you are not sure, ask your family members, including parents, grandparents, uncles, aunts, and cousins if possible. What steps can you take to protect your future children from a hereditary disease? Include specifics about diseases that run in your family, if any.

5. Many strains of bacteria are becoming resistant to the antibiotics used to treat them. One reason for this is that people pressure their health care providers for antibiotics when they do not have bacterial illnesses. Also, some people stop taking antibiotics before their physician says they should. Both these situations provide an opportunity for resistant strains of bacteria to develop and replicate. Do you practice either of these behaviors? If so, why? What have you learned in this chapter that may cause you to change those behaviors?

References

Associated Press. (December 15, 1999). Boy cured of sickle cell anemia. *San Diego Union-Tribune,* A-9.

Centers for Disease Control and Prevention. (1999). Achievements in public health, 1900–1999. Control of infectious diseases. *Morbidity and Mortality Weekly Report, 48*:621–629.

Centers for Disease Control and Prevention. (2000). *Tracking the hidden epidemics: Trends in STDs in the United States, 2000.* Atlanta, GA: Centers for Disease Control and Prevention. Retrieved from http://www.cdc.gov/nchstp/dstd/Stats_Trends/Trends2000.pdf.

Centers for Disease Control and Prevention. (2002). Nonoxynol-9 spermicide contraception use—United States, 1999. *Morbidity and Mortality Weekly Report, 51*:389–392.

Centers for Disease Control and Prevention (CDC). (2003). *Can I get infected with HIV from mosquitoes?* Retrieved from http://www.cdc.gov/hiv/pubs/faq/faq32.htm.

Centers for Disease Control and Prevention. (2004). *Sexually transmitted disease surveillance, 2003.* Atlanta, GA: U.S. Department of Health and Human Services.

Cooper, E. R., Nugent, R. P., Diaz, J. P., Hanson, C., Kalish, L. A., Mendez, H., Zorrilla, C., Hershow, R., Moye, J., Smeriglio, V., & Fowler, M. G. (1996). After AIDS clinical trial 076: The changing pattern of zidovudine use during pregnancy, and the subsequent reduction in the vertical transmission of human immunodeficiency virus in a cohort of infected women and their infants. *Journal of Infectious Diseases, 174*:1207–1211.

Edwards, S., & Crane, C. (1998). Oral sex and transmission of viral STIs. *Sexually Transmitted Infections, 74*(1):6–10.

Hutton, N., Wilson, M. H., Mellits, E. D., Baumgardner, R., Wissow, L. S., Bonuccelli, C., Holtzman, N. A., DeAngelis, C. (1991). Effectiveness of an antihistamine-decongestant combination for young children with the common cold: A randomized, controlled clinical trial. *Journal of Pediatrics. 118*:125–130.

Kochanek, K. D., & Smith, B. L. (2004). Deaths: Preliminary data for 2002. *National Vital Statistics Reports, 52*(13):1–48.

Langenberg, A. (2004). Interrupting herpes simplex virus type 2 transmission: The role of condoms and microbicides. *Herpes, 11*(Suppl 3):147A–154A.

Marwick, C. (1995). Trial halted as sickle cell treatment proves itself. *Journal of the American Medical Association, 273*:611.

National Institutes of Health. (2004, July). *Facts and figures: HIV/AIDS.* Retrieved from http://www.niaid.nih.gov/factsheets/aidsstat.htm.

Pereira, C. F., & Paridaen, J. T. (2004). Anti-HIV drug development—an overview. *Current Pharmaceutical Design, 10*:4005–4037.

Shugars, D. C. (1999). Endogenous mucosal antiviral factors of the oral cavity. *Journal of Infectious Diseases, 179*(Suppl 3):S431–435.

Sintchenko, V., & Dwyer, D. E. (1999). The diagnosis and management of influenza: An update. *Australian Family Physician, 28*:313–317.

United Nations Programme on HIV/AIDS. (2004). *2004 Report on the global HIV/AIDS epidemic: Fourth global report.* Geneva, Switzerland: Author.

Yang, Q. (2004). Eradication of HIV in infected patients: Some potential approaches. *Medical Science Monitor, 10*(7):RA155–165.

What You'll Learn

http://healthyliving.jbpub.com

The Web site for this book offers many useful tools and is a great source for supplementary health information for both students and instructors. Visit the site at http://healthyliving.jbpub.com for information on these topics:

Aging
Diversity in Health: Hunting for Supercentenarians
Dying
Death

Chapter Overview

The status of aging Americans

Why we age

The effects of aging on health and well-being

The spiritual and emotional aspects of dying

The options for terminal care

The definition of death

How to prepare for death

 Diversity in Health
Hunting for Supercentenarians

 Consumer Health
Choosing a Long-Term Care Facility

 Managing Your Health
After the Death of a Loved One

Across
THE LIFESPAN

Dying and Death

Student Workbook

Self-Assessment: Preparing for Aging and Death

Changing Health Habits: Can Changing a Habit Extend Your Life?

Do You Know?

· *Who was the oldest person to ever live?*

· *What happens to your body as you age?*

· *How to increase your chances of living a long and healthy life?*

Aging, Dying, and Death

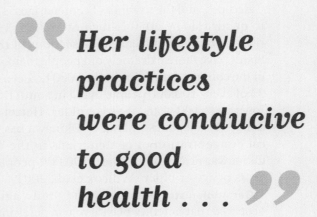

Mary Lombardo Blum enjoys watching television, reading the newspaper, discussing current events, and visiting with her family. If you have the opportunity to meet her, you'll immediately be drawn to her bright blue eyes, warm friendly smile, and pleasant personality. Her skin is so smooth and clear, it's hard to believe she's a *centenarian*, a person who is at least 100 years old. "Oh, I don't wear any makeup," she laughs. "I just powder my nose once in a while to get rid of the shine."

Why are Mary and other centenarians able to live such long lives? Lifestyle, environmental, and social factors are known to influence longevity, but genetic background largely determines whether a person lives to be at least 100 (Friedrich, 2002). In Mary's case, genetics may play a role in her longevity. Although she's lived longer than her parents and siblings, some of her closest relatives lived well into their 80s and early 90s. Additionally, her lifestyle practices were conducive to good health. She did not use tobacco products and she avoided alcohol, except for an occasional glass of beer. Throughout her life, she maintained a healthy body weight, enjoyed good health, and rarely needed medical care. According to a group of researchers who studies centenarians, Mary is an "escaper," a very aged person who survived because she did not develop chronic diseases such as heart disease, cancer, stroke, and diabetes that prematurely end the lives of most Americans (Evert et al., 2003). As you have learned from reading earlier chapters in this textbook, lifestyle is associated with the development of these deadly diseases.

> **Her lifestyle practices were conducive to good health . . .**

The ways individuals manage stressful life events can also influence their longevity. Mary demonstrated an ability to cope effectively with difficult situations early in her life. When she was only 4 years old, her mother died, and the little girl had to live with her grandmother. "I didn't have much of a childhood," she recalls. While in the fourth grade, Mary dropped out of school to care for her ailing grandmother. At the age of 16, she moved in with her father and stepmother, and although she worked long hours cleaning houses and sewing clothes to earn money, she remembers that time as a happy one.

Regardless of one's age, having a strong social network is an important element of good health. As a younger woman, Mary's relatives provided her with love and emotional support. After getting married, she stopped working, and she and her husband raised a daughter and enjoyed their relationship until he died after 44 years of marriage. Today Mary lives with and is taken care of by her daughter and son-in-law. Additionally, she has several grandchildren and great-grandchildren who live nearby and are concerned about her health and well-being. Frequent family gatherings for events such as birthdays and holidays are an important aspect of her social life.

In older persons, religiousness and spirituality are positively associated with well-being (Wink & Dillon, 2003). Indeed Mary credits her deep religious faith with helping her cope with the sad and distressing times in her life. A devout Catholic, she prays every day and reads the Mass from her prayer book. She's too frail to go to church, but she takes Communion at home whenever her parish priest visits. When asked about her long life, she smiles and says, "God is the one who is allowing me to live on this Earth."

gerontologist (JER-on-TOL-oh-jist) a scientist who studies aging.

aging the sum of all changes that occur in an organism during its life.

Mary is one of an estimated 50,000 Americans who are 100 or more years old; most centenarians are women. Today in the United States, more people are living to be 100 years old than in past decades, and the number of centenarians is predicted to quadruple by 2050 (Krach & Velkoff, 1999). For reasons that are unclear, some sections of the United States have more extremely old people than other parts of the country. According to the 2000 U.S. census, about 33 of every 100,000 people living in South Dakota and Iowa were 100 years of age or older (Hetzel & Smith, 2001). The Japanese island of Okinawa has the highest concentration of centenarians in the world. In Okinawa, nearly 34 of every 100,000 people are 100 years of age or older (Willcox et al., 2001).

Gerontologists, scientists who study aging, have observed that heredity plays a role in determining how long people can live. Nevertheless, individuals who have the genetic potential to live longer than average often eliminate this advantage by adopting unhealthy lifestyles, such as using tobacco and being physically inactive (Kahana et al., 2002). Therefore, an important key to enjoying a long and healthy life is taking actions *now* to improve your health and well-being.

For humans, growing old is a natural and universal process. The prospect of aging and dying, however, has troubled people for centuries. Instead of dreading this time of life, many elderly Americans are busy pursuing a variety of enjoyable and rewarding activities. Healthy people do not let the aging process interfere with their active lifestyles.

The Across the Lifespan sections of each chapter of this textbook highlight specific health concerns of elderly persons. This chapter provides more detailed information concerning the aging process, including ways to enjoy good health and a positive sense of well-being while growing old. Additionally, this chapter examines dying and death as well as ways of coping with loss and grief. To determine if you are prepared for aging and death, answer the questions in the assessment activity for this chapter that is in the student workbook.

■ Aging

We can define **aging** as the sum of all changes that occur in an organism during its life. The **life span** is the maximum number of years that members of a species can live when conditions are optimal. The life span of an adult mayfly is a few days; the life span of a human is 122 years. In 1997 Jeanne Calment of Marseilles, France, died at the age of 122. According to official records, Ms. Calment lived longer than any other person (Figure 15-1). However, very few people live longer than 105 years. Contrary to popular belief, there are no regions of the world where populations usually live more than 100 years (see the Diversity in Health feature "Hunting for Supercentenarians" on page 425).

Figure 15-1 Jeanne Calment.

Medical experts customarily divide the human life span into stages or periods (see Chapter 1, Table 1-5). Most people reach physical maturity or adulthood by the time they are 25 years old, but *adulthood* usually refers to the period spanning 21 through 65 years of age. Older adulthood or **senescence** is the stage of life that begins at 65 years of age and ends with death. In this chapter, the terms *growing old, aging,* and *elderly* are interchangeable with senescence. The ages that define these life stages are arbitrary; there are no obvious physical signs that indicate the precise ages when one passes from young adulthood into middle age or from middle age into senescence.

Life Expectancy

Life expectancy is the average number of years that an individual who was born in a particular year can expect to live. In the United States, life expectancies vary according to age, sex, and socioeconomic status. Overall, American females outlive American males by about 5 years (Kochanek & Smith, 2004). As a result, the elderly population consists of about one-third more women than men. White Americans outlive African Americans by about 6 years. The reasons for these differences are unclear, but hormonal, genetic, and socioeconomic factors are thought to influence life expectancy.

As mentioned in Chapter 1, life expectancies increased dramatically during the twentieth century, especially for people who live in developed countries. In the United States, for example, individuals born in 1900 could expect to live 47 years; individuals born in 2002 can expect to live

life span the maximum number of years that members of a species can expect to live when conditions are optimal.

senescence (seh-NES-ens) the stage of life that begins at age 65 and ends with death.

life expectancy the average number of years that an individual who was born in a particular year can expect to live.

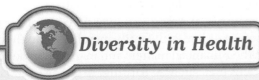

Diversity in Health

Hunting for Supercentenarians

Despite the high standard of living and excellent quality of medical care in the United States, few Americans live to be 100 years old. According to verifiable records, no one in the United States has lived longer than 120 years. Yet in certain isolated parts of the world, hundreds of people claim to be more than 120 years old (supercentenarians). Do people who live in these places actually live longer than Americans or the rest of the world's population?

In the first half of the twentieth century, reports emerged concerning the extreme longevity of people living in the Hunza area of Northern Pakistan, in the village of Vilcabamba in Ecuador, and in the Caucasus region in the Eastern European country of Georgia. Scientists visited these regions to question the very old people and determine factors that were associated with their extreme longevity. After interviewing the oldest people in these regions, some experts concluded that living in an isolated and unpolluted rural environment, eating a simple nutritious diet, avoiding the use of alcohol and tobacco, and maintaining an active daily schedule were the keys to superlongevity.

By the 1970s, however, the real story began to unfold concerning the existence of the so-called supercentenarians. As some investigators returned to locate and interview the same old people that they had met previously, their elderly subjects gave ages that did not match. For example, if 5 years had lapsed since the first interview, instead of being 5 years older, the old person reported being 7 or

10 years older. It did not take researchers long to realize that these elderly people typically inflated their ages. How could so many people have been fooled into believing that supercentenarians existed?

It is difficult to verify the ages of very old individuals who live in rural, underdeveloped places. During the 1800s birth records that could document the ages of very elderly persons were not kept, or they were destroyed. In some cases, investigators initially believed the authenticity of an extremely old individual's birth record, but later rejected it after determining that the person shared the name of a long-dead ancestor who was the rightful owner of the document. Even if individuals who claim to be extremely old have their birth records, the documents' value is questionable because birth dates can be altered.

Why would elderly people add years to their actual ages? In many isolated and impoverished places, conditions are not ideal for enjoying a lengthy life. Aged members of these populations know that the longer they live, the more fame, respect, and status they can expect to receive from younger members of the population. Government officials often do little to refute citizens' astounding superlongevity claims because the notoriety attracts a steady stream of curious international visitors whose money supports the local economy.

Scientists who study individuals who claim to be supercentenarians think that their subjects are old, but not that old. They may be over 80 years of age, but few are over age 90. Thus, no convincing evidence exists that supports the amazing longevity claims of supercentenarians. Many people, however, persistently believe stories that there are concentrations of extremely old people living in certain regions of the world.

77.4 years (Kochanek & Smith, 2004). An increase in life expectancy generally occurs when fewer people die during the earlier stages of life rather than in the later ones.

In the first part of the twentieth century, people lived past 65 years of age, but so many younger individuals died from serious injuries, infections, and in childbirth that these statistics lowered overall life expectancy. By the 1950s advances in scientific and medical technology significantly reduced the number of deaths from these conditions. Today, a greater proportion of the American population lives beyond age 65 than in the past, and the number of Americans who are in this age group is expected to increase over the next 30 years. Figure 15-2 shows estimates of the number of Americans who are or will be 65 to 84 years of age and 85 and more years of age in 2010, 2020, and 2030.

Scientists are learning more about the causes of aging and are seeking ways to extend life expectancy. Their efforts have led to the development and testing of new therapies for today's major killers: cancer and cardiovascular disease. Advances in genetic engineering offer ways to prevent and treat inherited disorders that can lead to disability and premature death. Additionally, organ transplantation gives thousands of dying individuals the opportunity to survive by replacing their failing organs with healthy ones. Living longer, however, does not necessarily mean living better.

Preserving the quality of life becomes increasingly important as people grow older. By the time Americans reach 65 years of age, chronic illnesses and disabilities often reduce their quality of life. A measurement called "years of healthy life" estimates the negative impact that quality of life can have on life expectancy. A broad goal of *Healthy People 2000* (U.S. Department of Health and Human Services [USDHHS], 1991) was to increase years of healthy life from 64 years to at least 65 years. Presently, Americans can still expect to live in good health for about 64 years.

The Characteristics of Aged Americans

In 2000, 12.4% of the U.S. population was 65 years of age and older (Administration on Aging [AOA], 2002). Between the mid-1940s and the mid-1960s, the birthrate was unusually high in the United States. As a result, experts estimate that 20% of the U.S. population will be 65 years and older by the year 2030.

The majority of Americans over 65 years of age own their homes or live with family members, and they can handle their financial matters and manage various daily living activities such as bathing, dressing, and cooking. Most elderly Americans suffer from at least one chronic health problem such as arthritis, hypertension, hearing or vision impairments, heart disease, or diabetes. Many older adults with mild physical disabilities live independently by making some adaptations to their homes. For example, installing elevated toilets, grab-bars, and shower seats makes it easier for people with physical conditions such as arthritis to take care of their personal hygiene (Figure 15-3). In 2001 4.5% of Americans 65 years of age and older lived in extended-care facilities, often referred to as nursing homes, but almost 20% of people older than 85 years lived in these places (Hetzel & Smith, 2001).

In 1999 about 1 million Americans were 90 years of age or older; this population is increasing so rapidly, experts think 10 million will be in this age group by 2050 (Glass et al., 1999). People who are 85 years old and older, the "oldest of the old," are more likely to be severely disabled than the "young old" who are 65 to 74 years of age. Nearly half of American centenarians live in extended-care facilities.

A significant number of the elderly are independent and financially secure, often because they planned for their retirement needs when they were young. Today, fewer older Americans live in poverty than in the late 1960s, thanks largely to federal programs such as Social Security, Medicaid, and Medicare. Nevertheless, many elderly people must live on lower incomes than when they were younger. In 2000 10% of older adults lived

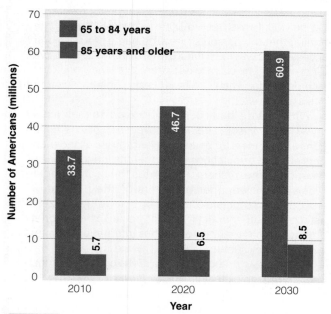

Figure 15-2 **Estimates of the U.S. Population 65 Years of Age and Older in 2010, 2020, and 2030.** The number of people living in the United States is expected to increase significantly in the next 30 years. Source: National Center for Health Statistics. *Health, United States, 1999.* Hyattsville, MD: U.S. Department of Health and Human Services.

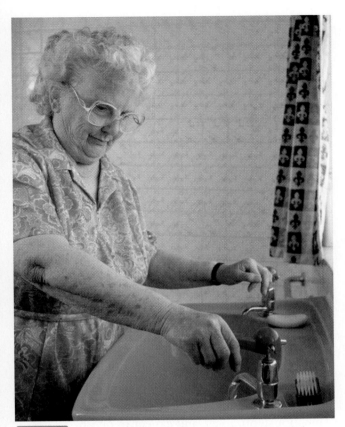

Figure 15-3 **Independent Living.** By adding certain features to their homes, such as these adaptive handles, older adults with physical disabilities are able to live independently.

in families with incomes that were less than the federal government's poverty line (AOA, 2002). Elderly members of minority groups, particularly African Americans and Latinos, are more likely to have lower retirement incomes and live in poverty than elderly white people.

While some of their expenses are less because they are no longer working, health care costs of retirees are generally higher than those of younger individuals. People who are 65 years of age and older constitute less than 13% of the population but account for 35% of personal health care expenditures in the United States (Desai & Zhang, 1999). *Medicare*, a federal health insurance program that provides benefits for people over 65 years of age, does not pay for every medical expense. Thus, elderly people must often buy additional health insurance. The cost of health care is not a barrier to health care for most elderly Americans. However, people with low incomes and less education are more likely to report difficulty paying for medical expenses not covered by insurance (Kamimoto et al., 1999). Without adequate insurance, serious chronic

health conditions can drain the financial resources of older adults and their families.

Why Do We Age?

People age at different rates. A person's *chronological age*, as measured in years, may not match his or her *physiological age*, as measured in functional ability. For example, some 50-year-old people experience the physical changes of aging earlier than average; they look, act, and feel older than others who are the same age. Inheritance accounts for some of this variation because a person's *genes* determine when certain physiological events occur. *Genes* are hereditary material located on *chromosomes* within a cell's nucleus. Genes provide chemical instructions for the production of vital proteins that are needed for cellular activities. For example, most body cells can divide to form new cells. A cell's genes control the number of times it can divide. After dividing its maximum number of times, the cell dies. Most tissues produce a surplus of cells, so they can afford the death of some cells. As people age, however, the rate of new cell production in tissues normally slows and the number of living cells declines as existing cells die.

The results of recent scientific research suggest that *telomeres* play a major role in the aging process by serving as biological clocks that control the number of times cell division can occur (Wai, 2004). Telomeres are structures that form the tips of chromosomes. Each time a normal cell divides, its telomeres shorten. When telomeres reach a certain length, they cannot become shorter and chemical processes that initiate cellular death occur. Theoretically, people who inherit instructions to produce chromosomes with longer telomeres have the genetic potential to live longer than those who inherit instructions to produce shorter telomeres. More research, however, is needed to determine the role of telomere length in the human aging process.

External factors such as environment and lifestyle also influence the aging process. For example, exposure to certain environmental conditions can damage genes. Damaged genes make mistakes in copying and transferring information concerning protein production. Young cells can correct many of these errors, but aging cells are less efficient at correcting such mistakes. When the parts of cells that manufacture proteins receive faulty instructions from the genes, they are unable to produce these compounds. Without an adequate supply of proteins, the affected cells eventually die.

An organ fails if it does not contain enough functioning cells. The systems of the body are interrelated, so when the organs of one system fail, the organs of the other systems soon lose their functional capacities. For example, when a heart that has been weakened by disease cannot pump blood efficiently, the lungs and kidneys are not able to function properly. As a result, other organs fail to perform their jobs, and death occurs.

Radiation, pollution, and some drugs and viruses may damage genes, thereby accelerating the rate of aging and shortening life expectancy. By limiting contact or exposure to these agents, you may be able to lengthen your life expectancy. Furthermore, adopting lifestyles that include regular exercise and that avoid smoking can reduce your risk of heart disease, stroke, and cancer. Eating more fruits and vegetables may lower your risk of cancer also. The Changing Health Habits feature of this and the other chapters can help you identify and change unhealthy practices (see student workbook).

The Effects of Aging on Physical Health

People begin to experience a gradual and irreversible decline in the functioning of their bodies when they are about 30 years old. Even healthy people experience this progressive decline as they grow older. Some common signs of aging, such as menopause, delayed sexual responsiveness, graying and thinning hair, loss of height, and *presbyopia,* the inability to see close

objects clearly, reflect normal changes associated with growing old. Table 15-1 describes some significant physical changes that are associated with normal senescence. As you can see, growing old affects every system of the body.

Aging is an individual process. There is no timetable that specifies at what age people can expect a particular physical change to occur. The rate at which these alterations occur, however, accelerates after 65 years of age. As a result of these normal changes, the aging body is less able to adapt to stress, repair itself, and resist or fight infection. Infections and accidents that were minor health problems when a person was young can become disabling or deadly experiences when a person is old. Compared to young adults, elderly people are more likely to develop nutritional deficiencies, especially of vitamins D and B_{12}, because aging bodies are less able to absorb or use certain nutrients. Additionally, people over 65 years of age are more likely than younger people to have at least one serious health problem, such as cardiovascular disease, hypertension, osteoporosis, or cancer. These disorders are associated with lifestyles and are preventable to some extent. Previous chapters discuss cardiovascular disease, hypertension, osteoporosis, and cancer in depth.

Although certain chronic health problems such as macular degeneration, cataracts, glaucoma, arthritis, and urinary incontinence commonly affect elderly

Table 15-1	Biological Effects of Normal Aging
System	Normal Changes
Cardiovascular	Heart function remains normal, but the heart muscle thickens; arterial walls thicken; pulse rate declines
Skeletal	Bone loss occurs, which can be abnormal if excessive (osteoporosis)
Nervous	Brain weight decreases, especially in the cerebral cortex; neurotransmitter levels decline, nervous message transmission and muscular responses slow; short-term memory becomes less efficient; visual and hearing ability decreases; the ability to taste bitter and salty foods declines; sleep disturbances, such as taking longer to fall asleep and frequent awakening during the night, often occur
Immune	Immune response against pathogens or developing cancer cells declines
Endocrine	Many hormone levels decline, including insulin (regulates carbohydrate metabolism), aldosterone (regulates sodium metabolism), and thyroid, estrogen, and growth hormones
Digestive	Tooth loss becomes more likely as gums recede; levels of stomach acid drop; intestinal absorption of calcium is less efficient; constipation can occur, often the result of medications or poor diet
Muscular	Muscle mass declines, resulting in less strength; stamina reduction occurs
Reproductive	Menopause occurs in women, resulting in thinning of vaginal lining, less vaginal lubrication, and shrinkage of reproductive organs; breast tissue shrinks; prostate gland enlarges in men; sexual responsiveness slows so that it takes longer for erections to occur; orgasms are shorter and less intense
Urinary	Kidneys become less efficient at filtering wastes from the blood
Skin (integument)	Skin becomes drier and less elastic, resulting in wrinkles; scalp hair growth slows, and its loss increases; hair growth in the nose and ears increases; fingernails often become yellow, develop ridges, and split

people, they are not normal aspects of aging. These ailments may not be life threatening, but they frequently reduce the quality of life.

Age-Related Macular Degeneration In the United States, macular degeneration is the leading cause of irreversible blindness for people age 65 and older (Hyman & Neborsky, 2002). The *macula* is a small region in the eye that enables you to see objects in your central line of vision clearly. As many people age, the light-sensitive cells in the macula gradually die, resulting in distorted, blurry, or lost central vision. People with macular degeneration have difficulty reading, driving, and viewing television or a computer monitor. In about 10% of cases, tiny blood vessels form under the macula and leak fluid and bleed, causing severe vision loss ("wet" macular degeneration). Medication and laser surgery can stop the bleeding in early stages of wet macular degeneration, but these treatments cannot restore lost vision. There is no effective treatment for the "dry" form of macular degeneration. Therefore, preventing the disease is important.

Aging people who smoke and have a family history of macular degeneration have a high risk of developing the condition. Other risk factors include hypertension and heart disease. Eating a diet that contains plenty of dark green leafy vegetables, such as spinach, collard, and mustard greens, may protect against macular degeneration. For people who have been diagnosed with the disease, zinc and antioxidant supplements may slow the deterioration of the macula. However, these dietary substances can be toxic and should not be taken without consulting a physician.

Cataracts Although the reasons for their occurrence are unclear, **cataracts** are common in people over 50 years of age. A cataract forms when the normally transparent lens of the eye becomes cloudy and opaque with aging. Clouded lenses scatter light as it enters the eyes, making it difficult to see images clearly. Symptoms of cataracts include blurry and double vision, sensitivity to bright light, and seeing halos around objects. Without surgery to remove damaged lenses, cataracts can lead to blindness. In many cases, surgeons can replace natural lenses with artificial ones; in others, they remove the damaged lenses and prescribe eyeglasses or contact lenses.

Some medical experts think that exposure to ultraviolet light can cause cataracts. You may be able to prevent cataracts by wearing sunglasses to shield your eyes.

Glaucoma **Glaucoma** is another ailment that frequently affects the vision of aged people. In this condition, an abnormal amount of fluid accumulates in the eyeball.

Over time, the high fluid pressure causes vision loss by permanently damaging the optic nerve, the nerve that transmits visual information to the brain. Eye pain, headache, and loss of peripheral vision are symptoms of glaucoma. Risk factors for developing glaucoma include family history, African ancestry, diabetes, and cardiovascular disease. In most cases, placing medicinal drops into the eyes can control the condition.

Glaucoma may not produce noticeable symptoms; therefore, early detection is the best way to control the effects of the disorder. A simple, painless screening test is available that can identify the disease before serious damage to the optic nerve occurs. Thus, you can prevent the irreversible effects of glaucoma by having a physician or optometrist perform periodic screenings.

Arthritis **Arthritis** is a broad group of chronic joint diseases characterized by inflammation, pain, swelling, and loss of mobility ("stiffness") of affected joints. According to the Centers for Disease Control and Prevention, nearly 70 million Americans suffer from arthritis or other chronic joint symptoms. In 1999, arthritis was the leading cause of disability among American adults (CDC, 2001). In *osteoarthritis*, the cartilage that protects the ends of bones and keeps them from rubbing together at joints wears away and breaks down. As a result, tiny bits of cartilage or bone float in the fluid that fills the joint and the joint becomes misshapen (Figure 15-4). People often confuse osteoarthritis with *osteoporosis*, a different condition that affects older adults. Information about osteoporosis is in Chapter 9.

cataracts
a chronic condition in which the lens of the eye becomes cloudy and opaque, impairing vision.

glaucoma
(glaw-KO-mah) a chronic ailment that occurs when fluid pressure increases in the eye.

arthritis
a group of diseases characterized by inflammation of the joints.

Figure 15-4 **Effects of Arthritis on the Hands.** Arthritis damages joint tissue, resulting in deformities and the loss of flexibility.

Aging is the strongest risk factor for osteoarthritis (Hinton et al., 2002). Joints simply wear out as a person ages. Other contributing factors include heredity, overuse, injury, and obesity. Overuse and injury of joints can occur when performing sports or jobs that place stress on joints. Obese older adults have a high risk of developing osteoarthritis, because carrying around extra weight stresses joints, especially the knees.

The symptoms of osteoarthritis tend to come and go. Treatment includes medications to relieve inflammation and pain, and exercises to strengthen muscles and improve or maintain joint mobility. Losing weight reduces stress on weight-bearing joints in obese people. In some cases, surgery is necessary to replace damaged joints with artificial implants.

Urinary Incontinence **Urinary incontinence**, the inability to control the flow of urine from the bladder, is an embarrassing and costly problem for millions of Americans. As people age, the muscles that control bladder emptying weaken, making it easier for urine to leak out when people move, sneeze, cough, or lift heavy things. Additionally, many older adults experience involuntary contractions of their bladders that cause some urine to be eliminated unexpectedly. Medications, infections, strokes, tumors, history of childbirth in women, and enlargement of the prostate gland in men can contribute to urinary incontinence.

urinary incontinence the inability to control the flow of urine from the bladder.

The fear of leaking urine accidentally while in public often makes many incontinent people avoid social situations. In severe cases, family members cannot manage the incontinent elderly relative, and they find it necessary to place him or her in a nursing home.

The majority of individuals who experience urinary incontinence can benefit from treatment, such as behavioral techniques that enable one to be more aware of the bladder's state of fullness. By learning to empty the bladder more frequently, a person may be able to avoid the leakage. Furthermore, people can learn and practice a series of exercises that strengthen the pelvic muscles that control urination. These exercises, called *Kegel exercises*, involve imitating the same muscular movements that individuals make when they voluntarily stop urinating. Incontinent people can also wear absorbent pads and undergarments designed to prevent embarrassing incidents of urine leakage. Medication and surgery may alleviate incontinence. Embarrassment or concerns about surgery, however, keep many incontinent people from discussing this common problem with health care practitioners.

Alzheimer's Disease You cannot find your keys; you forget an appointment; you sometimes call your child by your cat's name. Do you ever have the feeling that you are losing your mind? It may be reassuring to know that everyone has these and other similar annoying experiences from time to time, but many middle-aged Americans worry that instances of forgetfulness are early symptoms of Alzheimer's disease (AD).

An estimated 2.3 million Americans, mostly elderly, have AD, a severe degenerative disorder that affects the brain (Cummings & Cole, 2002). By the year 2050, experts predict that 1 in 45 Americans will suffer from this dreaded disorder. AD is the most common form of *age-related dementia*; strokes and Parkinson's disease are also major causes of age-related dementia. Memory loss, mental confusion, and loss of control over behavior and body functions are characteristics of AD.

The incidence of AD increases with advancing age. An estimated 5% to 7% of people over 65 years of age have the condition; this percentage increases to 40% of people over 85 years old (Howarth et al., 1999). Although the disease is common among the elderly, it is not a normal feature of growing old. What are the signs of AD? Is it preventable?

In the early stages of Alzheimer's, affected people may notice lapses in their memories and intellectual (*cognitive*) abilities. For example, they may have unusual difficulty remembering events that happened recently, learning new information, and using information to make reasonable conclusions. These symptoms typically begin between 40 and 60 years of age. Over time, people with the disease become increasingly forgetful, confused, disoriented, restless, and moody. Communicating becomes difficult as their speech deteriorates; depression is common. These changes are distressing to patients with AD, their family members, and their associates. One woman recalls her affected mother-in-law's gradual loss of cognitive functioning:

The first time I had a feeling that my elderly mother-in-law might have a serious problem with her memory occurred in April when she got lost while driving to our house. We live close to her and she had made the short trip dozens of times. When I told my husband that this was unusual behavior for her and could be a sign of a memory problem, he disagreed and said it was "easy" to make a wrong turn on the way to our house. A few months later, I was driving Mother to a store when she insisted that I should be making a right turn instead of a left one at a familiar intersection in our town. When I told her she was wrong, she became angry and argued with me about the directions to the store. When I finally reached the store, she recognized the place but didn't apologize for her behavior. At Christmas, Mother was very quiet and seemed to be in a fog. My husband and his sister finally recognized that she was "not herself," and they took her to the doctor's for an evaluation. After a series of medical tests to rule out minor strokes and other causes of brain damage, her condition was diagnosed as mild-to-moderate Alzheimer's disease.

Mother now takes two medications that seem to help her memory a little. At this point, she is not supposed to drive and she needs help with housework. She still cooks, but I'm concerned she'll forget that she's making something and she'll start a fire in her kitchen. My husband and his sister are thinking about selling Mother's house and placing her in a special group home for people with this terrible disease. I dread the day when my husband greets his mother and she doesn't recognize him.

As AD progresses, its victims neglect their personal hygiene, and they exhibit inappropriate and unpredictable behaviors such as undressing in public and attacking caretakers. In the terminal stages, individuals with this devastating illness require constant care. They are bedridden, and unable to talk and eat. Nothing can be done to stop the relentless progression of the disease. After diagnosis, the affected person can expect to survive only about 8 to 12 years. Death often results from pneumonia and starvation as the degenerating brain is unable to control vital functions such as breathing, swallowing, and digestion. In 2002 more than 58,000 Americans died of AD, making it the eighth leading cause of death (Kochanek & Smith, 2004).

The factors that cause AD are unclear, and many health experts think that the condition cannot be prevented. At least two forms of the disorder are inherited. Although genetic testing is available to determine whether relatives of patients with AD have the genes associated with the condition, many people who test positive do not develop the disease. Other forms of AD may be the result of slow-acting brain viruses, brain injury, or exposure to pollutants. At one time, scientists thought that aluminum poisoning caused the disease because higher than normal amounts of this metal are found in the brains of patients who died of Alzheimer's. Many people are concerned about the safety of using aluminum cookware and the natural presence of this element in drinking water. However, most experts think that the unusual concentration of aluminum in the brains of persons with AD is a result, not a cause, of the disorder.

Dietary factors may play a role in the development of AD. People with increased blood levels of homocysteine, a toxic amino acid, have a higher than normal risk of AD. On the other hand, eating fish and drinking moderate amounts of wine are associated with lower risks of the disease. Although the reasons are unclear, people who take nonsteroidal anti-inflammatory agents, medication to control hypertension, and statins, a class of medications used to treat elevated blood cholesterol levels, have a lower risk of

Table 15-2	Simple Memory Test for Identifying Dementia

Ask the person

1. His or her age
2. His or her date of birth
3. The time to the nearest hour
4. His or her address
5. The current year
6. Where he or she is
7. The names of two people who are pictured in family photos
8. The years of World War II
9. The name of the current president of the United States
10. To count backwards from 100 to 1
11. His or her phone number

Source: Adapted from Wattis, J. (1996). What an old age psychiatrist does. *British Medical Journal, 313*:101–104.

AD than people who do not take these drugs (Cummings & Cole, 2002).

Physicians often diagnose AD when patients cannot answer questions like those listed in Table 15-2. Until recently, the only way to confirm the diagnosis was by examining the patient's brain after death. Upon microscopic examination, the affected regions of the brain usually contain abnormal protein deposits called *senile plaques* and nerve cells with tangled masses of useless material. Brain imaging techniques such as magnetic resonance imaging (MRI) scans can now detect shrinkage in areas of the cerebral cortex, the thinking part of the brain (Fox et al., 2001). Such brain shrinkage is a sign of AD.

Although AD is incurable, a few medications can slow decline in cognitive functioning, control certain inappropriate behaviors of patients with the disease, and improve their mood. Researchers are testing the usefulness of other treatments, such as anti-inflammatory agents, including herbal supplements. In one study of over 240 Alzheimer's patients, extracts made from the gingko tree did not slow or stop the disease's progression (Van Dongen, 2003). In another study involving nearly 5,400 men and women, high intakes of vitamin E and C from foods (but not from supplements) were associated with a reduced risk of AD (Engelhart et al., 2002). More research, however, is needed to determine the effectiveness of certain diets and herbal supplements in preventing this disease (Martin, 2003).

Patients with Alzheimer's often live at home until they reach the terminal stage and require the care provided in a skilled nursing care facility. Living with an affected loved one can be emotionally stressful and physically demanding. While caring for a patient with this disease, family members must try to maintain their own health and well-being. To provide assistance, many communities have special "adult day care" centers where persons with AD can spend a few hours during the day before returning to their homes. Not every community offers this service, so if you need help caring for someone with AD, check with your local mental health association or Alzheimer's Association for information about adult day care centers in your area. The Analyzing Health-Related Information feature on pages 434 to 435 involves evaluating excerpts of an article about AD.

The Effects of Aging on Psychological Health

As they approach the end of middle age, most employed people face retirement, and many aging parents have grown children with families who have moved away. If older adults equate retirement from jobs and separation from their families with being old and useless, they may experience serious psychological distress. Additionally, the dramatic reduction of financial resources that often accompanies retirement can mean a serious loss of economic stability.

Many older adults began planning for their future financial security while they were young. Therefore, not every older adult dreads the prospect of retiring from job and family responsibilities. Many people approach retirement with a positive outlook and look forward to this time of life. Retired individuals often find pleasure from traveling, volunteering in their communities, caring for their grandchildren, and exploring new interests. Other retirement-age adults choose to continue working, especially if they enjoy what they do and their work is intellectually stimulating and personally fulfilling. The elderly often have a wealth of knowledge and experience that they can share with younger members of society.

Elderly people, especially those over 85 years of age, frequently experience deteriorating health, difficult social circumstances, and poor economic conditions. Deaths of spouses and friends, separations from family, and reductions in financial resources create emotional stress. As a result, the elderly often suffer depression. Regardless of one's age, depression is associated with an increased risk of suicide; suicide rates

ageism
a bias against elderly people.

are high among older Americans. Divorced or widowed elderly persons are more likely to kill themselves than married elderly persons (U.S. Surgeon General, 1999). Additionally, poor health is a risk factor for suicide. Results of a Canadian study indicated that elderly people suffering from cancer, chronic lung disease, and depression were more likely to commit suicide than those who did not have these conditions (Quan et al., 2002).

Like younger people, depressed or isolated aged individuals can benefit from participation in social and physical activities. In addition, antidepressant medications or psychotherapy may be necessary to help them regain and maintain their emotional balance.

The Effects of Aging on Social Health

Although a large segment of the U.S. population is over 65 years old, our society is highly youth-oriented. Not surprisingly, middle-age Americans often worry that aging will mean losing their jobs to younger people, being forced into early retirement, becoming widowed, and suffering from debilitating illnesses. Growing old in America can have serious social impacts on the elderly; they may be ignored, neglected, and abused by younger members of the population.

Some people in our society have negative attitudes toward the elderly. For example, they stereotype elderly people as poor, sick, useless, and dependent. Additionally, some young adults believe that the elderly demand too much from the rest of society. **Ageism** is a bias against the elderly. Ageism creates conflict between the generations because the old do not trust the young and vice versa. To combat ageism, people need to recognize that growing old does not always mean having poor health, living in an institution, depending on public support, and being useless.

Elderly Americans represent a valuable social asset that is not well used. Aging parents and grandparents often have experience and wisdom that they can share with younger family members. Additionally, many retirees have a variety of talents and special organizational skills that enable them to serve as consultants, managers, or advisors in business, governmental, or educational settings. Both young and old benefit when each accepts, values, and trusts the other.

Successful Aging

Many people would like to believe that it is possible to prevent aging or delay the process. The modern search for a "fountain of youth" has resulted in the promotion of pills, potions, diets, or treatments that are touted as having "anti-aging" or "life-extending" capabilities.

Contrary to the claims of advertisers, none of these substances or regimens prevents or slows aging.

Instead of searching for magic formulas to extend your life, you can take various actions while you are young to increase your chances of aging *successfully*. People who age successfully are independent, socially active, and in good health (Glass, 2003). Furthermore, the final stage of their lives is productive, enjoyable, and satisfying.

To increase your chances of aging successfully, evaluate your health status and lifestyle, identify specific unhealthy or risky behaviors, and then work at changing those behaviors. Although modifying all unhealthy behaviors is commendable, certain practices are associated more closely with lengthening one's life span than others.

Scientists who conduct aging research on animals have consistently found that restricting the animals' caloric intakes without creating nutritional deficiencies slows their rate of aging (Heibronn & Ravussin, 2003). In humans, excess body fat is associated with the increased risk of premature death (Peeters et al., 2003). Thus, it is extremely important for you to eat a nutritious, low-fat diet and maintain a weight that is appropriate for your height and body build.

Physically active people live longer than people who are sedentary or become sedentary as they age (Erikssen, 2001). Engaging in regular exercise throughout your life will help you control your body weight as well as improve your circulation, strengthen your heart, and maintain your muscle and bone mass. People over 65 years of age who perform regular exercise improve their physical strength and flexibility, features that can enhance their quality of living (Mazzeo et al., 1998). Aerobic exercise can even improve some cognitive abilities of aging adults, such as memory, but more research is needed to further support these findings (Kramer et al., 1999).

After studying more than 2,700 older adults, Thomas Glass and colleagues (1999) report that aging people can derive significant health benefits from engaging in social and productive activities such as attending religious services and participating in group shopping trips. According to the results of Glass's study, aging adults live longer and better when they are involved in social and meaningful activities.

Table 15-3 lists some basic recommendations for enhancing your health and quality of life as you age, such as managing stress, maintaining relationships, and developing a positive attitude. The other chapters of this textbook provide more detailed information about these recommendations. It is worth remembering the words of Eubie Blake, a jazz musi-

| Table 15-3 | Tips for Successful Aging |

Taking the following actions now, while you are still young, may help you enjoy a healthier, longer life:

- Maintain a healthy weight and eat a nutritious, low-fat diet that includes plenty of whole grains, fruits, and vegetables.
- Be physically active; exercise daily.
- Do not smoke, drink too much alcohol, or abuse other drugs.
- Manage stress; take time to relax daily.
- Have regular physical examinations.
- Adopt safer sex practices.
- Do not drive while under the influence of alcohol or other drugs; always wear a seat belt in vehicles.
- Protect your skin and eyes from sunlight.
- Obtain enough sleep.
- Be concerned about your safety at home, work, or play.
- Maintain social networks with your family and friends.
- Be flexible; expect changes.
- Develop a positive attitude; have a sense of humor.
- Find opportunities to learn new skills or information.
- Get involved with living while accepting your mortality.

Sources: Adapted from Kerschner, H., & Pegues, J. A. (1998). Productive aging: A quality of life agenda. *Journal of the American Dietetic Association, 98*:1445–1448; and Turner, L. W., Sizer, F. S., Whitney, E. N., & Wilks, B. B. (1992). *Life choices: Health concepts and strategies.* Minneapolis: West Publishing Co.

cian who died in 1983 at the age of 100, "If I had known that I was going to live this long, I would have taken better care of myself."

Healthy Living Practices

- Planning for your future financial needs while you are still young can help you enjoy your retirement years.
- To age successfully, evaluate your present health and lifestyle, identify risky behaviors, and then consider changing those behaviors.

Dying

Many Americans, including health professionals, fear dying and death, especially the possibility that dying will be premature and painful. Fearing death makes it difficult to be around someone who is dying. One reason many Americans fear dying and death is that few have had contact with dying persons or dead bodies. Usually an ambulance rushes the critically

CRITICAL THINKING

The following article is an abbreviated version of "Alzheimer's: Few Clues on the Mysteries of Memory" that appeared in *FDA Consumer* magazine. Read the article and evaluate it using the model for analyzing health-related information. The main points of the model are noted below; the model is fully explained on pages 13–15.

Alzheimer's

Few Clues on the Mysteries of Memory

by Audrey T. Hingley

It happened some years ago but the memory is still firmly implanted in my mind. One sunny afternoon I heard the sound of a car pulling into our driveway, peered out of my living room window, and saw one of my father's friends, Sam (not his real name), then in his early 80s. Sam got out of his car and walked just a few steps. I watched as he stood for a few moments, gazing at our house with an expressionless face. Then he silently returned to his car, got in, and drove away, without ever knocking on our door or communicating with us in any way.

I thought the incident puzzling, but it wasn't until months later that I learned the reason for it. Sam had Alzheimer's, a progressive disease in which nerve cells in the brain degenerate and brain substance shrinks.

A widower living alone, Sam clearly was in a dangerous position. Once he was followed home by a police officer, who told his grown children he had found Sam stopped by the side of the road, not able to remember how to get home by himself.

Sam's story is being played out in the lives of up to 4 million Americans who suffer from Alzheimer's disease. The disease plays no favorites, attacking rich and poor, famous and ordinary. Among its most famous sufferers: former President Ronald Reagan.

With an average lifetime cost of care per patient of $174,000, it is the third most expensive disease in America, following only heart disease and cancer. But perhaps even more staggering than the monetary costs are the emo-

tional and psychological costs borne by both patients and their families.

"People are very frightened of the possibilities because they know it represents a loss of one's self," says Steven T. DeKosky, M.D., director of the Alzheimer's Disease Research Center at the University of Pittsburgh and a practicing neurologist. "It's a very frightening prospect to see a loved one who looks the same but doesn't talk or act the same."

"I Have Lost Myself"

Alzheimer's disease, a progressive, degenerative disease attacking the brain and resulting in impaired thinking, behavior and memory, was first described by Alois Alzheimer, M.D., in 1906. German researchers recently found an important set of notes from Alzheimer's journal of the world's first documented case of the disease. The patient exhibited many of the symptoms seen in Alzheimer's patients today. But perhaps most poignant of all is the patient's own description of the disease: "I have lost myself."

In Alzheimer's, nerve cells in the part of the brain responsible for memory and other thought processes degenerate for still-unknown reasons. Some of the most severely affected cells normally use acetylcholine, a brain chemical, to communicate. Tacrine (brand name Cognex, also called THA), the first drug approved by the Food and Drug Administration specifically to treat Alzheimer's disease, works by slowing the breakdown of acetylcholine. This results in relieving some memory impairment.

Tacrine does not cure Alzheimer's or slow the disease's progression. It has only been studied in those with mild to moderate Alzheimer's disease who were otherwise in generally good health. Because tacrine can increase the blood levels of a liver enzyme that can indicate liver damage, regular monitoring is necessary. Other side effects include nausea, vomiting, diarrhea, abdominal pain, skin rash, and indigestion.

Aricept (generic name donepezil hydrochloride, also called E2020), approved by the FDA in 1996, is by far the most used drug for Alzheimer's treatment. Like tacrine, Aricept inhibits the breakdown of acetylcholine but does not cause the kind of increase in liver enzymes that tacrine does. It can also cause diarrhea, vomiting, nausea, fatigue, insomnia, and anorexia, but in most cases, such side effects are mild and decline with continued use of the drug. Again, the drug helps only those patients with mild to moderate symptoms of Alzheimer's and does not stop or slow the disease's progression.

Forgetfulness or Alzheimer's?

While most people understand at least some of the horrifying aspects of Alzheimer's disease, DeKosky says a big challenge is educating people regarding the widely held assumption that people are supposed to have memory impairment as they age.

"There's this huge prejudice where we think people should have severe mental impairment as they get older," he says. Memory loss, disorientation, and confusion are not part of the normal aging process, he explains. They are symptoms of dementia, and the most common form of dementia is Alzheimer's.

"You need to look at the functional consequences of what someone cannot remember," DeKosky says. "If mom forgets where she put her car in the parking lot at the mall, that's not abnormal. But if she walks home from the mall because she forgot she took her car, that's not normal. Memory is the first and worst change, but you will also see social withdrawal and less willingness to interact with others."

The Need for Answers

Although no cure for Alzheimer's is available now, planning and medical/social management can help ease the burden on both patient and family members. Physical exercise, good nutrition, and social activities are important. A calm, structured environment may also help the person to continue functioning.

At some point, however, people with Alzheimer's require 24-hour care. The financing of such care, including diagnosis costs, treatment, and paid care, is estimated to be $100 billion annually, according to the Alzheimer's Association. The federal government covers $4.4 billion and the states another $4.1 billion, with much of the remaining costs borne by patients and their families.

"It's a national imperative to find effective means to diagnose, treat and prevent this disease," says David Banks, R.Ph., a public health specialist in the FDA's Office of Special Health Issues. "When you look at it demographically, the nearly 80 million baby boomers living in the United States . . . now have an average life expectancy of approximately 78 years. One in five Americans could be age 65 or older by 2030, and tens of millions of baby boomers will live into their 80s. The Alzheimer's Association projects that as many as 14 million Americans could have Alzheimer's disease in 2050. When viewed in the context of accelerating Social Security and Medicare costs . . . , the future monetary costs of Alzheimer's disease may be unsustainable. The human costs could be even greater."

Note: Audrey T. Hingley is a freelance writer in Mechanicsville, Virginia.

1. Which statements are verifiable facts, and which are unverified statements or value claims?
2. What are the credentials of the woman who wrote the article? If this information is available, do her background and education qualify her as an expert in the topic area?
3. What might be the motives and biases of the woman who wrote the article? State reasons for your answer.
4. Which information in the article is relevant to the topic? Which information is irrelevant?
5. Is the source reliable? Does it have a reputation for publishing misinformation?
6. Does the article attack the credibility of conventional scientists or medical authorities?

Based on your analysis, do you think that this article is a reliable source of health-related information? Explain why you think it is or is not. Summarize your reasons for coming to this conclusion.

Figure 15-5 **Intensive Care.** Treatment of a critically injured or terminally ill person may include being connected to a variety of life-support machines in a hospital's intensive care unit.

injured or terminally ill person to a hospital, where he or she is connected to a variety of life-support machines and placed in an intensive care unit (Figure 15-5). Most hospitals permit family members to visit the seriously ill patient for only a few minutes each hour. In other instances, elderly or incurably ill patients die in nursing homes with few or no family members present. In the United States, dying often becomes a mechanized, isolated, and depersonalized process.

Dying was very different a hundred years ago. In that era, nearly everyone died at home, surrounded by family and friends. Shortly after death, the body was cooled, and it often remained in the home for the funeral ceremony. It was even customary for people to have photographs taken of their deceased loved ones to remember them (Figure 15-6). These practices helped survivors accept dying and death as a part of life.

Figure 15-6 **Remembrance Photo, Circa 1895.** A hundred years ago, nearly everyone died at home, surrounded by their families and friends. It was customary for people to have photographs taken of their deceased loved ones to remember them.

The Spiritual Aspects of Dying

Some people who have been revived after being unresponsive describe "near-death" experiences and relate them as spiritually uplifting events. They report that they were aware of what was happening before they recovered consciousness. They often recall feeling temporarily disengaged from their bodies and having unusual but peaceful sensations. Accounts of near-death experiences often include some features of the person's spiritual or religious beliefs. People who have been in these situations are often profoundly affected by their experiences, but scientists have no ways of verifying their stories.

People who believe in an afterlife may have less fear of dying and death. Many people believe that a soul exists, which leaves the body after death and goes to heaven or hell. Others believe in *reincarnation,* coming back to life as another person or organism after death. Some individuals are not concerned with what happens to them after death. In many instances, cultural and religious backgrounds provide the foundation for a person's feelings about life after death.

The Emotional Aspects of Dying

Although coping with the death of a beloved person is one of life's most difficult experiences, knowing that your own death is near is especially difficult. In the late 1960s, Elisabeth Kübler-Ross, a psychiatrist at the University of Chicago Billings Hospital, pioneered efforts to understand the psychological processes of dying and death (Kübler-Ross, 1969). After interviewing more than 200 terminally ill patients, she formulated a five-stage model to describe the emotional responses that people often experience as they face their deaths (Table 15-4).

The first stage of this coping process is *denial.* People in denial may act shocked after receiving news of their terminal condition. Frequently, they do not believe their physician's prognosis. While in denial, dying individuals may ignore their troublesome symptoms or seek more optimistic outlooks from other health care practitioners. Some dying patients completely lose faith in the value of conventional medical care; some maintain hope of "beating this thing" by using untested alternative treatments.

As the dying begin to accept their situation, they may enter the second stage, *anger.* In this stage, dying people are provoked easily; they may lash out at loved ones, medical staff, and anything or anybody. They often demand to know "Why me? Why not someone else?" It is important for people who care for or visit

Table 15-4 — Kübler-Ross's Stages of Emotional Responses to Dying

Stage	Typical Responses
Denial	Feels emotionally numb, avoids thinking about his or her condition, ignores the reality of his or her condition
Anger	Lashes out at health care practitioners and loved ones
Bargaining	Makes deals with health care practitioners, loved ones, or God to live long enough to do special things or experience certain events
Depression	Mourns his or her impending death, withdraws socially
Acceptance	Realizes that his or her condition is terminal, gives away cherished items, makes funeral plans

Source: Compiled with information from Kübler-Ross, E. (1969). *On death and dying.* New York: Macmillan Co.

dying individuals to expect this reaction and not take such anger personally.

The third emotional stage of dying is *bargaining.* Incurably ill individuals may make deals with medical staff or God, promising to exchange exceptionally good behavior for a few more years of life or a painless death. In the fourth stage, *depression,* dying people become increasingly aware that their condition will not improve. Terminally ill individuals mourn for themselves after realizing that they will not live long enough to enjoy experiences such as watching their children mature or playing with their grandchildren.

The final emotional stage of dying is *acceptance.* Although terminally ill people continue to hope for cures, they accept the possibility that nothing can be done to save them. Friends, family members, and caretakers can help maintain the self-esteem and dignity of the dying by visiting and touching them, as well as by listening to their concerns.

Critics of Kübler-Ross's research charge that she focused on people who were dying prematurely of chronic illnesses and had time to experience each stage. Therefore, her findings may have been different if she had studied people who were dying of acute illnesses or very sick elderly persons. Some people, particularly the elderly, may not experience all five stages of dying. Additionally, aged people who are terminally ill may accept their impending deaths more readily than people who face the prospect of dying while they are still young. The Kübler-Ross model, however, is useful for understanding the complex emotions of dying people.

Dying people are usually under extreme emotional distress. They often feel helpless and hopeless, and they have difficulty relaxing. Treatments such as surgery, chemotherapy, or radiation add to their discomfort. Some terminally ill people fight the prospect of dying; others accept what is happening to them and choose to make the most out of the time they have remaining. In modern societies, death can be the final stage of personal fulfillment if dying people have opportunities to satisfy their social and emotional needs. Thus, some terminally ill people choose to spend more time with their friends and families; others travel far from home.

As the end of life nears, terminally ill people may become more detached from others and the environment. They tend to sleep more often and may lapse in and out of consciousness. When awake or conscious, dying persons may not want to talk as much as they did before reaching this stage. According to Kübler-Ross, dying individuals are almost without feelings; most die without fear. Although the biological mechanisms are not known, some terminally ill people seem to be able to control the timing of their deaths (Phillips & Smith, 1990).

When you know that a beloved person is dying, you may experience a variety of intense emotions. You may be afraid of enduring the emotional pain of watching a close friend or relative die. You may be angry at the dying person, physicians, or God because you feel they are responsible for the impending death, or they are unable or unwilling to prevent it. You may feel guilty about your feelings toward the dying individual. Recognizing that someone is terminally ill forces us to face the reality that we will someday die.

Family and friends of a dying person typically feel helpless and intensely sad. As a result, they may avoid the person because such feelings are difficult to hide and uncomfortable to bear. This reaction does little to boost the dying person's dignity and sense of well-being. Being avoided makes the dying person feel isolated and rejected at a time when he or she usually has a high need for the compassionate support and comfort of others.

Physicians and family members have become increasingly aware that positive thinking, including hopefulness, can improve the well-being of the dying. Meeting the emotional and spiritual needs of terminally ill persons can help them live better while dying. Many physicians actively seek the participation of their seriously ill patients and their families in decisions concerning treatment. Health care practitioners can enhance the dignity and self-worth of dying patients by discussing the serious nature of their conditions with them, listening carefully to their concerns, and allowing them to make decisions regarding their medical care.

Terminal Care: The Options

The majority of Americans die in hospitals or extended-care facilities such as nursing homes. The goal of hospital-based health care is to provide technologically sophisticated medical care that enables sick people to become well. Since hospital care is costly, elderly patients who are too ill or frail to return home often move into nursing homes. These extended-care facilities offer less comprehensive medical care than hospitals, but they are designed and equipped to manage the long-term care of people recovering from surgery or illness. Not every condition is curable; many chronically ill patients die while residing in these care centers.

Choosing to place an aged parent or relative into a nursing home is often an emotionally difficult decision. Family members may have to select an available

hospice
(HOS-piss) health care specifically designed to give emotional support and pain relief to terminally ill people in the final stage of life.

facility quickly and without researching their options. The Consumer Health feature "Choosing a Long-Term Care Facility" lists some important questions to answer when selecting a residential facility that provides long-term nursing care.

When patients have only a few months to live, their personal physicians may refer them to **hospice**. Hospice is health care specifically designed to give emotional support and pain relief to terminally ill people in the final stage of life (*palliative care*). This care may be provided in the patient's home or in a hospice center. The primary goal of hospice care is not to save dying patients with aggressive treatments but to relieve their discomfort. Hospice physicians often prescribe powerful medications to keep terminally ill patients as free from pain as possible. Freedom from extreme pain permits the dying person to manage his or her activities more effectively and die with dignity.

Hospice staff receive specialized training to work closely with and to provide emotional and spiritual support to dying patients and their families. Staff encourage patients and their relatives to participate in decision making regarding care. Most terminally ill people and their families can obtain hospice services

---

$ Consumer Health

Choosing a Long-Term Care Facility

The most important feature to consider when choosing a residential facility is the quality of medical care that it provides. Before making this decision for a loved one, visit a few facilities, observe the condition of the buildings, its rooms, and residents, and answer the following questions:

1. Is the facility licensed by the state?
2. Is the facility clean, well maintained, and free of objectionable odors?
3. Are staff members friendly, helpful, and respectful to visitors and residents?
4. Are the rooms clean, comfortably furnished, well lit, and cheerful?
5. Do the residents appear to be appropriately dressed, clean, and well groomed? Do they appear to be alert?
6. Are there enough staff members to take care of the number of residents?
7. Are there handrails along the hallways and grab-bars in the bathrooms?

8. Does the facility have rehabilitation and exercise areas, a quiet place with reading material, and a chapel?
9. Does the facility have an activities director and scheduled social events that are appropriate for elderly people?
10. Are the dining room and kitchen clean?
11. Are menus nutritious? Do menus indicate that a variety of foods are offered? Can you sample a meal? How are the special dietary needs of patients handled?
12. If you have an opportunity, ask some residents and staff (privately) what they like and dislike about the facility.
13. What are the monthly fees? Can you afford this facility?
14. Contact your state's Division of Aging to obtain information about the facility's inspection reports.

Before making a final decision, visit the facility at least one additional unscheduled time to make another set of observations.

Source: Adapted from Goldsmith, S. B. (1990). *Choosing a nursing home.* New York: Prentice-Hall.

in their homes from a team of medical professionals. Family members are taught simple medical procedures such as care of surgical wounds or maintenance of feeding tubes. Hospice nurses make home visits to check patients' conditions and are available to answer questions concerning their care. Dying at home allows patients to remain in a comfortable and familiar environment where they can participate in holiday and other family-oriented events.

Some dying patients receive hospice care in clinical settings that have rooms designed to look more like patients' homes than hospitals. The staff encourage patients to decorate their rooms with favorite possessions to foster a homelike environment. Visiting family and friends provide additional social, emotional, and spiritual support and often participate in caring for their ill loved ones. Regardless of whether the terminally ill person dies at home or in a hospice center, hospice staff provide grief counseling services for survivors.

As the popularity of hospice care in the United States grows, many nursing homes and hospitals are offering hospice services that are covered by health insurance plans. To find such resources in your community, contact local hospitals or check the Yellow Pages under Hospice. Social workers in these facilities can provide information about local support groups for the terminally ill and their families. The National Hospice and Palliative Care Organization can also provide information about hospice programs in your area; this group's toll-free phone number is 800-658-8898.

■ Death

Many people have a difficult time thinking about and discussing death. For example, they may avoid using the term *died*, preferring to use euphemisms such as *passed away*. Whether people believe in an afterlife or not, most are reluctant to handle matters concerning their own dying and death, such as preparing a will or signing an organ donor card.

What Is Death?

Death, the cessation of life, occurs when the heart or lungs stop functioning. When this happens, no oxygen is available for metabolism, and brain cells begin to die. Within 4 to 5 minutes, the dying person loses consciousness. As remaining body cells die, other signs of death become obvious.

When a person dies, the muscles that control voluntary and involuntary movements no longer function. As a result, the body eliminates the contents of the bladder and rectum, and reflexes are absent. *Reflexes*

are neuromuscular responses that do not require thinking, such as eye blinking. Gradually, skeletal muscles become rigid, and body temperature cools until it matches that of the environment. Unless the body is chilled or treated with embalming chemicals, it decomposes rapidly. Decomposition occurs because the immune system no longer prevents bacteria and other microorganisms from breaking down the organic material of the body.

The physician who attended the dying patient is usually responsible for certifying that the patient has died. Then the medical staff informs family members. In most cases, they deliver the body to a funeral home or medical school, according to the deceased person's wishes. If there are any questions or suspicions about the cause of death, the family, physicians, or coroner can request an **autopsy**. During an autopsy, a specially trained physician conducts various medical examinations and tests that usually determine the cause of death.

In 1968 a team of experts at the Harvard Medical School (Ad Hoc Committee, 1968) defined death according to four irreversible physical criteria:

- The absence of electrical activity in the brain
- No spontaneous muscular movements, including breathing
- No reflexes
- No responses to the environment

death the cessation of life, which occurs soon after a person's heart or lungs stop functioning.

autopsy various medical examinations and tests that usually can determine the cause of death.

These criteria define what is commonly referred to as *brain death*. The majority of state laws recognize these criteria as the basis for defining death. A legal definition of death is important for criminal cases that involve murder. Defining death is necessary for physicians who need to establish that patients are dead before removing tissues or organs for transplantation.

Since the 1980s advances in medical technology have made it necessary for medical experts to reconsider the traditional definition of death. By using cardiopulmonary resuscitation (CPR), respirators (devices that assist breathing), and feeding machines, physicians can often save the lives of certain seriously ill persons, and in some instances, may sustain patients who have virtually no chance of recovering.

Cerebral Death The *cerebral cortex* of the brain controls thoughts, interprets sensory information, and integrates voluntary muscular activities. Individuals who experience severe damage to the cerebral cortex are *comatose*, that is, unresponsive to their environments. If the damage is irreversible, it is unlikely that the person will regain consciousness. In some comatose patients, the areas of the brain that control and regulate vital activities, including digestion and breathing, continue to function. Although their conditions do not meet the standard criteria for brain death, such individuals have experienced *cerebral death*. With specialized care, a person with a nonfunctioning cerebral cortex can exist in an irreversible coma, a *persistent vegetative state,* for years.

euthanasia
(YOU-thah-NAY-zhe-ah) the practice of allowing a permanently comatose or an incurably ill person to die.

The level of care required to maintain patients in persistent vegetative states is stressful for their families, as well as expensive. Under what circumstances can physicians remove life-sustaining care from a patient in an irreversible coma? The U.S. Supreme Court decision in the Quinlan case provides an answer.

In 1975 Karen Ann Quinlan, a 21-year-old New Jersey woman, was hospitalized in an unconscious state after allegedly consuming a combination of alcohol and tranquilizers. After realizing that she would not recover, Ms. Quinlan's parents requested that the medical staff and hospital administrators allow their daughter to die by disconnecting her respirator. However, the administrators and attending physicians denied the parents'

request, noting that the young woman was not dead according to established criteria.

After lower state courts supported the hospital's position, the Quinlans took their daughter's case to the New Jersey Supreme Court. In 1976 this court ruled that since Karen had previously told her mother and some friends that she would not want to live in a persistent vegetative state, her parents had the right to ask physicians to remove her respirator. After being removed gradually from the ventilation device, Karen was able to breathe without the machine's assistance, but she continued to be fed through tubes. The Quinlans moved their comatose daughter to a nursing home, where she died 10 years later.

Since the Quinlan case, several states have passed laws that establish steps for withholding or removing life-sustaining care in similar cases involving the terminally ill. A later section of this chapter describes how you can inform other people in advance about your wishes concerning such medical care.

Euthanasia and the Right to Die

Euthanasia is the practice of allowing permanently comatose or incurably ill persons to die. In cases of *active* euthanasia, physicians hasten the deaths of dying people by giving them large doses of pain-relieving medications that can completely suppress breathing. *Passive* euthanasia involves cases in which terminally ill people die because health care practitioners do not provide life-sustaining treatments, or they withdraw such care.

Since the Quinlan case, the courts have decided several right-to-die cases, particularly those involving people who were seriously ill but not dying. Some

chronically ill individuals decide that life is not worth living, or that they are tired of living in pain. To hasten death, these people may refuse life-prolonging medical treatment, demand that it be withdrawn, or remove it themselves. In recent years, the courts often have made or upheld decisions that give such seriously ill people the right to die. After physicians discontinued their life support, many of these patients died naturally within a couple of weeks.

In some instances, the seriously ill person is too physically or mentally incapacitated to actively end his or her life.

Figure 15-7 **Terri Schiavo.** These photographs show Terri before and after a heart attack deprived her brain of oxygen and resulted in a persistent vegetative state.

Concerned relatives, friends, or caregivers risk criminal prosecution by helping people commit suicide. Although most physicians strive to preserve life, some assist in the suicides of dying patients by prescribing overdoses of certain drugs. In the 1990s retired Michigan physician Jack Kevorkian focused national attention on the controversial practice of physician-assisted suicide by helping more than 100 people end their lives. In 1999 a Michigan judge sentenced Kevorkian to prison for injecting a deadly dose of drugs into a man who was suffering from an incurable deadly disease. Oregon is the only state that allows physicians to prescribe lethal doses of drugs to terminally ill patients so they can end their lives. Between 1998 and 2003, 171 Oregonian patients chose to end their lives by taking a prescribed dose of deadly medications (Oregon Department of Human Services, 2004).

In 1990 26-year-old Terri Schiavo's heart failed and the young woman's body entered a persistent vegetative state after a significant number of her brain cells died from the lack of nutrients and oxygen (Figure 15-7). For several years, Terri's parents fought legal battles with her husband over their desire to keep her alive in a long-term care facility by providing nourishment through tube feedings. Terri's husband contended that her life-supporting care should be withdrawn, because before her heart attack, she had indicated to him that she would not want to be kept alive in such a manner if she were incapacitated. By spring of 2005, the parents' legal options were exhausted after courts ruled consistently in Terri's husband's favor. When the comatose woman's feeding tube was removed, the tragic case made headline news in the United States and around the world, rekindling debate over euthanasia. Terri died almost 2 weeks after her feeding tube was withdrawn.

Preparing for Death

Young adults may see the need to plan for a comfortable retirement, but planning for a *good death* seems too morbid to consider. A dying person has a good death if he or she maintains a high degree of dignity and experiences little physical and emotional pain during the dying process. Additionally, a good death causes minimal amounts of emotional trauma for the person's survivors. Figure 15-8 shows the Dying Person's Bill of Rights, which, when honored, helps a person die with dignity.

Not everyone has time to prepare for a good death; death can be premature and unexpected, such as in cases of homicides or fatal accidents. Healthy people, however, can make various legal, financial, emotional, and spiritual preparations for their deaths. Such planning can reduce their survivors' confusion and anxiety.

The Dying Person's Bill of Rights

I have the right

- to be treated as a living human being until I die.
- to maintain a sense of hopefulness, however changing its focus may be.
- to be cared for by those who can maintain a sense of hopefulness, however challenging this might be.
- to express my feelings and emotions about my approaching death in my own way.
- to participate in decisions concerning my care.
- to expect continuing medical and nursing attention even when the "cure" goals must be changed to "comfort" goals.
- to not die alone.
- to be free from pain.
- to have my questions answered honestly.
- not to be deceived.
- to have help from and for my family in accepting my death.
- to die in peace and dignity.
- to retain my individuality and not be judged for my decisions, which may be contrary to the beliefs of others.
- to discuss and enlarge my religious or spiritual experiences, whatever these may mean to others.
- to expect that the sanctity of the human body will be respected after death.
- to be cared for by caring, sensitive, and knowledgeable people who will attempt to understand my needs and will be able to gain some satisfaction in helping me face my death.

Figure 15-8 **The Dying Person's Bill of Rights.** By honoring the Dying Person's Bill of Rights, people who care for the terminally ill can help them die with dignity. Source: Donovan, M. I., & Girton, S. E. (1984). *Cancer care nursing.* East Norwalk, CT: Appleton-Century-Crofts Publishing Company. Reprinted with permission.

Advance Directives The Patient Self-Determination Act gives people the right to prepare *advance directives* that indicate their wishes concerning treatment if they become incapacitated. The act also allows physicians and administrators of certain medical facilities to withhold or remove life-support care from comatose patients who have no hope of regaining consciousness and who would not want to be kept alive in such condition.

A living will or a durable power of attorney document can specify your wishes concerning your medical care in the event that you become permanently incapacitated. Figure 15-9 shows a sample *living will.* Not every state honors such documents. For example, your state may exclude the right to have artificial feeding and hydration (water) tubes removed, regardless of your wishes.

Although some states do not sanction living wills, they allow other advance directives such as a *durable power of attorney.* In this document, you identify a

FLORIDA LIVING WILL

Declaration made this ___ day of _____ , 20 ___ .

I, _____ willfully and voluntarily make known my desire that my dying not be artificially prolonged under the circumstances set forth below, and I do hereby declare:

If at any time I have a terminal condition and if my attending or treating physician and another consulting physician have determined that there is no medical probability of my recovery from such condition, I direct that life-prolonging procedures be withheld or withdrawn when the application of such procedures would serve only to prolong artificially the process of dying, and that I be permitted to die naturally with only the administration of medication or the performance of any medical procedure deemed necessary to provide me with comfort care or to alleviate pain.

It is my intention that this declaration be honored by my family and physician as the final expression of my legal right to refuse medical or surgical treatment and to accept the consequences of such refusal.

In the event that I have been determined to be unable to provide express and informed consent regarding the withholding, withdrawal, or continuation of life-prolonging procedures, I wish to designate, as my surrogate to carry out the provisions of this declaration:

Name: _____

Address: _____

_____ Zip Code: _____

Phone: _____

© 1996 CHOICE IN DYING, INC.

FLORIDA LIVING WILL—PAGE 2 of 2

I wish to designate the following person as my alternative surrogate, to carry out the provisions of this declaration should my surrogate be unwilling or unable to act on my behalf:

Name: _____

Address: _____

_____ Zip Code: _____

Phone: _____

Additional instructions (optional): _____

_____

_____

I understand the full import of this declaration, and I am emotionally and mentally competent to make this declaration.

Signed: _____

Witness 1:

Signed: _____

Address: _____

Witness 2:

Signed: _____

Address: _____

© 1996 CHOICE IN DYING, INC.

Courtesy of Choice In Dying, Inc.
200 Varick Street, New York, NY 10014 212-366-5540

Figure 15-9 **A Living Will.** While still able, a person can sign a living will to specify wishes concerning medical care in the event that he or she becomes permanently incapacitated. Source: Reprinted by permission of Partnership for Caring.

mentally competent individual to serve as a health care surrogate or proxy. A health care proxy will make decisions concerning your care if you become unable to do so. Additionally, you may indicate which life-prolonging medical actions are acceptable or necessary under certain circumstances. The results of surveys indicate that most Americans would want limited care if they became incapacitated. Few Americans, however, have prepared living wills or other advance directives.

Before preparing an advance directive, it is a good idea to discuss your wishes with family and address their concerns. Your physician can probably answer questions that you or your family may have about life-support care. Family members or the person who agrees to serve as your health care surrogate and your health care practitioner will need copies of these documents. It is a good idea to store your copy along with your other important documents in a safety deposit box.

Estate Management In addition to an advance directive, it is important to have a *will,* a legal document that specifies how you want your property to be distributed after your death. To prepare a formal will, it is a good idea to consult an attorney, preferably one who specializes in estate administration. For the will

to be valid, you must be of "sound mind" (aware of your actions) when you write and sign your will, and the document must be signed and witnessed by at least two people.

Most Americans die without having a will. When this happens, probate courts follow state laws concerning the division and distribution of the deceased person's estate. An estate includes the individual's sources of money, such as checking and savings accounts, life insurance policies, and retirement plans. In addition, possessions that can be sold, such as jewelry, real estate, furniture, and collectibles, are part of one's estate. A carefully constructed will can ensure that these assets go to whomever you want, and not to whom the courts choose. Furthermore, a will can eliminate much unhappiness, stress, and confusion among your survivors. If family members feel that provisions stated in your will unfairly distribute the estate, they can contest it in court.

In addition to making a will, it is a good idea to appoint an executor to manage your estate after your death. The executor uses income from the estate to pay your debts and funeral costs. If you have young children, it is important to identify and ask a person who will act as their legal guardian in case they become orphans. Most people choose a guardian who is a close relative or friend to whom they can entrust the care of their children.

In addition to having a will and an executor, you can protect your survivors' assets by having enough health and life insurance to cover your final medical and funeral expenses. The best time to buy life and health insurance is while you are young and healthy.

Organ Donation In dying, people can make a priceless contribution to the living by donating their tissues or organs. Soon after death, a donor's kidneys, skin, heart, and corneas can be removed and transplanted into people whose organs or tissues are failing. Many seriously ill patients who would have died without receiving donated organs are able to live nearly normal lives after having the procedures.

In 2004, over 87,000 people in the United States were on waiting lists to receive organ transplants (United Network for Organ Sharing, 2004). In the U.S., over 25,450 organ transplant operations occurred in 2003. Unfortunately, the demand for organs is greater than the supply. Over 6,000 Americans died while waiting for matching organs to become available for transplantation in 2002 (USOPTN/SRTR, 2003). Although people may express an interest in having their organs donated if they die, they often do not make their wishes known or document them formally. For example, potential donors may fail to inform family members of their decision or sign organ donor cards. In most states, family members can override the deceased person's wishes concerning organ donation.

People can help those who need healthy tissues and organs by completing and signing uniform donor cards like the one shown in Figure 15-10 . This card should be kept in a person's wallet. Additionally, people can fill in and sign the organ donor declaration on the back of their drivers' licenses. Additionally, individuals who would like to become organ donors when they die should inform their relatives of their wishes. Although there are no guarantees that surgeons will be able to transplant a person's tissues after death, it may be reassuring for some people to know that, even after death, they might be able to help others.

Some Final Thoughts on Death

Funeral and memorial services can help friends and family members deal with the loss of a loved one. You can ease some of the emotional and financial burdens of your survivors by planning your funeral arrangements. A funeral can be very costly, and it is often a difficult emotional task for families to make such arrangements when a loved one dies.

NATIONAL KIDNEY FOUNDATION

Please keep this card in a safe place and inform your family of your wishes to be a donor.

This is to inform you that, should the occasion ever arise, I would like to be an organ and tissue donor. Please see that my wishes are carried out by informing the attending medical personnel that I have indicated my wishes to become a donor. Thank you.

_____

Signature   *Date*

For further information contact:

NATIONAL KIDNEY FOUNDATION

(800) 622-9010 • www.kidney.org

- -

ORGAN AND TISSUE DONOR CARD

_____

Of _____

(print or type name of donor)

In the hope that I may help others, I hereby make this anatomical gift, if medically acceptable, to take effect upon my death. The words and marks below indicate my wishes.

I give: ☐ any needed organs or tissues

☐ only the following organs or tissues

_____

(specify the organ[s], tissue[s])

for the purposes of transplantation, therapy, medical research or education;

☐ my body for anatomical study if needed.

Limitations or special wishes, if any: _____

- -

Signed by the donor and the following two witnesses in the presence of each other:

Signature of Donor	*Date of Birth of Donor*
Date Signed	*City and State*
Witness	*Witness*

This is a legal document under the Anatomical Gift Act or similar laws.

☐ Yes, I have discussed my wishes with my family. For further information consult your physician or

NKF National Kidney Foundation
30 East 33rd Street, New York, NY 10016

Figure 15-10   **A Uniform Donor Card.** By completing and signing a donor card like this one, people can help others who need healthy tissues and organs. Source: The National Kidney Foundation, Inc. Copyright ©2002. Reprinted with permission.

Many mortuaries offer prearranged funerals that enable you to specify the kind of funeral you want and the most affordable services. For example, you could choose to have a simple memorial service, your body cremated (burned), and your ashes placed in a container and given to your survivors. You can contact mortuaries in your area for more information about making funeral and burial prearrangements.

In addition to making funeral and burial arrangements, you can prepare spiritually for your death. One spiritual arrangement you can make in preparation for death is to write your own obituary or death notice. Many obituaries include a brief biography. If you prepare these documents, you can give copies of them to your survivors and let them know where to send them. Newspapers, college alumni associations, and professional organizations usually print death notices.

After a beloved person dies, survivors often experience confusion and distress because they cannot locate the deceased person's will and other important documents. To reduce the likelihood that this situation will occur after your death, share copies of these personal papers with your spouse, adult children, the executor, and the individual who has the power of attorney. A safety deposit box is a safe place to store such documents. To help your survivors find these important papers, you can keep a small card in your wallet that lists their location.

Healthy Living Practices

- If you would like to be an organ donor when you die, complete a uniform donor card or sign the declaration on the back of your driver's license. Inform your relatives of this decision.
- Preparing a will can help your survivors manage your estate.
- To convey your wishes concerning treatment in case you become severely disabled and cannot communicate, consider preparing an advance directive.

Grief

Grief is the emotional state that nearly everyone experiences when they lose something special or someone with whom they enjoyed a close relationship. Losing someone you love is one of the most significant emotional events that can occur during your life. Some of life's losses are predictable, such as the death of beloved grandparents, parents, and spouses. Unexpected or premature losses, such as the death of a child or the sudden death of a spouse, can be emotionally devastating to the surviving parents, spouse, and other family members. Regardless of the circumstances surrounding a death, resolving the grief that follows the loss of a loved one (*bereavement*) involves regaining emotional balance and stability. Mourning, the culturally defined way in which survivors observe bereavement, can be a difficult and lengthy process.

The emotional and physical reactions to the death of a beloved person vary; some people have a more difficult time coping with the loss than others. People's emotional reactions are usually more severe after unexpected deaths than anticipated deaths. Typically, the initial responses of survivors are psychological shock, disbelief, and denial. They next enter the acute mourning stage, which is characterized by crying, withdrawal, and other symptoms of depression. In many societies, people in mourning are expected to display their grief, for example, by crying and by wearing somber clothing. After mourning, survivors are often able to accept the death of their loved one, recognize that they have grieved, and regain a sense of emotional balance.

The most intense period of grieving normally lasts about 4 to 6 weeks after the death. It is not uncommon for people to continue mourning for a year or longer after the loss. Some people experience psychological and physical problems if they are unable to resolve their feelings of grief.

Much of the research that examines the impact of grieving on health involves people whose spouses have recently died. Most widowed people experience some signs and symptoms of depression, such as sadness, withdrawal, and sleep disorders. With the support of family and friends, however, grieving individuals can often regain their emotional balance within a few months. Survivors may become saddened again over the loss of a spouse, especially on anniversaries, on holidays, and during family reunions. An estimated 10% to 20% of widowed people suffer severe depression that lasts a year or more after their spouses die. The Managing Your Health feature "After the Death of a Loved One" on page 445 contains some suggestions that can help people endure the first year after the death of a spouse or other beloved individual.

In addition to affecting emotional health, bereavement often influences the physical health of survivors. Most grieving people are emotionally distressed, and such stress often has a negative impact on their immune systems. Individuals who have weakened immune systems are at risk of developing frequent infections and chronic health problems such as cardiovascular disease. Additionally, grieving people may not take good care of themselves; for example, they may not eat nutritious foods or exercise, and some may abuse drugs, including alcohol.

People who undergo an abnormal grieving process may have had a poor relationship with the deceased person. According to Kübler-Ross, grief includes some degree of anger that is directed toward the dead individual. Survivors may hide their anger; others may express it by lashing out at someone else or by grieving for an unusually long period. Table 15-5 lists the signs of abnormal grieving. People with these signs may need professional counseling.

Managing Your Health

After the Death of a Loved One

The "Managing Grief" sections of this box provide some suggestions that may help you cope with the death of a beloved individual. The "Managing Legal, Social, and Financial Concerns" sections provide some actions that you can take to manage various concerns that often arise after the death of a spouse or other beloved person.

Immediate Actions and Concerns

Managing grief
- Resolve to survive the first few days of the sorrowful event.
- Accept the support and company of clergy, friends, and family.
- Permit yourself to vent your feelings, for example, to cry or to feel anger.

Managing legal, social, and financial concerns
- Notify your attorney; obtain the deceased person's will and make several photocopies of it.
- Order many (12) copies of the death certificate; the funeral director may do this for you.

Within the First Four Weeks

Managing grief
- Acknowledge those who sent food or flowers or who made memorial donations. Consider responding to those who visited or sent cards. This is an emotionally difficult task, but the process may be beneficial in itself.
- Anticipate feelings of grief: the tears, anger, guilt, and blame. Delayed or prolonged absence of grief may lead to negative physical and psychological consequences.
- If troubled by sleeplessness, nightmares, agitation, headaches, and even skin rashes, consult your physician for help to alleviate these conditions.
- Note changes in your appetite.

Managing legal, social, and financial concerns
- Notify relevant government agencies and other organizations of the death, such as the Social Security Administration, Veterans' Administration, and insurance companies.
- Submit insurance claims and apply for refunds and benefits where applicable. Keep records of all response letters from agencies and organizations.
- Notify your banks, credit card accounts, custodians of mutual funds and annuities, and accountant of the death.

Within Six Months

Managing grief
- Join a grief support group. For information concerning support groups in your area, contact social workers at a local hospital or hospice or your local United Way.
- Adapt to lifestyle changes. You may need to learn how to do unfamiliar chores such as maintaining the house, tracking investments, cooking meals, or paying bills.
- Continue previous activities such as participating in hobbies or clubs if they are satisfying.
- Participate in healthful physical activities such as walking, swimming, or golfing. Join a health spa or similar organization.

Managing legal, social, and financial concerns
- Share meals with friends and accept the invitations of others to dine out with them.
- Update your will: change beneficiaries, trustees, or executors if necessary.
- Consult your accountant; your tax situation may have changed.

Long-Term

Managing grief
- Establish your own identity to function independently. Your degree of dependence and attachment to the deceased may determine the time needed for adjustment.
- Establish new relationships; continue existing relationships.
- Consider participating in activities or organizations that help others.

Managing legal, social, and financial concerns
- Plan for the future. Do not rush into making major changes or decisions.

Professional counseling to handle grief may be necessary if the grieving person

- Doubts that his or her grieving is normal
- Experiences frequent outbursts of anger
- Finds little or no pleasure in life and has persistent suicidal thoughts
- Is preoccupied with thinking about the deceased loved one, or has hostile or guilty feelings that persist for more than a couple of years
- Experiences significant weight loss, weight gain, or persistent insomnia
- Begins engaging in risky behaviors such as abusing drugs or practicing unsafe sex
- Loses interest in taking care of personal hygiene for more than two weeks

Source: Adapted from Kouri, M. K. (1991). *Keys to dealing with the loss of a loved one.* Hauppauge, NY: Barrons Educational Series, Inc.

Healthy Living Practices

- Consider seeking professional counseling if your grief is severe or does not subside after the death of a loved one.

Across
THE LIFESPAN

Dying and Death

In the United States, parents often find it difficult to discuss death with their children until someone or something, such as a pet, is dying or has died. Young children have difficulty grasping the concepts of dying and death. For example, if a 4-year-old child attends a funeral and views a loved one's body, the youngster may think this person is asleep.

Children as young as 2 years old miss a familiar person who has died, especially if the deceased was a parent. Preschool-aged children, however, do not express grief as older children or adults do. At this age, children typically grieve differently than adults; they may act unconcerned about the death and become intensely involved in play activities or misbehave.

School-age children are able to understand that dead things do not come back to life, and they respond to the loss much like adults: crying, withdrawing, or being angry. Older children often associate death with being old, particularly if they have experienced the death of a grandparent. Thus, they may have a great deal of difficulty coping when a peer dies.

Adults need to be honest and straightforward when discussing terminal illness and death with children. They should consider the child's ability to understand the meaning of death. Frequently, children begin to understand and accept death when caring people share what is happening with them. Adults need to allow grieving children to express their concerns and feelings about dying and death. Professional counseling may be necessary if the child's responses are excessive, if the young person becomes preoccupied with death, or if the child becomes depressed.

Healthy Living Practices

- If your child becomes preoccupied with death or depressed after someone or something has died, professional counseling can help your child deal with the loss.

CHAPTER REVIEW

Summary

Aging is the sum of all changes that occur in an organism over its life span. The human life span is divided into stages. The final stage, senescence, generally refers to the stage of life that begins at 65 years of age.

The overall life expectancy of Americans has increased since 1900. In the United States, a person born in 2002 can expect to live for more than 77 years. Life expectancies, however, vary according to age, sex, and socioeconomic status. For example, American females outlive American males by about 5 years.

As of 2000, 12.4% of the U.S. population was 65 years of age and older. By the year 2030, nearly 20% of Americans will be in this age group. This segment of the American population is increasing at a rapid rate.

Aged people must often live on incomes that are lower than when they were younger. In the United States, elderly members of certain minority groups are more likely to have lower retirement incomes and live in poverty than are white aged persons. With appropriate financial planning, Americans who have adequate incomes when they are young may be able to maintain adequate incomes during their retirement years.

A gradual and irreversible decline in the functioning of the human body begins to occur around 30 years of age. People, however, age at different rates. Genetic, environmental, and lifestyle factors influence the rate of aging.

Some of the physical changes associated with the aging process, such as gray hair, presbyopia, and menopause, are normal and inevitable. Other age-related physical changes such as heart disease, cancer, and osteoporosis are not normal and are signs of disease processes. People who modify their lifestyles while they are young may be able to prevent or delay such conditions.

According to Kübler-Ross, the typical emotional responses to dying include denial, anger, bargaining, depression, and acceptance. However, death can be the final stage of personal fulfillment if dying people have opportunities to satisfy their social and emotional needs. Family, friends, and health care practitioners can help terminally ill individuals live better while dying by taking steps to enhance their dignity and self-worth.

Death occurs when the heart or lungs cease functioning and cells in the brain do not receive oxygen. The criteria for brain death include no brain waves, no spontaneous muscular movements, no reflexes, and no responses to the environment. A brain-dead person can exist in a persistent coma for years as long as the heart is functioning, nutritional needs are met, and the supply of oxygen to the heart is maintained by the use of a respirator. Euthanasia is the practice of allowing a permanently comatose or an incurably ill person to die.

The Patient Self-Determination Act gives people the right to prepare advance directives, documents that indicate a person's wishes concerning life-support measures if the individual becomes incapable of making such decisions.

Nearly everyone experiences grief with the loss of something special or someone with whom he or she enjoyed a close relationship. Although it is normal to grieve after such a loss, grief can have negative effects on health. To resolve grief, a person accepts the death of a loved one, recognizes that he or she has grieved for this person, and regains a sense of emotional balance. An individual who grieves for a prolonged period may require professional counseling.

Preschool children do not understand the concept of death, yet they still experience distress over the missing loved one. At this age, children may mourn by acting disinterested about the death or by misbehaving. Older children often grieve like adults by crying, withdrawing, and being angry. Grieving youngsters need to express their concerns and feelings about death. Like adults, children may need professional counseling if their emotional responses to death are severe or prolonged.

Applying What You Have Learned

1. Develop a will that reflects your wishes concerning the distribution of your assets after death. **Application**
2. Analyze how your present lifestyle may affect your life span. **Analysis**
3. Propose a special program that would prevent ageism by promoting understanding and cooperation between young and old members of your community. **Synthesis**
4. Choose a position concerning the issue of euthanasia. How would you defend your position? **Evaluation**

Key

Application	using information in a new situation.
Analysis	breaking down information into component parts.
Synthesis	putting together information from different sources.
Evaluation	making informed decisions.

Reflecting on Your Health

1. How do you feel about growing old? Are you undergoing the age-related changes that Table 15-1 describes? Which age-related changes trouble you the most? Are you making any lifestyle changes that will increase your chances of living a long and healthy life? If you answered yes to the previous question, what changes are you making, and how do you think they will affect your longevity?
2. If you suffered severe brain damage in an accident, would you want to be maintained in a persistent vegetative state? Why or why not? If so, for how long would you want to be kept alive? Why?

3. Do you intend to donate your organs if you die in an accident? Why or why not? Have you signed an organ donor card or the back of your driver's license, enabling survivors to donate your organs when you die? If you have not signed an organ donor card on the back of your license, explain why.
4. Have you ever known someone who knew he or she was dying? If so, describe any stages of Kübler-Ross's emotional responses to dying that you observed in that person.
5. If someone you loved has died, how did the grieving process affect your psychological, social, and spiritual health? What did you do to overcome the grief?

References

Ad Hoc Committee of the Harvard Medical School to Examine Brain Death. (1968). A defintion of irreversible coma. *Journal of the American Medical Association, 205*:337–340.

Administration on Aging. (2002). *A profile of older Americans: 2001.* Retrieved May 28, 2002, from http://www.aoa.dhhs.gov/aoa/stats/profile/2001/2.html.

Centers for Disease Control and Prevention. (2001). Prevalence of disabilities and associated health conditions among adults—United States, 1999. *Mortality and Morbidity Weekly Report, 50*(7):120–125.

Cummings, J. L., & Cole, G. (2002). Alzheimer disease. *Journal of the American Medical Association, 287*(18):2335–2338.

Desai, M. M., & Zhang, P. (1999). Surveillance for morbidity and mortality among older adults—United States, 1995–1996. *Morbidity and Mortality Weekly Report, 48*(SS-8):7–25.

Engelhart, M. J., Geerlings, M. I., Ruitenberg, A., van Swieten, J. C., Hofman, A., et al. (2002). Dietary intake of antioxidants and risk of Alzheimer disease. *Journal of the American Medical Association, 287*(24):3223–3229.

Erikssen, G. (2001). Physical fitness and changes in mortality. *Sports Medicine, 31*(8):571–576.

Evert, J., Lawler, E., Bogan, H., & Perls, T. (2003). Morbidity profiles of centenarians: survivors, delayers, and escapers. *Journals of Gerontology Series A: Biological Sciences and Medical Sciences, 58*(3):232–237.

Fox, N. C., Crum, W. R., Scahill, R. I., Stevens, J. M., Janssen, J. C., & Rossor, M. N. (2001). Imaging of onset and progression of Alzheimer's disease with voxel-compression mapping of serial magnetic resonance images. *Lancet, 358*(9277):201–205.

Friedrich, M. J. (2002). Biological secrets of exceptional old age. *Journal of the American Medical Association, 288*(18):2247–2253.

Glass, T. A. (2003). Assessing the success of successful aging. *Annals of Internal Medicine, 139*(5):382–383.

Glass, T. A., Mendes de Leon, C., Marottoli, R. A., & Berkman, L. F. (1999). Population-based study of social and productive activities as predictors of survival among elderly Americans. *British Medical Journal, 319*:478–483.

Heilbronn, L. K., & Ravussin, E. (2003). Calorie restriction and aging: review of the literature and implications for studies in humans. *American Journal of Clinical Nutrition, 78*(3):361–369.

Hetzel, L., & Smith, A. (2001). *The 65 years and older population: 2000* (Publication No. C2KBR/01-10). U.S. Census Bureau, Washington, DC: U.S. Government Printing Office.

Hinton, R., Moody, R. L., Davis, A. W., & Thomas, S. F. (2002). Osteoarthritis: Diagnosis and therapeutic considerations. *American Family Physician, 65*(5):841–848.

Howarth, D. F., Heath, J. M., & Snope, F. C. (1999). Beyond the Folstein: Dementia in primary care. *Primary Care, 26*(2):299–314.

Hyman, L., & Neborsky, R. (2002). Risk factors for age-related macular degeneration: An update. *Current Opinion in Ophthalmology 13*(3):171–175.

Kahana, E., Lawrence, R. H., Kahana, B., Kercher, K., Wisniewski, A., Stoller, E., Tobin, J., & Stange, K. (2002). Long-term impact of preventive proactivity on quality of life of the old-old. *Psychosomatic Medicine, 64*(3):382–394.

Kamimoto, L. A., Easton, A. N., Maurice, E., Husten, C. G., & Macera, C. A. (1999). Surveillance for five health risks among older adults—United States, 1993–1997. *Morbidity and Mortality Weekly Report, 48*(SS-8):89–124.

Kochanek, K. D., & Smith, B. L. (2004). Deaths: Preliminary data for 2002. *National Vital Statistics Reports, 52*(13):1–48.

Krach, C. A., & Velkoff, V. A. (1999). *Centenarians in the United States* (Current Population Reports, Series P23-199RV). Washington, DC: U.S. Government Printing Office.

Kramer, A. F., Hahn, S., Cohen, N. J., Banich, M. T., McAuley, E., Harrison, C. R., Chason, J., Vakil, E., Bardell, L., Boileau, R. A., & Colcombe, A. (1999). Aging, fitness, and neurocognitive function. *Nature, 400*(7643):418–419.

Kübler-Ross, E. (1969). *On death and dying.* New York: Macmillan.

Martin, A. (2003). Antioxidants vitamins A and C and risk of Alzheimer's disease. *Nutrition Reviews, 61*(2):69–79.

Mazzeo, R. S., Cavanagh, P., Evans, W. J., Fiatarone, M., Hagberg, J., McAuley, E., & Startzell, J. (1998). ACSM position stand on exercise and physical activity in older adults. *Medicine & Science in Sports & Exercise, 30*(6):992–1008.

Oregon Department of Human Services. (2004). *Sixth annual report on Oregon's Death with Dignity Act.* Retrieved November 18, 2004, from http://www.ohd.hr.state.or.us/chs/pas/arresult.cfm#lethal.

Peeters, A., Barendregt, J. J., Willekens, F., Mackenbach, J. P., et al. (2003). Obesity in adulthood and its consequences for life expectancy: A life-table analysis. *Annals of Internal Medicine, 138*(1):24–32.

Phillips, D. P., & Smith, D. G. (1990). Postponement of death until symbolically meaningful occasions. *Journal of the American Medical Association, 263*(14):1947–1951.

Quan, H., Arboleda-Florez, J., Fick, G. H., Stuart, H. L., & Love, E. J. (2002). Association between physical illness and suicide among the elderly. *Social Psychiatry and Psychiatric Epidemiology, 37*(4):190–197.

United Network for Organ Sharing. (2004). Retrieved November 18, 2004, from www.unos.org/.

U.S. Organ Procurement and Transplantation Network and the Scientific Registry of Transplant Recipients. (2003). *OPTN/SRTR annual report: Organ donation and transplantation trends in the United States, 2003.* Retrieved November 19, 2004, from http://www.optn.org/AR2003/default.htm.

U.S. Department of Health and Human Services. (1991). *Healthy People 2000: National health promotion and disease prevention objectives.* U.S. Public Health Service, Washington, DC: U.S. Government Printing Office.

U.S. Surgeon General. (1999). *The Surgeon General's call to action to prevent suicide.* Retrieved May 28, 2002, from http://www.surgeongeneral.gov/library/calltoaction/fact2.htm.

Van Dongen, M., van Rossum, E., Kessels, A., Sielhorst, H., & Knipschild, P. (2003). Ginkgo for elderly people with dementia and age-associated memory impairment: A randomized clinical trial. *Journal of Clinical Epidemiology, 56*(4):367–376.

Wai, L. K. (2004). Telomeres, telomerase, and tumorigenesis. *Medscape General Medicine, 6*(3):19.

Willcox, B. J., Willcox, D. C., & Suzuki, M. (2001). *Evidence-based extreme longevity: The case of Okinawa, Japan.* Scientific abstract of research presented at the Presidential Poster Session of the American Geriatrics Society Annual Meeting, 2001. Retrieved May 29, 2002, from http://okinawaprogram.com/evidence.html.

Wink, P., & Dillon, M. (2003). Religiousness, spirituality, and psychosocial functioning in late adulthood: Findings from a longitudinal study. *Psychology and Aging, 18*(4):916–924.

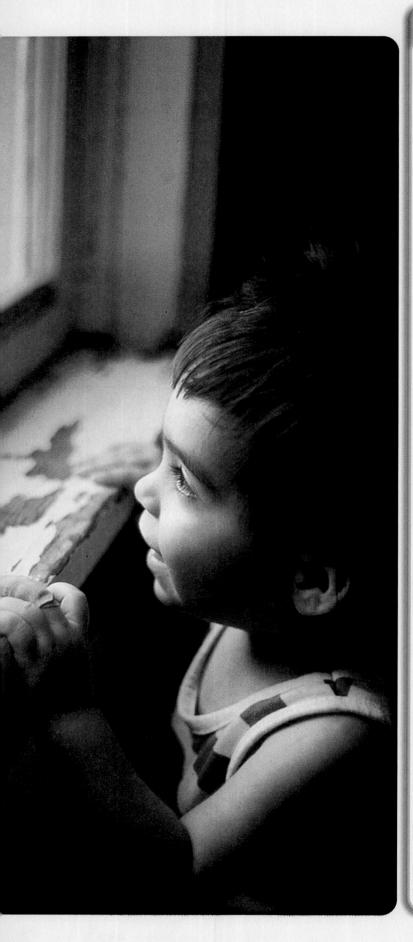

Chapter Overview

Which types of poisoning are prevalent in the United States?

How to avoid poisoning in the home

Which toxic chemicals are prevalent in the workplace?

What factors contribute to indoor air pollution?

How water supplies become contaminated

Why air pollution is a threat to health

How noise pollution affects hearing

Diversity in Health
Hunger, the Environment, and the World's Population

Consumer Health
Carbon Monoxide Detectors: Are They Reliable?

Managing Your Health
Tips on Reducing the Incidence of Poisoning in the Home | Avoiding ELF Radiation | Reducing Pesticide Levels in the Food You Eat

Across
THE LIFESPAN

Environmental Health

Student Workbook

Self-Assessments: Poison Lookout Checklist | Checklist for the Prevention of Carbon Monoxide Poisoning

Changing Health Habits: Can You Reduce Environmental Threats to Your Health?

Do You Know?

· *If you work or go to school in a "sick" building?*

· *If you are in danger of pesticide poisoning?*

· *If your house or apartment is painted with lead-based products?*

Environmental Health

chapter

16

Azarcon, greta, and pay-loo-ah . . . if you have Hispanic or Asian ancestry, the names of one or more of these traditional ethnic remedies may be familiar to you. Greta and azarcon are Mexican remedies for empacho, a colicky digestive disorder. Pay-loo-ah is a Southeast Asian tonic for rash or fever. All three are fine powders and may be given as a tea, or a pinch may be added to a baby's bottle. They also can be mixed with milk or sugar and administered by teaspoon. Family members who rely on folk medicine give these remedies regularly to children.

Many folk remedies contain substances that are useful in medical practice. In fact, pharmaceutical companies often start looking for new drugs by chemically analyzing the herbs and other plants used in many traditional folk remedies that have been part of a culture for generations. However, some remedies, like those mentioned above, can cause harm. Azarcon, greta, and pay-loo-ah all contain high levels of lead, as can ayurvedic medications (Centers for Disease Control and Prevention [CDC], 1993; CDC, 2004b; Saper et al., 2004). Ayurveda is a type of traditional or folk medicine practiced in India and other South Asian countries. Ayurvedic medications are used for conditions such as rheumatoid arthritis, infertility, diabetes, and menstrual problems.

Lead is only one of the many substances in our environment that can cause serious illness. The major ways in which U.S. children are poisoned by lead are by eating lead-based paint chips and by inhaling lead particles in contaminated dust or soil (CDC, 2000). In adults in the United States, 95% of lead poisoning occurs from occupational exposure, such as the mining and smelting of lead ore, the manufacture of batteries, and construction work involving lead-based products (CDC, 2004a). Nonetheless, folk remedies containing lead pose a serious health risk for both children and adults.

" . . . children are poisoned by lead . . . by eating lead-based paint chips . . . "

The study of the effects of environmental factors on humans and the effects of humans on their environments is called **environmental health**. People often affect the environment in ways that later influence their health. For example,

451

people emitted chlorofluorocarbons (CFCs) into the atmosphere when they used certain spray can propellants prior to their being banned in 1979. CFCs contribute to the depletion of the ozone layer in the upper atmosphere. These depleted areas are commonly referred to as **ozone holes**. The upper atmospheric ozone layer protects people from some of the sun's harmful ultraviolet (UV) radiation, which can cause skin cancer. (Chapter 13 discusses the relationship between the depletion of the ozone layer and skin cancer.) Many automobile air conditioners still contain chemicals harmful to the ozone layer. In another example, people in industrialized countries such as the United States produce millions of tons of **municipal solid waste** per year—all of those items that trash collectors pick up from homes and offices each week. This waste is usually placed in landfills. Along with running out of space for this trash, a problem with landfills is that chemicals may seep into the ground from these massive waste sites and pollute water supplies. We discuss water pollution from various sources later in this chapter.

Many **toxic chemicals** present in the home, workplace, or outdoor environments affect human health. They may be in the form of dusts, fumes, particles, or liquids and are found in a wide variety of substances, such as household products, plants, products manufactured or used in the workplace, and prescription and illegal drugs. (The adverse effects of drug abuse are described in Chapter 7, and of alcohol abuse in Chapter 8. The hazardous substances in tobacco products are also discussed in Chapter 8.) Additionally, toxic chemicals are present in the air we breathe and the water we drink.

Toxic chemicals result in poisoning, or **toxicity**, which damages body tissues and affects bodily functioning in various ways. Toxins may affect chemical reactions of the body. They may also hinder the normal functioning of body cells. Additionally, toxins may cause cells in the body to release chemicals that may have an adverse effect on certain body structures. The consequences of these effects are a variety of conditions such as dermatitis (inflammation of the skin), asthma, lung disease, and immune system disorders.

environmental health the effects of environmental factors on humans and the effects of humans on their environments.

ozone holes depleted areas of the ozone (O_3) layer in the upper atmosphere.

municipal solid waste nonhazardous refuse generally collected from homes and offices.

toxic chemicals poisonous substances present in the home, workplace, or outdoor environments that affect human health.

toxicity (tok-SIH-si-tea) poisonous quality.

■ Environmental Health in and Around the Home

Poisoning

The Toxic Exposure Surveillance System (TESS) is composed of participating poison centers that report on human poisoning incidents. Begun in 1983, TESS grew from 16 participating centers to a high of 73 centers in 1991; currently, TESS is made up of 64 centers. TESS data are compiled by the American Association of Poison Control Centers (AAPCC). Because the number of centers composing TESS has changed from year to year, the data from 1983 to the present cannot be used to determine a trend in human poisoning incidents. In 2003, TESS reported nearly 2.4 million human poisonings (Watson et al., 2004).

Most human poisonings in 2003—about 93%—occured in the home. About 2% occured in workplaces, 1.5% in schools, and less than 1% each in health care facilities and restaurants. Nearly 85% of poisonings were unintentional, which included medication errors, bites and stings, food poisonings, and occupational mishaps. Nearly 12% were intentional and included suicides and drug abuse. The remaining 3% were due to causes such as malicious intent and adverse reactions to drugs or food. Only about 0.05% of all human poisoning incidents in 2003 were fatal. Fifty-eight percent of poisoning fatalities occurred in adults aged 20 to 49 years (Watson et al., 2004).

Most poisonings, however, are not fatal. Nonfatal poisonings are most often caused by the ingestion of household products and over-the-counter or prescription drugs. They occur in children under the age of 6 approximately 52% of the time (Watson et al., 2004). Table 16-1 lists the substances most frequently involved in the poisoning of children under 6 years. Table 16-2 lists substances that are usually not toxic. See the self-assessment "Poison Lookout Checklist" in the student workbook to determine whether your home is free of substances that can lead to poisoning.

Unless a child or adult is observed ingesting a toxic substance, it may be difficult to determine if he or she is poisoned. Poisoning does not always start the moment exposure occurs. Also, symptoms vary depending on the substance and how it entered the body, which can occur by ingestion, inhalation, or skin contact (Figure 16-1).

Suspect poisoning in a person who becomes suddenly ill with symptoms that affect many systems of the body, appears drowsy and indifferent, or exhibits bizarre behavior. Also, consider poisoning as a possibility in children or young adults with chest pain; they may have ingested poison or an overdose of drugs. If poisoning may have occurred, call the local poison control center immediately. If the suspected poisoning victim is experiencing severe symptoms such as unconsciousness, seizures, intense chest pain, or repeated vomiting, he or she should be rushed to the emergency room of the closest hospital. Follow the tips in the Managing Your Health box on page 455 entitled "Tips on Reducing the Incidence of Poisoning in the Home" to lessen the chances of being accidentally poisoned.

Table 16-1	Substances Most Frequently Involved in the Poisoning of Children Under 6 Years Old	
Substance	**Number**	**%***
Cosmetics and personal care products	166,874	13.4
Cleaning substances	121,048	9.7
Analgesics	97,463	7.8
Foreign bodies	92,166	7.4
Topicals	92,091	7.4
Cough and cold preparations	68,493	5.5
Plants	57,778	4.6
Pesticides	50,938	4.1
Vitamins	45,352	3.6
Antimicrobials	35,152	2.8
Antihistamines	32,622	2.6
Arts/crafts/office supplies	31,211	2.5
Gastrointestinal preparations	29,770	2.4
Hormones and hormone antagonists	23,787	1.9
Electrolytes and minerals	22,337	1.8

Note: Despite a high frequency of involvement, these substances are not necessarily the most toxic, but rather may only be the most accessible.
*Percentages are based on the total number of exposures in children under 6 years, rather than the total number of substances.
Source: Watson, W. A., Litovitz, T. L., Klein-Schwartz, W., Rodgers, G. C., Youniss, J., Reid, N., Rouse, W. G., Rembert, R. S., & Borys, D. (2004). 2003 annual report of the American Association of Poison Control Centers Toxic Exposure Surveillance System. *American Journal of Emergency Medicine, 22*:335–404. Reprinted with permission by The American Association of Poison Control Centers. All rights reserved.

Toxic Plants Toxic (poisonous) plants can be the source of poisoning emergencies, especially in children. A wide variety of plants have parts that are poisonous and parts that are not. For example, tomatoes are not poisonous, but the stems and leaves of tomato plants are. Some common plant parts that are poisonous include holly berries, morning-glory seeds, narcissus and daffodil bulbs, rhubarb leaves, and sweet pea seeds. The entire hemlock, jimson weed, dieffenbachia, philodendron, and mountain laurel plants are poisonous. Some plants are so poisonous that drinking the water from a vase in which their cut flowers were kept can result in poisoning.

Although many plants are not poisonous—including the poinsettia, which for years has been inaccurately reported to be toxic—house plants and cut flowers should be kept out of reach of children under 5 years old, and all children should be instructed that eating house and yard plants can make them sick. Many plants, such as the poinsettia, may be highly irritating when ingested, even if they are not poisonous. If a child ingests a plant, call the local poison control center and describe the plant, where it was growing,

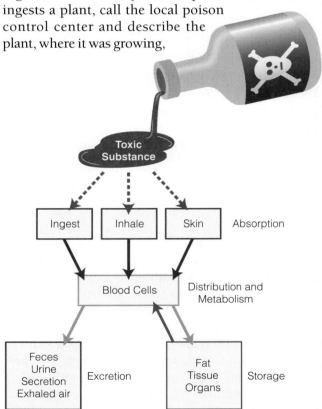

Figure 16-1 **The Path of Toxic Substances Through the Body.** The body absorbs toxic substances via the digestive system if they are ingested, or via the respiratory system if they are inhaled. Some toxic substances can be absorbed through the skin. Once in the body, toxic substances reach the blood and lymph, which brings them to all the cells. Body cells (principally the liver) metabolize toxins; the products of metabolism are stored or excreted.

Table 16-2 Frequently Ingested Products That Are Usually Nontoxic[a]

Abrasives	Fabric softeners	Perfumes
Antacids	Fertilizer (if no insecticides or herbicides added and no caution label)	Petroleum jelly
Antibiotics		Play-Doh
Ballpoint pen inks	Fish bowl additives	Polaroid picture coating fluid
Bathtub floating toys	Glues and pastes	Porous tip ink marking pens
Bath oil (castor oil and perfume)	Golfball (child may choke on core)	Putty (less than 2 oz)
Body conditioners	Greases	Rubber cement[b]
Bubble bath soaps	Hair products (dyes, sprays, tonics)	Sachets (essential oils, powder)
Calamine lotion	Hand lotions and creams	Shampoos (regular, not treated)
Candles (beeswax or paraffin)	Hydrogen peroxide (medicinal, 3%)	Shaving creams and lotions
Caps (toy pistol) (potassium chlorate)	Incense	Soap and soap products (hand soaps)
Chalk (calcium carbonate)	Indelible markers	Spackling compound
Cigarettes or cigars (small amounts of nicotine)	Laxatives (small amounts)	Suntan preparations
	Lipstick	Sweetening agents (Saccharin, aspartame)
Clay (modeling)	Lubricant	Teething rings (water sterilized)
Contraceptives	Lubricating oils	Toilet water
Cosmetics	Matches	Toothpaste (with or without fluoride)
Crayons (marked A.P., C.P., C.S. 130–46)	Mineral oil	Vitamins (without fluoride or iron)
Dehumidifying packets (silica or charcoal)	Motor oil	Water colors
Detergents (phosphate type, anionic)	Newspaper	Zinc oxide
Deodorants	Paint (indoor or latex)	Zirconium oxide
Deodorizers (spray and refrigerator)	Pencil (lead-graphite, coloring)	
Etch-A-Sketch		

[a]In the event that large quantities of any of these substances are ingested, consult a poison control center.
[b]May cause acute poisoning if inhaled in a closed area.
Source: Mofenson, H. C., Greensher, J., & Caraccio, T. R. (1984). Ingestions considered nontoxic. *Clinics in Laboratory Medicine, 4*:587–602. Reprinted with permission from Elsevier Science.

and what part of the plant the child ate. If possible, take a leaf from the plant for identification when seeking emergency medical treatment. Only plant experts should rely on their knowledge of whether the plant is poisonous.

In addition to plants, approximately 1% to 2% of mushroom species are poisonous. (Mushrooms are not plants, but fungi.) One type of mushroom is so poisonous that eating one-third of its cap can be lethal.

Symptoms of mushroom poisoning may occur immediately after ingestion and may include increased salivation, tearing, increased urination, diarrhea, difficulty breathing, and an abnormal heartbeat. Other mushroom species have toxins that produce symptoms 12 to 24 hours after ingestion that include headache, jaundice (a yellowish cast to the skin), confusion, convulsions, and possible coma. Because poisonous mushrooms can be lethal or cause severe poisoning,

do not eat any mushrooms that you find growing wild. Only a person trained in mushroom identification should attempt to distinguish between mushrooms that are safe to eat and those that are not.

Ingestion of Household Cleaning Aids, Medications, and Vitamins

Children under the age of 5 years are most in danger of being poisoned from household cleaning aids and from over-the-counter and prescription drugs and vitamins. The Federal Hazardous Substances Act, passed into law by the Consumer Product Safety Commission in 1966, has been helpful in lowering the incidence of poisoning in children by controlling the concentration of toxic chemicals in household products. The Poison Prevention Packaging Act of 1972 established standards for the packaging of potentially harmful household products and medications by requiring child-resistant caps and packaging on products that present a serious danger to children. The intent of this packaging is to

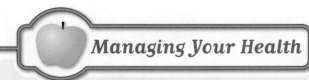
Tips on Reducing the Incidence of Poisoning in the Home

If there are children in the home:

- Store all medications and household cleaning aids in locked cabinets and away from food.
- Replace child-resistant caps securely after use.
- Replace medications and household cleaning items in their locked cabinets immediately after use. If the phone or doorbell rings when you are using a toxic chemical or medication, take it with you.
- Never refer to medicines as candy when administering drugs to children.
- Never take medicines in front of small children or make light to them of taking medicine.
- Keep plants away from children or others likely to ingest them. Many plants are poisonous.
- Educate children about the dangers of poisons in the home.
- Use adhesive stickers showing Mr. Yuk, or similar characters, to help children identify dangerous substances.

In all homes:

- Store all medications and household chemicals separately from each other and away from food.

- Periodically check and discard medications and household cleaning aids you no longer use. Flush the product down the toilet and then rinse the containers before discarding them.
- Work with household chemicals only in well-ventilated areas.
- Do not mix chemicals (e.g., bleach and toilet bowl cleaner) unless specifically directed to do so. They can react, emitting dangerous fumes.
- Keep all medications and toxic substances in their original containers. Never store such items in soda bottles, food containers, or any other unmarked containers.
- In houses built prior to 1978, check for peeling paint or loose plaster, both of which can be a significant source of lead poisoning.
- Never operate fuel-consuming engines, kerosene heaters, or charcoal fires in poorly ventilated areas.
- Develop a plan of action in case a poisoning should occur. Right now, look up important phone numbers (local poison center, doctor, pharmacist, emergency rescue squad, etc.) and record these by the phone.
- Stock emergency antidotes (activated charcoal and syrup of ipecac). Call the local poison control center for guidance as to when to administer these substances because they can cause serious problems when administered under inappropriate conditions.

Source: Adapted from Gossel, T. A., & Bricker, J. D. (1990). *Principles of clinical toxicology* (2nd ed.). New York: Raven Press, pp. 13–14.

make it difficult for children to open toxic substances so that adults will discover their attempts before they are successful. The use of blister packs in which pills are individually encased is another approach to lessen a child's ability to remove pills from packaging.

Although warning stickers such as Mr. Yuk (Figure 16-2) are available for placing on hazardous substances, the results of research suggest that their use does not lower the incidence of poisoning in children (Fergusson et al., 1982; Vernberg et al., 1984). Therefore, since child-resistant packaging *can* be opened by children (although with difficulty) and since warning stickers do not appear to deter children from investigating package contents, all dangerous household substances, including medications and cleaning aids, should be locked in cabinets. Special child-proof locks are available that enable an adult to open a cabinet easily but bar the child from doing so. Placing items on high shelves is not a good substitute and is not safe;

children easily stack items and climb on them to reach these substances.

Never suggest to a child that any medication or vitamin pill is candy because the child will seek out the pills at another time. Additionally, never take med-

Figure 16-2 **Poison Prevention Symbols.** The skull and crossbones is the traditional warning of poison. Mr. Yuk is a warning label designed for children, but using such labels is an unreliable deterrent. Lock all toxic substances in cabinets, away from children.

ication or vitamins in front of a young child who may think that it is candy or food and try to do the same.

Children become poisoned by vitamins and mineral supplements due to accidental overdose, but adults become poisoned by intentional overdose. Megadosing with vitamins (taking much greater amounts than that recommended per day) has become a popular practice but may cause health problems. Vitamin overdosing in adults most often occurs with vitamins A and D, two fat-soluble vitamins that are readily stored in the body. Daily overdoses of most fat-soluble vitamins build up, resulting in chronic intoxication. Daily doses of 3 to 10 times the recommended amount of vitamin A over a few months to a few years produce toxic symptoms. Accutane, a form of vitamin A taken to treat skin conditions, can cause vitamin A toxicity when taken by mouth. Daily doses of 10 times the recommended amount of vitamin D over 6 months to a year produce toxic symptoms as well. Minerals that most commonly cause poisoning are iron, selenium, and zinc. Chapter 9 discusses vitamins and minerals and their roles in the body in more detail. Table 9-7 lists vitamin toxicity symptoms and Table 9-9 lists mineral toxicity symptoms.

Lead Poisoning Lead poisoning is still a health problem in children in the United States even though many sources of lead poisoning have been eliminated in this country: leaded gasoline, leaded solder in food and soft drink cans, and leaded paint. (Solder is a metal that is heated and then used, when soft, to join other metals. It hardens on cooling and makes the joint solid.)

Even though many sources of lead have been removed from the environment, leaded dangers still exist. Ceramicware that is poorly made can have very high levels of leaching lead (that is, lead that dissolves out of the dishes and passes into food). Car batteries contain lead and should be brought to collection centers for proper disposal or recycling. Some pipes that bring water to homes contain lead-based solder. Additionally, the soil surrounding roads and highways often contains lead from years-past auto emissions.

Houses and apartments built before 1978 were often painted with lead-based paint (Office of Pollution Protection and Toxics [OPPT], 1997). Although layers of nonleaded paint may cover leaded paint, the top coats of paint can chip. The exposed leaded paint creates leaded dust that may be inhaled, or the leaded paint may chip and children may eat it. Leaded paint on the exterior of homes and apartments often contaminates the surrounding soil in which children may play.

lead poisoning
a toxic condition that affects the central nervous system, caused by the ingestion or inhalation of the metallic element lead.

Figure 16-3   **Lead Paint Removal.** These experts are removing lead paint from an old home in Nashua, New Hampshire. They are using a specialized vacuum cleaner and are wearing protective clothing and respirators.

Many cases of lead poisoning occur when older homes are remodeled without attention to the containment of leaded dust and paint chips. When doing such work, use a high-efficiency particulate air filter–equipped vacuum cleaner, properly fitted respirators, wet sanding equipment, and protective clothing (Figure 16-3). Seal off work areas with heavy-duty polyethylene plastic sheeting, and keep all nonworkers away from the area (OPPT, 1997).

Lead poisoning is serious because it affects the central nervous system and can cause coma, convulsions, and even death. Today, deaths resulting from lead poisoning are rare in the United States (CDC, 2001). Nonetheless, many children are severely affected by this toxin. While adults absorb about 11% of lead reaching the digestive tract, children absorb from 30% to 75%. When lead is inhaled, up to 50% is absorbed (Farley, 1998).

Low levels of lead in the blood (10 micrograms per deciliter [μg/dl]) are associated with decreased intelligence, learning disabilities, impaired development of the nervous system, and delayed or stunted growth. Behavioral disorders also have been linked to lead poisoning. At slightly higher levels of lead poisoning, the body does not metabolize certain vitamins properly or manufacture red blood cells correctly.

A child with high blood levels of lead (70 μg/dl) will show some of the following symptoms: decreased appetite, vomiting, abdominal pain, constipation, drowsiness, and indifference. Children who have even higher blood levels will exhibit some of the signs and symptoms of degenerative brain disease: coma, seizures, bizarre behavior, impaired muscular coordination, and vomiting. Either situation is a medical emergency and the child should be hospitalized. Tests should be performed to determine the child's lead blood level, and medications will be administered to reduce that level. However, the most important therapy is removing sources of lead from the child's environment. Call the National Lead Information Center at 800-424-LEAD for more information on how to avoid lead poisoning.

Carbon Monoxide Poisoning Carbon monoxide (CO) is a colorless, odorless, tasteless gas that can kill. In fact, unintentional CO poisoning causes approximately 500 deaths in the United States per year (CDC, 2004c). Carbon monoxide is produced by the incomplete combustion of carbon-containing fuels such as oil, coal, wood, natural gas, charcoal, and gasoline. Fires are a major source of **carbon monoxide poisoning**; persons caught in a fire often die from inhaling carbon monoxide and other toxic gases rather than from the fire. Firefighters also are at risk for carbon monoxide poisoning. Other primary sources of carbon monoxide poisoning are automobile exhaust, malfunctioning furnaces, charcoal fires, gasoline-powered tools, wood stoves, fireplaces, unvented kerosene and gas space heaters, gas cooking stoves and ovens, and tobacco smoking. See the self-assessment "Checklist for the Prevention of Carbon Monoxide (CO) Poisoning" in the student workbook to determine if your home, auto, cabin, or camper are as safe as they can be.

The proper maintenance and use of tools and appliances that burn fuel cuts down on the amount of CO they produce; these levels are usually not hazardous. Improper maintenance and incorrect use often result in dangerous levels of CO. To protect against these dangers, be certain that home heating stoves or furnaces are vented properly and are inspected regularly for carbon monoxide leakage. Use charcoal grills and gas-powered tools only in well-ventilated areas. (Don't use your charcoal grill in your garage or in a tent while camping.) Additionally, do not leave a car running in an attached garage where fumes can leak into the house. Run the car engine outdoors only. Carbon monoxide can also leak into a car if the exhaust system is faulty.

Carbon monoxide sensors are available for home use. These products are designed to sound an alarm when indoor air contains dangerously high levels of this toxin. Research results show that the use of carbon monoxide detectors could reduce by half the number of unintentional deaths by CO poisoning in the home (Yoon et al., 1998). (See the Consumer Health box "Carbon Monoxide Detectors: Are They Reliable?")

Carbon monoxide kills because it binds to the oxygen-carrying molecule hemoglobin. When CO is bound to hemoglobin, oxygen cannot bind and the person dies of suffocation. Before carbon monoxide poisoning kills, however, it produces signs and symptoms that become more severe as blood levels of this gas increase. At first, a person may have a slight headache that worsens as blood levels rise. (This level of poisoning can even occur if you jog near rush-hour traffic.) Fatigue sets in and the poison victim may become dizzy. As the poisoning continues, nausea, vomiting, a cherry-red skin color, and blurry vision result. Eventually the person collapses, may have convulsions, and dies.

Carbon monoxide poisoning is an emergency; immediately get the victim to fresh air and seek medical help. Health care practitioners treat CO poisoning victims with oxygen and test them for other medical problems that may have occurred at the time of the poisoning (such as a blow to the head in a fall). In some circumstances, the poisoning victim is placed in a hyperbaric (pressure) chamber and administered oxygen.

Inhalation of Asbestos Fibers

Asbestos is a fiberlike mineral that resists damage by fire and other natural processes. Because of these qualities, asbestos has been used in the manufacture of products exposed to fire, such as stoves, furnaces, and appliances; insulation in walls and ceilings; insulation surrounding pipes; patching compounds and textured paints (as a binding compound and texturizer); roofing and siding materials; and vinyl flooring (as a strengthener).

Asbestos-containing products came into use beginning in the 1920s, but by the early 1970s scientists discovered that long-term inhalation of microscopic asbestos fibers can result in **asbestosis** as well as cancer of the lungs and stomach. During asbestosis, scar

carbon monoxide poisoning a toxic condition that affects red blood cells' ability to carry oxygen, caused by the inhalation of the gas carbon monoxide.

asbestosis (AS-bes-TOE-sis) a condition in which scar tissue forms in the lungs as a response to irritation by asbestos.

Carbon Monoxide Detectors: Are They Reliable?

Carbon monoxide (CO) detectors should be thought of only as a back-up to proper use and maintenance of fuel-burning appliances. The technology of these detectors is still developing, and a variety of types are available for home use. However, none is considered to be as reliable as home smoke detectors.

The U.S. Environmental Protection Agency reports that CO detectors have been laboratory tested with varying results. Some performed well, others failed to alarm at high CO levels, and still others alarmed at low levels that do not pose an immediate health risk. Because CO is invisible and odorless, it is hard to tell if an alarm is false or a real emergency.

When purchasing a CO detector, research the features of various models and brands and use this knowledge, not the price, as your basis for selection. Carefully follow the manufacturer's instructions for its placement, use, and maintenance. If your CO detector goes off:

- Make certain it is the CO detector alarm and not the smoke detector alarm.
- Seek medical help for anyone experiencing CO poisoning symptoms.
- Ventilate the home with fresh air and turn off all potential sources of CO.
- Have a qualified technician inspect all fuel-burning appliances and chimneys to make sure they are operating correctly and that there is nothing blocking fumes from being vented.

Adapted from U.S. Environmental Protection Agency, Indoor Environments Division, Office of Air and Radiation. (1996, October). *Protect your family and yourself from carbon monoxide poisoning.* EPA-402-F-96-005. Available at http://www.epa.gov/iaq/pubs/coftsht.html. Updated 2003.

---

tissue forms in the lungs as a response to irritation by asbestos fibers. The patient experiences shortness of breath, which progresses to a fatal lack of oxygen or heart failure. Because of the danger that asbestos exposure poses to humans, the U.S. Environmental Protection Agency (EPA) banned the use of various asbestos-containing products during the 1970s and 1980s. In 1989 the EPA announced a ban on all asbestos products by 1996 (U.S. Consumer Product Safety Commission, 1989).

Aside from the danger to those who mine asbestos, those in primary danger of asbestos exposure are people who live in homes built between 1920 and 1978. Various asbestos products were developed at different times during those years and were used in home construction. Asbestos was also widely used in schools built between 1950 and 1973. Intact asbestos products do not pose a hazard. Danger exists when asbestos fibers are released from the products of which they were a part and become airborne. Asbestos fibers are released from products that are deteriorating; banged, rubbed, or handled frequently; or disturbed during home remodeling. Asbestos fibers are also released when asbestos-containing flooring is sanded or seriously damaged.

To protect against the inhalation of asbestos fibers, avoid disturbing this material. Do not vacuum particles that may be asbestos-laden; vacuuming them releases microscopic asbestos fibers that are inhaled. If possible, contact the contractor who built the home to determine if asbestos was used. If this is not possible, contact a certified professional trained in asbestos removal and repair to determine if the home contains asbestos. Sometimes materials must be sent to a laboratory to assess their content. If so, use a laboratory accredited to perform asbestos analysis. If removal, repair, or sealing of the material is necessary, hire only trained, certified personnel who can do this job safely and properly.

Electromagnetic Radiation

Are computer screens, television sets, electric blankets, microwave ovens, cell phones, or electric appliances health hazards? Are people putting their health at risk if they live near high-tension electric power lines or electrical distribution substations? A variety of studies have been conducted regarding the effects on the body of extremely low frequency (ELF) radiation, which is emitted by these sources. ELF radiation has been associated with negative effects such as risk of cancer, DNA damage, and changes in human brain electrical activity. One positive effect appears to be the inhibition of cancer cell growth in the laboratory (Cook et al., 2004; Ivancsits et al., 2003; Traitcheva et al., 2003). So far, however, most scientists see no major negative effects and no reason to recommend extreme caution. However, taking reasonable preventive measures against undue exposure may be prudent.

Extremely low frequency radiation is a type of *electromagnetic radiation*—electric and magnetic fields of energy that travel at the speed of light through the atmosphere. Sunlight, for example, is electromagnetic energy. Other forms of electromagnetic radiation include x rays, ultraviolet light, infrared light, and radio waves.

The electric fields of extremely low frequency radiation are not as potentially problematic as are their magnetic fields. Although the strength of both the electric and magnetic fields decreases dramatically and quickly as a person moves away from the source, magnetic fields penetrate the walls of buildings that electric fields cannot.

Computer monitors (video display terminals [VDTs]) produce radiation that spans the electromagnetic spectrum from x rays to radio waves. However, these terminals are manufactured with protective shielding to prevent most of the radiation from escaping. The small amount that does escape results in electric and magnetic fields in the atmosphere surrounding the VDT user, but the level of radiation where the user sits is well below occupational and exposure limits recommended by governmental and industrial safety standards (Sisto et al., 1999). Additionally, the levels of electromagnetic radiation emitted by newer models of

VDTs are generally lower than older models, reducing the health hazard further.

Cell phones and microwave ovens emit a form of electromagnetic radiation called nonionizing radiofrequency (RF) energy. At high enough levels, RF energy can heat living tissue; this is the principle used in microwave cooking. A person using a microwave often stands away from the oven, and results of studies show that radiation exposure from microwaves during regular use is unlikely to be harmful (Alhekail, 2001).

The heat generated by cell phones is small in comparison to that generated by microwave ovens. A cell phone's main source of RF energy is its antenna. The closer the antenna is to the user's head, the higher the user's exposure to the phone's RF energy. Therefore, cell phones (and lower-energy cordless home phones) with antennas mounted away from the user are considered safe.

Many experts say that a cell phone's power is too low to affect health, even if the phone is held to the head. Results of a recent analysis of nine studies, however, concluded that there is evidence of enhanced cancer risk associated with mobile phone use (Kundi et al., 2004). Many health researchers suggest that studies be conducted on long-term cell phone use and health.

Regarding exposure to ELF radiation of all types, medical researchers have adopted the position of "prudent avoidance" until research data indicate that another course of action should be taken. The Managing Your Health box entitled "Avoiding ELF Radiation" gives some tips.

Managing Your Health

Avoiding ELF Radiation

- Do not sleep or sit for a long time near electric devices, particularly those with motors.
- Sit a minimum of 18 inches (at arm's length) from your computer screen.
- Turn off your computer monitor when it is not being used.
- Sit several feet away from the back or sides of a computer monitor or television. Follow this rule even if the TV or monitor is in another room; magnetic fields travel through walls.
- Adults and especially children should sit several feet away from a television screen.

- Turn on your waterbed heater or electric blanket before going to bed. Unplug them when you get into bed.
- Use a mobile phone in the car with an antenna located outside the vehicle, or use a cell phone with a headset.

Sources: Adapted from Lamarine, R. J., & Narad, R. A. (1992). Health risks associated with residential exposure to extremely low frequency electromagnetic radiation. *Journal of Community Health*, 17:291–301.
Frumkin, H., Jacobsen, A., Gansler, T., & Thun, M. J. (2001). Cellular phones and risk of brain tumors. *CA: A Cancer Journal for Clinicians*, 51:137–141.

Irradiation of Food: The Debate

Many types of organisms contaminate the food supply. *E. coli* (a common intestinal bacterium) can be found in such foods as hamburger and unpasteurized apple juice. A particularly deadly strain of *E. coli* (0157:H7) has caused illness and death. *Salmonella* bacteria are common contaminants of poultry. Certain insects and their larvae contaminate wheat and wheat flour. A wide range of organisms cause not only food-borne illness but the spoilage of food.

One method of killing organisms in food is irradiation; that is, treating food with radiation. Radiation is the emission of energy by the unstable nuclei of certain atoms in the form of rays or waves. Food is irradiated in its packaging by either exposing it to gamma (γ) rays (a form of electromagnetic radiation similar to x rays) or to high-energy electron beams produced by electron accelerators. Radiation is harmful to living tissue, so it kills living organisms in the food as the energy passes through it, much like microwaves pass through food in a microwave oven. And just as a dentist's x ray does not make your teeth radioactive, irradiation does not make food radioactive.

Food irradiation is a process that was patented in the United States in 1921, but was not approved for use on the first food products (wheat, wheat flour, and white potatoes) by the Food and Drug Administration (FDA) until the early 1960s. Since then, whether or not to irradiate food in the United States has been a contentious issue. Approximately 40 years after its approval, irradiation remains in limited use, although the FDA has since approved the use of irradiation on fresh produce, herbs, spices, pork, poultry, and red meat.

So what is the debate about? Numerous national and international organizations (such as the American Medical Association and the World Health Organization) as well as many university-based research institutes endorse the irradiation of food. Supporters point out that irradiation has been shown to be the only way to rid ground beef of *E. coli* 0157:H7 before cooking. (Cooking ground beef thoroughly also kills this pathogen.) Irradiation also kills other bacteria, as well as insects and fungi that can make people sick or spoil food. Additionally, irradiating food can inhibit the sprouting of vegetables and delay the ripening of fruits. Food irradiation proponents hold, therefore, that using this process would make the food supply safer, would provide a better quality of food, and would extend the "shelf life" of food.

The opposition to food irradiation comes primarily from consumers and consumer groups. They point out that irradiation induces chemical changes in the nutrients that compose food (lipids, proteins, carbohydrates, water, and vitamins). Therefore, opponents argue, these changes can affect the color, odor, and texture of food, and could result in unidentified toxins remaining in food that might be harmful to humans and might even cause cancer. Additionally, opponents charge that irradiation lowers the nutritional value of food; some vitamins, for example, are affected by radiation. Some persons simply oppose technologies that involve radiation, citing problems such as nuclear waste.

The Analyzing Health-Related Information activity on pages 461 to 462 contains a newspaper article on this topic that discusses the process of food irradiation and the debate surrounding this issue.

Healthy Living Practices

- Teach children not to ingest house or yard plants because they may be poisonous. In homes with young children, substitute safe plants for poisonous ones.
- Eat only mushrooms that you are certain are nonpoisonous.
- In homes with small children, store all dangerous household substances, including medications and cleaning aids, in locked cabinets.
- Never suggest to a child that medications or vitamin pills are candy.
- Do not take large doses of fat-soluble vitamins except under the direction of a physician.
- If you live in a house or apartment built before 1978, be certain that children do not ingest peeling paint. Consult a professional to test for lead, and, if lead is present, to minimize its release into the home.
- To avoid carbon monoxide poisoning, maintain and use fuel-burning tools and appliances properly, be certain that heating stoves and furnaces are correctly vented, and warm up the car outside rather than in the garage.
- Seek medical assistance immediately for anyone who exhibits symptoms of carbon monoxide poisoning.
- Do not disturb asbestos that is deteriorating.
- Seek professional help for asbestos cleanup.

The following newspaper article discusses food irradiation and various points of view regarding this process. Read the article and evaluate it using the model for analyzing health-related information. The main points of the model are noted below; the model is fully explained on pages 13–15.

1. Which statements are verifiable facts, and which are unverified statements or value claims?
2. What are the credentials of the woman who wrote the article? If this information is available, do the author's background and education qualify her as an expert in the topic area?
3. What might be the motives and biases of the person who wrote the article? State reasons for your answer.
4. Which information in the article is relevant to the topic? Which information is irrelevant?
5. Does the article attack the credibility of conventional scientists or medical authorities?

Based on your analysis, do you think that this article is a reliable source of health-related information? Summarize your reasons for coming to this conclusion.

A bug-zapper for food

Many health experts say irradiation is not only safe but needed

Jill Burcum; Staff Writer

Salmonella. Listeria. E. coli. Campylobacter.

If there were a most-wanted list of culprits causing gastric distress and worse, these bacteria, or "bugs," would top it. Each year, they sicken millions and kill thousands of people, according to the Centers for Disease Control and Prevention. And during this decade, they've been responsible for some of the biggest and deadliest outbreaks of foodborne illness in U.S. history.

But if these bugs are the supercriminals of food safety, many experts believe there's a supercop available—irradiation—to stop these and other perpetrators. Approved by the federal government for use in a variety of foods, irradiation is a process in which food is zapped briefly with low levels of radiation to kill virtually all pathogens it may contain.

Nevertheless, the role irradiation will play in protecting the food supply is not yet clear. Although the most prestigious well-known health organizations favor irradiation, irradiated foods aren't yet sold on a widespread basis. In addition, a small but vocal group of activists who say the process is dangerous have added to consumer concerns.

What is clear, according to those on both sides of the issue, is the need for public education. "The best thing consumers can do is find out more information about it to help make the right decision for themselves," said Donald Derr, a Maryland-based food safety consultant.

Straightforward method

Irradiation may sound like a complex, futuristic innovation, but neither the concept nor the technology is new.

Scientists long have known that irradiation can sterilize and help preserve food, according to the International Food Information Council, in Washington, D.C. Its development began in the early part of the century and gained momentum in the 1950s as scientists sought peaceful applications of nuclear research.

In the early 1960s, the Food and Drug Administration approved the use of irradiation for white flour and potatoes. Two decades passed before the FDA approved irradiation of pork in 1985 and spices and fresh produce in 1986. In the meantime, use of irradiation grew to disinfect medical supplies, cosmetics, contact lens solution and baby pacifiers. In the 1990s, the FDA added poultry to the list of approved foods and in November 1997, red meat. Internationally, irradiated food is sold in more than 40 countries.

Both food and nonfood items undergo essentially the same process during irradiation, according to Dennis Olson, professor of animal science at Iowa State University (ISU), in Ames, and head of its irradiation center, which is the only such facility in the Upper Midwest.

In both its design and the way it works, the ISU facility is typical of many commercial operations, Olson said. It has three parts—a receiving room for the goods to be irradiated, a chamber in which they are exposed to radiation and then an area in which the products are picked up and transported away.

The foods are put in carts on a conveyor belt and moved automatically through the building.

Radiation is generated by a machine that accelerates electrons to 99 percent of the speed of light, according to Olson. Food passes through the electron beam thus produced. Other radiation sources approved for food use at other facilities include gamma rays, which are produced by the radioisotopes cobalt-60 or cesium-137, and machine-generated x rays.

'Nuked,' not radioactive

No matter what the source of radiation, pathogens in food are killed in the same way, according to Craig Hedberg, an epidemiologist with the Minnesota Department of Health.

Pathogens—which include bacteria, viruses and fungi—are both alive and replicating themselves, he said. Radiation exposure causes the pathogens' DNA, the double helix-shaped structure containing a cell's genetic material, to break, disabling the pathogens' ability to reproduce, so their populations rapidly wane.

Other types of contaminants, such as insect larvae, are eliminated the same way. So are the molds and fungi that play a role in ripening and spoilage in fruits and vegetables—one reason why irradiation can prolong the shelf life of many foods.

Irradiated food does not become radioactive, according to Olson and other experts. The reasons are that food is simply exposed to radiation, and approved doses don't cause changes at the atomic level that would result in radioactivity.

It's no more cosmic than a trip to the dentist, said Derr. "After you have an x ray, you don't think that you're radioactive, do you?"

Opposing views

Opponents of food irradiation point out that some molecular changes do occur after irradiation. Chemical bonds are broken during the process and new compounds, called radiolytic compounds, are produced.

Food and Water, a Vermont-based activist group, says some of these compounds never have been seen before, much less studied. Michael Colby, the group's executive director, said the safety of these compounds and other effects of irradiation, therefore, is not known.

The Internet has dozens of antifood-irradiation sites. Another group, the Center for Science in the Public Interest, doesn't oppose irradiation, but it worries that food handlers will rely on irradiation to sterilize food processed under filthy conditions.

Most-studied option

More traditional health organizations have endorsed the use of food irradiation, including the World Health Organization, the American Medical Association, the American Dietetic Association and the American Gastroenterological Association. The head of the FDA also has stated he is satisfied that the process doesn't change the nutritional content of food, its flavor or aroma.

Many proponents feel the safety issue is moot from a scientific point of view. "All questions about the safety of irradiated foods have been answered," said Derr.

Former Minnesota epidemiologist Michael Osterholm agreed, noting that studies on irradiation safety have been conducted for decades.

"It is the most extensively studied food safety technology in our history," said Osterholm, who has long advocated food irradiation. "There's more data on this than freezing, drying and canning combined."

Osterholm said radiolytic compounds do occur in irradiated food, but said the same ones occur in foods that are cooked, canned or exposed to sunlight.

Osterholm said irradiation complements other measures to ensure food safety, and it is more effective than any of them in preventing pathogens in food. Delaying its use, he said, costs lives.

"We are not going to get to the next level of food safety without irradiation," he said.

Will it sell?

The question is: Will consumers buy irradiated products? Because regulations require irradiated food to be labeled with a readily recognized symbol, consumers will know if the product they're buying has been irradiated by a symbol of a circle with a plant inside. But most consumers thus far have not had a choice.

Even though food irradiation has been approved for years, few supermarkets—none in Minnesota, according to the state's Department of Health—carry irradiated produce.

That may be changing. While polls in the 1980s showed that a majority of consumers would not buy irradiated products, recent studies by advocates suggest that consumers may be more likely to buy them if they are told about irradiation's benefits.

Nationally, trade organizations for supermarkets, restaurants and meat producers greeted with enthusiasm the FDA's approval of red meat in November 1997. In Minnesota, Cargill has said it hopes to have a meat irradiation facility in a year. SuperValu, the Eden Prairie-based food wholesaler and retailer, and the Minnesota Department of Health also are working together to introduce irradiated ground beef. However, experts say that a shortage of irradiation facilities in this region may prevent treated products from reaching shelves soon.

Despite the controversy over food irradiation, many experts predict that it eventually will become as widespread and accepted as milk pasteurization, a heating process that kills pathogens but was itself controversial when first begun.

"Twenty years from now, we're going to look back and say 'What was the discussion about?'" Osterholm said.

Environmental Health in the Workplace

Exposures to some toxins can occur both at home and at work, depending on one's occupation. Accidental carbon monoxide poisoning, for example, is certainly a hazard for automobile mechanics if car exhaust is not properly vented, but carbon monoxide poisoning more frequently occurs in the home. Pesticides are another group of toxic substances that persons may accidentally ingest at home if these chemicals are placed in unlabeled containers. However, pesticide poisoning more frequently occurs on the job in people who manufacture or apply pesticides. Poisoning by exposure to certain solvents, metals, plastics, and adhesives generally occurs only during their manufacture.

Figure 16-4 **Protection Against Pesticides.** This worker is properly protecting his skin and respiratory passageways from the pesticide spray.

Pesticide Poisoning

Pesticides are chemicals that kill plant and animal pests; they are used on farms and in homes and businesses to control insects, rodents, and weeds. People rarely become poisoned from spraying pesticides in their homes or yards; however, they should be cautious, spray downwind, and protect their skin and eyes. Occasionally, people accidentally drink or eat pesticides (or other toxic chemicals) stored in unmarked food containers in storage areas. For this reason, pesticides always should be kept in clearly marked containers. A person who has ingested pesticides should receive immediate medical attention.

People also ingest pesticides in the food they eat. These pesticides are not simply what is sprayed on fruits and vegetables but are found in fish, seafood, and meat. Animals often ingest foods sprayed with pesticides. Marine and freshwater organisms also eat food contaminated with pesticides when rain washes chemicals from the land into the water. Animals store certain pesticides they eat (and other toxic chemicals such as heavy metals) in their tissues, especially in fat.

Although many harmful pesticides, such as DDT, have been banned in the United States, these toxic chemicals, as well as pesticides being manufactured today, persist in the food chain. In addition, certain harmful pesticides such as DDT are still used in other countries on crops that are imported to the United States. However, pesticide levels in humans from eating supermarket produce are not considered toxic. The FDA, EPA, and Food Safety and Inspection Service of the U.S. Department of Agriculture together ensure that the levels of pesticides in food are not hazardous to the health of consumers. Data collected by the FDA

over a 7-year period show that pesticide residues on infant foods and adult foods that infants and children eat are almost always *well below* the highest levels legally allowed by the EPA (and that includes testing foods such as bananas without washing and peeling them) (Foulke, 1993). See the Managing Your Health feature for tips on reducing the level of pesticides in your food.

Most often, pesticide poisoning occurs in workers who manufacture or apply pesticides (Figure 16-4). These people inhale or have their skin exposed to toxic chemicals over a period of time if their skin and respiratory passageways are not properly protected. The signs and symptoms of poisoning in such cases may be vague and nonspecific at first: headache, intermittent dizziness, and general discomfort. As the poisoning worsens, the symptoms progress to include insomnia, nausea, increased sweating, involuntary eye movements, double or blurred vision, ringing in the ears, and involuntary body movements. If exposure continues, the poisoning victim may have convulsions. Treatment of chronic pesticide poisoning requires careful medical evaluation and is individualized for each patient.

pesticides
chemicals that kill plant and animal pests and that can cause poisoning when ingested.

Exposure to and Inhalation of Other Toxic Chemicals

A *solvent* is a liquid in which another substance is dissolved. Solvents are varied and perform a broad range of tasks in business and industry, such as removing unwanted substances (e.g., dry-cleaning solvents remove stains from clothing) or adding coatings such as paints and sealers to surfaces. (In the latter case, the

Reducing Pesticide Levels in the Food You Eat

- Scrub all fruits and vegetables with water for at least 20 seconds.
- Remove and discard the outer leaves of leafy vegetables.

- Trim the fat from red meats.
- Remove the skin and underlying fat from fish and poultry.
- Discard pan drippings and broths from animal products.

coating is dissolved in the solvent, which then evaporates upon drying.)

Exposure to most solvents slows nerve transmission in the brain and spinal cord, resulting in slowed movements and thought processes. Continued solvent exposure can lead to unconsciousness. Some solvents are irritants that can cause fluid to collect in the lungs or cause the skin to redden. Chronic exposure to solvents can also cause cracking or scaling of the skin.

Metals (such as aluminum, tin, copper, and iron) are elements that are usually shiny, are good conductors of heat and electricity, and can be melted, fused, hammered into thin sheets, or drawn into wires. Metals are extracted from ores by various processes. During these processes, ores are crushed, melted, and poured, which results in the production of metal dusts and vapors (Figure 16-5). Processing metal ores sometimes uses toxic and caustic chemicals such as sulfuric acid or cyanide, and often produces other toxic gases such as carbon monoxide and sulfur dioxide (see pages 466–467). Various industries use metals in the manufacture of products such as bearings, solder, batteries, cutting tools, plumbing, cookware, and roofing materials.

Exposure to heavy metals results in a variety of signs and symptoms depending on the metal and how it enters the body. Inhaling metal dusts or fumes, for example, can cause a variety of lung disorders such as lung scarring, fluid in the lungs, and emphysema (a lung disease in which the air sacs break apart and breathing is difficult). Inhaling fumes of heavy metals can also irritate the eyes and mouth, damage the kidneys, and damage the brain and spinal cord, especially with exposure to lead, mercury, or manganese. Skin contact with fumes can cause burns, rashes, reddening, swelling, and itching. Exposure to many heavy metals also causes cancer.

Adhesives are used to join substances during assembly operations. In order to join parts, other processes may also be used, such as etching, roughening, or solvent cleaning. Each of these processes may introduce its own specific hazards.

In most cases, the U.S. Occupational Safety and Health Administration (OSHA) of the U.S. Department of Labor regulates procedures in industries to protect the health of workers. However, many small companies, such as auto repair shops, are not regulated by OSHA.

Indoor Air Pollution

As people became concerned about the excessive use of energy in the 1970s and started creating "tighter" buildings to conserve energy in heating and cooling, they also became concerned about the quality of indoor air. Numerous studies have been conducted during the past two decades to address this concern and determine the cause of "sick building syndrome."

Figure 16-5 **Processing Steel.** This woman is working at a blast furnace in a steel mill. She is wearing an asbestos suit for protection as she opens the furnace with a long tool to release the molten steel. In the process, she is exposed to metal vapor.

Sick building syndrome refers to a variety of symptoms reported by occupants of large buildings. Buildings are identified as problems when a large proportion (sometimes as many as 30%) of their occupants complain about the same vague health-related problems, such as headaches; unusual fatigue; eye, nose, and throat irritation; and shortness of breath.

The results of studies of sick buildings show the predominant problem to be inadequate ventilation. A less frequent cause of health problems is chemical contamination from a variety of sources such as building materials, carpets, and plastic panels used as office dividers (Sundell, 2004). Other sources of contamination of indoor air include asbestos and combustion-generated pollutants (discussed earlier in this chapter), radon, and formaldehyde (Bardana, 2001).

Formaldehyde is a chemical used in the manufacture of many building materials and furnishings, which then release formaldehyde into the air. Specific products that are most frequently responsible for high levels of formaldehyde in indoor air are pressed wood products such as fiberboard, particleboard, and hardwood plywood paneling and urea-formaldehyde foam, which is usually used to insulate walls.

Formaldehyde irritates the eyes, nose, and sinuses; people who inhale formaldehyde may have difficulty breathing, experience chest pain, and begin to wheeze. Some people experience headaches, fatigue, nausea, and have difficulty sleeping, while others exhibit gastrointestinal disturbances such as vomiting and diarrhea. Formaldehyde's role in the development of asthma and cancer is controversial.

If formaldehyde contamination occurs in a home or public building (as noted by occupants' symptoms), the source must be determined and removed, or other measures must be taken to reduce the level of this gas in the indoor air. This process may be difficult and expensive. Removing urea-formaldehyde foam insulation from walls is costly and damages the walls. (However, urea-formaldehyde foam insulation installed 5 to 10 years ago is unlikely to still release formaldehyde.) Paneling may need to be removed or furniture discarded. Alternatives are to install an air ventilation system designed to remove toxic substances such as formaldehyde from the air, bring large amounts of fresh air into the building, or seal the surfaces of the formaldehyde-containing products.

Radon gas may also contaminate indoor air. Radon is present in the rocks and soils in many areas in the United States. People who live in these regions may be exposed to radon gas if it leaks through cracks in basement walls and collects in their homes. Chapter 13 contains a discussion of this colorless and odorless gas and its relationship to lung cancer.

■ Environmental Health in the Outdoors

Water Pollution

People get the water they drink from underground reservoirs called *aquifers* and from above-ground sources: lakes, rivers, and man-made reservoirs. Both sources of water can become contaminated with toxic chemicals. Surface water, however, can also become contaminated with pathogens, plant fertilizers, sediments (soil), radioactivity, and heat.

In developed countries, waterborne pathogens are infrequently a cause of disease because sewage plants treat wastewater so it will not contaminate water supplies. Additionally, public drinking water is chlorinated to kill pathogens. However, infection can occur when water purification and supply systems break down. Waterborne infectious disease is a widespread problem in developing countries, which have no water purification systems.

Plant fertilizers, sediments, and heat, which often contaminate surface waters, do not generally harm humans. The radioactivity emitted by nuclear power plants that enters the water supply is thought to be so low as to be harmless to humans. However, chemical contaminants such as toxic chemical compounds

sick building syndrome a variety of vague health-related problems reported by many occupants of large buildings.

formaldehyde (form-AL-de-hide) a chemical used in the manufacture of certain building materials and furnishings; may cause health problems when released into indoor air.

radon gas a substance present in the rocks and soils in many areas in the United States; may seep through cracks in basements and cause health problems.

(including pesticides), heavy metals (such as mercury and lead), and acids (from acid precipitation; see the "Air Pollution" section) can cause noninfectious diseases and poisoning.

Chemical contaminants pollute both groundwater (aquifers) and surface water. Such pollutants enter surface water when industries spill waste chemicals into waterways, mining wastes flow into rivers, pesticides wash into rivers and lakes during a rain, and salt used to de-ice roads washes into rivers and streams during spring rains.

Heavy metals can also contaminate surface water. Metals enter the water when they are dumped into rivers and streams from industrial sources. However, the Clean Water Act of 1972 and the Federal Water Pollution Control Act of 1972 and their amendments have all been instrumental in prohibiting industry from discharging such toxic chemicals into surface water. Metals also get into drinking water on its way to homes by leaching from lead solder in water pipes. (Leaching is the removal of the dissolvable parts of a substance as water moves through or over it.) The Safe Drinking Water Act and its 1986 amendments authorize the EPA to monitor the safety of drinking water and requires the use of lead-free solder in plumbing pipes.

hazardous waste toxic chemical refuse.

acid precipitation rain, snow, or fog combined with sulfur dioxide from fossil fuel emissions.

Groundwater becomes polluted from deteriorating underground petroleum storage tanks at gasoline stations, chemicals from road salting, or agricultural chemicals that leach into the ground. However, **hazardous waste** (toxic chemical waste) is the primary source of groundwater pollution as toxic chemicals leach into aquifers.

In 1980 Congress passed a toxic waste clean up bill and allocated funds to clean up hazardous substances. Known as the Superfund, it provides money to find the parties guilty of dumping toxic waste at specific sites and forces them to pay clean up costs. If the government cannot find the guilty parties, it pays to have the sites cleaned up. Since 1980 the Superfund program has fostered the cleanup of hundreds of hazardous waste sites nationwide. At the end of 2004, the EPA reported that cleanup was completed on approximately 61% of the sites listed as national priorities. The EPA estimates that 85% of national priority sites will be cleaned up by 2008.

To ensure the safety of drinking water, purification methods in the United States often involve chlorination to kill unwanted pathogens. In fact, 75% of the nation's drinking water is treated with chlorine. In 1974, however, scientists realized that this chemical interacts with other chemicals in drinking water to form new compounds such as chloroform. Since this discovery, scientists have been studying whether these compounds are associated with the incidence of cancer. A recent review of data from multiple studies concluded that the compounds formed from chlorine in drinking water, at normal levels of consumption, are not likely to produce cancer (Fawell, 2000). Additionally, reviews have found the reliability of data showing a link between ingestion of water disinfectant by-products and miscarriages or birth defects to be mixed, inconsistent, or weak (Graves et al., 2001; Nieuwenhuijsen et al., 2000). Researchers suggest that tolerable daily intake levels of water disinfectant by-products should be developed.

Becoming aware of the potential for water pollution is only the first step in protecting against the short-term and long-term health effects of drinking contaminated water. Tap water can be tested to be sure that it does not contain toxic or other unwanted chemicals. If it does, it can be treated using various methods such as carbon filtration. Carbon filters remove many carbon-containing compounds and chlorine from the water, improving its taste, odor, and color. The filters are not useful for all water-treatment needs. Some persons choose to use only bottled water for cooking and drinking. However, bottled water is not necessarily better than tap water. To judge its purity, have your bottled water tested for the presence of toxic chemicals, or write to the International Bottled Water Association (IBWA), 1700 Diagonal Road, Suite 650, Alexandria, VA 22314 for information regarding a specific bottler. Their information hotline is 800-WATER-11.

Air Pollution

Air pollution is also a threat to health. The primary substances in the air that harm humans are sulfur dioxide (SO_2), nitrogen dioxide (NO_2), carbon monoxide (CO), ozone (O_3), and particulates. These substances are formed when fossil fuels are burned. Fossil fuels are carbon-containing substances formed over time and under pressure from once-living organisms (both plants and animals). Gasoline, coal, natural gas, and oil are all fossil fuels.

The two main contributors to air pollution are automobiles and coal-fired power plants. The use of small gasoline-powered machines such as leaf blowers, chain saws, weed cutters, and snow blowers also contributes to air pollution.

Coal-fired power plants generate particulates and sulfur dioxide as their primary pollutants. People who live downwind of such power plants experience the greatest impact from these pollutants. Sulfur dioxide combines with water in the atmosphere to produce sulfuric acid, the major component of **acid precipitation**. Acid precipitation (rain, snow, and fog) damages both living and nonliving things, and acidifies surface water. When it falls in cities, it can harm vegetation as well as damage stone statues and buildings, as shown in Figure 16-6 . Acid water in reservoirs leaches metals from pipes carrying the water into the drinking water supplies. The regions of the United States affected most heavily by acid precipitation are the Great Lakes area and New England. Southern Canada also experiences the effects of American power plant emissions.

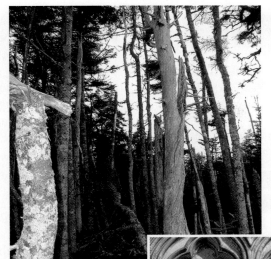

(a)

(b)

Figure 16-6   **The Effects of Acid Rain.**
Many of the trees in this Maine forest have been damaged by acid rain (a) as have statues at Salisbury Cathedral in England (b).

Sulfur oxides and particulates also combine with atmospheric moisture to form a haze called **smog** (smoke plus fog). Smog can harm the lungs. Cities with sulfur oxide smog are usually located in cold, moist climates and rely on coal and oil for electricity and home heating.

Of the sulfur oxides and particulates in smog, particulates do the most damage to the lungs. *Particulates* are small particles that are dispersed in the air. Although nasal hairs and mucus in the nose and throat trap large particles, particulates reach the lungs and accumulate over time. Eventually, this material irritates the lungs and blocks their microscopic air sacs, making breathing more difficult. Particulates in the air passageways and lungs can also be a factor in the development of respiratory diseases such as bronchitis, emphysema, and asthma. They also make existing respiratory illness worse.

Sulfur dioxide in the air irritates the mucous lining of the eyes and lungs. Like particulates, sulfur dioxide worsens respiratory illness. Together, particulates and sulfur dioxide have a greater effect on respiratory problems than if only one of these pollutants were present. At highest risk are the elderly and people with chronic lung and/or heart disease.

Carbon monoxide (see page 457), nitrogen dioxide, and ozone are produced primarily as a result of emissions from vehicles. Nitrogen dioxide is formed when nitrogen gas in the air chemically combines with oxygen during the combustion of fuel. This compound irritates the eyes, lungs, and other mucous membranes. It also reacts with hydrocarbons (the hydrogen and

carbon in fuel) in the presence of sunlight to produce a secondary pollutant—ozone. In the upper atmosphere, ozone protects us from the sun's damaging ultraviolet rays. But when it is in the air we breathe, ozone is irritating to the lungs. Cities polluted primarily by the emissions of automobiles, or photochemical smog, are located primarily in the western United States.

The **Air Quality Index (AQI)** is a means by which the public is informed of air quality. Levels of five major air pollutants (CO, NO_2, O_3, SO_2, and particulates) are monitored and used to determine AQI values (Figure 16-7). The descriptor for air quality (good, moderate, unhealthful, and so forth) is determined by the highest concentration of each pollutant in the air. When the air is unhealthful or worse, the AQI cautionary statements should be heeded; many elderly persons and those with chronic lung or heart conditions can die during times of unhealthful and hazardous air quality. Since strict amendments to the Clean Air Act were passed in 1970 and even tougher standards were set with the pas-

smog
(smoke and fog) a haze in the atmosphere formed by various pollutants.

Air Quality Index (AQI)
a guide to air quality that uses levels of various pollutants to determine its values.

Air Quality Index (AQI) Values	Levels of Health Concern	Colors
When the AQI is in this range:	...air quality conditions are:	...as symbolized by this color:
0 to 50	Good	Green
51 to 100	Moderate	Yellow
101 to 150	Unhealthy for Sensitive Groups	Orange
151 to 200	Unhealthy	Red
201 to 300	Very Unhealthy	Purple
301 to 500	Hazardous	Maroon

Figure 16-7 The Air Quality Index (AQI). Source: United States Environmental Protection Agency. (2000). *Air Quality Index: A guide to air quality and your health.*

sage of amendments in 1990, the quality of the air in the United States has improved greatly, but many cities and areas of the country still have high levels of pollution.

Noise Pollution

Noise pollution can have a negative effect on health, but it is unlike any of the environmental dusts, fumes, vapors, gases, and liquids discussed previously. Noise is composed of sound waves. If sound waves were visible, they would look much like ripples on water— areas of compressed air molecules followed by areas in which the molecules are more spread out. These waves in the air are the result of the vibration of an object disturbing the air around it.

The human ear detects these sound vibrations in the air as they hit the eardrum, causing it to vibrate. The vibrating eardrum moves the tiny bones of the middle ear, which, in turn, cause the fluid of the inner ear to move across delicate hairs. The hairs of the inner ear are connected to nerves that send messages to the brain. These messages are interpreted as sound. The fragile hairs, however, can be permanently injured by sound waves that are too loud.

How loud are everyday sounds? Table 16-3 lists some everyday sounds and their loudness. Sound intensity, or loudness, is expressed in *decibels* (dB). The faintest sound a human can hear is considered zero (0) dB. As the intensity of sound increases on the decibel scale, each 10-dB increase means a tenfold increase in the intensity of the sound. Therefore, a 50-dB sound is 10 times louder than a 40-dB sound.

Sounds that are considered quiet or soft are 50 dB or less. The National Institute on Deafness and Other Communication Disorders (NIDCD) states that sounds of less than 75 dB are unlikely to cause hearing loss.

When sounds get as loud as 80 dB, they begin to be annoying and can be harmful over time. At 85 dB, hearing is at risk of permanent damage. Pain sets in at 120 dB.

The EPA estimates that 40% of the U.S. population is exposed to enough noise to cause permanent hearing loss. The average person can damage his or her hearing if he or she

- uses a power lawn mower (90 dB) for 8 hours.
- is at a loud party (90 dB) for 6 to 8 hours.
- uses a chain saw (100 dB) for 2 hours.
- uses a gasoline-powered leaf blower (110 dB) for 30 minutes.
- is at a dance club or rock concert (115 dB) for 15 minutes.

Although you may not be at one party for 8 hours, damage to hearing from loud sounds is cumulative. That is, the effects add up. These effects can be devastating; the National Institutes of Health have determined that permanent hearing loss *will* result from years of exposure, 8 hours per day, to 85-dB and louder sounds. Permanent deafness may result from such continual exposure and can also result from a single exposure, such as being close to an explosion of 140 dB.

How do people know if they are losing their hearing? First, a person may lose the ability to hear high-frequency sounds. He or she may be unable to hear occasional words in conversation or have difficulty hearing on the telephone. Additionally, people with partial hearing loss often experience ringing or roaring in their ears, called *tinnitus*. Tinnitus makes hearing even more difficult. Hearing aids may be helpful

Table 16-3 Loudness of Some Everyday Sounds

Sound Loudness	(dB)
Rustling leaves	10
Normal conversation	50
Suburban neighborhood noise	52
Vacuum cleaner	70
City noise; busy traffic	80
Inside a passenger jet (takeoff)	78–83
Heavy trucks at 50 feet	76–88
Home shop tools	65–110
Subway noise	80–114
Nearby jet airplane	150
Shooting a gun	150–170

to the person with partial hearing loss but cannot totally compensate for the problem.

Total or partial hearing loss is only one of the effects of listening to sounds that are too loud. Parts of the body other than the ear react to noise. Researchers have shown that exposure to 70-dB noise results in an increase in the heart rate and a rise in blood pressure; muscles tighten and breathing patterns change. Exposure to noise also increases the rate at which stress-related hormones are secreted into the bloodstream. Even moderate daytime noise levels have been shown to increase anxiety and hostile behavior in some persons. In a variety of studies, environmental noise exposure has also been linked to impaired learning ability and performance in school (Staples, 1996).

Paying attention to the noise in your environment will help save your hearing. For example, many health clubs blast loud music as an aerobics instructor yells commands. Often, these sounds top 110 dB. Request that the volume be turned down. If you wear ear protection, use only materials and items manufactured to reduce sound; placing cotton or tissue in your ears does not do an adequate job of protecting your ears.

If you attend loud concerts, check your hearing when you leave. Set your car or home radio to a level at which you can barely hear the words. Then, as soon after the concert as possible, turn on the radio. Can you hear the words? If not, you have sustained short-term hearing loss from the loudness of the music. Frequently listening to such loud music could result in a permanent hearing problem.

Healthy Living Practices

- To avoid hearing loss and the other effects of noise pollution, avoid situations in which the sound is over 80 dB. Pay attention to noise levels and complain if they are too high.
- If you must work or be temporarily in an environment with noise over 80 dB, wear ear protection.

Across THE LIFESPAN

Environmental Health

Environmental health hazards are a risk for all segments of the population. However, young children are most at risk for unintentional poisoning by ingestion of toxic substances because they lack understanding that these materials are harmful and they put most things in their mouths; this is a normal exploratory behavior for small children. Additionally, carbon monoxide and lead are particularly injurious to fetuses and young children because their brains and nervous systems are still developing. Also extremely susceptible to carbon monoxide poisoning or air pollutants are the elderly and persons with chronic lung or heart disease, whose lung function may be impaired.

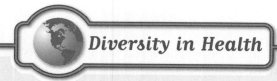
Hunger, the Environment, and the World's Populations

Nearly one of six people in the world suffers from acute or chronic hunger. Hunger is more than appetite, the psychological desire for food, or feeling hungry after not eating for a few hours. Acute hunger, or starvation, is a condition in which a person has not eaten for a prolonged period and will eventually die from lack of food. Chronic hunger refers to a long-term condition in which food intake is inadequate. People who experience chronic hunger are undernourished (see Chapter 9) and do not have the nutrients they need for proper growth, development, and body function.

Although many of the factors that lead to hunger are political, social, and economic, environmental conditions play a role in the many perceived causes of world hunger. Overpopulation, environmental limits to food production, and land use problems are factors that scientists debate with regard to their roles in hunger. In fact, many scientists assert that there is no global hunger problem. Instead, they assert, regional hunger problems exist, each with diverse causes.

The world population is approximately 6.4 billion people, increasing at a rate of approximately 100 million per year. Various experts in the United Nations predict that the world population will level off, reaching its carrying capacity between 12.4 billion and 14 billion people. The carrying capacity is the maximum number of individuals that can be supported by the available resources. However, scientists disagree as to whether the global food output can support that many individuals. Many scientists calculate that even with the use of the best agricultural technologies, the carrying capacity of the earth will be limited to 7.5 billion people.

Scientists disagree as to whether the increase in food production during the 1980s kept up with the need for food worldwide. They also disagree as to whether technological advances in various areas of agriculture, such as changes in machinery, seed varieties, fertilizers, pesticides, and management practices, as well as the genetic engineering of plants to resist certain crop pests, will allow the world's farmers to produce greater and greater crop yields. Many scientists assert that to increase sufficiently the amount of food produced around the world, farmers must increase the amount of land they cultivate. However, using marginal land (land not well suited for cultivation) may increase the danger of erosion, landslides, and floods. Marginal land is also likely to produce lower crop yields than land already in cultivation. Additionally, the limited availability of water in many regions may constrain agricultural expansion.

Many parts of the earth cannot support the population that now exists on their lands. A country is overpopulated when its natural resources cannot sustain its people. An example of such overpopulation is Africa, the continent with the fastest population growth in the world. More than 50% of the African population is under the age of 15. Therefore, the size of this population will increase in the next decade and beyond because a large proportion of the population will be in its reproductive years. Much of the land in Africa has a low natural carrying capacity. Additionally, its climate is highly changeable and therefore unreliable for growing crops.

The problem of world or regional hunger is serious. Environmental issues such as overpopulation, methods of food production, and approaches to land use interact with political, cultural, social, and economic issues to create situations that can affect the health of many peoples throughout the world.

CHAPTER REVIEW

Summary

In general, environmental factors that are the sole cause of disease are toxic chemicals. Such substances damage body tissues and affect bodily functioning; they are present in the home, workplace, and environment. Toxic chemicals are found in a wide variety of substances, such as household products, plants, products used in the workplace, and prescription and illegal drugs.

Toxic (poisonous) plants can be the source of poisoning emergencies, especially in children. Although many plants are not poisonous, house plants and cut flowers should be kept out of reach of children under 5 years old. In addition to plants, approximately 1% to 2% of mushroom species are poisonous.

Children under the age of 5 years are those most in danger of being poisoned from household cleaning aids and from over-the-counter and prescription drugs and vitamins. Special packaging that makes it difficult for young children to open hazardous products has lowered the incidence of poisoning in this age group. Nevertheless, such substances should be locked in cabinets in homes in which young children reside or visit often.

Lead poisoning is still a health problem in children in the United States even though many sources of lead poisoning have been eliminated in this country. Lead poisoning is serious because it affects the central nervous system and can cause coma, convulsions, and death. Children can exhibit a wide range of symptoms of lead poisoning, depending on the level of lead in the blood. It is extremely important to remove sources of lead, such as lead-based paint, from a child's environment.

Carbon monoxide poisoning can occur when levels of this gas build up in an enclosed environment. Major sources of carbon monoxide poisoning are fires, automobile exhaust, malfunctioning furnaces, charcoal fires, gasoline-powered tools, woodstoves, fireplaces, unvented kerosene and gas space heaters, gas cooking stoves and ovens, and tobacco smoke. To avoid this hazard, properly maintain and use tools and appliances that burn fuel, avoid running the car in the garage, vent home heating stoves and furnaces properly, and use charcoal grills and gas-powered tools only in well-ventilated areas.

Extremely low frequency (ELF) radiation is emitted by computer screens, microwave ovens, cell phones, television sets, electric blankets, electric appliances, high-tension electric power lines, and electrical distribution substations. ELF radiation has been associated with negative effects such as risk of cancer, DNA damage, and changes in human brain electrical activity. Nonetheless, scientists have seen no major negative effects and see no reason to recommend extreme caution. Medical researchers suggest, however, that people avoid being unnecessarily close to products and power lines that emit ELF radiation.

Many types of environmental hazards exist in the workplace. Common workplace hazards include exposure to pesticides while manufacturing or applying them, and exposure to toxins in the industrial manufacture and use of certain solvents, metals, plastics, and adhesives. People who work with toxic chemicals should protect themselves from damage to their skin and eyes and should assess the danger from toxic fumes that may be created as a result of their work.

Indoor air may be contaminated with pollutants such as formaldehyde, asbestos, and combustion-generated products. Some buildings have poor ventilation systems, which are the primary cause of vague health-related symptoms in building occupants.

The air we breathe and the water we drink are also contaminated with toxins to a greater or lesser degree in various parts of the United States. Contaminated drinking water can result in both short-term and long-term health effects. The air is contaminated with emissions from coal-fired power plants and vehicles. When the air is unhealthful, the elderly and those with respiratory illness are most at risk for further damage to their health.

Noise pollution can have a negative effect on health. Sounds of less than 75 dB are unlikely to cause hearing loss. To avoid hearing loss and other negative health effects of noise pollution, avoid situations in which the sound is over 80 dB or wear specially designed ear protection in such situations.

Applying What You Have Learned

1. Your 4-year-old cousin is coming to visit for the summer. What steps would you take to make your house or apartment safe for your cousin? **Application**
2. List and then analyze your interactions with the environment in the last 24 hours. Develop a list of environmental threats to your health from these interactions. **Analysis**
3. You have just moved to a part of the country that is new to you. Develop a plan to assess whether you are being exposed to hazardous chemicals and toxins and to evaluate which health hazards might be present, if any. **Synthesis**

4. Develop a fictitious set of at least three outcomes based on question 3. What will be your course of action to diminish or eliminate these threats to your health? **Evaluation**

Key

Application	using information in a new situation.
Analysis	breaking down information into component parts.
Synthesis	putting together information from different sources.
Evaluation	making informed decisions.

Reflecting on Your Health

1. Do you take steps to protect your hearing? If so, what do you do? Do you think about possible hearing loss when you are in noisy environments? Describe three situations in which you regularly are exposed to harmful noise levels and discuss what you can do to avoid hearing loss in these situations.
2. Go through your house or apartment and identify environmental health risks. What can you do to reduce these risks to health?
3. Do you ever put yourself or others at risk for carbon monoxide poisoning? If so, describe your risky behaviors and what you can do to eliminate the risk. If not, identify behaviors in others that you have observed that put people at risk for carbon monoxide poisoning. How might you help others avoid such risks?

4. Find out about environmental risks in your area. For example, is your tap water chlorinated to levels that are worrisome? Do you live in a region of the country in which water comes to your home in lead pipes? What might you do in either of these situations to reduce or eliminate your health risks from water? Investigate air pollution in your area. How can you protect your respiratory health in the region in which you live? Describe any environmental health risks that affect your community and suggest what you might do to reduce health risks to yourself and your family.
5. Do you ever discard toxic waste improperly, such as putting old batteries (especially car batteries), solvents, or paints in the trash? If so, describe the proper disposal methods for these substances in your city or town.

References

Alhekail, Z. O. (2001). Electromagnetic radiation from microwave ovens. *Journal of Radiological Protection, 21*:251–258.

Bardana, E. J. (2001). Indoor air pollution and its impact on respiratory health. *Annals of Allergy, Asthma, & Immunology, 87*(suppl):33–40.

Centers for Disease Control and Prevention. (1993). Lead poisoning associated with use of traditional ethnic remedies—California, 1991–1992. *Morbidity and Mortality Weekly Report, 42*:521–524.

Centers for Disease Control and Prevention. (2000). Recommendations for blood lead screening of young children enrolled in Medicaid: Targeting a group at high risk. *Morbidity and Mortality Weekly Report, 49*(RR-14):1–13.

Centers for Disease Control and Prevention. (2001). Fatal pediatric lead poisoning—New Hampshire, 2000. *Morbidity and Mortality Weekly Report, 50*:457–459.

Centers for Disease Control and Prevention. (2004a). Adult blood lead epidemiology and surveillance—United States, 2002. *Morbidity and Mortality Weekly Report, 53*(26):578–582.

Centers for Disease Control and Prevention. (2004b). Lead poisoning associated with ayurvedic medication—five states, 2000–2003. *Morbidity and Mortality Weekly Report, 53*(26):582–584.

Centers for Disease Control and Prevention. (2004c). *Carbon monoxide poisoning.* Retrieved from http://www.bt.cdc.gov/disasters/pdf/carbonmonoxide.pdf.

Cook, C. M., Thomas, A. W., & Prato, F. S. (2004). Resting EEG is affected by exposure to a pulsed ELF magnetic field. *Bioelectromagnetics, 25*:196–203.

Farley, D. (1998). Dangers of lead still linger. *FDA Consumer, 32*(1):16–21.

Fawell, J. (2000). Risk assessment case study—chloroform and related substances. *Food & Chemical Toxicology, 38*(1 suppl):S91–S95.

Fergusson, D. M., Horwood, L. J., Beautrais, A. L., & Shannon, F. T. (1982). A controlled field trial of a poisoning prevention method. *Pediatrics, 69*:515–520.

Foulke, J. E. (1993). FDA reports on pesticides in foods. *FDA Consumer, 27*(5):29–32.

Graves, C. G., Matanoski, G. M., & Tardiff, R. G. (2001). Weight of evidence for an association between adverse reproductive and developmental effects and exposure to disinfection by-products: A critical review. *Regulatory Toxicology & Pharmacology, 34*:103–124.

Ivancsits, S., Diem, E., Jahn, O., & Rüdiger, H. W. (2003). Intermittent extremely low frequency electromagnetic fields cause DNA damage in a dose-dependent way. *International Archives of Occupational and Environmental Health. 76*:431–436.

Kundi, M., Mild, K., Hardell, L., & Mattsson, M. O. (2004). Mobile telephones and cancer—a review of epidemiological evidence. *Journal of Toxicology and Environmental Health Part B: Critical Reviews, 7*:351–384.

Nieuwenhuijsen, M. J., Toledano, M. B., Eaton, N. E., Fawell, J., & Elliott, P. (2000). Chlorination disinfection byproducts in water and their association with adverse reproductive outcomes: A review. *Occupational & Environmental Medicine, 57*:73–85.

Office of Pollution Prevention and Toxics. (1997). *Reducing lead hazards when remodeling your home.* Washington, DC: U.S. Environmental Protection Agency.

Saper, R. B., Kales, S. N., Paquin, J., Burns, M. J., Eisenberg, D. M., Davis, R. B., & Phillips, R. S. (2004). Heavy metal content of ayurvedic herbal medicine products. *Journal of the American Medical Association, 292*:2868–2873.

Sisto, R., Casciardi, S., Giliberti, C., & Moleti, A. (1999). Electromagnetic radiation from VDT units: Study of the effectiveness of an active shielding device. *American Industrial Hygiene Association Journal, 60*:111–115.

Staples, S. L. (1996). Human response to environmental noise. *American Psychologist, 51*:143–150.

Sundell, J. (2004). On the history of indoor air quality and health. *Indoor Air, 14*(Suppl 7):51–58.

Traitcheva, N., Angelova, P., Radeva, M., & Berg, H. (2003). ELF fields and photooxidation yielding lethal effects on cancer cells. *Bioelectromagnetics, 24*:148–150.

U.S. Consumer Product Safety Commission. (1989). *Asbestos in the home.* Washington, DC: U.S. Environmental Protection Agency.

Vernberg, K., Culver-Dickinson, P., & Spyker, D. A. (1984). The deterrent effect of poison-warning stickers. *American Journal of Diseases of Children, 138*:1018–1020.

Watson, W. A., Litovitz, T. L., Klein-Schwartz, W., Rodgers, G. C., Youniss, J., Reid, N., Rouse, W. G., Rembert, R. S., & Borys, D. (2004). 2003 annual report of the American Association of Poison Control Centers Toxic Exposure Surveillance System. *American Journal of Emergency Medicine, 22*:335–404.

Yoon, S. S., Macdonald, S. C., & Parrish, R. G. (1998). Deaths from unintentional carbon monoxide poisoning and potential for prevention with carbon monoxide detectors. *Journal of the American Medical Association, 279*:685–687.

Healthy People 2010 Leading Health Indicators

Healthy People 2010 Leading Health Indicators: United States, Selected Years 1990–2002, and 2010 Target

Leading Health Indicators, Measures, and *Healthy People 2010* Objective Numbers	1990	1995	1998	1999	2000	2001	2002	2010 Target
Physical Activity								
1a. Adolescents in grades 9–12: percent who engaged in 20 minutes or more of vigorous activity 3 or more days per week (obj 22–07)	---	64	---	65	---	65	---	85
1b. Adults age 18 years and over: age-adjusted percent who engaged in moderate activity (at least 30 minutes, 5 days per week) or vigorous activity (at least 20 minutes, 3 days per week) (obj 22–02)[1]	---	---	30	30	32	32	33	50
Overweight and Obesity[2]								
2a. Overweight or obese children and adolescents, age 6–19 years: percent who are at or above the sex- and age-specific 95th percentile of Body Mass Index (BMI) based on CDC Growth Charts: United States (obj 19–03c)	11	---	---	---	15	---	---	5
2b. Obese adults age 20 years and over: age-adjusted percent with BMI of 30 Kg/m^2 or more (obj 19–02)	23	---	---	---	31	---	---	15
Tobacco Use								
3a. Adolescents in grades 9–12: percent who smoked cigarettes one or more days in the past 30 days (obj 27–02b)	---	35	---	35	---	28	---	16
3b. Adults age 18 years and over: age-adjusted percent who smoked more than 100 cigarettes in their lifetime and now report smoking on some days or every day (obj 27–01a)[1]	25	25	24	23	23	23	22	12
Substance Abuse[3]								
4a. Adolescents age 12–17 years: percent who reported no use of alcohol or illicit drugs in the past 30 days (obj 26–10a)	---	---	---	80	80	---	---	89
4b. Adults age 18 years and over: percent who reported illicit drug use in the past 30 days (obj 26–10c)	---	---	---	5.8	5.9	6.6	---	2.0
4c. Adults age 18 years and over: percent who reported binge drinking in the past 30 days (obj 26–11c)	---	---	---	21	22	22	---	6
Responsible Sexual Behavior								
5a. Adolescents in grades 9–12: percent who are not sexually active or sexually active and used condoms (obj 25–11)	---	83	---	85	---	86	---	95
5a1. Never had intercourse	---	47	---	50	---	54	---	...
5a2. Used a condom at last intercourse	---	21	---	21	---	19	---	...
5a3. No sexual intercourse in past 3 months	---	15	---	14	---	12	---	...
5b. Sexually active unmarried women age 18–44 years: percent who reported condom use by partners (obj 13–06a)	---	23	---	---	---	---	---	50
5c. New cases of gonorrhea per 100,000 population (obj 25–02) (supplemental measure)	277	149	132	132	129	129	---	19

Continued.

Healthy People 2010 **Leading Health Indicators: United States, Selected Years 1990–2002, and 2010 Target (continued)**

Leading Health Indicators, Measures, and *Healthy People 2010* Objective Numbers	1990	1995	1998	1999	2000	2001	2002	2010 Target
Mental Health								
6a. Adults age 18 years and over: percent with recognized depression who received treatment (obj 18–09b)[4]	---	23	---	---	---	---	---	50
6b. Age-adjusted suicide rate per 100,000 standard population (obj 18–01) (supplemental measure)[5,6]	12.5	11.8	11.1	10.5	10.4	10.7	---	5.0
Injury and Violence								
7a. Age-adjusted death rate for motor vehicle traffic-related injuries per 100,000 standard population (obj 15–15a)[5]	18.0	15.9	15.3	14.7	14.9	14.9	---	9.2
7b. Age-adjusted homicide rate per 100,000 standard population (obj 15–32)[5,6]	9.4	8.3	6.4	6.0	5.9	7.1	---	3.0
Environmental Quality								
8a. Percent of population exposed to ozone above EPA standard (obj 08–01a)	---	---	43	43	43	41	---	0
8b. Persons age 4 years and over: age-adjusted percent of nonsmokers exposed to environmental tobacco smoke (obj 27–10)[2]	88.1	---	---	---	53.9	---	---	45
8c. Persons under age 18 years: hospital admissions for asthma per 10,000 population (obj 01–09a) (supplemental measure)	---	---	---	25.5	---	21.4	---	17.3
Immunization								
9a. Children age 19–35 months: percent who received all DTaP, polio, MMR, Hib, and HepB vaccines (obj 14–24a)	---	---	73	73	73	74	75	80
9b. Adults age 65 years and over: age-adjusted percent who received influenza vaccine in the past 12 months (obj 14–29a)[1]	---	59	64	66	65	63	66	90
9c. Adults age 65 years and over: age-adjusted percent who ever received pneumococcal vaccine (obj 14–29b)[1]	---	35	46	50	53	54	55	90
Access to Health Care								
10a. Persons under age 65 years: age-adjusted percent with health insurance (obj 01–01)[1]	---	84	83	84	83	84	84	100
10b. Persons of all ages: age-adjusted percent with a specific source of ongoing primary care (obj 01–04a)[1]	---	87	87	86	87	88	88	96
10c. Pregnant women: percent who received prenatal care in the first trimester (obj 16–06a)	76	81	83	83	83	83	---	90

--- Data not available.

... Data not applicable.

[1] Data for 1997 and later years are not strictly comparable with data for earlier years due to the 1997 questionnaire redesign. Data for 2002 are provisional.

[2] NHANES data for 1990 are for the period 1988–1994. NHANES data for 2000 are for the period 1999–2000 and are based on a smaller sample size and therefore are subject to greater sampling error than the estimate for 1988–1994.

[3] In a major redesign of the survey in 1999, the sample size, mode of administration, and survey content changed. Data are not shown for 1998 and earlier years because only limited comparisons can be made between data from the redesigned surveys (1999 onward) and data obtained from surveys prior to 1999.

[4] Baseline year 1997 and baseline value 23 percent are shown in 1995.

[5] Population estimates used to compute rates for 1991–2000 differ from those used previously. Starting with *Health, United States, 2003*, rates for 1991–1999 were revised using intercensal population estimates based on Census 2000. Rates for 2000 were revised based on Census 2000 counts. Rates for 2001 were computed using 2000-based postcensal estimates.

[6] Figures for 2001 include September 11–related deaths for which death certificates were filed as of October 24, 2002.

Note: Data are based on interviews and examinations of samples of the civilian noninstitutionalized population or special population subgroups; information from death certificates and birth certificates; and air quality measurements.

Data sources: Youth Risk Behavior Surveillance System (YRBSS), CDC, NCCDPHP: measures 1a, 3a, and 5a; National Health Interview Survey (NHIS), CDC, NCHS: measures 1b, 3b, 9b, 9c, 10a, and 10b; National Health and Nutrition Examination Survey (NHANES), CDC, NCHS: measures 2a, 2b, and 8b; National Household Survey on Drug Abuse (NHSDA), SAMHSA: measures 4a, 4b, 4c, and 6a; National Survey of Family Growth (NSFG), CDC, NCHS: measure 5b; Sexually Transmitted Diseases (STD) Surveillance System, CDC, NCHSTP: measure 5c; National Vital Statistics System (NVSS), CDC, NCHS: measures 6b, 7a, 7b, 10c; Aerometric Information Retrieval System (AIRS), EPA, OAR: measure 8a; Healthcare Cost and Utilization Project (HCUP), AHRQ: measure 8c; National Immunization Survey (NIS), CDC, NIP and NCHS: measure 9a.

Source: Fried, V. M., Prager, K., MacKay, A. P., & Xia, H. (2003). *Health, United States, 2003, with Chartbook on Trends in the Health of Americans.* Hyattsville, MD: National Center for Health Statistics.

Injury Prevention and Emergency Care

■ Injury Prevention

During the next hour, at least 11 people will die in the United States from unintentional injuries. The causes will be diverse, including automobile crashes, drownings, poisonings (see Chapter 16), and fires. Some of those who die this hour will probably be children, because unintentional, preventable injury is the number one killer of children (through young adulthood, from 1 through 21 years old) in the United States. In fact, unintentional injuries kill more children than all childhood diseases combined.

Until recently, the number of fatal unintentional injuries had been steadily declining, reaching a 68-year low of approximately 89,000 in 1994. However, that number has been rising annually since then. In 2002, slightly more than 102,300 people died from unintentional injuries. This appendix will alert you to the most prevalent types of unintentional injuries and deaths in the United States today, and discusses their causes, prevention, and emergency treatment.

Automobile Safety

Motor vehicle crashes are the greatest cause of preventable death due to injuries. In 2002, 45,380 people died on America's roads and highways. Nearly half of them were driving while intoxicated or were killed by drunk drivers. In addition to deaths, motor vehicle accidents are the leading cause of unintentional injury in the United States. To keep yourself and others safe while riding in automobiles, heed the following recommendations. For general vehicle safety:

- Never drink and drive or take other drugs that impair your ability to drive.
- Always wear your seat belt; this practice reduces by half your chance of injury or death in a motor vehicle crash.
- Slow down and prepare to stop as you approach yellow lights. Many people cause automobile crashes because they try to "beat" the light.
- Yield the right of way at intersections.
- Don't tailgate; allow at least one car length for each 10 mph (e.g., stay four car lengths behind the car ahead if you are traveling at 40 mph).
- Know the traffic laws of the state in which you are driving and obey these laws.

- Read and heed traffic signs, especially railroad warning signals and gates. Always proceed cautiously across railroad tracks. Not all railroad crossings have gates or sound warnings to signal oncoming trains.
- Obey the speed limit.

Children and Automobile Safety To protect children while they are passengers in automobiles, follow these safety recommendations:

- Place infants in properly secured rear-facing safety seats until they are 1 year of age and weigh at least 20 lb.
- Always put rear-facing child safety seats in the back seat. Deploying passenger-side air bags in the front seat can injure or kill infants in rear-facing seats.
- Properly restrain all children in safety seats, lap belts, or lap and shoulder belts. Children should be restrained in car seats until they weigh 40 lb. and then should be in booster seats until they are about 8 years old and weigh 80 lb.
- An infant's or child's car seat needs to be secured so tightly that it will not move more than one inch from side to side. Locate a certified Child Passenger Safety Seat Technician in your area to check the installation of your child's safety seat.
- It is best to have children of any age ride in the back seat to avoid injury from a deploying air bag. If a child must ride in the front, push the seat back as far as possible to create distance between the child and the bag.
- Never leave a child alone in the car.

Pedestrian Safety

Pedestrians accounted for 11% of preventable deaths involving motor vehicles in the United States and approximately 4% of motor vehicle–related injuries in 2002. Not only are drunk drivers often a cause of these injuries and deaths, but intoxicated pedestrians put themselves at increased risk. Other high-risk groups for sustaining unintentional pedestrian–automobile injuries and deaths are the elderly and young children. Children are most frequently hit when they dart into traffic from between parked cars. Children younger than 10 years old do not have fully developed cognitive, developmental, behavioral, physical, and sensory abilities to be safe pedestrians on their own. To help prevent pedestrian injuries, practice these safety steps:

- Help children develop injury-prevention skills by modeling proper safety behaviors such as those listed here.

- Be sure that children younger than 10 years of age are accompanied by an older person when they cross the street.
- Cross at marked crosswalks and at corners whenever possible. Do not assume that drivers will stop because you are in a crosswalk.
- Stop, look both ways, and listen before deciding that it is safe to cross. Continue to look and listen as you cross.
- Cross only on a green light or a "walk" signal.
- Never cross between parked cars.
- Never run into the street.
- Walk on sidewalks whenever possible. If you must walk in the street, walk to the left facing traffic.
- When walking at dusk or at night, wear light colors and some type of reflective device. Walk with someone, not alone.
- Do not allow children to play in driveways, in adjacent unfenced yards, in streets, or in parking lots.

Water Safety

In 2002, slightly more than 3,400 people died from drowning. Drowning is the second leading cause of injury-related death for children aged 1 through 14 years, the highest rates being for children aged 1 through 4 years. (Fatalities involving automobiles is the leading cause of injury-related death for children.) Most drownings of children happen in pools, hot tubs, or spas owned by their parents, relatives, or friends, and they happen within five minutes of the child's being missing from sight. Children usually drown silently, so don't think that splashing or screaming will alert you to the danger.

Safety for Small Children To protect small children from drowning in residential pools or other accessible bodies of water, follow these safety practices:

- Provide barriers to water, such as fences and walls. If the house is part of the barrier, install door alarms so you know when the child has gone outside, and install a power safety cover over the pool, hot tub, or spa.
- Fence gates should be self-closing and self-latching. The latch should be out of a child's reach.
- Never prop open the fence gate.
- Instruct babysitters about pool hazards for young children.
- If a young child is missing, check the pool first.
- Do not assume that children will not drown because they know how to swim.

- Never leave a child unsupervised near a pool, and while at the pool, watch small children continuously; do not become preoccupied with something else.
- Children can drown in the bathtub, in a bucket of water, or in the toilet. Never leave children alone, even for a minute, when they are in or near any type of water.

Safety for Swimmers Even good swimmers have accidents in the water and drown. For safety in the water, follow these guidelines:

- Never swim alone.
- Don't push or jump on others.
- Check water depth before you dive or jump into the water.
- Never swim in unsupervised areas such as quarries, canals, or ponds.
- Don't swim or use a hot tub or spa while drinking alcoholic beverages or taking other drugs that could impair your judgment, impair your ability to swim, or make you drowsy. (Alcohol is involved in 25% to 50% of adolescent and adult deaths associated with water recreation.)

Bicycle Safety

In the United States in 2002, approximately 550 people died in traffic-related bicycle crashes. Seventy-five percent of such deaths are usually due to head injuries. Supporters of wearing bicycle helmets contend that 40% to 75% of head-injury deaths could be prevented if riders wore helmets. Opponents suggest that these statistics are unreliable and that most bicycle fatalities involve a crash with an automobile, a situation in which a helmet cannot protect the bicyclist. Those who take a middle stance suggest that it is prudent to wear helmets because they protect the head in many types of falls and make bicyclists more visible to automobile drivers.

By the end of 2003, 19 states, the District of Columbia, and 144 local governments had enacted legislation about bicycle helmets. Most of these laws pertain to children and adolescents. In 1999, the U.S. Consumer Product Safety Commission issued a new safety standard for bike helmets.

Bicycle helmets are designed to absorb much of the impact when the head hits another object like a car or the road. Oftentimes, a cyclist hits a car and then the road, so the helmet needs a strap to ensure that it stays on during multiple hits. Also, it should not be covered with any material that can catch on something during a fall and twist the cyclist's head. When purchasing a helmet, make sure that it is level on the head, covers the top of the forehead, touches all around, and is comfortably snug. Many sellers and manufacturers of helmets offer instructions about the proper fit of helmets.

Bicycle injuries are a leading cause of preventable death in children, exceeding the death rate from poisonings, falls, and firearm injuries combined. Most bicycle-related deaths occur from head trauma and are not caused by colliding with cars. Rather, children fall from their bikes or lose control of their bikes and collide with objects such as curbs and trees. Therefore, all children benefit from wearing helmets while bicycling. They should also wear helmets while being carried as passengers on adults' bikes. Have a pediatrician check a toddler's helmet, however, because the neck muscles of toddlers are weak and may be unable to properly support a helmeted head.

Bicycle Safety Rules For bicycling safety, follow these simple rules:

- Make yourself or your children visible with light-colored clothing and reflective tape.
- Be certain that your bicycle horn or bell is working properly.
- Drive on the right-hand side of the road in single file, obeying all traffic signs and signals. Small children should ride their bikes on the sidewalk.
- When cycling in the road, leave a distance of about 3 feet between you and parked cars. You will be more noticeable to drivers and will not be knocked off your bike by the opening doors of parked cars.
- Walk your bike at busy street corners in pedestrian crosswalks.
- Never carry a passenger on your bicycle unless you have a tandem bike or are carrying a child in a properly mounted child seat.
- When exiting a driveway into a lane of traffic, stop, look both ways, and listen to determine that it is safe to enter.
- Before turning, use hand signals and look in all directions.
- Don't ride your bike on rainy nights. Your chances of being involved in a crash are 30 times greater than on a dry night because roads are slippery, wet bicycle brakes do not work well, and automobile drivers cannot see bicyclists well in the rain.
- If you are falling off your bike, tuck and roll rather than extending an arm to break your fall.
- Children should not ride in the street until they are 10 years old, demonstrate good riding skills, and are able to observe the basic rules of the road.

Fire Prevention

Although the number of residential fires has declined about 30 percent since 1980, every year there are still over 400,000 residential fires (one every 70 seconds) in which more than 3,500 people die. Most fires are started by home cooking equipment. However, residential fires caused by lit cigarettes, cigarette lighters, or matches are the leading cause of fire-related death. A fewer number of fires are ignited by faulty electrical wiring or supplemental home heating devices such as wood stoves, kerosene heaters, gas-fired space heaters, and portable electric heaters.

The number of supplemental home heaters has decreased in recent years, as has the number of fires associated with them. However, supplemental heaters still cause about 22% of residential fires. Additionally, thousands of people are burned each year by coming into contact with the hot surfaces of these devices, and hundreds are poisoned by their carbon monoxide emissions (see Chapter 16).

Home Heaters Some safety recommendations for the use of supplemental home heaters include the following:

- Be certain that any supplemental heater is properly installed and meets building codes.
- Inspect wood stoves according to the manufacturer's directions (usually twice monthly) and have chimneys inspected and cleaned by a professional chimney sweep.
- Use a floor protector designed for use under the type of supplemental heater you have. It should extend 18 inches beyond the heater on all sides.
- Follow directions regarding how far the heater must be from combustible walls and other materials such as draperies.
- Never burn trash in a wood-burning stove because this practice could cause overheating.
- Never use gasoline to start a wood fire.
- Use only the fuel(s) the manufacturer has designated as safe in the heater.
- If using a liquid fuel, be certain that its container is well marked and is out of the reach of children.
- Place kerosene heaters out of the path of traffic and where they cannot be knocked over.
- Always fill a kerosene heater outdoors and when the heater is not operating.
- Kerosene heaters are not usually vented; therefore, keep a window ajar for ventilation.
- Use unvented gas heaters only in large, open areas that are well ventilated; do not operate vented styles unvented.

- Do not use supplemental heating devices while you are sleeping or not at home; many fires and deaths occur at these times from the unsupervised use of supplemental heaters.
- With electric heaters, follow the manufacturer's recommendations regarding the type of power cord to use. Avoid using extension cords, but if you do, be certain that it is marked with a power rating at least as high as that of the heater itself. Keep the cord stretched out and do not place anything on top of the cord.

General Fire Prevention Many residential fires could have been prevented with little trouble. To decrease your risk of fire, take the following precautions:

- Keep matches and cigarette lighters away from children.
- Do not store food items such as candy or other items attractive to children above the stove.
- Always check ashtrays to be certain that cigarettes are out. After a party or other gathering, check under and between the cushions of upholstered furniture to make sure that no smoldering ashes are present.
- Never place ashtrays on the arms of furniture, especially upholstered furniture that is likely to ignite from lit cigarettes or their ashes.
- Avoid placing lit candles near draperies or other flammable materials. Be certain that they do not tip easily and are not positioned where they can be easily knocked over.
- Consider purchasing clothes made out of fabrics that are difficult to ignite and tend to self-extinguish, such as 100% polyester, nylon, wool, and silk. Cotton, cotton/polyester blends, rayon, and acrylic ignite easily and burn rapidly.
- Store flammable liquids, such as gasoline and paint thinners, outside the house. They produce invisible explosive vapors.
- Install at least one smoke detector on each floor of your home and near the bedrooms. Replace the batteries annually or when they make a chirping sound.
- Plan an escape route from each room in the house. Have each family member rehearse the plan often. Designate a safe place to meet if you have to escape a fire in your home. This helps firefighters determine if there are people in a burning building.

Source of statistics for injury prevention: Centers for Disease Control and Prevention, National Center for Injury Prevention and Control.

Emergency Care

When to Call for Help

Know the emergency number in your area; in most areas that number is 9-1-1. Calling for help in a medical emergency is important and may save a person's life. When a serious situation occurs, call for emergency medical help *first*. Do not call your doctor, the hospital, a friend, relatives, or neighbors. Calling anyone else first only wastes time.

Call for emergency help in the following situations:

- Fainting
- Chest or abdominal pain or pressure
- Sudden dizziness, weakness, or change in vision
- Difficulty breathing, shortness of breath
- Severe or persistent vomiting
- Sudden, severe pain anywhere in the body
- Suicidal or homicidal feelings
- Bleeding that does not stop after 10 to 15 minutes of pressure
- A gaping wound with edges that do not come together
- Problems with movement or sensation following an injury
- Cuts on the hand or face
- Puncture wounds
- The possibility that foreign bodies such as glass or metal may have entered a wound
- Most animal bites and all human bites
- Hallucinations and clouding of thoughts
- A stiff neck in association with a fever or a headache
- A bulging or abnormally depressed fontanel (soft spot) in infants
- Stupor or dazed behavior accompanying a high fever that is not alleviated by acetaminophen or aspirin
- Unequal pupil size, loss of consciousness, blindness, staggering, or repeated vomiting after a head injury
- Spinal injuries
- Severe burns
- Poisoning
- Drug overdose

When in doubt, CALL.

Good Samaritan Laws

States have enacted laws to protect physicians and other medical personnel from legal actions that may arise from emergency treatment they give while not on duty.

Although Good Samaritan laws cover medical personnel primarily, several states have expanded them to include laypersons who, in good faith, help others in emergency situations. Unless a person acts in a reckless or wantonly negligent manner when trying to voluntarily assist another, he or she is usually immune from conviction in a legal action. These laws vary from state to state; find out about your state's Good Samaritan laws by contacting a legal professional or checking with your local library.

Heart Attack

For information on recognizing the signs of a possible heart attack and on how to respond, see Chapter 12, especially page 323.

Poisoning

For information on preventing poisonings and how to treat a person who has been poisoned, see Chapter 16, especially pages 452 to 457.

Bleeding

If a person is bleeding heavily from a wound, it is important to stop the bleeding as quickly as possible. First, take the following action, then call for help or take the person to an emergency room.

- Protect yourself from disease by wearing medical exam gloves.
- Expose the wound by removing or cutting the clothing to see where the blood is coming from.
- Place a sterile gauze pad or a clean cloth (such as a washcloth or towel) over the entire wound and apply direct pressure with your fingers or the palm of your hand.
- If the bleeding is from an arm or leg, while still applying pressure, elevate the injured area above heart level to reduce blood flow.
- When the bleeding stops, wrap a roller gauze bandage tightly over the dressing to hold it in place and prevent further bleeding.

Breathing Emergencies

Signs of inadequate breathing include a rate of breathing significantly less than 12 times per minute (for adults), skin that is pale or bluish and cool, and nasal flaring, especially in children. Ask someone to call for emergency care, and then if the person is *not* breathing:

- Tilt the head back and lift the chin to open the airway.
- Pinch the victim's nose shut, take a deep breath, and make a tight seal around the victim's mouth with your mouth.

- Slowly blow air into the victim's mouth until you see the chest rise.
- Remove your mouth to allow the air to come out, and turn your head away as you take another breath.
- Repeat one more breath.
- Check the victim for signs of circulation (breathing, coughing, or movement). If the victim is not breathing and has signs of circulation:
  - Give one breath about every 4 to 5 seconds for an adult.
  - Recheck for signs of circulation about every minute.
  - Continue this process as long as the person has signs of circulation, until help arrives.

If the first breath does not go in, retilt the victim's head and try a second breath. If the second breath does not go in, use the procedure to aid a choking victim.

Choking

You can tell if a person is choking if he or she is unable to speak, breathe, or cough or breathes with a high-pitched wheezing. A choking victim may instinctively reach up and clutch his or her neck. To help, first tell someone to call for emergency care. Then do the following:

- Stand behind the choking person.
- Wrap your arms around the victim's waist. (Do not allow your forearms to touch the ribs.)
- Make a fist with one hand and place the thumb side just above the victim's navel.
- Grasp your fist with your other hand.
- Press your fist into the victim's abdomen with quick inward and upward thrusts.
- Continue thrusts until the object is removed or the victim becomes unresponsive.

Each thrust should be a separate and distinct effort to dislodge the object.

Burns

If a person is burned by fire and his or her clothing is on fire, have the victim roll on the ground using the "stop, drop, and roll" method. You can also smother the flames with a blanket or douse the victim with water. Ask someone to call for emergency help. Then do the following:

- Remove jewelry and hot or burned clothing immediately, but *do not* remove clothing stuck to the skin.
- Cool the burn. Use large amounts of cool water, not ice. Immerse the burn in cool water if possible.

- Apply a thin layer of antibiotic ointment and cover the burn with dry, sterile dressings or clean cloths.
- Wait for help or transport the person to the emergency room of the local hospital.

Heat-Related Emergencies

Everyone is susceptible to heat illness if environmental conditions overwhelm the body's temperature-regulating mechanisms. Such illnesses are progressive conditions, and could become life threatening. Therefore, it is important to recognize heat-related illness early and treat it immediately.

Heat cramps are painful muscular spasms that happen suddenly, usually in the legs and abdomen. If someone has heat cramps, have him or her

- rest in a cool place,
- drink lightly salted cool water ($\frac{1}{4}$ tsp. salt per quart of water) or a commercial sports drink diluted to half strength, and
- lightly stretch and gently massage the cramped muscle.

Heat exhaustion is another heat-related emergency. It is characterized by heavy perspiration with normal or slightly above normal body temperatures and is caused by water or salt depletion or both. To help a person with heat exhaustion, have him or her

- rest in a cool place,
- drink lightly salted cool water ($\frac{1}{4}$ tsp. salt per quart of water) or a commercial sports drink diluted to half strength,
- remove excess clothing, and
- lie down and raise the legs 8 to 12 inches, while keeping them straight.

Sponge the victim with cool water and fan him or her. If no improvement is seen within 30 minutes, seek medical attention.

In its advanced stages, heat exhaustion is called heatstroke and can cause death. It must be treated rapidly. Heatstroke is characterized by red, hot, dry skin and an altered mental state ranging from slight confusion and disorientation to coma. To treat heatstroke, send someone for emergency care and do the following:

- Have the person rest in a cool place.
- Remove clothing down to the victim's underwear.
- Keep the victim's head and shoulders slightly elevated.
- Cool the person by placing ice bags wrapped in wet towels on the wrists, ankles, groin, and neck, and in the armpits.
- Fan the person.

Appendix C

Food and Nutrition Board, National Academy of Sciences—National Research Council
Dietary Reference Intakes for Certain Nutrients* (Abridged)

Designed for the maintenance of good nutrition of practically all healthy people in the United States

Life Group Stage	Protein‡ (g)	Vitamin A (µg RE)	Vitamin E (mg α-TE)	Vitamin D (µg)	Vitamin C (mg)	Thiamin (mg)	Niacin (mg)	Vitamin B₆ (mg)	Vitamin B₁₂ (µg)	Folate (µg)	Iron (mg)	Calcium (mg)	Zinc (mg)	Selenium (µg)
Infants														
0–6 mo	13	400	4	5	40	0.2	2	0.1	0.4	65	0.27	210	2	15
7–12 mo	14	500	5	5	50	0.3	4	0.3	0.5	80	11	270	3	20
Children														
1–3 y	16	300	6	5	15	0.5	6	0.5	0.9	150	7	500	3	20
4–8 y	24	400	7	5	25	0.6	8	0.6	1.2	200	10	800	5	30
Males														
9–13 y	45	600	11	5	45	0.9	12	1.0	1.8	300	8	1300	8	40
14–18 y	59	900	15	5	75	1.2	16	1.3	2.4	400	11	1300	11	55
19–30 y	58	900	15	5	90	1.2	16	1.3	2.4	400	8	1000	11	55
31–50 y	63	900	15	5	90	1.2	16	1.3	2.4	400	8	1000	11	55
51–70 y	63	900	15	10	90	1.2	16	1.7	2.4	400	8	1200	11	55
>70 y	63	900	15	15	90	1.2	16	1.7	2.4	400	8	1200	11	55
Females														
9–13 y	46	600	11	5	45	0.9	12	1.0	1.8	300	8	1300	8	40
14–18 y	44	700	15	5	65	1.0	14	1.2	2.4	400	15	1300	9	55
19–30 y	46	700	15	5	75	1.1	14	1.3	2.4	400	18	1000	8	55
31–50 y	50	700	15	5	75	1.1	14	1.3	2.4	400	18	1000	8	55
51–70 y	50	700	15	10	75	1.1	14	1.5	2.4	400	8	1200	8	55
>70 y	50	700	15	15	75	1.1	14	1.5	2.4	400	8	1200	8	55
Pregnant														
19–50 y	60	770	15	5	85	1.4	18	1.9	2.6	600	27	1000	11	60
Lactating														
19–50 y	65	1300	19	5	120	1.4	17	2.0	2.8	500	9	1000	12	70

*For more information about the DRIs, go to http://www.nal.usda/gov/fnic/etext/000105.html.
‡RDA values.
Source: Adapted from National Academy of Sciences. (2001). *Dietary Reference Intakes: Applications in dietary assessment.* Washington, DC: National Academy Press.

MyPyramid

Food Intake Patterns

The suggested amounts of food to consume from the basic food groups, subgroups, and oils to meet recommended nutrient intakes at 12 different calorie levels. Nutrient and energy contributions from each group are calculated according to the nutrient-dense forms of foods in each group (e.g., lean meats and fat-free milk). The table also shows the discretionary calorie allowance that can be accommodated within each calorie level, in addition to the suggested amounts of nutrient-dense forms of foods in each group.

Daily Amount of Food From Each Group

Calorie Level[1]	1,000	1,200	1,400	1,600	1,800	2,000	2,200	2,400	2,600	2,800	3,000	3,200
Fruits[2]	1 cup	1 cup	1.5 cups	1.5 cups	1.5 cups	2 cups	2 cups	2 cups	2 cups	2.5 cups	2.5 cups	2.5 cups
Vegetables[3]	1 cup	1.5 cups	1.5 cups	2 cups	2.5 cups	2.5 cups	3 cups	3 cups	3.5 cups	3.5 cups	4 cups	4 cups
Grains[4]	3 oz-eq	4 oz-eq	5 oz-eq	5 oz-eq	6 oz-eq	6 oz-eq	7 oz-eq	8 oz-eq	9 oz-eq	10 oz-eq	10 oz-eq	10 oz-eq
Meat and Beans[5]	2 oz-eq	3 oz-eq	4 oz-eq	5 oz-eq	5 oz-eq	5.5 oz-eq	6 oz-eq	6.5 oz-eq	6.5 oz-eq	7 oz-eq	7 oz-eq	7 oz-eq
Milk[6]	2 cups	2 cups	2 cups	3 cups	3 cups	3 cups	3 cups	3 cups	3 cups	3 cups	3 cups	3 cups
Oils[7]	3 tsp	4 tsp	4 tsp	5 tsp	5 tsp	6 tsp	6 tsp	7 tsp	8 tsp	8 tsp	10 tsp	11 tsp
Discretionary calorie allowance[8]	165	171	171	132	195	267	290	362	410	426	512	648

[1] **Calorie Levels** are set across a wide range to accommodate the needs of different individuals. The attached table "Estimated Daily Calorie Needs" can be used to help assign individuals to the food intake pattern at a particular calorie level.

[2] **Fruit Group** includes all fresh, frozen, canned, and dried fruits and fruit juices. In general, 1 cup of fruit or 100% fruit juice, or 1/2 cup of dried fruit can be considered as 1 cup from the fruit group.

[3] **Vegetable Group** includes all fresh, frozen, canned, and dried vegetables and vegetable juices. In general, 1 cup of raw or cooked vegetables or vegetable juice, or 2 cups of raw leafy greens can be considered as 1 cup from the vegetable group.

[4] **Grains Group** includes all foods made from wheat, rice, oats, cornmeal, barley, such as bread, pasta, oatmeal, breakfast cereals, tortillas, and grits. In general, 1 slice of bread, 1 cup of ready-to-eat cereal, or 1/2 cup of cooked rice, pasta, or cooked cereal can be considered as 1 ounce equivalent from the grains group. **At least half of all grains consumed should be whole grains.**

[5] **Meat & Beans Group** in general, 1 ounce of lean meat, poultry, or fish, 1 egg, 1 Tbsp. peanut butter, 1/4 cup cooked dry beans, or 1/2 ounce of nuts or seeds can be considered as 1 ounce equivalent from the meat and beans group.

[6] **Milk Group** includes all fluid milk products and foods made from milk that retain their calcium content, such as yogurt and cheese. Foods made from milk that have little to no calcium, such as cream cheese, cream, and butter, are not part of the group. Most milk group choices should be fat-free or low-fat. In general, 1 cup of milk or yogurt, 1 1/2 ounces of natural cheese, or 2 ounces of processed cheese can be considered as 1 cup from the milk group.

[7] **Oils** include fats from many different plants and from fish that are liquid at room temperature, such as canola, corn, olive, soybean, and sunflower oil. Some foods are naturally high in oils, like nuts, olives, some fish, and avocados. Foods that are mainly oil include mayonnaise, certain salad dressings, and soft margarine.

[8] **Discretionary Calorie Allowance** is the remaining amount of calories in a food intake pattern after accounting for the calories needed for all food groups—using forms of foods that are fat-free or low-fat and with no added sugars.

Vegetable Subgroup Amounts are Per Week

Calorie Level	1,000	1,200	1,400	1,600	1,800	2,000	2,200	2,400	2,600	2,800	3,000	3,200
Dark green veg.	1 c/wk	1.5 c/wk	1.5 c/wk	2 c/wk	3 c/wk	3 c/wk	3 c/wk	3 c/wk	3 c/wk	3 c/wk	3 c/wk	3 c/wk
Orange veg.	.5 c/wk	1 c/wk	1 c/wk	1.5 c/wk	2 c/wk	2 c/wk	2 c/wk	2 c/wk	2.5 c/wk	2.5 c/wk	2.5 c/wk	2.5 c/wk
Legumes	.5 c/wk	1 c/wk	1 c/wk	2.5 c/wk	3 c/wk	3 c/wk	3 c/wk	3 c/wk	3.5 c/wk	3.5 c/wk	3.5 c/wk	3.5 c/wk
Starchy veg.	1.5 c/wk	2.5 c/wk	2.5 c/wk	2.5 c/wk	3 c/wk	3 c/wk	6 c/wk	6 c/wk	7 c/wk	7 c/wk	9 c/wk	9 c/wk
Other veg.	3.5 c/wk	4.5 c/wk	4.5 c/wk	5.5 c/wk	6.5 c/wk	6.5 c/wk	7 c/wk	7 c/wk	8.5 c/wk	8.5 c/wk	10 c/wk	10 c/wk

Estimated Daily Calorie Needs

To determine which food intake pattern to use for an individual, the following chart gives an estimate of individual calorie needs. The calorie range for each age/sex group is based on physical activity level, from sedentary to active.

	Calorie Range	
Children	Sedentary* ⟶	Active[†]
2–3 years	1,000 ⟶	1,400
Females		
4–8 years	1,200 ⟶	1,800
9–13	1,600 ⟶	2,200
14–18	1,800 ⟶	2,400
19–30	2,000 ⟶	2,400
31–50	1,800 ⟶	2,200
51+	1,600 ⟶	2,200
Males		
4–8 years	1,400 ⟶	2,000
9–13	1,800 ⟶	2,600
14–18	2,200 ⟶	3,200
19–30	2,400 ⟶	3,000
31–50	2,200 ⟶	3,000
51+	2,000 ⟶	2,800

*Sedentary means a lifestyle that includes only the light physical activity associated with typical day-to-day life.

[†]Active means a lifestyle that includes physical activity equivalent to walking more than 3 miles per day at 3 to 4 miles per hour, in addition to the light physical activity associated with typical day-to-day life.

Sample Menus for a 2000 Calorie Food Pattern

Averaged over a week, this seven day menu provides all of the recommended amounts of nutrients and food from each food group.

Food Group	Daily Average Over One Week	
Grains	Total Grains (oz eq) 6.0	
	Whole Grains 3.4	
	Refined Grains 2.6	
Vegetables*	Total Veg* (cups) 2.6	
Fruits	Fruits (cups) 2.1	
Milk	Milk (cups) 3.1	
Meat and Beans	Meat/Beans (oz eq) 5.6	
Oils	Oils (tsp/grams) 7.2 tsp/32.4 g	

*Vegetable subgroups	(weekly totals)
Dk-Green Veg (cups)	3.3
Orange Veg (cups)	2.3
Beans/ Peas (cups)	3.0
Starchy Veg (cups)	3.4
Other Veg (cups)	6.6

Nutrient	Daily Average
Calories	1994
Protein, g	98
Protein, % kcal	20
Carbohydrate, g	264
Carbohydrate, % kcal	53
Total fat, g	67
Total fat, % kcal	30
Saturated fat, g	16
Saturated fat, % kcal	7.0
Monounsaturated fat, g	23
Polyunsaturated fat, g	23
Linoleic acid, g	21
Alpha-linolenic acid, g	1.1
Cholesterol, mg	207
Total dietary fiber, g	31
Potassium, mg	4715
Sodium, mg*	1948
Calcium, mg	1389
Magnesium, mg	432
Copper, mg	1.9
Iron, mg	21
Phosphorus, mg	1830
Zinc, mg	14
Thiamin, mg	1.9
Riboflavin, mg	2.5
Niacin equivalents, mg	24
Vitamin B_6, mg	2.9
Vitamin B_{12}, mcg	18.4
Vitamin C, mg	190
Vitamin E, mg (AT)	18.9
Vitamin A, mcg (RAE)	1430
Dietary folate equivalents, mcg	558

* Starred items are foods that are labelled as no-salt-added, low-sodium, or low-salt versions of the foods. They can also be prepared from scratch with little or no added salt. All other foods are regular commercial products which contain variable levels of sodium. Average sodium level of the 7 day menu assumes no-salt-added in cooking or at the table.

(Italicized foods are part of the dish or food that preceeds it.)

Day 1

BREAKFAST

Breakfast burrito
1 flour tortilla (7" diameter)
1 scrambled egg (in 1 tsp soft margarine)
*1/3 cup black beans**
2 tbsp salsa
1 cup orange juice
1 cup fat-free milk

LUNCH

Roast beef sandwich
1 whole grain sandwich bun
3 ounces lean roast beef
2 slices tomato
1/4 cup shredded romaine lettuce
1/8 cup sauteed mushrooms (in 1 tsp oil)
1 1/2 ounce part-skim mozzarella cheese
1 tsp yellow mustard
3/4 cup baked potato wedges*
1 tbsp ketchup
1 unsweetened beverage

DINNER

Stuffed broiled salmon
1 ounce bread stuffing mix
1 tbsp chopped onions
1 tbsp diced celery
2 tsp canola oil
1/2 cup saffron (white) rice
1 ounce slivered almonds
1/2 cup steamed broccoli
1 tsp soft margarine
1 cup fat-free milk

SNACKS

1 cup cantaloupe

Day 2

BREAKFAST

Hot cereal
1/2 cup cooked oatmeal
2 tbsp raisins
1 tsp soft margarine
1/2 cup fat-free milk
1 cup orange juice

LUNCH

Taco salad
2 ounces tortilla chips
2 ounces ground turkey, sauteed in
2 tsp sunflower oil
*1/2 cup black beans**
1/2 cup iceberg lettuce
2 slices tomato
1 ounce low-fat cheddar cheese
2 tbsp salsa
1/2 cup avocado
1 tsp lime juice
1 unsweetened beverage

DINNER

Spinach lasagna
1 cup lasagna noodles, cooked (2 oz dry)
2/3 cup cooked spinach
1/2 cup ricotta cheese
*1/2 cup tomato sauce tomato bits**
1 ounce part-skim mozzarella cheese
1 ounce whole wheat dinner roll
1 cup fat-free milk

SNACKS

1/2 ounce dry-roasted almonds*
1/4 cup pineapple
2 tbsp raisins

Day 3

BREAKFAST

Cold cereal
1 cup bran flakes
1 cup fat-free milk
1 small banana
1 slice whole wheat toast
1 tsp soft margarine
1 cup prune juice

LUNCH

Tuna fish sandwich
2 slices rye bread
3 ounces tuna (packed in water, drained)
2 tsp mayonnaise
1 tbsp diced celery
1/4 cup shredded romaine lettuce
2 slices tomato
1 medium pear
1 cup fat-free milk

DINNER

Roasted chicken breast
*3 ounces boneless skinless chicken breast**
1 large baked sweetpotato
1/2 cup peas and onions
1 tsp soft magarine
1 ounce whole wheat dinner roll
1 tsp soft margarine
1 cup leafy greens salad
3 tsp sunflower oil and vinegar dressing

SNACKS

1/4 cup dried apricots
1 cup low-fat fruited yogurt

Day 4

BREAKFAST

1 whole wheat English muffin
2 tsp soft margarine
1 tbsp jam or preserves
1 medium grapefruit
1 hard-cooked egg
1 unsweetened beverage

LUNCH

White bean-vegetable soup
1 1/4 cup chunky vegetable soup
*1/2 cup white beans**
2 ounce breadstick
8 baby carrots
1 cup fat-free milk

DINNER

Rigatoni with meat sauce
1 cup rigatoni pasta (2 ounces dry)
*1/2 cup tomato sauce tomato bits**
2 ounces extra lean cooked ground beef (sauteed in 2 tsp vegetable oil)
3 tbsp grated Parmesan cheese
Spinach salad
1 cup baby spinach leaves
1/2 cup tangerine slices
1/2 cup chopped walnuts
3 tsp sunflower oil and vinegar dressing
1 cup fat-free milk

SNACKS

1 cup low-fat fruited yogurt

Day 5

BREAKFAST

Cold cereal
1 cup puffed wheat cereal
1 tbsp raisins
1 cup fat-free milk
1 small banana
1 slice whole wheat toast
1 tsp soft margarine
1 tsp jelly

LUNCH

Smoked turkey sandwich
2 ounces whole wheat pita bread
1/4 cup romaine lettuce
2 slices tomato
*3 ounces sliced smoked turkey breast**
1 tbsp mayo-type salad dressing
1 tsp yellow mustard
1/2 cup apple slices
1 cup tomato juice*

DINNER

Grilled top loin steak
5 ounces grilled top loin steak
3/4 cup mashed potatoes
2 tsp soft margarine
1/2 cup steamed carrots
1 tbsp honey
2 ounces whole wheat dinner roll
1 tsp soft margarine
1 cup fat-free milk

SNACKS

1 cup low-fat fruited yogurt

Day 6

BREAKFAST

French toast
2 slices whole wheat French toast
2 tsp soft margarine
2 tbsp maple syrup
1/2 medium grapefruit
1 cup fat-free milk

LUNCH

Vegetarian chili on baked potato
*1 cup kidney beans**
*1/2 cup tomato sauce w/ tomato tidbits**
3 tbsp chopped onions
1 ounce lowfat cheddar cheese
1 tsp vegetable oil
1 medium baked potato
1/2 cup cantaloupe
3/4 cup lemonade

DINNER

Hawaiian pizza
2 slices cheese pizza
1 ounce canadian bacon
1/4 cup pineapple
2 tbsp mushrooms
2 tbsp chopped onions
Green salad
1 cup leafy greens
3 tsp sunflower oil and vinegar dressing
1 cup fat-free milk

SNACKS

5 whole wheat crackers*
1/8 cup hummus
1/2 cup fruit cocktail (in water or juice)

Day 7

BREAKFAST

Pancakes
3 buckwheat pancakes
2 tsp soft margarine
3 tbsp maple syrup
1/2 cup strawberries
3/4 cup honeydew melon
1/2 cup fat-free milk

LUNCH

Manhattan clam chowder
3 ounces canned clams (drained)
3/4 cup mixed vegetables
*1 cup canned tomatoes**
10 whole wheat crackers*
1 medium orange
1 cup fat-free milk

DINNER

Vegetable stir-fry
4 ounces tofu (firm)
1/4 cup green and red bell peppers
1/2 cup bok choy
2 tbsp vegetable oil
1 cup brown rice
1 cup lemon-flavored iced tea

SNACKS

1 ounce sunflower seeds*
1 large banana
1 cup low-fat fruited yogurt

* Starred items are foods that are labeled as no-salt-added, low-sodium, or low-salt versions of the foods. They can also be prepared from scratch with little or no added salt. All other foods are regular commercial products which contain variable levels of sodium. Average sodium level of the 7 day menu assumes no-salt-added in cooking or at the table.

CANADA'S
Food Guide
TO HEALTHY EATING

Enjoy a variety of foods from each group every day.

Choose lower-fat foods more often.

Grain Products
Choose whole grain and enriched products more often.

Vegetables & Fruit
Choose dark green and orange vegetables and orange fruit more often.

Milk Products
Choose lower-fat milk products more often.

Meat & Alternatives
Choose leaner meats, poultry and fish, as well as dried peas, beans and lentils more often.

Different People Need Different Amounts of Food

The amount of food you need every day from the four groups and other foods depends on your age, body size, activity level, whether you are male or female, and if you are pregnant or breast-feeding. That's why the Food Guide gives a lower and higher number of servings for each food group. For example, young children can choose the number of servings, while male teenagers can go to the higher number. Most other people can choose servings somewhere in between.

Grain Products

5–12

SERVINGS PER DAY

Vegetables and Fruit

5–10

SERVINGS PER DAY

Milk Products

SERVINGS PER DAY
Children 4–9 years: 2–3
Youth 10–16 years: 3–4
Adults: 2–4
Pregnant and Breast-feeding
Women 3–4

Other Foods

Taste and enjoyment can also come from other foods and beverages that are not part of the 4 food groups. Some of these foods are higher in fat or calories, so use these foods in moderation.

Meat and Alternatives

2–3

SERVINGS PER DAY

Enjoy eating well, being active and feeling good about yourself. That's *VITALIT*

Source: © Minister of Public Works and Government Services Canada, 1997.

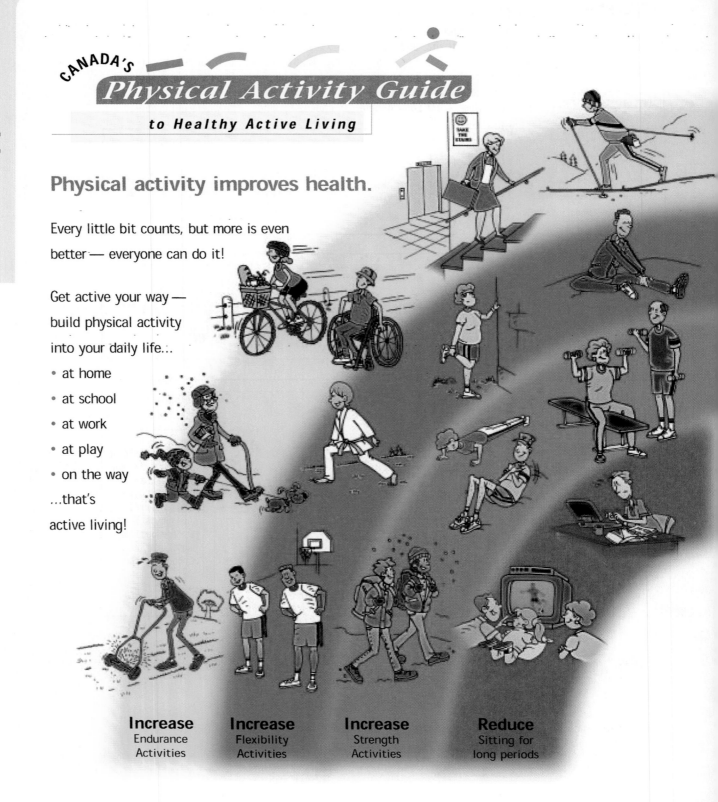

Physical Activity Guide
to Healthy Active Living

Physical activity improves health.

Every little bit counts, but more is even better — everyone can do it!

Get active your way — build physical activity into your daily life...
- at home
- at school
- at work
- at play
- on the way

...that's active living!

Increase
Endurance
Activities

Increase
Flexibility
Activities

Increase
Strength
Activities

Reduce
Sitting for
long periods

Health Canada   Santé Canada

Canadian Society for Exercise Physiology

Choose a variety of activities from these three groups:

Endurance

4–7 days a week
Continuous activities for your heart, lungs, and circulatory system

Flexibility

4–7 days a week
Gentle reaching, bending, and stretching activities to keep your muscles relaxed and joints mobile

Strength

2–4 days a week
Activities against resistance to strengthen muscles and bones and improve posture

Starting slowly is very safe for most people. Not sure? Consult your health professional.

For a copy of the *Guide Handbook* and more information: **1-888-334-9769**, or **www.paguide.com**

Eating well is also important. Follow *Canada's Food Guide to Healthy Eating* to make wise food choices.

Get Active Your Way, Every Day—For Life!

Scientists say accumulate 60 minutes of physical activity every day to stay healthy or improve your health. As you progress to moderate activities you can cut down to 30 minutes, 4 days a week. Add up your activities in periods of at least 10 minutes each. Start slowly... and build up.

Time needed depends on effort

Very Light Effort	Light Effort *60 minutes*	Moderate Effort *30–60 minutes*	Vigorous Effort *20–30 minutes*	Maximum Effort
• Strolling • Dusting	• Light walking • Volleyball • Easy gardening • Stretching	• Brisk walking • Biking • Raking leaves • Swimming • Dancing • Water aerobics	• Aerobics • Jogging • Hockey • Basketball • Fast swimming • Fast dancing	• Sprinting • Racing

Range needed to stay healthy

You Can Do It – Getting started is easier than you think

Physical activity doesn't have to be very hard. Build physical activities into your daily routine.

- Walk whenever you can—get off the bus early, use the stairs instead of the elevator.
- Reduce inactivity for long periods, like watching TV.
- Get up from the couch and stretch and bend for a few minutes every hour.
- Play actively with your kids.
- Choose to walk, wheel, or cycle for short trips.

- Start with a 10 minute walk—gradually increase the time.
- Find out about walking and cycling paths nearby and use them.
- Observe a physical activity class to see if you want to try it.
- Try one class to start — you don't have to make a long-term commitment.
- Do the activities you are doing now, more often.

Benefits of regular activity:	Health risks of inactivity:
• better health • improved fitness • better posture and balance • better self-esteem • weight control • stronger muscles and bones • feeling more energetic • relaxation and reduced stress • continued independent living in later life	• premature death • heart disease • obesity • high blood pressure • adult-onset diabetes • osteoporosis • stroke • depression • colon cancer

No changes permitted. Permission to photocopy this document in its entirety not required.
Cat. No. H39-429/1998-1E ISBN 0-662-86627-7

Source: © Minister of Public Works and Government Services Canada, 1997.

Index

Terminal care options, 438–439
Terrorism, 83
Testes, 96
Testicular cancer, 343–344, 369–370
Testicular self-examination (TSE), 369–370
Testosterone, 134, 136, 175, 261, 297
Thalidomide, 103
THC (tetrahydrocannabinol), 174, 175
Theories
 about love, 145–146
 of personality development, 30–31
 set point, 266
Thermic effect of food (TEF), 262
Throat, sore, 396
Thrombus, 319
Thrush, 400
Thymus, 391–392
Thyroid gland, 261
Ticks, 387, 388
Tobacco
 See also Smoking
 clove cigarettes (Kreteks) and bidis, 206
 diseases caused by, 208–212
 drinking, 208
 products, types of, 205
 reasons for using, 205–208
Tolerance, drug, 167, 192, 193
Tonsils, 391
Total mastectomy, 365
Toxic chemicals, 452, 463–464
Toxic Exposure Surveillance System (TESS), 452
Toxic plants, 453–454
Toxic shock syndrome (TSS), 102
Toxins, 387–388
Training effect, 289
Tranquilizers, 172
Transcendental meditation (TM), 66
Trans fatty acids, 234, 334–337
Transient ischemic attacks (TIAs), 324, 325
Transmission, 385, 387–389
Transmyocardial laser revascularization (TMLR), 321
Transsexuals, 141
Trichomonas vaginalis infections, 410
Triglycerides, 232, 326
Trisomy 21, 381
Trust, 30
TRUSTe, 13
Tubal ligation, 120, 121–122
Tuberculosis, 385
Tumors
 benign, 344, 345
 malignant, 344
Tumor-suppressor genes, 344–345

Ulcers, 59, 383
Ultrasound, 104
Ultraviolet radiation, cancer and, 367–368
Underwater weighing, 264
U.S. Department of Health and Human Services (HHS), 164
 Public Health Service of, 4, 6
 web site, 13
Urethra, 99
Urethritis, 99, 408
Urinary incontinence, 430
 Urinary system, effects of aging on, 428
Urinary tract infection (UTI), 99, 408
Uterine tubes, 99
Uterus, 99
 cancer, 348

Vaccines, 385, 394, 395
Vacuum aspiration, 122–123
Vagina, 99
Vaginal ring, contraceptive, 120
Vaginal sex, 143
Vaginismus, 138–139
Valerian, 61
Value, 139
Varicose veins, 317
Vas deferens, 96, 97
Vasectomy, 120, 121–122
Vasocongestion, 136
Vector, 389
Vegetarianism, 236
Veins, 317
Ventricles, 316
Venules, 317
Viagra, 138
Vicodin, 174
Violence
 affects on health, 76
 assessing your risk of, 83–84
 causes of, 76–77
 community (gang), 81–82
 defined, 75, 76
 family (domestic), 78–80
 institutional (school), 82–83
 intergenerational, 76
 preventing and avoiding, 84–87
 reporting, 87
 sexual, 77–81
 stalking, 81
 statistics, 75
 terrorism, 83
 workplace, 83
Viral infections, cancer and, 365–366
Virginity, 140
Viruses, 386–387
 sexually transmitted infections caused by, 398–406
Vision, effects of aging on, 429

Vitamins, 226, 237–239
 cancer and, 355
 cardiovascular health and, 330
 poisoning from, 454–456
 supplements, 246–247, 248
Voice box, cancer of the, 357
Vulva, 99

Waist-to-hip circumference ratio (WHR), 264–265
Warts, genital, 405–406
Waste
 hazardous, 466
 solid, 452
Wasting syndrome, 401
Water
 accidents and alcohol consumption, 202
 bottled, 466
 as a nutrient, 226, 242
 pollution, 465–466
 safety, 478
Web sites, 13, 20, 155
Weight
 cycling, 270
 gaining, 276
 loss aids, 178
 management, 268–277, 329
 reduction diets, 268–279, 272
 strategies for losing, 274–276
 tables, 258, 259
Wellness, 2–3
Wernicke-Korsakoff syndrome, 197
 White blood cells, immunity and, 391
Whites
 cystic fibrosis and, 380
 life expectancy and, 425
 malignant melanoma and, 367–368
 prostate cancer in, 369
 sexuality, 153
 testicular cancer in, 369
Wills, 442–443
Withdrawal
 alcohol and, 197
 birth control method, 115–116
 drug, 167
 nicotine, 209
Workplace violence, 83
World Health Organization (WHO), 2
World Trade Center, 83
Worms, 387

Xenical, 273

Yeast infections, 410–411
Yoga, 67–68
Yogurt, 247
Yohimbe, 19

Zinc, 240
Zone therapy, 18

Vegetarian Diet Pyramid